**Biosynthesis
of Heme
and Chlorophylls**

Biosynthesis of Heme and Chlorophylls

Harry A. Dailey

Department of Microbiology
University of Georgia
Athens, Georgia

McGraw-Hill Publishing Company

New York St. Louis San Francisco Auckland Bogotá
Caracas Hamburg Lisbon London Madrid Mexico
Milan Montreal New Delhi Oklahoma City
Paris San Juan São Paulo Singapore
Sydney Tokyo Toronto

Library of Congress Cataloging-in-Publication Data

Biosynthesis of heme and chlorophylls.

Bibliography: p.
Includes index.
1. Heme—Synthesis. 2. Chlorophyll—Synthesis.
I. Dailey, Harry A.
QP671.H45B56 1990   574.19′297   89-12283
ISBN 0-07-015088-5

1234567890   DOC/DOC   8965432109

ISBN 0-07-015088-5

The editor for this book was Jennifer Mitchell, and the production
supervisor was Suzanne W. Babeuf. It was set in Century Schoolbook by
Science Typographers, Inc.

Printed and bound by R.R. Donnelley & Sons Company.

Contents

v

ABOUT THE AUTHOR

Harry A. Dailey is Associate Professor and Acting Head of the Department of Microbiology at the University of Georgia in Athens. His research interests have included work on the terminal, membrane-bound enzymes of the heme biosynthesis pathway in eukaryotic organisms. Dr. Dailey received his Ph.D. at the University of California at Los Angeles.

Contributors

Tamara L. Andrew Department of Microbiology, University of Georgia, Athens, Ga. (CHAP. 4)

Samuel I. Beale Division of Biology and Medicine, Brown University, Providence, R.I. (CHAP. 7)

Stanley B. Brown Department of Biochemistry, University of Leeds, Leeds, U.K. (CHAP. 11)

Timothy M. Cox Department of Haematology, Royal Postgraduate Medical School, Hammersmith Hospital, London, U.K. (CHAP. 8)

Harry A. Dailey Department of Microbiology, University of Georgia, Athens, Ga. (CHAPS. 3 AND 4)

Peter Dierks Department of Biology, University of Virginia, Charlottesville, Va. (CHAP. 5)

Jean-Charles Deybach French Porphyria Center, University of Paris 7, Hospital Louis Mourier, Colombes, France (CHAP. 10)

Jennifer D. Houghton Department of Biochemistry, University of Leeds, Leeds, U.K. (CHAP. 11)

Peter M. Jordan Department of Biochemistry, School of Biochemical and Physiological Sciences, The University of Southampton, Bassett Crescent East, Southampton, U.K. (CHAP. 2)

Pierre Labbe Laboratoire de Biochimie des Porphyrines, Institut Jacques Monod, Université Paris, Paris, France (CHAP. 6)

Rosine Labbe-Bois Laboratoire de Biochimie des Porphyrines, Institut Jacques Monod, Université Paris, Paris, France (CHAP. 6)

Michael R. Moore University Department of Medicine, Western Infirmary, Glasgow, Scotland (CHAP. 1)

Yves Nordmann French Porphyria Center, University of Paris, Hospital Louis Mourier, Colombes, France (CHAP. 10)

Prem Ponka Departments of Physiology and Medicine, McGill University, Montreal, Quebec and the Lady Davis Institute for Medical Research of the Sir Montimer B. Davis–Jewish General Hospital, Montreal, Quebec, Canada (CHAP. 8)

Pascale G. Riley Department of Microbiology, University of Georgia, Athens, Ga. (CHAP. 4)

Herbert M. Schulman Departments of Physiology and Medicine, McGill University, Montreal, Quebec, Canada (CHAP. 8)

Ann Smith   School of Basic Life Sciences, Division of Structural and Systems Biology, University of Missouri, Kansas City, Mo. (CHAP. 9)

Jon D. Weinstein   Department of Biological Sciences, Clemson University, Clemson, S.C. (CHAP. 7)

Angela Wilks*   Department of Biochemistry, University of Leeds, Leeds, U.K. (CHAP. 11)

---

*Present address: Department of Pharmaceutical Chemistry, University of California at San Francisco, Calif.

Preface

The fields of heme and chlorophyll biosynthesis have always been fascinating, although frustrating, to those individuals involved in research of these ubiquitous biological compounds. Yet in spite of their obvious importance, tetrapyrroles remain a poorly appreciated biological subject of research. This is unfortunate since the biosynthetic pathway offers opportunities to researchers whose interests vary from stereochemistry to biomedical genetics.

In assembling this book I have had two goals. The first was to provide a vehicle for the first major presentation of significant new areas of research concerning heme and chlorophyll metabolism. The second goal was to produce a work that could serve as a solid introduction into this interesting field for researchers new to tetrapyrroles, and toward this end we have included fairly extensive reference lists for each chapter. The first of these tasks, I feel, has been achieved by the contributed chapters on yeast, molecular biology of 5-aminolevulinate synthase, iron metabolism, and tetrapyrrole transport. Whether the second goal is met can only be measured with time and the infusion of new researchers into tetrapyrrole research.

Acknowledgments

As with any book, there are a number of individuals to whom I owe some debt. The first of these must be June Lascelles, my doctoral mentor. I remember with some fondness my introduction to microbial heme biosynthesis at UCLA by the master of "la belle" *Rhodobacter sphaeroides* and her hand-held spectrophotometer and Australian wit.

Second, I must acknowledge Ann Smith, who told me that, because there was not a complete recent text on this subject, I should write one myself. Her constant encouragement provided motivation as well. To my occasionally abandoned graduate students and technicians I give my sincere thanks for their patience and help. In particular, I owe a great debt to Tammy Andrew, who not only kept my lab running, but also served as a buffer to colleagues and salespersons while I was locked away. In addition, her good nature and quick smile, along with Karen Proulx's jokes, probably did more to lift my spirits than the occasional receipt of a chapter draft. I would also like to extend my greatest thanks to Ms. Pat Bates, who managed to read my handwriting and undertook revisions rapidly and without a harsh word.

My contributors, while occasionally tardy, made this entire work possible. Their enthusiasm and hard work are responsible for the success of this volume. I sincerely thank them for their efforts and completeness in reviewing their topics.

Finally, I would like to dedicate this volume to my mother and father, who always loved and believed in their son.

Harry A. Dailey
ACTING HEAD *and*
ASSOCIATE PROFESSOR OF MICROBIOLOGY

Nomenclature Conventions

As in any field of biological science today, the common nomenclature frequently differs from that which is scientifically acceptable. This is certainly true in the field of tetrapyrrole metabolism, where several generally utilized terms may be used for a single enzyme and one term (such as heme) may be used in a highly generic manner. As an aid to readers not intimately familiar with this field, there follows a list of some of the more frequently used terms with brief descriptions where necessary. It will also be found that some authors in their chapters have made an effort to define terms that are of particular significance to their topic.

Heme—This is perhaps the most frequently generalized term in the field. The word heme is usually used as a generic term to identify iron protoporphyrin IX (unless otherwise specified) regardless of the oxidation or ligation state of the chelated iron. Properly, heme refers only to ferro-protoporphyrin whereas ferri-protoporphyrin is called hemin. Hemin, which has a net positive charge, is usually isolated with a counterion, frequently chloride.

Pathway enzymes—Due to changes in nomenclature and a reluctance to accept proper E.C. names, there exists a variety of commonly used names for some pathway enzymes. Although efforts toward uniformity have been made in the text, there still exists some variety (especially in author-prepared tables and figures) that is only natural in a multiauthor volume such as this. All of the biosynthetic pathway enzymes along with common abbreviations and frequently used common names are given in the following list:

1. 5-aminolevulinate synthase—ALAS, ALA synthetase (improper)
2. Porphobilinogen synthase—ALA dehydratase, ALA dehydrase, PBG synthase

3. Porphobilinogen deaminase—PBGD, hydroxymethylbilane synthase, uro I synthase

4. Uroporphyrinogen III synthase—Uro III synthase, uro III cosynthase

5. Uroporphyrinogen III decarboxylase—Uro D, uro'gen decarboxylase

6. Coproporphyrinogen III oxidase—CPO, copro'gen oxidase, coproporphyrinogenase (old)

7. Protoporphyrinogen IX oxidase—PPO, proto'gen oxidase

8. Ferrochelatase, Fc, protoheme ferrolyase, heme synthase, heme synthetase (improper)

1

Historical Introduction to Porphyrins and Porphyrias

Michael R. Moore

I. Introduction

Porphyrins are intriguing compounds. Among the areas in which they are used biologically, those related to the processes of energy capture and utilization have had the greatest impact. It has been suggested that abiotic formation of porphyrins, in particular uroporphyrinogen, would have provided the first pigments necessary for the eventual synthesis of the chlorophylls. This would have facilitated the emergence of simple photosynthetic organisms in primordial Earth through enhanced efficiency of energy capture. It is but a small step to perceive that such compounds will also enhance the efficiency of the reverse reaction—to provide energy.

$$\text{Carbon dioxide} + \text{Water} \underset{\text{Hemoproteins}}{\overset{\text{Chlorophyll}}{\rightleftharpoons}} \text{Carbohydrates}$$

Photosynthesis (top), Biological Oxidation (bottom)

The porphyrias provide examples of the derangement of the pathway which synthesizes these tetrapyrroles. From the outset, the name "porphyria" described not the diseases but the lustrous purple-red crystalline porphyrins—they are named from the Greek,

πορφυροσ

[porphuros or purple].

The allusions to porphyrins, around 1840, by Lecanu and other workers, preceded the first clinical presentations of porphyria by Schultz and Baumstark by 30 years. In the years that followed to the present time, knowledge of the clinical aspects of the porphyrias and the scientific advances made in their comprehension have existed in an elegant symbiosis. The porphyrias belong to that larger group of diseases described by Garrod as "inborn errors of metabolism." They demonstrate a unique combination of neurological and dermatological features, which show characteristic variations from one condition to another, the reasons for which may be sought in enzymic change within the heme biosynthetic pathway. Toxic compounds such as lead and ethanol can also be shown to inhibit the activity of many of these enzymes. The error is now recognized to lie in either the imperfect synthesis of enzymes having an aberrant structure or in the slowed synthesis of the perfect enzyme protein. Both situations have been shown to exist in the porphyrias. The history of various aspects of the porphyrias and porphyrin metabolism has been recorded by Goldberg and Rimington (1962), Florkin and Stotz (1979), Dolphin (1979), and With (1980).

II. Structure

The basic porphyrin nucleus is a unique biological structure. It consists of a macrocycle of four pyrrole rings linked by four methene bridges (Fig. 1.1). This is a rigid planar structure onto which eight side chains can be attached at positions 1 through 8 in the Fischer nomenclature. The type of side chain determines the physical characteristics of the porphyrin.

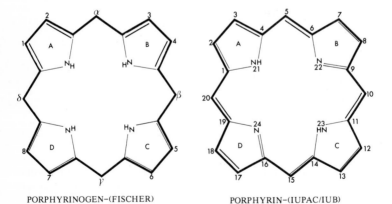

PORPHYRINOGEN–(FISCHER)   PORPHYRIN–(IUPAC/IUB)

Figure 1.1 The structures of porphyrin and porphyrinogen showing the numeration of the four pyrrole rings according to Fischer, in the conventional nomenclature, and that of the International Union of Pure and Applied Chemistry and the International Union of Biochemistry.

The four pyrrole rings are designated A, B, C, and D and the four methene bridges α, β, γ, and δ. The more recent IUPAC-IUB nomenclature has defined a new numbering system for porphyrins (IUPAC-IUB, 1980). The normal biological intermediate is not this highly conjugated porphyrin, but the hexa-hydro porphyrin, the porphyrinogen in which each of the methene bridges is reduced. Porphyrinogens are colorless and unconjugated in comparison with the conjugated and brightly colored porphyrins, which fluoresce red in light at a wavelength around 400 nm. The chemistry of these compounds is well described by Falk (1964), Marks (1969), Smith (1975), and Dolphin (1979).

An important feature of this complex ring structure is its metal-binding capability. The most common bound metals are iron and magnesium. In this form the metalloporphyrins reach their true apotheosis. Heme, an iron-containing complex usually bound to various proteins, is central to all biological oxidations, especially those associated with drugs (Fig. 1.2). Hemoproteins are also used as oxygen carriers. The chlorophylls are the magnesium-porphyrin compounds, which are central in solar energy utilization in the biosphere. Thus, all known photosynthetic organisms show porphyrin-dependent metabolism. Organisms which have lost the ability to complete the synthesis of heme are, therefore, dependent upon host cells for their existence.

As well as the systematic formation of porphyrins by biological systems, abiotic synthesis of porphyrins has been described in which a primitive chemical system has produced porphyrin-like compounds through the high entropy of their formation (Hodgson and Baker, 1967). Such synthesis was important in the ontogenesis of terrestrial life, since it would have facilitated the emergence of life forms on primordial Earth by increasing the efficiency of oxido-reductive processes as well as of energy capture (Mercer-Smith and Mauzerall, 1984; Mercer-Smith et al.

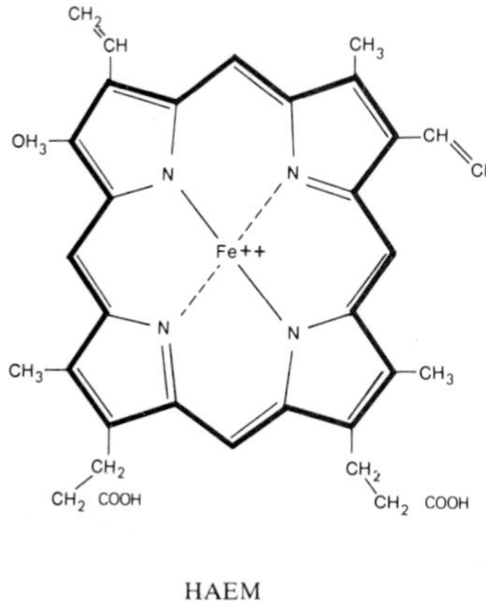

Figure 1.2   The structure of heme (ferroprotoporphyrin 9).

1985). As a consequence, porphyrins are found in fossil life forms (Bonnett and Czechowski, 1984) and have even been identified in rocks from the moon (Hodgson, 1972).

III. Chemistry and Biochemistry

A. Early studies

The history of the porphyrins begins with the work of Lecanu (1837), Berzelius (1840), Scherer (1841), and Mülder (1844). Scherer added concentrated sulfuric acid to dried and powdered blood and washed the precipitate free of iron. The iron-free residue was then heated with alcohol which took on a blood-red color. He thus had shown that the red coloration of blood was not due to iron. In Mülder's study, he described a "purple-red fluid" without any iron, which he named "Eisenfreises hämatin" (iron-free hematin). This red substance was called "cruentine" by Thudichum (1867) in a report to the Privy Council of Great Britain. He defined its spectrum, which was shown in full color in these early Victorian plates in that publication, and noted that "it fluoresced with a splendid blood-red color." Thus, in porphyrin chemistry, descriptive and structural studies came first and provided eventually, through the work of Nencki, Küster, Willstätter, and Fischer, a firm foundation in terms of chemical constitution and physical properties (Fig. 1.3).

Contemporaneously, the first tentative efforts were being made to understand the part played by the tetrapyrroles in living organisms. In 1871, Hoppe-Seyler found that "iron-free hematin" was a mixture of two

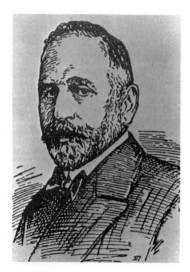

Figure 1.3 Willstätter—Nobel laureate (courtesy of the Nobelstiftelsen).

substances, the main constituent of which he called "hämatoporphyrin." Three years later, Schultz (1874) published the clinical details of a case of so-called "Pemphigus Leprosus" for his doctoral thesis. The patient was a 33-year-old weaver who had suffered from skin photosensitivity since the age of 3 months. His spleen was enlarged and he passed a wine-red urine; this urine was thoroughly investigated by Baumstark (1874) who named two pigments derived from it—"urorubrohematin" and "urofuscohematin." He thought that the spectrum of an acid solution of urorubrohematin resembled that of Hoppe-Seyler's acid hematoporphyrin, although he did not regard these two substances as identical. The importance of his observations was in his interpretation that the source of the porphyrin pigments was from an error of biosynthesis. Although it was suggested that this was a case of leprosy, it is clear that the case of Schultz and Baumstark was a description of congenital porphyria. This was the first association of this class of pigments in urine with a disease in humans. The diagnosis is almost certainly confirmed by the autopsy record record of intense red-brown discoloration of the skeleton, a feature of this disease in both animals and humans.

In 1880, MacMunn, who later discovered the cytochromes in 1884, described a dark pigment excreted in the urine of a patient who had been taking sodium salicylate. MacMunn called this pigment "urohematin," but later, he renamed it "urohematoporphyrin" because "it bears a very striking resemblance to hematoporphyrin." Hoppe-Seyler (1879) studied the porphyrin in chlorophyll and rediscovered the property of red fluorescence first seen by Thudichum. He named it "phylloporphyrin." The term "porphyrin" was used by others such as Church (1892) in his description of the porphyrin from Turaco feathers (turacin). Finally, the major spectroscopic feature of porphyrins, the strong absorptions lying around 400 nm was described for hemoglobin by Soret (1883). This absorption band for porphyrins is still called the Soret band.

B. Biochemical developments

A true biology of the porphyrins could not at that time be formulated because the exact route to their biosynthesis, together with their relationship within intermediary metabolism, were lacking. Many erroneous views were propounded during this period concerning the origins and interrelationships of the porphyrins, views which obfuscated and retarded progress in the biological sphere. It was thought, for example, that porphyrins arise as degradation products of hemoproteins, such as hemoglobin, by removal of iron and the protein moiety and that protoporphyrin, so formed, was "detoxicated" by progressive carboxylation providing, in uroporphyrin, a more hydrophylic molecule for urinary excretion. These mistaken assumptions inevitably confused any understanding of the porphyrias, although Günther's (1911) clinical classification helped to resolve some of the misunderstanding. One may also admire Baumstark's foresight in 1874. He believed the urinary pigments of Schultz's case (1874) arose by an error in the biosynthesis of hemoglobin and not by any fault in its degradation, a concept that was not confirmed for another 50 years.

The chemical excreted in the porphyrias remained a matter of debate. The urinary pigment had been thought to be hematoporphyrin but clearly this was not so (Hammarsten, 1891; Stokvis, 1895; Salkowski, 1891). Garrod (1892) showed that the absorption spectra of the urinary porphyrins were being masked by other chromophores in the urine, but it was not until the time of Fischer (1915) that "urineporphyrin" was shown to be quite discrete from "hematoporphyrin." Nencki and his co-worker, Sieber, contributed to the knowledge of the time by showing, first, that hematoporphyrin was a dicarboxylic porphyrin, both carboxyls of which could be esterified (1888). A new porphyrin was also found which was named "mesoporphyrin" (Zaleski, 1903). Saillet (1896) prepared "urospectrine" from urine which was subsequently named "coproporphyrin" (Fischer and Zerweck, 1924b) and also showed the presence of this compound in urine as a colorless chromogen (probably "coproporphyrinogen"). "Protoporphyrin" was also prepared unknowingly at this time by Laidlaw (1904). The correct structure of heme was first proposed by Küster (1912) but subsequently rejected by other workers, of greater stature, such as Willstätter and Fischer. Following

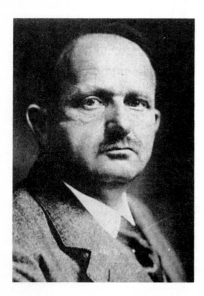

Figure 1.4   Hans Fischer—Nobel laureate (courtesy of the Nobel-stiftelsen).

the separation studies of Willstätter and co-workers (1906, 1913), Fischer began a series of studies which continued for 30 years until his death in 1945. During this time, he was awarded the Nobel prize for chemistry in 1930 (Fig. 1.4).

1. Mathias Petry and Hans Fischer. Mathias Petry was one of Günther's cases of congenital hematoporphyria. At that time there was some competition between the various labs working on porphyrins, including those of Günther, Schumm, and Fischer, to attract Petry to work with them. His eventual move to Munich was reputed to have been as much for the famous Münchener beer as for any other considerations. Petry became both laboratory aide and source of porphyrins for Fischer. Fischer worked with him until Petry's death in January 1925 when Fischer undertook a chemicopathological autopsy which he published under the name of "Porphyrinurie" (Fischer et al., 1925), whereas the extensive pathological autopsy was published later by Borst and Königsdörffer (1929). Many stories are told of Fischer's chemical abilities but that which is most attractive to the traditional chemist is reputed to have come from Müller, a professor of medicine in Munich,

Der Mench, er spukt in die hand; es kristallisiert sofort aus
(That man—he spits in his hand and it crystallizes right out)

By this research the naturally occurring porphyrins of excreta, uroporphyrin and coproporphyrin, were found to differ structurally from hematoporphyrin, which was considered to be a chemical artifact. Laidlaw (1904), Fischer (1915), and Schumm (1924) differentiated the naturally occurring porphyrin of heme itself from hematoporphyrin and the name "protoporphyrin" was suggested for this substance by Fischer (Fischer and Orth, 1937).

It was during the 1930s that the next generation started their work. During this time, some key names and prominent contributions emerged: the discovery of Ehrlich's positive chromogen in the urine of patients with acute porphyria in attack (Sachs, 1931); Rimington's work in South Africa on congenital porphyria in cattle and on turacin; the copper complex of "uroporphyrin III" found in the feathers of the Cape Lowry (Fig. 1.5). Fischer's laboratory was host during this time to two workers of note—Waldenström and Watson (Watson, 1965). Waldenström went on to clinical investigations in Sweden of what was to be called "acute intermittent porphyria" (Fig. 1.6). He studied Sachs' Ehrlich's positive chromogen, which, together with Vahlquist, he named "porphobilinogen" (Waldenström and Vahlquist, 1939). Watson founded the school in Minneapolis, which numbered among its successes the development of a screening test for porphobilinogen (Watson and Schwartz, 1941).

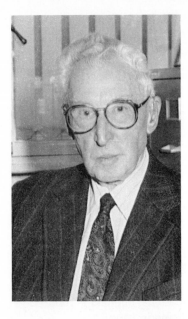

Figure 1.5 Claude Rimington.

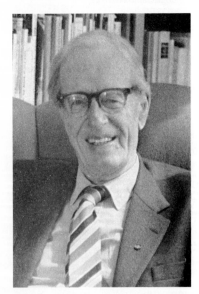

Figure 1.6 Jan Waldenström.

C. Heme biosynthetic pathway

The next milestone in the development of this subject rested upon the emergence of a systematic biochemical description of the pathway of heme biosynthesis. The names most commonly associated with this are Shemin and Neuberger (Fig. 1.7). Their work encompassed the early description of how ^{15}N-glycine was incorporated into heme by humans and animals (Shemin and Rittenberg, 1946; Shemin and Wittenberg, 1951; Shemin et al., 1955; Gray, 1952; Grinstein et al., 1949, 1950; Muir and Neuberger, 1950). This led, first, to the realization that ALA was a precursor of porphyrins (Shemin and Russell, 1953; Neuberger and Scott, 1953) and at the same time that the monopyrrole, porphobilinogen, was, indeed, the precursor of uro-, copro-, protoporphyrin, and heme (Falk et al., 1953). It was in 1945 that Shemin and Rittenberg and, subsequently, Neuberger and his co-workers, showed, by use of the new technique of isotopic labeling, that glycine was one of the precursors of the heme of hemoglobin and when, later, the use of ^{14}C-labeled acetate by Shemin established the contribution of the tricarboxylic acid cycle to the complete biosynthesis of the protoporphyrin molecule, that the way was opened for a rational theory of porphyrin biosynthesis and a description made of the relationship of the individual porphyrins, one to another.

A "pyrrolic intermediate" was postulated as a vital step in the biosynthesis of the tetrapyrrole ring, but the precise structure it would possess was uncertain. The decisive contribution came in 1952 when the substance called porphobilinogen, excreted by patients suffering from acute intermittent porphyria, was shown to be a monopyrrole (Westall, 1952; Cookson and Rimington, 1954) (Fig. 1.8). This satisfied the requirements for the intermediate in Shemin's scheme. It was shown to give rise, enzymatically, to uroporphyrinogen when incubated with a hemolysate of chicken red cells (Falk et al., 1953). Uroporphyrinogen

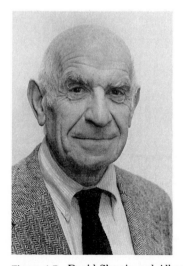
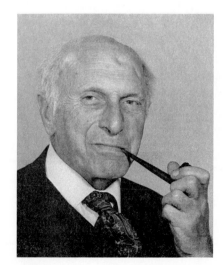

Figure 1.7 David Shemin and Albert Neuberger.

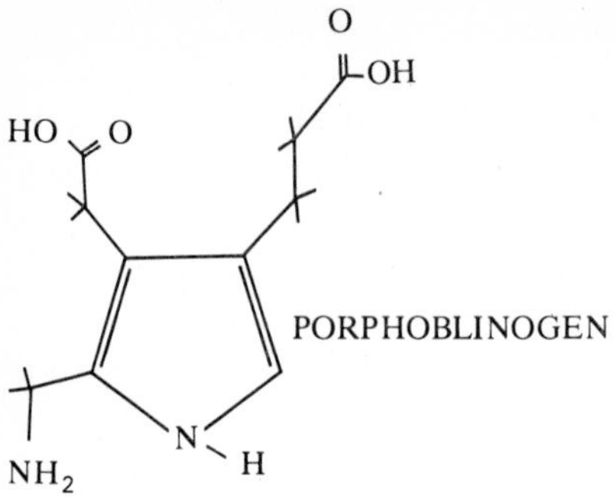

O

$\parallel$—OH

HO   O

PORPHOBLINOGEN

N—H

NH$_2$

Figure 1.8   Porphobilinogen.

was, thus, clearly established as the first tetrapyrrole to be produced biosynthetically. It is interesting to note that as early as 1949, Lemberg and Legge had suggested that this was the order of events.

The provision of authentic uroporphyrin III by removal of copper from turacin made it possible to investigate further the biosynthetic sequence (Rimington, 1939). These attempts failed until it was realized that it was the porphyrinogens, the reduced forms of the porphyrins, and not the porphyrins themselves, which were the actual intermediate substrates (Bogorad, 1955) (Fig. 1.9).

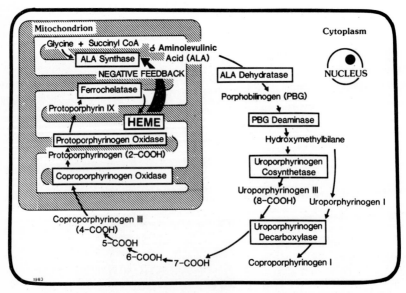

Figure 1.9   The heme biosynthetic pathway, showing negative feedback control by heme which is a feature of hepatic biosynthesis.

IV. Early Description of Porphyria

After sulfonal was introduced as a hypnotic by Kast in 1888, Stokvis (1889) reported that an elderly woman who had taken sulfonal excreted a dark-red urine and had later died. He considered that the pigment in this urine, producing coloration resembling port wine, was similar to, but not identical with, hematoporphyrin. A fatal case of an unusual form of nervous disturbance associated with dark-red urine in a 27-year-old woman was reported by Harley (1890); this woman had been given sulfonal and presented many of the neurological features of porphyria. Ranking and Pardington (1890) described two woman who excreted "hematoporphyrin" and who exhibited the gastrointestinal and neurophychiatric manifestations of acute intermittent porphyria. Their patients had not taken sulfonal. However, it appeared that between 5 and 10% of women treated with sulfonal developed porphyria (Geill, 1891; Fehr, 1891). The terms "porphyria" and "porphyrinuria" emerged gradually and slowly replaced "hematoporphyria" and "hematoporphyrinuria." In the next 20 to 30 years, many other cases were recorded of "hematoporphyrinuria." Günther (1911, 1922) listed these individual cases. Sometimes sulfonal or the allied drugs, tetronal and trional, had been taken for variable periods prior to the onset of symptoms. Other cases had no obvious relationship to drugs and, presumably, were precipitated by unknown causes. When barbiturates were introduced into medicine in 1903, it was not long until a report of an acute porphyric attack, precipitated by diethyl barbituric acid, was reported (Dobrschansky, 1906). With the use of porphyrin in chemical nomenclature in the subsequent two decades, so it was that the diseases of porphyrin metabolism came to be termed "porphyrias," rather than "hämatoporphyrie" as introduced by Günther in 1911. One may note that the term "porphyrinurie" had already been in use for some time (Ellinger, 1916; Noorden, 1916). Günther, however, adhered to his original term "hematoporphyria."

A. Drugs and chemical porphyria

The earliest evidence that we have for the drug-related development of porphyria occurred when the drug sulfonal induced the first published example of an attack of acute porphyria (Stokvis, 1889). Since that time, as well as numbers of commonly used drugs being linked with the development of acute attacks of these diseases, workers have used the ability of certain compounds to increase porphyrin synthesis in experimental animals as a means of examining the processes of heme biosynthesis (De Matteis, 1967; Marks, 1981; Smith and De Matteis, 1980). It was hoped that by mimicking the natural diseases, one might relate structure to activity and gain insight into the control of porphyrin metabolism (Seuberg et al., 1985). Had the reports emanating at the beginning of the century implicating sulfonal as a porphyrinogenic agent not been so confusing, the role of experimental porphyria could have been established at an earlier date. Experimentation with animals added much to this area of knowledge, but, confusingly, some drugs produced different patterns of porphyrin excretion in different species due to differences in response and susceptibility. Some investigators maintained that drugs merely precipitated attacks in patients already suffering from acute porphyria inherited genetically, while others disputed this. The studies of the Danish workers Geill and Fehr had shown that sulfonal porphyria was indeed a toxic porphyria, but they were published in Danish and largely overlooked (With, 1980).

1. Allyl compounds. Experiments in the 1950s were stimulated by a previous report from Duesberg (1932) that a patient treated with large quantities of allylisopropylacetylcarbamide had developed porphyria. This work developed rapidly. Schmid and Schwartz (1952) found that the hypnotic compound Sedormid (allylisopropyl acetylurea) could produce a porphyria in laboratory rodents, which was in some ways chemically similar to acute intermittent porphyria in humans. Allylisopropylacetamide (AIA), a structural analogue of Sedormid, and many other drugs were soon found to be equally effective porphyrinogenic agents (Goldberg and Rimington, 1955, 1962) (Fig. 1.10).

2. DDC. A chance observation by Solomon and Figge (1959) revealed that the substituted dihydropyridine, 3,5-diethoxycarbonyl-1,4 dihydro-

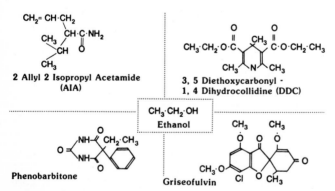

Figure 1.10 The structures of some porphyrinogenic chemicals and drugs.

collidine (DDC) caused an experimental porphyria (Fig. 1.10). The porphyrins were primarily excreted in the bile and the experimental porphyrinuria, thus produced, was similar to that of variegate porphyria. Mention must be made of the work of Tephly et al. (1979, 1980, 1981), De Matteis and Marks (1983), and others on the chemical events following experimental administration of the porphyrinogenic drug, DDC. Stimulation of ALA synthase occurs due to inhibition of hepatic ferrochelatase and consequently diminished heme-mediated feedback repression of the enzyme. The result is a hepatic porphyria. DDC is metabolized by the lipid-soluble drug-oxidizing systems mediated by the hepatic cytochrome P450. It has been shown that the N-alkylated protoporphyrins are the immediate inhibitors of ferrochelatase and that they originate from the heme of the P450 cytochrome, DDC being the methyl donor.

3. Fungicides. Another compound, hexachlorobenzene, has been shown to cause experimental porphyria in humans. An outbreak of cutaneous porphyria in Turkey (Cam 1957; Cam and Nigogosyan, 1963; Cetingil and Ozen, 1960) was related to the ingestion of seed-wheat treated with hexachlorobenzene as a fungicide, which initiated the work which continues to the present into the effects of polyhalogenated hydrocarbons on heme biosynthesis (Elder, 1976; Strik and Koeman, 1979; Morris and Cabral, 1986). Another therapeutic fungicide, griseofulvin, was also shown to be porphyrinogenic (De Matteis and Rimington, 1963; Lochhead et al., 1967) (Fig. 1.10).

The mode by which these compounds initiate induction of heme synthesis is quite different, but they provided a means of studying the processes of regulation of heme biosynthesis. This was no more evident than in the laboratories of Granick and co-workers where, following their experiments in 1963 using DDC, they were able to show that the primary regulatory role in heme biosynthesis lay at the level of ALA synthase (Fig. 1.11). The means by which each of these three compounds, AIA, DDC, and hexachlorobenzene, influence the biosynthetic pathway are of interest since they provide a useful pointer to the diversity of influence of chemical compounds upon the processes of control of heme synthesis and provide the rationale for development of the lists of drugs contraindicated for use in acute porphyria (Wetterberg, 1976; Moore, 1980; Moore and McColl, 1987).

V. Classification of Porphyrias

In two comprehensive papers published in 1911 and 1922, Günther was the first to classify the diseases of porphyrin metabolism (Table 1.1). In the first of these he quoted 14 cases from the literature in which acute symptoms of porphyria arose spontaneously, "haematoporphyria acuta," and 56 cases of "haematoporphyria acuta toxica," in which the symptoms were associated with the ingestion of sulfonal, trional, or veronal. He also defined and named, for the first time, the very rare condition, congenital porphyria, "haematoporphyria congenita," in which the predominating symptoms were due to skin photosensitivity. In Glasgow, McCall-Anderson (1898) had described two brothers, both of whom had solar sensitivity and excreted "hematoporphyrin" in the urine. He suggested that there was a "close connection between the cutaneous manifestations and the pigment in the urine." Meyer-Betz, who subsequently died during World War I, was the first of Fischer's co-workers. He injected 200 mg of hematoporphyrin into his own veins in 1913. Knowing the marked photodynamic effect of this substance on mice, paramecia, and erythrocytes, from the studies of Hausmann (1908, 1911), he intended to remain indoors and expose himself very cautiously to light. However, he was a practicing physician and soon after the injection he received an urgent message from a sick patient and he felt obligated to make a house call. It was a sunny day and though he strove to avoid direct exposure, in this he was unsuccessful. Shortly thereafter, he developed an extreme solar urticaria of the hands and face. This experiment revealed the potent photosensitizing influence of this particular porphyrin.

Günther's classification also included a group of cases called "haematoporphyria chronica," which showed some resemblance to haematoporphyria congenita, but in which the photosensitization occurred later in life. There is in Günther's description of congenital

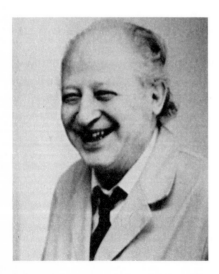

Figure 1.11   Sam Granick (courtesy of S. Sassa).

porphyria the realization that the disease persists throughout life and Gaarod (1923) credits Günther with the first recognition that this disease was an "inborn error of metabolism." In Günther's second work in 1922, he elaborated on his first thesis, quoting further cases. He noted the possibility that acute hematoporphyria might be hereditary and suggested that people liable to develop acute or congenital hematoporphyria had a "porphyrism" with certain notable physical and mental characteristics—neurosis, insomnia, dark hair, and pigmented skin. In a survey of the clinical features of acute hematoporphyria, he described a triad of symptoms which were commonly present, namely abdominal pain, constipation, and vomiting.

A. Hepatic and erythropoietic classification

Waldenström (1937) made a clinical survey of 103 cases of acute porphyria found in Sweden. He reviewed some previously published cases of chronic hematoporphyria (Günther's classification) in which light sensitivity occurred some years after birth, at times associated with abdominal pain. For these cases, he substituted the name "porphyria cutanea trada" (Table 1.1). He later revised this to include both symptomatic (porphyria cutanea tarda symptomatica) and hereditary (porphyria cutanea tarda hereditaria, "protocoproporphyria") forms of the disease (Waldenström, 1957). In 1954, Schmid and co-workers classified the porphyrias on the basis of the porphyrin content of the livers and bone marrows of 31 cases. In two cases of congenital porphyria they found porphyrins concentrated in the bone marrow, particularly in the normoblastic nucleus, and they, therefore, renamed the condition "porphyria erythropoietica." In the remaining 29 cases, porphyrins were found mainly in the liver and these were, therefore, called "porphyria hepatica." This included the typical "acute intermittent porphyria," a "mixed" type in which photosensitivity and acute symptoms may occur in the same patient and "porphyria cutanea tarda," a term they reserved for a group in which photosensitivity occurs later in life, unassociated with acute symptoms. This classification was further extended by Watson in 1960, Goldberg and Rimington in 1962, and Eales in 1979.

B. Classification into acute and nonacute porphyria

On the basis of studies such as these attempts have been made to provide a classification that would encompass all of their features. The general aim in most classifications was to provide a clinical basis consistent with the known biochemical features. The full elucidation had, however, to await the complete description of each of these diseases as a

TABLE 1.1 Classifications of Porphyria

A. Günther (1911)
  1. Haematoporphyria acuta
  2. Haematoporphyria acuta toxica
  3. Haematoporphyria chronica
  4. Haematoporphyria congenita

B. Waldenström (1937)
  1. Porphyria congenita
  2. Porphyria cutanea tarda
  3. Porphyria acute
     a. Latent porphyria
     b. Abdominal form
     c. Nervous form
     d. Classical acute porphyria
     e. Comatose form commencing as abdominal form

C. Schmid, Schwartz, and Watson (1954)
  1. Porphyria erythropoietica—congenital photosensitive porphyria, usually associated with hemolytic anemia and splenomegaly
  2. Porphyria hepatica—hepatic disease or functional impairment frequent
     a. Intermittent acute type—abdominal and/or nervous manifestations
     b. "Cutanea tarda" type—late appearance of photosensitivity without other manifestations
     c. "Mixed" type—photosensitivity with intermittent abdominal and/or nervous manifestations

D. Waldenström (1957)
  1. Congenital porphyria
  2. Porphyria cutanea tarda symptomatica, e.g., alcoholic cirrhosis, Bantu "cirrhosis," hepatoma
  3. Porphyria cutanea tarda hereditaria (protocoproporphyria)
  4. Acute intermittent porphyria

E. Watson (1960)
  1. Porphyria erythropoietica (recessive)
  2. Porphyria hepatica
     a. Hereditary acute intermittent (dominant)
        i. Manifest
        ii. Latent
     b. Hereditary, mixed, or "variegate" group (dominant)
        i. Cutaneous with little or no acute manifestations
        ii. Acute intermittent without cutaneous symptoms
        iii. Various combinations
        iv. Latent
     c. Hereditary cutaneous
     d. Constitutional or idiosyncratic (PCT)
        i. Chemicals, especially alcohol
        ii. Idiopathic
        iii. With systemic disease
     e. Acquired
        i. Secondary to hepatoma
        ii. Secondary to fungicide—Turkish epidemic

F. Goldberg and Rimington (1962)
  1. Congenital (erythropoietic) porphyria
  2. Acute intermittent porphyria
  3. Cutaneous hepatic porphyria
     a. Hereditary forms
        i. Porphyria cutanea tarda hereditaria or protocoproporphyria
        ii. Mixed porphyria
        iii. Porphyria variegata

TABLE 1.1   **Classifications of Porphyria** (*Continued*)

b. Acquired forms
   i. Porphyria cutanea tarda symptomatica
   ii. Bantu porphyria
   iii. Turkish porphyria
   iv. Porphyrin-producing hepatic adenoma
4. Experimentally induced porphyrias

G. Eales (1979)

Erythropoietic
1. Congenital erythropoietic porphyria (CEP), Gunther's disease
2. Congenital erythropoietic porphyria atypical variant (CEP/VAR)
3. Erythrohepatic protoporphyria (EHP), formerly erythropoietic protoporphyria
4. Erythrohepatic coproporphyria (EHC), formerly erythropoietic coproporphyria, coproporphyrinemia
5. Hepatoerythrocytic porphyria (HEP)

Hepatic
Hereditary forms
6. Acute intermittent porphyria (AIP), Swedish genetic porphyria, pyrrolia, pyrroloporphyria
7. Hereditary coproporphyria (HC), idiopathic coproporphyrinuria
8. Variegate porphyria (VP), South African genetic porphyria, mixed porphyria, porphyria cutanea tarda hereditaria, protocoproporphyria

Symptomatic forms
9. SP-A, SP associated with alcohol abuse and iron overload
10. SP-C, SP induced by chemicals, including hexachlorobenzene (HCB), pentachlorophenol, estrogens, and other hepatotoxic drugs and possibly bacterial and fungal metabolites
11. SP-D, SP associated with systemic disease, including a miscellaneous group of rare immunologically determined disorders (systemic lupus erythematosus, scleroderma, Felty's syndrome, Waldenstrom's macroglobulinemia)
12. Hepatic porphyrinoma

Combinations
Coincidental association of two discrete disorders

Modifications
Intercurrent liver disease in VP and HC may modify clinical presentation and the routes and patterns of porphyrin excretion

ALA-uric disorders simulating clinical AIP
ALA-uria and tyrosinosis (hereditary tyrosinaemia)
ALA-uria and Copro'uria (lead poisoning)

Secondary coproporphyrinurias (Copro'uria)

H. Moore, McColl, and Goldberg (1979)

Acute porphyria
   Acute intermittent porphyria
   Variegate porphyria
   Hereditary coproporphyria
   Plumboporphyria

Nonacute porphyria
Cutaneous hepatic porphyria
   i. Familial, including hepatoerythropoietic porphyria
   ii. Acquired, including toxic forms
Erythropoietic protoporphyria
Congenital porphyria

specific enzymic disorder of the heme biosynthetic pathway, a process that evolved over the years between 1955 and 1980. This included the later description of the diseases, hereditary coproporphyria (Berger and Goldberg, 1955), erythropoietic protoporphyria (Magnus et al., 1961; Langhof et al., 1961), and plumboporphyria (Bird et al., 1979; Doss et al., 1979).

The clinical manifestations of the porphyrias vary enormously. The traditional classification of the diseases as either hepatic or erythropoietic, dependent upon the primary site, or what was thought to be the primary site, of overproduction of the porphyrins, is inadequate. For that reason the additional classification into the acute and nonacute types of porphyria based upon the main clinical presentation offers a more satisfactory means of subdivision of this group of diseases.

The obvious feature of most of the porphyrias is skin photosensitization brought about by the action of light upon porphyrins in the skin. This is not found in acute intermittent porphyria, which is classified as one of the acute porphyrias, the other two being hereditary coproporphyria and variegate porphyria. The major feature of these diseases is that they may be provided into an acute attack with a neuropsychiatric or neurovisceral syndrome, associated with huge increases in production and urinary excretion of the porphyrin precursors ALA and PBG. The reasons for these changes have been sought in a number of theories which presently have settled upon either an excess of ALA, a deficiency of heme, or a combination of these two (Yeung-Laiwah et al., 1987). Hereditary coproporphyria and variegate porphyria, unlike acute intermittent porphyria, may also be present with cutaneous photosensitivity. The neuropsychiatric or neurovisceral syndrome is not present in the nonacute porphyrias, which consist of congenital erythropoietic porphyria, erythropoietic protoporphyria, and cutaneous hepatic porphyria. The primary presenting feature in the nonacute porphyrias in skin photosensitivity, although there may be other systemic features found in each of these diseases. Most of the porphyrias are in fact inherited as mendelian dominant autosomal characters, although congenital erythropoietic porphyria is inherited as mendelian recessive. Erythropoietic protoporphyria has been described as coming from a 3-allele defect and cutaneous hepatic porphyria exists in two forms—as a hereditary disease or as an acquired one. Some of these classifications are shown in Table 1.1 in historical sequence.

VI. Enzymes

With the description of the pathway sequence, the time was ripe for the elucidation of the catalytic steps—the enzymic description of the biosynthetic pathway. Steps in this direction had already been undertaken by the earlier pioneers, but it was not until the middle of the century, with the description of enzymes like the iron-incorporating enzyme, ferrochelatase, that the process gained momentum.

Thereafter, each of the stages of the pathway was exhaustively examined. This continues to the present day. The most important point in this sequence is the first one, the formation of ALA by ALA synthase. Granick provided the evidence from his studies that this was indeed the control point of the biosynthetic pathway (Granick, 1963, 1966; Granick and Sassa, 1971) which was supported by a number of other workers (Gibson et al., 1958; Kikuchi et al., 1958) and this control might relate to glycine availability (Neuberger, 1980). The last enzyme of the sequence to be described was protoporphyrinogen oxidase (Jackson et al., 1974; Poulson and Polglase, 1975). It was clear, however, that additional control points would have to be sought in the biosynthetic sequence. One such enzymic control point was demonstrated at porphobilinogen deaminase (PBG-D) (Elder, 1976; Brodie et al., 1977a). It was at this site in the pathway that the most obscure stage of the biosynthetic sequence, the formation of uroporphyrinogen III, was eventually elucidated by Jordan and Battersby during 1979 and 1980 (Fig. 1.12).

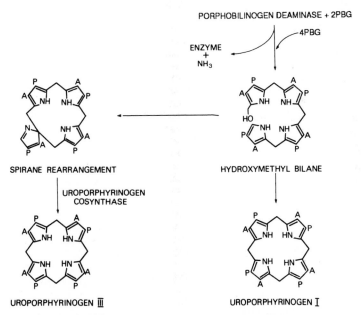

Figure 1.12 The synthesis of the macrocycle—formation of the asymmetric coproporphyrinogen III from porphobilinogen and hydroxymethylbilane requires that one ring (the D ring) is inverted through a spirane rearrangement catalyzed by uroporphyrinogen cosynthase (A, acetyl; P, propionyl).

A. Enzymic classification

All this new knowledge led to a profound advance in understanding of the porphyrias, the diseases in which porphyrins were produced in excessive amounts, but clarity in this field was still obscured by the attempts to classify and subdivide these diseases according, primarily, to their clinical manifestations. Much debate ensued which was of limited value until the individual biochemical errors in each porphyria could be ascertained.

Hepatic porphyrin biosynthesis is normally regulated by a negative feedback mechanism by heme on the initial and rate-limiting enzyme of synthesis, 5-aminolevulinate synthase. Deficiency of heme releases this repression. Such control does not occur in the erythropoietic system. The most important feature of current levels of understanding of the porphyrias is that the metabolic disorder can in all cases be localized to one specific enzyme within the heme biosynthetic pathway (Waldenström, 1956; Brodie et al., 1977a). Theoretically, such genetically defined alterations in enzyme activity should be expressed by all cells of the body, yet in practice there is considerable variation in the level of expression of such cellular defects in porphyria.

Thus, in the acute porphyrias the expression is largely hepatic. In acute intermittent porphyria, the defect has been shown to lie at the level of porphobilinogen deaminase (EC 4.3.1.8) where there is a deficiency of about 50% of normal enzyme activity. This defect is found in numerous tissues ranging from red cells to cultured fibroblasts. In each of the other acute porphyrias, the defect lies further along the pathway and as well as overproduction of the porphyrin precursors, there is excess production of porphyrins. In hereditary coproporphyria the defect lies at the level of coproporphyrinogen oxidase (EC 1.3.3.3); in variegate porphyria at protoporphyrinogen oxidase (EC 1.3.3.4) and in the exceptionally rare "plumboporphyria" at ALA dehydratase (EC 4.2.1.24). The resultant overproduction of coproporphyrinogen and protoporphyrin, respectively, in these diseases can account for their photocutaneous manifestations. There are in the acute porphyrias, however, some anomalies in the exact expression of enzyme deficiency. Although in each of these diseases the defect is as stated, other alterations in enzyme activity can also be observed in both hereditary coproporphyria and variegate porphyria, where there is a common finding of diminished activity of porphobilinogen deaminase, whereas in variegate porphyria, ferrochelatase activity and uroporphyrinogen decarboxylase activity have also been found to be lower than normal. The precise reasons for these additional changes is unclear, but their existence is reflected by the alterations in the patterns of production and excretion of porphyrins and their precursors.

In the nonacute porphyrias, the expression is both hepatic and erythropoietic. The deficient enzymes are as follows: in congenital erythropoietic porphyria, uroporphyrinogen cosynthetase (EC 4.2.1.75), which normally acts concertedly with porphobilinogen deaminase to produce the series III isomer porphyrins from hydroxymethylbilane (Fig. 1.10); erythropoietic protoporphyria, ferrochelatase (EC 4.99.1.1); and cutaneous hepatic porphyria, uroporphyrinogen decarboxylase (EC 4.1.1.37). A classification based upon these enzymic lesions may have merit, but there are logistical problems in the application of such a classification, not the least of which is the difficulty in reproducible measurement of enzyme activities and the nonavailability of biopsy material upon which the estimations might be carried out. These problems will probably be resolved following the rapid developments in molecular biology and molecular genetics. At present, the classification, based on the acute and nonacute porphyrias, brings together both the clinical and biochemical aspects of these diseases and differences between them and allows a ready differential diagnosis of the different porphyrias on the basis of a combination of clinical and biochemical features.

1. Molecular genetics.   Molecular genetics have allowed a more fundamental recognition of the nature of the genetic defects in these diseases. The early concept that was shown to be true for *Staphylococcus aureus* was that the genes would all lie on one chromosome and be cotransducible; that is, unfortunately, not so. In humans, the early investigations in this sphere have shown clearly that they are not clustered in the human genome, but dispersed among different chromosomes. Five different chromosomal locations have now been demonstrated: uroporphyrinogen decarboxylase on 1; ALA synthase on 3; ALA dehydratase and coproporphyrinogen oxidase on 9; and porphobilinogen deaminase on 11. The other genes will certainly be located in the near future, by resolving the problem of how the processes of enzyme-protein synthesis are coordinated. From the work thus established, cDNA probes have been synthesized for some of these proteins which are facilitating further investigation of the molecular defect and of the familial association of these diseases.

VII. Acute Porphyria

Waldenström's studies in Sweden were greatly aided by the presence in his patients' urines of porphobilinogen which gives a red color with Ehrlich's aldehyde reagent (an acidic solution of paradimethyl-amino-benzaldehyde). It is the precursor of most of the uroporphyrin found in these urines. As early as 1890, Harley had noted that the urine of a case of sulfonal-induced acute porphyria contained a chromogen which, when oxidized, became a red pigment. Such a substance in the urine of a patient with acute porphyria gave a red coloration, insoluble in chloroform, with Ehrlich's aldehyde reagent and which was, therefore, not urobilinogen (Sachs, 1931). Waldenström (1937) showed that this was not only excreted in the urine of every one of his patients with acute porphyria, but that some apparently healthy relatives of these patients also excreted it. The idea of a "latent porphyria" was thus conceived. On the basis of his work, he suggested that acute porphyria was transmitted as a mendelian dominant characteristic. Later, Waldenström and Vahlquist (1939) considered that the Ehrlich-reacting chromogen, which they named porphobilinogen and partly purified, was a dipyrrolmethane.

The liver and kidney of fatal cases of acute porphyria contained porphobilinogen (Prunty, 1945; Gray, 1950), which was isolated from the urine of a patient with acute porphyria in University College Hospital in London (Westall, 1952), Cookson and Rimington (1954) showed it to be a monopyrrole and Haeger (1958) found that two-thirds of patients with latent or manifest acute intermittent porphyria excreted excess 5-aminolevulinic acid (ALA) in addition to increased porphobilinogen.

A. Concurrent porphyria

Concurrent porphyria has been defined as two differing types of porphyria occurring in the same individual (Moore et al., 1987). Since there is concurrent inheritance of more than one genetic defect there is more than one enzymic defect (McColl et al., 1985; Qadiri et al., 1986). A large kindred in Chester have been described, with excretion and enzymic patterns of both acute intermittent porphyria and variegate porphyria (both PBG-deaminase and protoporphyrinogen oxidase with low activity). In another study, Day et al., (1982) reported 25 patients with a variant of variegate porphyria combined with porphyria cutanea tarda which they called "dual porphyria." These were patients who belonged to families with well-documented variegate porphyria and who were found to have the porphyrin excretion pattern of CHP superimposed on that of variegate porphyria. Studies performed in six of these dual porphyria patients by Meissner et al. (1985) showed that erythrocyte uroporphyrinogen decarboxylase activity was reduced as was protoporphyrinogen oxidase activity. A similar case was presented by Vaidya and Kanan (1987). Such parallel inheritance need not imply that there is further genetic disadvantage since the effects of multiple enzyme inhibition in the pathway are not necessarily additive, as is shown by the example of lead poisoning (Moore and Goldberg, 1985). This is not the case for homozygous porphyrias in which the dermatological and other features are usually severe (Grandchamp et al., 1977; Kordac et al., 1984; Murphy et al., 1986; and Mustajoki et al., 1987).

B. Neuropathy

The acute porphyrias have in common the features of acute abdominal pain, limb weakness, and neurophychiatric presentation. This symptomatology can be explained on a neurogenic basis. Despite advances in genetics and biochemistry, the link between these biochemical abnormalities and the neuropathological and clinical manifestations remains unclear. The earliest case of acute porphyria examined pathologically was that of Campbell in 1898 who failed to find any nervous system abnormality. However, in 1903, Erbslöh described features of axonal demyelination in the femoral nerve from a porphyric patient who had died after treatment with sulfonal. Several case reports followed and when the subject was reviewed by Mason and co-workers (1933) the most characteristic lesions were seen in the nervous system and affected peripheral nerves and sympathetic ganglia. On the basis of current evidence there are two rational hypotheses to explain these clinical manifestations. First, an intracellular deficiency of heme and, therefore, heme-containing compounds, such as the cytochromes, would link the clinical and biochemical findings. Second, an excess of 5-aminolevulinate could act pharmacologically on these systems (Fig. 1.13). These are not mutually exclusive and could act concurrently. Unfortunately, these have as yet been inadequately tested and only formulated on isolated case reports (Yeung-Laiwah et al., 1987).

1. Psychiatric aspects

> ... and all her hair
> In one long yellow string I wound
> Three times her little throat around
> And strangled her ...
> ... Fear death?—to feel the fog in my throat
> The mist in my face.
>
> from *Porphyria's Lover* by Robert Browning

When Robert Browning wrote these words the porphyrias had not been described, yet alone named. In that verse, however, he associated, by chance, porphyria and psychiatry. The acute attack may reveal a variety of psychiatric manifestations, including anxiety, depression, and frank psychosis (Table 1.2). The literature on the psychiatric features is sparse, although the earliest cases were described by Copeman in 1891 and by Campbell in 1898. It is clear that a frequent misdiagnosis of hysteria is made, although Brugsch (1959) recognized it as a distinct psychosis in his review of the literature. The available data show that the psychopathology is related to affective neurotic, rather than psychotic, features and a truly schizophreniform presentation has not been observed (Moore et al., 1987). All patients who had experienced an attack described a prodromal mood alteration with increased irritability, depression, and anxiety. It was also more common to find epileptiform seizures in those with a psychiatric history. This is in accordance with the findings of Stein and Tschudy (1970), who recorded an excess of subjects with an abnormal EEG in patients with psychiatric symptomatology. This was further amplified by the studies of Tishler and coworkers (1985) in 3867 psychiatric inpatients. They found that 0.2% of this population, 8 patients, who experienced episodic psychosis and depression, had confirmed acute intermittent porphyria. In general terms, the psychiatric phenomena may be expected in up to 70% of acute attacks. It is intriguing that disturbances of porphyrin metabolism have been observed in schizophrenics. Urinary ALA and coproporphyrin ex-

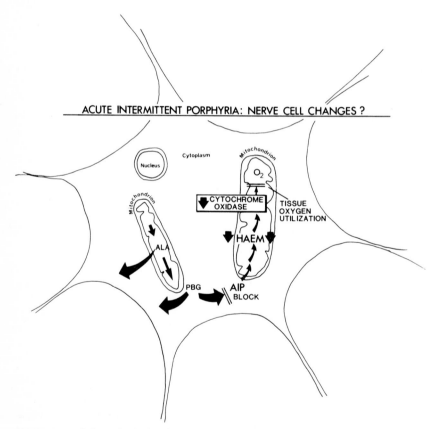

Figure 1.13 A hypothesis for the etiology of the neurological features of acute porphyria. This is due either to the pharmacological effects of excess 5-aminolevulinate (ALA) or to a decrease in heme and, therefore, hemoprotein synthesis. Heme deficiency would diminish the synthesis of a number of heme-containing proteins and thus alter oxidative processes such as terminal oxidation by cytochrome oxidase.

cretion rose, as did erythrocyte protoporphyrin, after a load of tryptophan and isoniazid were given to schizophrenics (Huszak and Durko,
1970).

VIII. Nonacute Porphyrias

A. Congenital Porphyria

Congenital porphyria is one of the rarest of the porphyrias, but was the
first recorded case of porphyria in the literature, probably because of the
severity and dramatic nature of its symptoms. The case was described by
Schultz in 1874. His patient was a 33-year-old weaver who had suffered
from photosensitivity of the skin from the age of 3 months. He had an
enlarged spleen, was anemic, and was mildly icteric. His urine was wine
red and contained pigments which resembled Hoppe-Seyler's acid

TABLE 1.2   Review of Reported Cases with Psychiatric Features

Reference	Case
Copeman, 1891	4 female patients—highly neurotic
Campbell, 1898	1 case—subacute mania
Günther, 1911	Attacks preceded by nervous tension—nervous constitution
Waldenström, 1937	No neurotic traits between attacks
Roth, 1945	10 patients—severe neurotic personality disorders
Schneck, 1946	1 case—hysterical personality
De Gennes et al., 1949	1 case—psychosis, delirium
Levy and Perry, 1949	1 case—psychotic episodes which remitted as urine regained normal color
Freeman and Kolb, 1951	1 case—psychiatric symptoms treated with electroshock
Olmstead, 1953	1 case—Rohrschach and Bender-Gestalt tests suggested strongly neurotic personality
Hare, 1953	3 cases 1. Anxiety or early schizophrenia—patient died 2. Postoperative anxiety, depression 3. Depression—patient died
Markowitz, 1954	5 cases—75% showed mental changes
Vischer and Aldrich, 1954	1 case—intensive psychotherapy
Cross, 1956	2 cases—psychiatric symptoms prominent
Goldberg, 1959	29 of 50 patients showed significant mental symptoms
Luby et al., 1959	6 patients—no consistent pattern in Minnesota multiphasic personality inventory test
Duret-Cosyns and Duret, 1959	6 cases—emotional stress associated with onset of attacks No evidence of neurotic trait preceding attack; hysterical signs and behavior varied with the metabolic disturbance
Eilenberg and Scobie, 1960	1 case—2 attacks brought on by stress, but many others unrelated to stressful situation
Holmberg, 1961	1 case—depressive illness, ECT precipitation of attack
Ackner et al., 1962	13 cases—no psychogenic factor in the etiology of the disorder or neurotic predisposition

TABLE 1.2   Review of Reported Cases with Psychiatric Features (*Continued*)

Reference	Case
Fiume and Vella, 1966	4 cases 1. "Acute hallucinatory delirium" (confusion) 2. "Acute hallucinatory delirium" (mania) 3. "Chronic delusions of persecution—and hallucinations 4. "Psychiatric symptoms"—died
Roth, 1968	5 cases—anxiety, melancholia, Meyer-Reichner-Korsakoff and Garcin-Lapresle syndromes 12 cases hysteria or conversion hysteria
Wetterberg and Osterberg, 1970	25 cases of AIP—no differences in Maudsley personality inventory
Carney, 1972	4 cases 1. Alcoholism and depression 2. Paranoid psychosis 3. Suspected psychopath 4. Acute phobic anxiety
Jancar, 1975	2 cases of manic depressive psychosis
Trafford, 1976	1 case—impulsive hysterical psychopath
Guidotti et al., 1979	1 case—Kluver-Bucy syndrome
Skulj, 1979	1 case—psychosis
Pepplinkhuizen et al., 1980	4 cases—all intermittent psychoses
Offenstadt et al., 1980	1 case—hereditary coproporphyria, catatonia, schizophrenia
Baruch et al., 1981	1 case—depressive syndrome
Goldberg and Stinnett, 1983	1 case of AIP, schizophrenic—psychotic
Bronckart and Troisfontaines, 1984	Review of psychiatric features
Barillari et al., 1984	1 case—psychosis without neuropathy
Kamal and Grivois, 1985	1 case—acute psychosis and use of psychotropic drugs
Urban, 1985	1 case—psychotic
Tishler et al., 1985	8 cases, 0.2% of a psychiatric inpatient population—psychosis and depression
Grabowski and Yergani, 1987	1 case—psychotic

hematoporphyrin. At autopsy, his bones were found to be dark brown in color. Further cases reports were made by other authors, such as those by Gagey in 1896, McCall-Anderson in 1898, and Vollmer et al. in 1903. The paper by McCall-Anderson was of interest since it described two brothers, fishermen from Stornoway, who had attended the Western Infirmary, Glasgow, since the age of 4 years because of solar sensitivity of the face, ears, and hands. Each summer the brothers would feel an itching and burning in these areas and within 12 hours blisters would arise. Their urine was burgundy red in color and probably due to porphyria. McCall-Anderson suggested that there was a close connection between the cutaneous manifestations and the urinary pigmentation. Günther (1911) defined and named the disease haematoporphyria congenita. One of Günther's cases of congenital porphyria was a man called Mathias Petry and it is from the study of this patient's excrete by

Fischer that much of our present knowledge of porphyrin chemistry is derived. When Petry died there was an exhaustive autopsy. On examining the bone marrow sections with a fluorescence microscope, Borst and Königsdörffer (1929) noted that the developing erythropoietic cells contained unusually large amounts of porphyrin. They also found porphyrins deposited, sometimes in crystalline form, in many organs of the body.

In subsequent autopsies of two cases of congenital porphyria, the porphyrins were found to be concentrated in the bone marrow rather than in the liver. Congenital porphyria was therefore renamed "porphyria erthyropoietica." In subsequent patients examined with fluorescence and absorption microscopy two different types of normoblast were found, an abnormal type which exhibited marked porphyrin fluorescence, apparently in the nuclei, and other normal normoblasts without such fluorescence. It was then thought that these abnormal normoblasts which carried the trait representing the inborn error of metabolism (Schmid et al., 1954, 1955). Fifty cases of congenital porphyria were listed by Goldberg and Rimington (1962) and since that time a number of publications have listed the features of this disease. It is, however, reasonably certain, on the basis of the studies carried out to date in humans, together with the evidence of the bovine disease, that this is inherited as a mendelian autosomal recessive trait. These studies also indicate that the recessive character is not sex-linked.

B. Cutaneous hepatic porphyria

The cutaneous hepatic porphyrias (CHP) or porphyria cutanea tarda (PCT) are the most common forms of porphyria. Patients present with cutaneous photosensitivity but do not experience attacks of neurovisceral dysfunction. CHP differs from the other porphyrias in that there is no clear pattern of inheritance in the majority of cases although, in some, familial transmission can clearly be established. Environmental factors play an important role. Tio in 1956 made clear the distinction between hereditary and nonhereditary cutaneous porphyria and Waldenström (1957) introduced the term "porphyria cutanea tarda" (PCT). The cause of the reduced uroporphyrinogen decarboxylase (URO-D) activity remains unclear, but appears to be the result of complex interactions of both genetic and acquired factors (Sweeney, 1986).

CHP is usually classified into two main types based on the relative importance of inherited and acquired factors (Tio, 1956). The majority of patients may be classified as *sporadic*. These patients have no family history of the disorder and its development appears largely related to chronic alcohol ingestion or the use of the contraceptive pill. Erythrocyte URO-D activity is normal in these patients although hepatic URO-D activity is depressed. In *familial CHP* evidence of heredity is usually obtained. There is a 50% reduction of URO-D activity in erythrocytes which is inherited in an autosomal dominant fashion. In the sporadic or toxic disease polyhalogenated hydrocarbons have been shown to be the etiological agent in some cases. The most common precipitant is, however, alcohol ingestion which is known to disturb porphyrin metabolism in normal subjects (Moore et al., 1984). Franke and Fikentscher (1935) noted that urinary coproporphyrin excretion doubled after drinking 1 L of beer or 90 mL of cognac and Sutherland and Watson (1951) found increased urinary coproporphyrin in chronic alcoholics with increased excretion of isomer III. Orten et al. (1963) studied the urinary excretion of porphyrins and precursors in chronic alcoholics and noted increased coproporphyrin excretion but no significant increase in excretion of uroporphyrin, ALA, or PBG.

1. Toxic porphyria. If one excludes the porphyria caused by sulfonal, toxic porphyria in humans only became clearly established after 1957 when there was a disastrous outbreak of porphyria among Turkish peasants who had inadvertently ingested the fungicide, hexachlorobenzene, with their wheat and bread (Cam, 1957; Cetingil and Ozen, 1960). Whereas the erythropoietic and hepatic types of human porphyria previously studied had all been genetically transmitted, either as recessive or dominant mendelian characters, inherited metabolic error or predisposition was absent in Turkish porphyria or at the most of secondary importance. In this Turkish population, Günther's postulate of "toxic porphyria" in his early classification was fully substantiated.

2. Hepatoerythropoietic porphyria. At present, 17 patients have been described with hepatoerythropoietic porphyria (1987). It is a homozygous form of familial CHP first reported by Pinol-Aguade in 1960. This topic is well reviewed by Smith (1986). All have exhibited severe mutilating photosensitivity from birth. In addition, there are hepatic changes and there is usually a mild normochromic normocytic anemia. Uroporphyrin is excreted in great excess in the urine and the excretion pattern may closely resemble that seen in CHP. Unlike CHP, erythrocyte protoporphyrin is markedly increased in hepatoerythropoietic porphyria. URO-D activity examined in erythrocytes and fibroblasts is markedly reduced to less than 10% of normal. The studies to date are consistent with hepatoerythropoietic porphyria, representing homozygosity for the gene associated with reduced URO-D activity.

All the above forms of CHP present with a similar clinical picture of cutaneous photosensitivity and an identical porphyrin excretion pattern due to reduced hepatic URO-D activity. However, the mechanism of the enzyme defect appears to vary, genetic factors being most important in the familial type and acquired factors in the sporadic or toxic type.

C. Erythropoietic protoporphyria

Erythropoietic protoporphyria is principally characterized by acute solar photosensitivity. The nature of the disease was first clearly established by Magnus et al. (1961) and Langhof et al. (1961) although there had been earlier reports (Kosenow and Treibs, 1953). At that stage, it was seen to be an erythropoietic porphyria, but it became clear from the investigations of Barnes et al. (1968) and other workers that there was also a significant hepatic component. Despite its late description this is a relatively common condition although its prevalence has not been precisely calculated. It was thought to be inherited in an autosomal dominant character with partial penetrance. The reasons for this were sought by Went and Klasen (1984) in a study of 91 families in the Netherlands. Their conclusion was that the disease itself was inherited as an autosomal recessive character whereas changes in porphyrin synthesis were inherited as an autosomal dominant character and, on the basis of these findings, it was hypothesized that a 3-allele system applied to this disease to account for the poor penetrance and limited expression of the condition. Decrease of ferrochelatase activity by up to 70% supports their findings. In one subject, the homozygous condition has been reported (Deybach et al., 1986). The age of onset is usually from birth, as with congenital porphyria, but onset may, occasionally, be much later and not necessarily include many of the described features of this disease (Murphy et al., 1985).

IX. Porphyrinurias and Pseudoporphyria

The heterogeneous group of diseases best described as porphyrinurias are those in which the disturbances of porphyrin metabolism have been brought about by endogenous and exogenous factors other than the genetic ones linked to the porphyrias. The porphyrin normally excreted in excess is coproporphyrin. This category includes lead poisoning, hereditary tyrosinemia (Gentz et al., 1969), ethanol abuse (Moore et al., 1984), myocardial infarction (Koskelo, 1956; Koskelo and Hiekkila, 1965), and the effects of drugs like carbamazepine (Yeung-Laiwah et al., 1983) and many other compounds such as polyhalogenated hydrocarbons (Marks, 1981). Coproporphyrinuria has also been reported in a number of condition such as liver disease and hepatocellular carcinoma (Fischer and Zerweck, 1924a; Udagawa et al., 1984). Porphyrins are probably hepatotoxic and may even be associated with the development of neoplasms (Tio et al., 1957). When Lithner and Wetterberg (1984) carried out a retrospective study of 20 years of the relationship between hepatocellular carcinoma and acute intermittent porphyria, they found this to be highly significant.

In addition to those porphyrinurias, there are changes in the pattern or porphyrin isomer excretion in the hyperbilirubinemias of the Dubin-Johnson syndrome and in the Rotor syndrome. In these two conditions the quantity of porphyrin synthesized and excreted is not necessarily in excess of normal upper limits, but they are associated with excess production of series I isomer porphyrin (Koskelo et al., 1967; Ben Ezzer et al., 1971; Cohen et al., 1986).

A. Lead

The connection between lead and porphyrin biosynthesis is reputed to have been first made by Binnendjik (cited by Stokvis, 1895), but the connection between this metal and anemia had been made very much earlier by Laennec in 1831. This was confirmed by Garrod in 1892 who observed abnormal porphyrin excretion in the urine of a patient with lead poisoning and then in 1895 by Stokvis who found that lead-poisoned rabbits excreted excess urinary porphyrins. Other effects of lead on the hemopoietic system were reported before the end of the century by Behrend (1899), who observed stippled basophils in the blood of a patient with lead poisoning.

1. Lead porphyrinemia and porphyrinuria. The crude compound that Garrod identified as hematoporphyrin was shown to be coproporphyrin III by Duesberg (1931). Liebig (1927) had suggested that it was produced by the action of lead on the bone marrow. By 1932, Grotepass had demonstrated elevated coproporphyrin in urine in lead poisoning, and Gould et al. (1937) discovered that, during treatment of cancer patients with lead, a progressive anemia could be found. One of the problems which beset this work was that it was realized that overexposure to lead did not invariably cause lead poisoning, although such effects in children were usually more marked (Albahary et al., 1965). This indicated the problem of differentiating between health effects that might be found in different sectors of the population (Moore and Goldberg, 1985).

The increased concentration of a free porphyrin in blood was identified by Hijmans van den Bergh et al. in 1932 as protoporphyrin IX located in the erythrocytes of subjects dosed with lead. In 1958, Gajdos recommended the routine determination of erythrocyte protoporphyrin (EPP) as an efficient method for discovering masked cases of lead overexposure. Finally, diminution of ALA dehydratase activity (ALA-D) was identified as a means of lead assessment (Gibson et al., 1955) and a European standardized method was introduced (Berlin and Schaller, 1974).

B. Pseudoporphyria

Poh-Fitzpatrick (1986) pointed out that the term "pseudoporphyria" had been used to describe a bullous dermatosis associated with a number of dermatological conditions that bear some resemblance to porphyria, often induced by many drugs but which were not porphyrias! In these conditions there is no alteration in porphyrin metabolism or excretion. It is, therefore, inappropriate to name any of them a porphyria. The term "pseudoporphyria" should not be used to describe them, but only to describe conditions in which alterations of porphyrin metabolism can be found, such as the bullous dermatosis of hemodialysis (Topi et al., 1980; Seubert et al., 1985).

X. Porphyrin Synthesis in the Animal Kingdom

Free porphyrins in varying amounts are found in widely, although somewhat erratically, distributed in most living organisms. It would have been surprising had it been otherwise since the tetrapyrrole ring system is central to the fabric of life. Indeed, anaerobes that have no cytochromes or other hemoproteins may perhaps be regarded as degenerate forms in which this biosynthetic ability has been lost. Microbial porphyrins represent a useful source of material for the examination of porphyrin synthesis (Vannotti, 1954), For example *Rhodobacter spheroides* was used by Lascelles (1964) in her studies of the control of porphyrin synthesis.

Among the mammals, a few genera appear to produce much more porphyrin than others; these belong to the family of rodents. The rat produces a relatively large quantity of protoporphyrin, by synthesis in the harderian glands. Squirrels also produce much porphyrin and their bones have a pale-brown color due to deposition of uroporphyrin and fluoresce pale red in ultraviolet light. This is most marked in the American fox squirrel, *Sciurus niger* (Rimington, 1955). The urine also contains appreciable quantities of porphyrin. Only *Tamias striatus* has this in common with *S. niger* (Turner, 1937). This condition has frequently been referred to as a "physiological porphyria." Levin and Flyger (1971) found reduced activity of the enzyme uroporphyrinogen III cosynthetase in hemolysates and tissue extracts from fox squirrels as compared with grey squirrels. An important factor here is that these squirrels show neither photosensitivity nor anemia, which means that no discernible metabolic, and hence, genetic disadvantage is likely to accrue from this inherited metabolic status. The animals appear in every way normal without untoward symptoms accompanying their high porphyrin production and must, therefore, be regarded as physiological examples of excess porphyrin synthesis. Analogous to this are the mollusks that deposit quantities of uroporphyrin in their shells (Kennedy, 1979), or, among other higher forms of animal life, the group of birds known as the touracos, or plantain eaters, who utilize the copper complex of uroporphyrin III, called turacin, for the deep-red areas of pigmentation in their flight feathers (Church, 1869, 1892; Fischer and Hilger, 1924). Some green pigmentation may be due to porphyrin radical formation (Blumberg and Peisach, 1965). There seems to be nothing otherwise unusual about the porphyrin metabolism of these birds. Other birds also have porphyrins in their feathers and down (With, 1978), and porphyrins are used in the coloration of eggs (With, 1973), probably by deposition within the oviduct (Derrien and Turchini, 1925). Such porphyrin synthesis has been linked with calcification processes (Vannotti, 1954).

1. Harderian gland. An interesting model of heme biosynthesis is the harderian gland, first described by Harder (1694) in red deer. It is found in many rodents and other terrestrial vertebrates, but not in primates (Brownscheidle and Niewenhuis, 1978). An orbital structure, it is associated with the nictitating membrane, but no specific function has yet been described for it. Potentially, it will provide lubrication for the eye, but it may also be part of the retinal-pineal axis and a site of immune response (Wetterberg et al., 1970). Its role as a source of pheromones and thermoregulatory lipids has also been investigated (Mueller et al., 1971; Thiessen et al., 1982).

The harderian gland in the golden hamster is an extremely rich source of porphyrins (Mindegaard, 1976). It has been extensively studied in this rodent. Although the female gland is arguably the richest natural source of porphyrins known, the male gland contains little porphyrin, possibly because the rate-limiting enzyme, 5-aminolevulinic acid (ALA) synthase is more active in the female than the male (Thompson et al., 1984). This sexual dimorphism points to hormonal control of porphyrin synthesis in the gland. Indeed, it has been shown that castration and ovariectomy (Payne et al., 1977, 1979; Spike et al., 1985) and other factors such as season, puberty, and pregnancy will alter gland porphyrin synthesis (Moore et al., 1980). All of these, including the role of hormone replacement (Spike et al., 1985), emphasize the role that steroids play in porphyrin synthesis and the activities of the enzymes of the biosynthetic pathway.

A. Porphyria in animals

1. Hepatic porphyria. Since acute intermittent porphyria is the most common of the porphyrias affecting humans, one might expect that cases of this condition would have been encountered in animals, but up to the present, no clear example of acute intermittent porphyria in animals has been reported. This might be explained by the difficulties in diagnosis of the disease, should it occur in animals. The symptoms of colic and of neuromuscular weakness which characterize attacks in humans would be difficult to perceive in animals. Moreover, in acute porphyria the freshly passed urine containing porphobilinogen may be normally colored and, as such, may elude detection. It is notable that only the cutaneous porphyrias such as congenital porphyria, erythropoietic protoporphyria, and possibly cutaneous hepatic porphyria have been unequivocally seen in animals (Ruth et al., 1978).

2. Congenital porphyria in cattle.   Several reports described the finding of chocolate or brown-colored bones in abattoir carcasses. The first such report was by Brouwier in 1884, followed a year later by one from Tappeiner (1885) of red-brown bones in swine. Mosselman and Hebrant (1898) were convinced that it was formed from hemoglobin while Ingier (1911) thought it to be melanin associated with another pigment derived from chlorophyll. As a result of intensive investigation, Poulsen (1910) came to the conclusion that the disease in animals was entirely different from human ochronosis and that the bone marrow of affected carcasses contained an iron-rich pigment, probably hemosiderin, together with an iron-free coloring matter which was the one responsible for the pigmentation. The latter could be extracted with acids, yielding a reddish-brown solution with spectral absorption reminiscent of that of acid solutions of hematoporphyrin. The similarly between this condition in animals and human congenital porphyria was recognized by Schmey (1913), who proposed for it the name "osteohemochromatosis" instead of the misleading "ochronosis" with which it had previously been known. Hausmann (1923) made similar findings. That the pigment in the bone was a porphyrin seems to have been first clearly realized by Möller-Sorensen (1920), who collected the literature on the disease up to that date. Credit for the suggestion of its hereditary nature should probably go to Witte (1914).

3. Studies in South Africa .   In 1936, a herd of grade shorthorn cattle was discovered in South Africa in which no fewer than 13 cases of congenital porphyria were seen (Rimington 1936, Rimington et al., 1938). One animal was killed and a complete biochemical examination was made which showed a close resemblance between this bovine case and the human subject, Petry. Excessive quantities of uroporphyrin I and coproporphyrin I were found in the organs and body fluids and there was definite evidence of photosensitization. The urine was wine red in color and was rich in uroporphyrin and coproporphyrin; the feces, erythrocytes, and plasma were also rich in coproporphyrin I. The entire skeleton was deep brown in color and afforded large quantities of uroporphyrin I. On cross section it showed rings of lesser and greater pigmentation

(Goldberg and Rimington, 1962). The inheritance was relatively easy to trace as autosomal recessive. The United Kingdom had no record of living cases of congenital porphyria in bovines until discovered by Ross (1957) and Amoroso et al. (1957).

4. Mycosis porphyria. In addition to hereditary porphyria in cattle, an acquired form has been described, attributable to a fungal infection. In cattle infected with *Candida guilliermondii* (Sutka and Durko, 1981), it was found that there was diminished red cell survival and that the porphyrin synthesized by this organism accumulated in certain organs. This was attributed to the lytic effects of porphyrin in the erythrocyte (Kaneko and Cornelius, 1970). Similar to this was the case reported by Lim et al. (1984) of a 24-year-old man who had increased fecal porphyrin excretion, resembling that seen in variegate porphyria. The abnormal fecal porphyrins were shown to be the result of excessive consumption of brewers yeast, which was shown to have a high porphyrin content. In this respect it is notable that anaerobic bacteria can contribute significantly to the fecal porphyrin production in normal subjects (Beukeveld et al., 1987).

5. Porphyria in pigs. As with cattle, dark-colored bones had been noticed in pig carcasses long before living cases of congenital porphyria were diagnosed (Tappeiner, 1885; Poulsen, 1910; Ingier, 1911; Schmey, 1913). The first living cases were observed in New Zealand, and the report by Clare and Stephens (1944) records an affected sow of mixed breed and five affected piglets, but information on the breeding of pigs was too incomplete to allow any assessment of inheritance. In Denmark, what appeared to be congenital porphyria in pigs, appeared in the Thisted district during 1951 and 1954. The inheritance could be traced to a particular board (Jørgensen, 1959). When the boar in question was excluded from breeding operations, the condition rapidly disappeared. Affected animals had discolored teeth displaying pinkish-red fluorescence in ultraviolet light. A closer study of the teeth showed that the porphyrin was not evenly distributed, but was mainly located in the dentine layer just below the enamel. Porphyrin deposition seemed to be associated with the formation of the enamel. None of the affected animals displayed photosensitivity (Jørgensen and With, 1965).

6. Cats and dogs. In 1964, a report appeared of a young kitten whose deciduous teeth were brownish with red fluorescence in ultraviolet light and whose urine had been blood-colored since the cat was 2 months old; it was otherwise normal. When the permanent teeth erupted they were lighter in color and devoid of fluorescence. A littermate and some kittens from a former litter of the mother also had discolored teeth, suggesting a dominant inheritance (Tobias, 1964). Breeding experiments were carried out in 1968 by Glenn and his co-workers. Mendelian dominant inheritance was supported. The skeletons of the affected kittens were brownish at birth and showed red fluorescence. The absence of skin photosensitivity, dominant inheritance, and decrease of porphyrin deposition with age is similar to the porphyria found in pigs. More recently, Haskin (personal communication) established a kindred of cats with dominant inheritance and features similar to acute porphyria.

In studies in Cape Town it has been shown that many dogs have abnormally high excretion of coproporphyrin in urine, which may relate to their carnivorous, rather than omnivorous, eating patterns. Owen et al. (1962) described a young dog with permanent teeth showing a transient pink color in ultraviolet light, but both disappeared after several months. The fluorescence seen in all the teeth was located in the dentine. No fluorocytes could be detected in bone marrow smears and autopsy studies were not performed. This example of a porphyric condition in a dog is reminiscent of porcine porphyria.

XI. Phototherapy and Cancer

The early foundation of photochemotherapy may be sought in the work of the 1903 Nobel laureate Neils Finsen. Thereafter, Hausmann in 1908 and 1911 showed that hematoporphyrin photosensitized both paramecia and mice. Normal human tissue also reacts in a pathological fashion when saturated with porphyrins and exposed to light, as was so clearly demonstrated by Meyer-Betz in 1913. It is a simple step to conclude that this photoreaction might be usefully employed in the destruction of pathological tissue. This was aided by the early description by Policard (1924) of the preferential uptake by rat sarcoma of hematoporphyrin. This was thought to be due to infecting bacteria, but Körbler (1931, 1932) found no evidence that bacteria were involved. That injected porphyrins accumulated in tumors were observed by Körbler (1931) and confirmed, through the ensuing years, by Bungeler (1937), Auler and Banzer (1942), and Figge et al. (1948). The work of both Schwartz and co-workers (1955) and Rassmussen-Taxdal et al. (1955) is of interest since it pointed the way for future work in humans.

A. Hematoporphyrin derivative

The foundation of the present use of hematoporphyrin derivative is based on the work of Lipson et al. (1961), who showed that some components of hematoporphyrin derivative (HPD) were better localized in malignant tissue than "crude" hematoporphyrin and in the development of lasers. Hematoporphyrin derivative is still produced in a fashion similar to that described by Lipson. Hematoporphyrin in crystalline form is dissolved in a mixture of glacial acetic acid and concentrated sulfuric acid which, after neutralization with sodium acetate, is redissolved in sodium hydroxide in saline. Such chemical treatment of the hematoporphyrin produces a complex mixture of substances, such as mono- and diacetates of hematoporphyrin, protoporphyrin, deuteroporphyrin, and, in particular, a dihematoporphyrin ether or ester (Kessel, 1982; Dougherty et al., 1984; Kessel and Chang, 1985). This may be the principal photoactive component of HPD.

The fundamental principle behind this therapy is that since tumor tissue will preferentially accumulate porphyrins, these may be used for both identification and therapy of neoplastic tissue. The obvious aim in therapy is to produce porphyrins with maximal quantum yield which will, consequently, produce the maximal tissue destruction. Unfortunately, other metabolically active tissue, such as liver and kidney, also accumulate porphyrins, but being remote from light sources these are relatively safe from the photodestructive effects of therapy. The red fluorescence seen in ultraviolet light of tumors after injection of various porphyrins has proved of help to the surgeon in the localization of neoplasms during an operation. This property of localization is common to any rapidly growing tissue. Normal cutaneous tissue also accumulates porphyrin and a serious side effect of therapy is continued light photosensitivity of exposed skin for a considerable time after treatment (Fig. 1.14).

This area of study is one of which work continues to seek better localizers and/or sensitizers, based either on specific synthesis of porphyrin derivatives or through the use of other naturally occurring porphyrins or synthetic porphyrins and in the development of better light sources. At the present time, the clinical interest in this subject has been stimulated by technological developments. These relate principally to the development of better laser light sources such as gold vapor lasers and other forms of tunable lasers and endoscopic probes.

XII. "Royal Malady"

The history of the porphyrias is naturally only truly reliable from the time at which there was concurrent medical observation and scientific mensuration. Any studies prior to the well-documented works at the end of the last century are, therefore, liable to be steeped in anecdotal inaccuracy. It is, however, of interest to consider the hypothesis propounded by MacAlpine and Hunter in 1964 that porphyria, possibly variegate porphyria, was presented in the Royal Houses of Stuart and Hanover in the United Kingdom (MacAlpine and Hunter, 1969). The ability to carry out such investigations depended not only on the inevitable extensive documentation of royalty, but also on the very precise descriptions conveyed to us over time by their physicians.

Of these, one of the more remarkable is that of Sir Theodore Turquet de Mayerne, physician to James, VI and I. He described one acute episode, following a hunting trip:

> On his return he passed blood red urine.... He also told me that he quite frequently passed water, red like Alicante wine but without attendant pain....

Mary Queen of Scots had suffered similarly to her son from acute

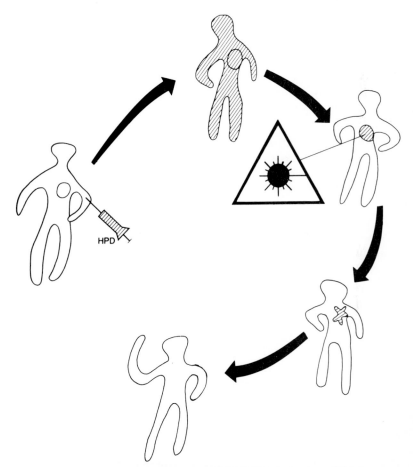

Figure 1.14 The mode of action of hematoporphyrin derivative (HPD) in cancer therapy. There is preferential update of HPD by metabolically active tissues such as neoplasms. When this is irradiated with light of an appropriate wavelength, as produced by a tunable laser, there is tissue necrosis and regression of the tumor.

attacks of abdominal colic, described as

> ...he labored under painful colic from flatus (an affliction from which his mother also suffered)...

The tale may then be followed through many of their descendants including Goeorge III, Frederic the Great of Prussia, and Kaiser Wilhelm II, all of whom evinced features consistent with those of acute porphyria. The greatest weakness in the argument is that no living relative has yet been shown to have porphyria. This hypothesis provoked considerable dispute, which is well described by Dean (1971). It is clear that when a personage or family of standing can be involved in a controversy such as this, the story will be espoused by the general population, often repeated, and bound to be believed by some, despite its lack of substance. However, it is noteworthy that no acceptable alternative suggestion in explanation of King George's illness, for example, has, as yet, been proposed by anyone who finds difficulty in accepting MacAlpine and Hunter's hypothesis.

The historical implications of these observations are profound and if true could imply that the loss of the power of the British and of the American Colonies could be ascribed to a genetic disease (Ware, 1968). Perhaps with the benefit of hindsight the best judgment on the "royal malady" must remain "not proven" (that equivocal Scottish legal term).

XIII. Werewolves

A bizarre suggestion has been that persons with congenital porphyria or hepatoerythropoietic porphyria or other of the homozygous porphyrias were the werewolves or vampires of legend. Lycanthropy (magical transformation of human to wolf) certainly did not take place, but the subjects' skin mutilation, hypertrichosis, and desire to eschew light exposure may had led the superstitious to this conclusion (Illis, 1964; Dolphin, 1985). The medieval descriptions of werewolves included: "pale yellowish excoriated skin"—explicable by hemolytic anemia and pruritis; reddish teeth—erythrodontia; and "habitation in isolated regions, such as Central European valleys"—familial association and inbreeding in such areas. There is no doubt that in the past the gross disfigurement associated with these diseases, particularly to the face and to the development of clawlike hands, could have been given a magical provenance. It is not easy to explain either fear of garlic or lust for blood. The effects of garlic might have related to the oxidative metabolism of dialkyl disulfide. The consequential loss of heme, as happens during drug metabolism, might have been replaced by heme from hemoglobin in the blood, to act as hematin does during therapy. In all of this the needs of the patient should be considered. The press hysteria in the United

TABLE 1.3   Selected Chronology of Porphyrins and Porphyria

1831	Laennec	Anemia of lead poisoning
1837	Lecanu	Acid extraction of hemin from blood
1841	Scherer	Hemin extraction—iron free
1844	Mülder	Purple-red fluid devoid of iron
1864	Hoppe-Seyler	Named hemoglobin
1867	Thudichum	Spectrum and red fluorescence of porphyrins
1871	Hoppe-Seyler	Prepared porphyrins from blood and showed they were pyrroles
1874	Schultz	Congenital porphyria—(pemphigus leprosus)
	Baumstark	Urinary porphyrin pigments—an error of biosynthesis
1879	Hoppe-Seyler	Chlorophyll tetrapyrrole, phylloporphyrin, structurally similar to heme
1880	McMunn	Salicylate-induced porphyrinogenesis
1883	Soret	Light absorption around 400 nm of hemin
	Krukenberg	Red fluorescence of eggshells
1884	McMunn	Discovery of cytochromes (myohematin)
	Brouwier	Chocolate-colored bones in abbatoir carcasses
1888	Nencki and Sieber	Hematoporphyrin dicarboxylic
1889	Stokvis	Sulfonal-induced acute porphyria
	McMunn	Porphyrins in echinoderms and the black slug, *Arion*
1890	Ranking and Pardington	Described the symptoms of acute porphyria
1891	Geill and Fehr	Induction of acute porphyria in women by sulfonal
	Copeman	Neurosis in female porphyrics
1892	Church	Turacin shown to be a porphyrin
1895	Stokvis	Animal porphyria
	Binnendijk	Excess porphyrins in urine of lead-poisoned patient
1896	Saillet	Coproporphyrin (urospectrine)
1903	Zaleski	Mesoporphyrin
	Erbslöh	Axonal degeneration in acute porphyria
1904	Laidlaw	Preparation of protoporphyrin
1906	Willstätter	Chlorophyll characterization commenced
	Dobrschansky	Barbiturate-induced porphyria
1908	Hausmann	Porphyrin photosensitization of mice
1911	Günther	First classification of porphyria
1912	Küster	Correct tetrapyrrolic structure of heme
1913	Meyer-Betz	Hematoporphyrin sensitization of skin
1915	Willstätter	Nobel prize for chlorophyll work
1923	Kämmerer	Porphyrin from putrefying meat—protoporphyrin
	Garrod	Porphyria—inborn error of metabolism
1924	Fischer and Kögl	Ooporphyrin (protoporphyrin) in eggshells
	Policard	Preferential uptake of hematoporphyrin by rat sarcoma
1925	Keilin	Rediscovers cytochromes
	Derrien and Turchini	Oviduct porphyrin deposition on eggshells Intense red fluorescence of harderian gland
1929	Fischer and Zeile	Hemin synthesis confirming Küster's structure Similarities of side chains of heme and chlorophyll
	Borst and Königsdörffer	Autopsy study of Petry
1930	Fischer	Nobel prize for porphyrin work
1931	Sachs	Chromogen giving red coloration with Ehrlich's reagent
	Körbler	Porphyrin uptake by tumors
1932	Grotepass	Urinary coproporphyrin III in lead poisoning
	Hijmans van den Bergh	Lead increase in erythrocyte protoporphyrin
1933	Watson	Stercobilins

TABLE 1.3   Selected Chronology of Porphyrins and Porphyria (*Continued*)

1933	Dhéré et al.	Studies of microbial porphyrins
1935	Franke and Fikentscher	Doubling of urinary coproporphyrin excretion after ethanol
1936	Dobriner	First case of what would be called hereditary coproporphyria
	Rimington	Congenital porphyria in cattle
1937	Waldenström	Review, naming of porphyria cutanea tarda and classification of acute porphyria
	Turner	Porphyrins in fox squirrels
	Guildemeister	Albumin binding of porphyrins
1939	Rimington and Hemmings	Coproporphyrinuria following use of sulfanilamide
	Waldenström	Isolation of porphobilinogen
1941	Watson and Schwartz	Simple test for urinary porphobilinogen
1944	Strong	Harderian gland porphyrin and carcinoma in mice
	Clare and Stephens	Congenital porphyria in pigs
1945	Barnes	Variegate porphyria in South Africa
1946	Shemin and Rittenberg	Isotopic study of porphyrin biosynthesis
	Corwin and Erdman	IR investigation of NH tautomerism
1948	Folkers and Smith	Isolation and characterizatiaon of vitamin B12
1949	Pauling and Itano	Sickle cell hemoglobin
	Lemberg and Legge	Description of biosynthetic sequence
1950	Neuberger et al. and Shemin et al.	Uroporphyrin first formed biosynthetically
	Rimington and Sveinsson	Spectral absorption of porphyrins
1951	Watson et al.	Erythropoietic and hepatic classification of porphyria
	Shemin and Wittenberg	Requirement for succinyl-CoA
1952	Westall	Isolation of PBG
1953	Shemin and Russell and Neuberger and Scott	Role of ALA in biosynthesis
	Kosenow and Treibs	Erythropoietic protoporphyria
1955	Goldberg and Rimington	Allylisopropylacetamide-induced experimental porphyria
	Hodgkin et al.	X-ray structure of vitamin B12
	Bogorad	Reduced porphyrins—porphyrinogens are biosynthetic intermediates
	Shemin	The succinate-glycine cycle
	Berger and Goldberg	Named hereditary coproporphyria
	Tio	Porphyria cutanea tarda associated with adenoma
	Schwartz et al. and Rassmussen-Taxdal et al.	Use of hematoporphyrin derivative on cancer
1956	Goldberg et al.	Ferrochelatase—the iron-incorporating enzyme
	Waldenström	Recognition that each porphyria can be localized to a defect in one enzyme
1957	Cam	Turkish porphyria—hexachlorobenzene-induced
	Lascelles and Schulman and Richert	ALA synthase—requirement for pyridoxal phosphate
	Haeger	ALA in urine in lead poisoning

TABLE 1.3   **Selected Chronology of Porphyrins and Porphyria** (*Continued*)

1958	Granick	ALA synthase the primary control point of heme biosynthesis
1959	Solomon and Figge	3,5-Dicarbethoxy-1,4-dihydrocollidine experimental porphyria
	Becker and Bradley	First application of nmr to porphyrin structure
1961	Calvin	Nobel prize for photosynthesis work
	Magnus et al. and Langhof et al.	Named and studied erythropoietic protoporphyria
	Lipson et al.	Use of purified hematoporphyrin derivative
	Gajdos et al.	Role of ATP in control of prophyrin synthesis
1962	Perutz and Kendrew	Nobel prize for x-ray structure of Hb
1964	Illis	Porphyria and the etiology of werewolves
	Heide et al.	Hemopexin a heme-binding β-globulin
	Dagg et al.	Similarities between acute porphyria and lead poisoning
1966	Macalpine and Hunter	"Royal malady"
1969	Pinol-Aguade et al.	Hepatoerythropoietic porphyria
	Gajdos et al.	Homozygous hereditary coproporphyria
	Romeo and Levin	Uro'gen III cosynthase and congenital porphyria
1970	Strand et al.	Acute intermittent porphyria related to deficiency of PBG deaminase
	Koskelo et al.	Binding of ^{14}C-porphyrins by hemopexin and albumin
1971	Bonkowsky et al.	Hematin use in acute porphyria
	Moore et al.	Ethanol inhibition of ALA dehydratase
1973	Beale et al.	ALA synthesis from glutamate, through DOVA
1974	Jackson et al.	Protoporphyrinogen oxidation enzymically controlled
1975	Bonkowsky et al. and Bottomley et al. and De Goeij et al.	Ferrochelatase and erythropoietic protoporphyria
1976	Elder	Hydroxymethylbilane synthase as secondary control stage
	Wetterberg	International review of drugs in porphyria
	Brodie et al. and Elder et al.	Coproporphyrinogen oxidase and hereditary coproporphyria
	Kushner et al.	Uro'gen decarboxylase and PCT
1977	Brodie et al.	Control of acute porphyrias by PBG deaminase
1979	Jordan et al. and Battersby et al.	Mechanism of formation of uroporphyrinogen III from hydroxymethylbilane (preuroporphyrinogen)
	Bird et al.	First description of plumboporphyria (ALA dehydratase deficiency)
	Moore et al.	Acute and nonacute classification of porphyria
	Tephly et al.	DDC forms N-alkylated porphyrins
1980	Meisler et al.	Gene for porphobilinogen deaminase on chromosome 11
	Brenner and Bloomer	Protoporphyrinogen oxidase and variegate porphyria
1981	Mustajoki and Anderson et al.	Immunological variants of PBG deaminase—CRIM positive and CRIM negative
1982	Day et al.	Concurrent (dual) variegate porphyria and PCT
	Nordmann et al.	Description of harderoporphyria
1983	Eiberg et al.	Gene for ALA dehydratase on chromosome 9
	Grandchamp et al.	Gene for coproporphyrinogen oxidase on chromosome 9
	Batlle et al.	Use of ALA dehydratase replacement therapy
1984	Kordác et al.	Homozygous variegate porphyria
	Grandchamp et al.	cDNA for PBG deaminase mRNA
	de Verneuil et al.	Gene for uroporphyrinogen decarboxylase on chromosome 1
1986	Deybach et al.	Homozygous erythropoietic protoporphyria
1987	Llewellyn et al.	DNA polymorphism for PBG deaminase

States, following these disclosures, established an inaccurate and unjustified perception of porphyria in the public mind and did considerable harm to the porphyric patient (Dresser, 1986).

XIV. Epilogue

In the evolution of understanding of heme biosynthesis, many factors have played a part. Not the least of these is serendipity. Would Fischer have been the giant that he was without Petry? Indeed would Petry have gone to Munich without the beer? It is informative to overview the developments of history as shown in Table 1.3 in order that the mistakes and stumbling blocks that occurred in the past are not repeated in the future.

Modern, molecular genetic methods have, as pointed out by Gajdos in 1986, opened up a new and promising field of porphyrin research. Chromosomal location of the gene encoding for the various enzymes participating in the synthesis of porphyrins has clearly shown that they are not clustered in the human genome, but dispersed among different chromosomes. This fact poses a lot of new problems concerning the coordinative mechanism of porphyrin biosynthesis and may further illuminate the characteristics of the individual porphyrias and certainly contribute to innovative developments in the measurement of enzyme activity and lead to an effective clinical use of the enzymic classification. The individual errors in the porphyrias have now been mapped so that bewilderment over their kaleidoscopic manifestations has given place to a more rational understanding of them. It is because porphyrins are photoactive that they play the part that they do in biological systems. It is, therefore, obvious that the toxic effects of excess porphyrin will relate to these same abilities. The central role that porphyrins play in biological energy entrapment and utilization ensures that the investigation of their chemistry and biology will continue and that further uses will be sought and found for their unique structures. As Claude Rimington said, "It is arguably true that the tetrapyrrole system is Nature's most remarkable creation."

REFERENCES

Ackner, B., Cooper, J. E., Gray, C. H., and Kelly, M. (1962). Acute porphyria: A neuropsychiatric and biochemical study, *J. Psych. Res.* **6**:1–24.

Albahary, C., and Martins, G. P. (1965). La nocivite hematologique du plomb. Bilan de 40 malades hospitalises pour saturnisme professionnel, *Nouv. Rev. Franc. Hematol.* **5**:689–695.

Amoroso, F. C., Loosmore, R. M., Rimington, C., and Tooth, B. (1957). Congenital porphyria in bovines: First living cases in Britain, *Nature (London)* **180**:230–231.

Anderson, P. M., Reddy, R. M., Anderson, K. E., and Desnick, R. J. (1981). Characterisation of the porphobilinogen-deaminase deficiency in acute intermittent porphyria, *J. Clin. Invest.* **68**:1–12.

Auler, H., and Banzer, G. (1942). Untersuchungen uber die rolle der porphyrine bei geschwulstkranken menschen und tieren, *Z. Krebs.* **53**:65–68.

Barillari, B., Zappoli-Thyrion, E., De Cesare, M., and Marinig, L. (1984). Severe psychic disorders without clinical signs of peripheral neuropathy in a subject with porphyria, *Riv. Neurobiol.* **30**:394–397.

Barnes, H. D. (1945). A note on porphyrinuria with a resume of 11 South African cases, *Clin. Proc.* **4**:269–275.

Barnes, H. D., Hurworth, E., and Millar, J. H. D. (1968). Erythropoietic porphyria hepatitis, *J. Clin. Pathol.* **21**:157–159.

Baruch, L., Krupa-Matusczyk, I., and Sobczyk, P. (1981). Zespol depresyjny w przbiegu porphyrii, *Przegl. Dermatol.* **68**:503–504.

Batlle, A. M. del C., Bustos, N. I., Stella, A. M., Wider, E. A., Conti, H. A., and Mendez, A. (1983). Enzyme replacement therapy in porphyrias. IV. First successful human clinical trial of 5-aminolaevulinate dehydratase-loaded erythrocyte ghosts, *Int. J. Biochem.* **15**:1261–1265.

Battersby, A. R., Fookes, C. J. R., Matcham, G. W. J., and McDonald, E. (1980). Biosynthesis of the pigments of life: Formation of the macrocycle, *Nature* **285**:17–21.

Baumstark, F. (1874). Zwei pathologische Harnfarbstoff, *Pflugers Arch. ges. Physiol.* **9**:568–584.

Beale, S. I., Gough, S. P., and Granick, S. (1975). Biosynthesis of delta-aminolevulinic acid from the intact carbon skeleton of glutamic acid in greening barley, *Proc. Nat. Acad. Sci. (U.S.A.)* **72**:2719.

Becker, E. D., and Bradley, R. B. (1959). NMR and porphyrin structure, *J. Chem. Phys.* **31**:1413.

Behrend, B. (1899). Uber endoglobulare Einschlusse volker Blutkorperchen, *Deutsch. Med. Wschr.* **25**:254.

Ben Ezzer, J., Rimington, C., Shani, M., Seligsohn, U., Sheba, C., and Szeinberg, A. (1971). Abnormal excretion of the isomers of urinary coproporphyrin by patients with Dubin-Johnson syndrome in Israel, *Clin. Sci.* **40**:17–30.

Berger, H., and Goldberg, A. (1955). Hereditary coproporphyria, *Brit. Med. J.* **11**:85–87.

Berlin, A., and Schaller, K. H. (1974). European standardised method for the determination of delta aminolaevulinic acid dehydratase activity in blood, *Z. Klin. Chemie Klin, Biochem.* **12**:389–390.

Berzelius, J. J. (1840). *Lehrbuch der Chemie*, Arnoldische Buchhandlung, Dresden and Leipzig, pp. 67–69.

Beukeveld, G. J. J., Wolthers, B. G., Van Saene, J. J. M., de Haan, T. H. I. J., de Ruyter-Buitenhuis, L. W., and Van Saene, R. H. F. (1987). Patterns of porphyrin excretion in faeces as determined by liquid chromatography: Reference values and the effect of flora suppression, *Clin. Chem.* **33**:2164–2170.

Bird, T. D., Hamernyik, P., Nutter, J. Y., and Labbe, R. F. (1979). Inherited deficiency of delta-aminolevulinic acid dehydratase, *Amer. J. Hum. Genet.* **31**:662–668.

Blumberg, W. E., and Peisach, J. (1965). Electron spin resonance of Cu URO III and other Turaco feather compounds, *J. Biol. Chem.* **240**:870–875.

Bogorad, L. (1955). Intermediates in the biosynthesis of porphyrins from porphobilinogen, *Science* **121**:878–879.

Bonkowsky, H. L., Bloomer, J. R., Ebert, P. S., and Mahoney, M. J. (1975). Haem synthetase deficiency in human protoporphyria: demonstration of the defect in liver and cultured skin fibroblasts, *J. Clin. Invest.* **56**:1139–1148.

Bonkowsky, H. L., Tschudy, D. P., Collins, A., Doherty, J., Bossenmaier, I., Cardinal, R., and Watson, C. J. (1971). Repression of the over-production of porphyrin precursors in acute intermittent porphyria by intravenous infusions of hematin, *Proc. Nat. Acad. Sci. (U.S.A.)* **68**:2725–2729.

Bonnett, R., and Czechowski, F. (1984). Metalloporphyrins in coal—gallium porphyrins in bituminous coal, *J. Chem. Sci.* **1**:125–132.

Borst, M., and Königsdörffer, H. (1929). *Untersuchungen uber porphyrie mit besonderer berucksichtigung der Porphyrie Congenita*, Hirzel, Leipzig.

Bottomley, S. S., Tanaka, M., and Everett, M. A. (1975). Diminished erythroid ferrochelatase activity in protoporphyria, *J. Lab. Clin. Med.* **86**:126.

Brenner, D. A., and Bloomer, J. R. (1980). The enzymatic defect in variegate porphyria, *N. Engl. J. Med.* **302**:765–769.

Brodie, M. J., Moore, M. R., and Goldberg, A. (1977a). Enzyme abnormalities in the porphyrias, *Lancet* ii:699–701.

Brodie, M. J., Thompson, G. G., Moore, M. R., Beattie, A. D., and Goldberg, A. (1977b). Hereditary coproporphyria, *Quart. J. Med.* **46**:229–241.

Bronckart, C., and Troisfontaines, B. (1984). Porphyries aigues et psychiatrie, *Acta Psych. Belg.* **84**:336–352.

Brouwier, L. (1884). Quelques observations recueilles dans le service d'inspection de l'abbatoir de Liege: Alteration des os, *Echo. Vet.* (*Liege*) 271–273.

Brownscheidle, C. M., and Niewenhuis, R. J. (1978). Ultrastructure of the Harderian gland in male albino rats, *Anat. Rec.* **190**:735–754.

Brugsch, J. (1959). *Porphyrine,* J. Ambrosius Barth, Leipzig.

Bungeler, W. (1937). Uber den einflub photosensibilisierender substanzen auf die entstehung von hautgeschwulsten, *Z. Krebs.* **46**:130–167.

Calvin, M. (1959). Evolution of enzymes and the photosynthetic apparatus, *Science* **130**:1170.

Cam, C. (1957). Report on few cases of congenital porphyria, *Nester* (*Instanbul*) **1**:2–6.

Cam, C., and Nigogosyan, G. (1963). Acquired toxic porphyria cutanea tarda due to hexachlorobenzene, *J. Amer. Med. Assoc.* **183**:88–91.

Campbell, K. (1898). A case of haematoporphyrinuria, *J. Men. Sci.* **44**:305–313.

Carney, M. W. P. (1972). Hepatic porphyria with mental symptoms—four missed cases, *Lancet* ii:100–101.

Cetingil, A. I., and Ozen, M. A. (1960). Toxic porphyria, *Blood* **16**:1002–1010.

Church, A. H. (1869). Researches in turacin, an animal pigment containing copper, *Phil. Trans. Roy. Soc.* **159**:627–636.

Church, A. H. (1892). Researches in Turacin an animal pigment containing copper II, *Philos. Trans. Roy. Soc. Lond. Ser. A* **183**:511–530.

Clare, T., and Stephens, E. H. (1944). Congenital porphyria in pigs, *Nature* (*London*) **153**:252–253.

Cohen, C., Kirsch, R. E., and Moore, M. R. (1986). Porphobilinogen-deaminase and the synthesis of porphyrin isomers in Dubin-Johnson syndrome, *S. Afr. Med. J.* **70**:36–39.

Cookson, G. H., and Rimington, C. (1954). Porphobilinogen, *Biochem. J.* **57**:476–484.

Copeman, S. M. (1891). Porphyrinuria, *Proc. Pathol. Soc. Lond. Lancet* i:197.

Cross, T. N. (1956). Porphyria—a deceptive syndrome, *Amer. J. Psych.* **112**:1010–1022.

Dagg, J. H., Goldberg, A., Lochhead, A., and Smith, J. A. (1964). The relationship of lead poisoning to acute intermittent porphyria, *Quart. J. Med.* **34**:163–175.

Day, R. S., Eales, L., and Meissner, D. (1982). Co-existent variegate porphyria and porphyria cutanea tarda, *N. Engl. J. Med.* **307**:36–41.

De Gennes, L., Bricaire, H., and Tubiana, M. (1949). La porphyrie aigue intermittente, *Ann. Med.* **50**:56–71.

De Goeij, A. F. P. M., Christianse, K., and Van Steveninck, J. (1975). Decreased haem synthetase activity in blood cells of patients with erythropoietic protoporphyria, *Eur. J. Clin. Invest.* **5**:397–400.

De Matteis, F. (1967). Disturbances of liver metabolism caused by drugs, *Pharm. Rev.* **19**:523–550.

De Matteis, F., and Marks, G. S. (1983). The effect of *N*-methylprotoporphyrin and succinylacetone on the regulation of haem biosynthesis in checken hepatocytes in culture, *FEBS Lett.* **159**:127–131.

De Matteis, F., and Rimington, C. (1963). Disturbance of porphyrin metabolism caused by griseofulvin in mice, *Brit. J. Dermatol.* **75**:91–104.

De Verneuil, H., Grandchamp, B., Foubert, C., Weil, D., N'Guyen, V. C., Gross, M. S., Sassa, S., and Nordmann, Y. (1984). Assignment of the gene for uroporphyrinogen decarboxylase to human chromosome 1 by somatic cell hybridization and specific enzyme immunoassay, *Hum. Genet.* **66**:202–205.

Dean, G. (1971). *The Porphyrias,* Pub Pitman, London.

Derrien, E., and Turchini, J. (1925). Sur les fluorescences rouges de certains tissus ou secreta animaux en lumiere ultraviolette—nouvelles observations de fluorescences rouges chez les animaux. *C. R. Soc. Biol.* (*Paris*) **92**:1028–1032.

Deybach, J. C., Da Silva, V., Pasquier, Y., and Nordmann, Y. (1986). Ferrochelatase in human erythropoietic protoporphyria—the first case of a homozygous form of the enzyme deficiency, *Porphyrins and Porphyrias* (Y. Nordmann, Ed.), Libbey, London, pp. 163–173.

Dhéré, C. (1933). Sur les spectres de fluorescence de l'hypericine et de la mycoporphyrine, *C. R. Acad. Sci. (Paris)* **197**:948–951.

Dobriner, K. (1936). Simultaneous excretion of coproporphyrin 1–III. In a case of chronic porphyria, *Proc. Soc. Exp. Biol. Med.* **35**:175–176.

Dobrschansky, M. (1906). Einiges uber malonal, *Wiener Med. Presse* **47**:2145.

Dolphin, D. (Ed.) (1979). *The Porphyrins*, Academic, New York, 7 volumes.

Dolphin, D. (1985). Werewolves and vampires, *Proc. Amer. Assoc. Adv. Sci.* May 1985

Doss, M., Von Tiepermann, R., Schneider, J., and Schmid, H. (1979). New type of hepatic porphyria with porphobilinogen synthase defect and intermittent acute clinical manifestation, *Klin. Woch.* **57**:1123–1127.

Dougherty, T. J., Potter, W. R., and Weishaupt, K. R. (1984). An overview of the status of photoradiation therapy, *Porphyrin Localisation and Treatment of Tumors* (T. J. Doiron and C. J. Gomer, Eds.), Alan R. Liss, New York.

Dresser, N. (1986). Vampires are in the headlines, but patients pay the price, Cal. Folk. Soc., Modesto, Calif.

Duesberg, R. (1931). Uber die anamien—1. Porphyrie und erythropoese, *Arch. Exp. Pathol.* **162**:249.

Duesberg, R. (1932). Toxische porphyrie, *Mun. Med. Wschr.* **79**:1821.

Duret-Cosyns, S., and Duret, R. L. (1959). Etude psychiatrique de la porphyrie essentielle, *Ann. Med. Psych.* **2**:193–211.

Eales, L. (1979). Clinical chemistry of the porphyrias, *The Porphyrias* (D. Dolphin, Ed.), Academic, New York, pp. 665–793.

Eiberg, H., Mohr, J., and Staub-Nielsen, L. (1983). Delta-aminolaevulinate dehydrase—syntegency with AB0-AK1-ORM and assignment to chromosome 9, *Clin. Genet.* **23**:150–154.

Eilenberg, M. D., and Scobie, B. A. (1960). Prolonged neuropsychiatric disability and cardio-myopathy in acute intermittent porphyria, *Lancet* **i**:858.

Elder, G. H. (1976). Acquired disorders of haem synthesis, *Essays Med. Biochem.* **2**:75–114.

Elder, G. H., Evans, J. O., Thomas, N., Cox, R., Brodie, M. J., Moore, M. R., Goldberg, A., and Nicholson, D. C. (1976). The primary enzyme defect in hereditary coproporphyria, *Lancet* **ii**:1217–1219.

Ellinger, H. (1916). Uber chronische trionalvergiftung, *Mun. Med. Wschr.* **63**:684.

Erbslöh, W. (1903). Zur pathologie und pathologischen anatomie der toxischer polyneuritis nach sulfonalgebrauch, *Deutsch. Z. Nervenheik* **23**:197–204.

Falk, J. E. (1964). *Porphyrins and Metalloporphyrins*, Elsevier, Amsterdam.

Falk, J. E., Dresel, E. I. B., and Rimington, C. (1953). Porphobilinogen as a porphyrin precursor and interconversion of porphyrins in a tissue system, *Nature* **172**:292.

Fehr, H. (1891). Et par tilfaelde af sulfonalforgiftning, *Hosp. Tidende* **9**:1122–1138.

Figge, F. H. J., Weiland, G. S., and Manganiello, L. O. J. (1948). Cancer detection and therapy: The affinity of neoplastic, embryonic and traumatized tissues for porphyrins and metalloporphyrins, *Proc. Roy. Soc. Exp. Biol. Med.* **68**:640–641.

Fischer, H. (1915). Uber das urinporphyrin. 1. Mitteilung, *Hoppe-Seyler's Z. Physiol. Chem.* **95**:34–60.

Fischer, H., and Hilger, J. (1924). Zur kenntnis der naturlichen porphyrine. 8 mitteilung. Uber das vorkommen von uroporphyrin (als kuppfersalz, Turacin) in den turakusvogeln und den nachweis von koproporphyrin in der hefe, *Hoppe-Seyler's Z. Physiol. Chem.* **138**:49–67.

Fischer, H., Hilmer, H., Lindner, F., and Putzer, B. (1925). Chemische befunde bei einem fall von porphyrie (Petry), *Hoppe-Seyler's Z. Physiol. Chem.* **150**:44–101.

Fischer, H., and Kögl, F. (1924). Uber ooporphyrin, *Hoppe-Seyler's Z. Physiol. Chem.* **138**:262–268.

Fischer, H., and Orth, H. (1937). *Chemie des Pyrrols*, Acad. Verlag, Leipzig.

Fischer, H., and Zerweck, W. (1924a). Uber den harnfarbstoff bei normalen und pathologis-chen verhaltnissen und seine lichtschutzende wirkung. Zugleich einige beitrage zur kenntnis der porphyrinurie, *Hoppe-Seyler's Z. Physiol. Chem.* **137**:176–241.

Fischer, H., and Zerweck, W. (1924b). Uber uroporphyrinogen heptamethylester und eine neue uberfuhrung von uro-koproporphyrin, *Hoppe-Seyler's Z. Physiol. Chem.* **137**:242–264.

Fiume, S., and Vella, G. (1966). Psychiatric features of porphyria, *Panmin. Medica* **8**:271–274.

Florkin, M., and Stotz, E. H. (1979). Biosynthesis of tetrapyrroles and of corrinoids, *Comprehensive Biochemistry: A History of Biochemstry*, Elsevier, Amsterdam, pp. 193–238.

Franke, K., and Fikentscher, R. (1935). Die bedeutung der quantitativen porphyrin bestim-mung mit der lumineszenzmessung fur die prufung der leberfunktion und fur er-nahrungsfrogen, *Mun. Med. Woch.* **82**:171–172.

Freeman, J. G., and Kolb, L. C. (1951). Acute intermittent porphyria—associated psychi-atric symptoms treated by electro-shock, *Proc. Staff Meetings Mayo Clin.* **26**:401–406.

Gagey, P. L. (1896). Un cas d'hemoglobinurie en cours d'un xeroderma pigmentosum, Thèse de Paris.

Gajdos, A. (1986). *Porphyrins and Porphyrias* (Y. Nordmann, Ed.), Libbey, London, pp. 11–13.

Gajdos, A., and Gajdos-Torok, M. (1958). Modification du taux de la protoporphyrine libre et de l'activite catalasique dans les globules rouge du lapin intoxiqué par le plomb ou par la phenylhydrazine, *Sang* **29**:27–33.

Gajdos, A., and Gajdos-Torok, M. (1961). The therapeutic effect of adenosine-5-monophos-phoric acid in porphyria, *Lancet* **ii**:175.

Gajdos, A., Weil, J., Gajdos-Torok, M., and Coupry, A. (1969). Une nouvelle variété de porphyrie: la coproporphyrie mixte ou variegata, *Rev. Franc. Clin. Biol.* **14**:279–282.

Garrod, A. (1892). On the occurrence and detection of haematoporphyrin in the urine, *J. Physiol.* **13**:598–620.

Garrod, A. E. (1923). *Inborn Errors of Metabolism*, 2nd ed., Hodder and Stoughton, London.

Geill, C. (1891). Sulfonal og sulfonalforgiftning, *Hosp. Tidende* **9**:797–812.

Gentz, J., Johansson, S., Lindblad, B., Lindstedt, S., and Zetterstrom, R. (1969). Excretion of delta-aminolaevulinic acid in hereditary tyrosinaemia, *Clin. Chim. Acta* **23**:257–263.

Gibson, K. D., Laver, W. G., and Neuberger, A. (1958). Initial stages in the biosynthesis of porphyrins. II. The formation of 5-ALA from glycine and succinyl CoA by particles from chicken erythrocytes, *Biochem. J.* **70**:71–76.

Gibson, K. D., Neuberger A., and Scott J. J. (1955). The purification and properties of delta-aminolaevulinic acid dehydratase, *Biochem. J.* **61**:618–629.

Gildemeister, H. (1937). Porphyrine und serumeiweiss, *Z. Exp. Med.* **102**:58–87.

Glenn, B. L., Glenn, H. G., and Omtvedt, I. (1968). Congenital porphyria in a domestic cat (*Felis catus*). Preliminary investigations on inheritance pattern, *Amer. J. Vet. Res.* **29**:1653–1657.

Goldberg, A. (1959). Acute intermittent porphyria: A study of 50 cases, *Quart. J. Med.* **28**:183–209.

Goldberg, A., Ashenbrucker, M., Cartwright, G. E., and Wintrobe, M. M. (1956). Studies on the biosynthesis of haem in vitro by avian erythrocytes, *Blood* **11**:821–833.

Goldberg, A., and Rimington, C. (1955). Experimentally-produced porphyria in animals, *Proc. Roy. Soc. Biol. Med.* **143**:257–280.

Goldberg, A., and Rimington, C. (1962). *Diseases of Porphyrin Metabolism*, Thomas, Springfield, Ill.

Goldberg, L. H., and Stinnett, J. L. (1983). Acute intermittent porphyria in schizophrenics, *Penn. Med.* **86**:52–53.

Gould, S. E., Kullman, H. J., and Shecket, H. A. (1937). *Amer. J. Med. Sci.* **194**:304–310.

Grabowski, J., and Yergani, V. K. (1987). Porphyria and psychosis: A case report, *Canad. J. Psych.* **32**:393–394.

Grandchamp, B., Phung, N., and Nordmann, Y. (1977). Homozygous case of hereditary coproporphyria, *Lancet* **i**:1348–1349.

Grandchamp, B., Romeo, P. H., Dubart, A., Raich, N., Rosa, J., Nordmann, Y., and Goossens, M. (1984). Molecular cloning of a cDNA sequence complementary to porphobilinogen deaminase mRNA from rat, *Proc. Nat. Acad. Sci. (U.S.A.)* **81**:5036–5040.

Grandchamp, B., Weil, D., Nordmann, Y., Van Cong, N., De Verneuil, H., Foubert, C., and Gross, M. S. (1983). Assignment of the human coproporphyrinogen oxidase to chromosome 9, *Hum. Genet.* **64**:180–183.

Granick, S. (1963). Porphyrin synthesis in erythrocytes. 1. Formation of 5-aminolaevulinic acid in erythrocytes, *J. Biol. Chem.* **232**:1101–1117.

Granick, S. (1966). The induction in vitro of the synthesis of delta-aminolaevulinic acid synthetase in chemical porphyria: A response to certain drugs, sex hormones and foreign chemicals, *J. Biol. Chem.* **241**:1359–1375.

Granick, S., and Sassa, S. (1971). Delta-aminolaevulinic acid synthetase and the control of haem and chlorophyll synthesis, *Metabolic Regulation* (H. J. Vogel, Ed.), Academic, New York, pp. 77–141.

Gray, C. H. (1950). Porphyria, *Arch. Intern. Med.* **85**:459–470.

Gray, C. H. (1952). Isotope studies in porphyria, *Brit. Med. Bull.* **8**:229.

Grinstein, M., Aldrich, R. A., Hawkinson, V., and Watson, C. J. (1949). An isotopic study of porphyrin and haemoglobin metabolism in a case of porphyria, *J. Biol. Chem.* **179**:963.

Grinstein, M., Wilkoff, H. M., Pimenta de Mello, R., and Watson, C. J. (1950). Isotopic studies of porphyrin and haemoglobin metabolism. II. The biosynthesis of coproporphyrin III in experimental lead poisoning, *J. Biol. Chem.* **182**:723.

Grotepass, W. (1932). Zur kenntnis des harn auftretenden porphyrins bei bleivergiftung. *Hoppe-Seyler's Z. Physiol. Chem.* **205**:193–197.

Guidotti, T. L., Charness, M. E., and Lamon, J. M. (1979). Acute intermittent porphyria and the Kluver-Bucy syndrome, *The Johns Hopkins Med. J.* **145**:233–235.

Günther, H. (1911). Die hamatoporphyrie, *Deutsch. Arch. Klin. Med.* **105**:89–146.

Günther, H. (1922). Die bedeutung der hamatoporphyrinurie in der physiologie und pathologie, *Ergebnisse der Allgemeinen Pathol. Pathol. Anat.* **20**:608–764.

Haeger, G. (1958). Urinary 5-aminolaevulinic acid and porphobilinogen in different types of porphyria, *Lancet* **ii**:606–607.

Hammarsten, O. (1891). Tva fall af hamatoporphyrin i urinen, *Uppsala Lak For. Forh.* **26**:259–288.

Harder, J. J. (1694). Glandula nova lacrymalis una cum ducta excretoria in cervis et damis detecta, *Acta Eruditorum Lipsiae* **11**:49–52.

Hare, E. M. (1953). Acute porphyria presenting with mental symptoms, *J. Men. Sci.* **99**:144.

Harley, V. (1890). Two fatal cases of an unusual form of nerve disturbance associated with red urine, probably due to defective tissue oxidation, *Brit. Med. J.* **11**:1169–1170.

Hausmann, W. (1908). Uber die sensibilisierende wirkung tierischer farbstoffe, *Anwendung. Biochem. Z.* **14**:275–283.

Hausmann, W. (1911). Die sensibilisierende wirkung des hamatoporphyrins, *Biochem. Z.* **30**:276–316.

Hausmann, W. (1923). *Grundzuge der lichtbiologie und lichtpathologie*, Urban and Schwartzenberg, Berlin.

Heide, K., Haupt, H., and Storiko, K. (1964). On the heme binding capacity of hemopexin, *Clin. Chim. Acta* **10**:460–469.

Hijmans van den Bergh, A. A., Grotepass, W., and Revers, F. E. (1932). Beitrag uber das porphyrin in Blut und Galle, *Klin. Wschr.* **11**:1534–1536.

Hodgkin, D. C., Pickworth, J. H., Trueblood, K. N., Prosen, R. J., and White, J. G. (1955). NH Tautomerism of porphyrins, *Nature* **176**:325.

Hodgson, G. W. (1972). Cosmochemical evolution of large organic molecules—illustrative laboratory simulations for porphyrins, *Ann. N.Y. Acad. Sci.* **194**:86–97.

Hodgson, G. W., and Baker, B. L. (1967). Porphyrin abiogenesis from pyrrole and formaldehyde under simulated geochemical conditions, *Nature* **216**:29–32.

Holmberg, M. B. (1961). Psychiatric aspects of acute porphyria, *Lancet* **i**:1226.

Hoppe-Seyler, F. (1871). Das hamatin, *Tubinger Med. Chem. Untersuchungen* **4**:523–533.

Hoppe-Seyler, F. (1879). Uber das chlorophyll der pflanzen, *Hoppe-Seyler's Z. Physiol. Chem.* **205**:193–197.

Huszak, I., and Durko, I. (1970). Disturbances of porphyrin metabolism in schizophrenia, *Acta Physiol. Acad. Sci. Hungar.* **38**:77–84.

Illis, L. (1964). On porphyria and the aetiology of werewolves, *Proc. Roy. Soc. Med.* **57**:23–26.

Ingier, A. (1911). Ochronose bei tieren, *Zieglers Beirage zur Pathol. Anat.* **51**:199–208.

IUPAC/IUB (1980). Joint Commission on Biochemical Nomenclature. Nomenclature of tetrapyrroles, *Eur. J. Biochem.* **108**:1–20.

Jackson, A. H., Games, D. E., Couch, P., Jackson, J. R., Belcher, R. B., and Smith, S. G. (1974). Conversion of coproporphyrinogen III to protoporphyrin IX, *Enzyme* **17**:81–87.

Jancar, J. (1975). Neurocutaneous disorder and mental functioning, *Brit. J. Psych.* **126**:105–113.

Jordan, P. M., Burton, G., Nordlov, H., Schneider, M. M., Pryde, L., and Scott, I. A. (1979). Pre-uroporphyrinogen—a substrate for uroporphyrinogen III cosynthetase, *J. Chem. Soc. Chem. Comm.* 204–205.

Jørgensen, S. K. (1959). Congenital porphyria in pigs, *Brit. Vet. J.* **115**:160–175.

Jørgensen, S. K., and With, T. K. (1965). Congenital porphyria in animals other than man, *Comparative Physiology and Pathology of the Skin* (A. J. Rook and G. S. Walton, Eds.), Blackwell, Oxford, pp. 317–331.

Kamal, S., and Grivois, H. (1985). Porphyrie aigue: Psychose aigue et psychose aigue et psychotropes (une cas), *Union Med. Canad.* **114**:330–331.

Kämmerer, H. (1924). Uber das durch darmbakterien gebildete porphyrin und die bedeutung der porphyrinprobe fur die beurteilung der darmfaulnis, *Deusch. Arch. Klin. Med.* **145**:257–284.

Kaneko, J., and Cornelius, C. E. (1970). *Clinical Biochemistry of Domestic Animals*, 2nd ed., Vol. 1. Academic Press, N.Y.

Kast, A. (1888). Uber die art der darreichung und verordnung des sulfonals. *Ther. Mh.* **11**:316–319.

Keilin, D. (1925). On cytochrome—a respiratory pigment common to animals, yeasts and higher plants, *Proc. Roy. Soc. Biol. Med.* **98**:312.

Kennedy, G. Y. (1979). Pigments of marine invertebrates, *Adv. Mar. Biol.* **16**:309–381.

Kessel, D. (1982). Components of hematoporphyrin derivatives and their tumor-localizing capacity, *Cancer Res.* **42**:1703–1706.

Kessel, D., and Cheng, M. L. (1985). Biological and biophysical properties of the tumor-localizing component of hematoporphyrin derivative, *Cander Res.* **45**:3053–3057.

Kikuchi, G., Shemin, D., and Bachmann, B. J. (1958). The enzymatic synthesis of 5-amino-levulinic acid, *Biochim. Biophys. Acta* **28**:219–220.

Körbler, J. (1931). Untersuchung von krebsgewebe im fluoreszenzerregenden licht, *Strahlentherapie* **41**:510–518.

Körbler, J. (1932). Rote fluoreszenz in krebsgeschwuren, *Strahlentherapie* **43**:317–326.

Kordäc, V., Deybach, J. C., Martasek, P., Seman, J., Da Silva, V., Nordmann, Y., Houstkova, H., Rubin, A., and Holub, J. (1984). Homozygous variegate porphyria, *Lancet* i:851.

Kosenow, W., and Treibs, A. (1953). Lichtuberempfindlichtkeit und porphyrinamie, *Z. Kinderkeikunde* **73**:82–92.

Koskelo, P. (1956). Studies of urinary coproporphyrin excretion in acute coronary diseases. *Ann. Med. Intern. Fenniae* (Supplement 24).

Koskelo, P., Bergrahm, B., and Toivonen, I. (1971). Observations in the binding of C-labelled porphyrins by human plasma proteins, *S. Afr. J. Lab. Clin. Med.* **17**:167–169.

Koskelo, P., and Heikkila, J. (1965). Urinary excretion of porphyrin precursors in myocardial infarction, *Acta Med. Scand.* **178**:681.

Koskelo, P., Toivonen, I., and Adlercreutz, H. (1967). Urinary coproporphyrin isomer distribution in the Dubin-Johnson syndrome, *Clin. Chem.* **13**:1006–1008.

Krukenberg, C. F. W. (1883). Die farbstoffe der vogeleierschalen, *Verh. Physik. Med. Ges.* (*Wurzburg*) **17**:109–118.

Kushner, J. P., Barbuto, A. J., and Lee, G. R. (1976). An inherited enzymatic defect in porphyria cutanea tarda: Decreased uroporphyrinogen decarboxylase activity, *J. Clin. Invest.* **58**:1089–1097.

Küster, W. (1912). Beitrage zur Kenntnis des Bilirubins und Hämins, *Hoppe Seyler's Z. Physiol. Chem.* **82**:463–483.

Laennec, R. T. M. (1831). *Traite sur l'auscultation mediate*, 4th ed, Chaude, Paris.

Laidlaw, P. P. (1904). Some observations on blood pigments, *J. Physiol.* **31**:464–472.

Langhof, H., Muller, H., and Rietschel, I. (1961). Untersuchungen zur familiaren protoporphyrinamischen lichurticaria, *Arch. Klin. Exp. Dermatol.* **212**:506–518.

Lascelles, J. (1957). Synthesis of porphyrins by cell suspensions of tetrahymena vorax, *Biochem. J.* **66**:65–72.

Lascelles, J. (1964). *Tetrapyrrole Biosynthesis and Its Regulation*, Benjamin, New York.

Lecanu, L. R. (1837). Etudes chimiques sur le sang humain (cited by Berzelius, 1840), 4° Paris No. 395.

Lemberg, R., and Legge, J. W. (1949). *Haematin Compounds and Bile Pigments*, Interscience, New York.

Levin, E. Y., and Flyger, V. (1971). Uroporphyrinogen, III. Cosynthetase activity in the fox squirrel (*Sciurus niger*), *Science* **174**:59–60.

Levy, S., and Perry H. A. (1949). Psychosis with haematoporphyrinuria, *Arch. Neurol. Psych.* **61**:699–407.

Liebig, N. S. (1927). Uber die experimentelle Bleihämatoporphyrie, *Arch. Exp. Pathol. Pharmacol.* **125**:16–27.

Lim, C. K., Rideout, J. M., and Peters, T. J. (1984). Pseudoporphyria associated with consumption of brewer's yeast, *Brit. Med. J.* **288**:1640.

Lipson, R. L., Baldes, E. J., and Olsen, A. M. (1961). The use of a derivative of hematoporphyrin in tumor detection, *J. Nat. Cancer Inst.* **26**:1–11.

Lithner, F., and Wetterberg, L. (1984). Hepatocellular carcinoma in patients with acute intermittent porphyria, *Acta Med. Scand.* **215**:272–274.

Llewellyn, D. H., Elder, G. H., Kalshekern, A., et al. (1987). DNA polymorphisms of human porphobilinogen-deaminase gene in acute intermittent porphyria, *Lancet* **ii**:706–708.

Lochhead, A. C., Dagg, J. H., and Goldberg, A. (1967). Experimental griseofulvin porphyria in adult and foetal mice, *Brit. J. Dermatol.* **79**:96–102.

Luby, E. D., Ware, J. G., Senf, R., and Frohman, C. E. (1959). Stress and precipitation of acute intermittent porphyria, *Psychosomat. Med.* **21**:34–48.

Macalpine, I., and Hunter, R. (1969). *George the III and the "Mad Business,"* Penguin, London.

MacMunn, C. A. (1880). Further researches into the colouring-matters of human urine, with an account of their artificial production from bilirubin, and from haematin, *Proc. Roy. Soc. Lond. Ser. B.* **31**:206–237.

MacMunn, C. A. (1884). On myohaematin: An intrinsic muscle pigment of vertebrates and invertebrates on histohaematin and on the spectrum of the suprarenal bodies, *J. Physiol.* **5**:24–26.

MacMunn, C. A. (1889). Contribution to animal chromatology, *Quart. J. Micro. Sci.* **30**:51–65.

Magnus, I. A., Jarret, A., Prankerd, T. A. J., and Rimington, C. (1961). Erythropoietic protoporphyria: A new porphyria syndrome with solar urticaria due to protoporphyrinaemia, *Lancet* **ii**:448–451.

Markowitz, M. (1954). Acute intermittent porphyria: A report of 5 cases and review of the literature, *Ann. Intern. Med.* **41**:1170–1188.

Marks, G. S. (1969). *Heme and Chlorophyll*, Van Nostrand Rheinhold, Princeton, N.J.

Marks, G. S. (1981). The effects of chemicals on hepatic heme biosynthesis, *TIPS* **2**:59–61.

Mason, V. R., Courville, C., and Ziskind, E. (1933). The porphyrins in human disease, *Medicine* **12**:355–439.

McCall-Anderson, T. (1898). Hydroa aestivale in two brothers, complicated with the presence of hematoporphyrin in the urine, *Brit. J. Dermatol.* **10**:1–4.

McColl, K. E. L., Moore, M. R., Thompson, G. G., Goldberg, A., Church, S. E., Qadiri, M. R., and Youngs, G. R. (1985). Chester porphyria: Biochemical studies of a new form of acute porphyria, *Lancet* **ii**:796–799.

Meisler, M., Wanner, L., Eddy, R. E., and Shows, T. B. (1980). The UPS locus encoding uroporphyrinogen-1 synthase is located on human chromosome II, *Biochem. Biophys. Res. Comm.* **95**:170–176.

Meissner, P. N., Sturrock, E. D., Moore, M. R., Disler, P. B., and Maeder, D. L. (1985). Protoporphyrinogen oxidase, porphobilinogen-deaminase and uroporphyrinogen decarboxylase in variegate porphyria. *Biochem. Soc. Trans.* **13**:203–204.

Mercer-Smith, J. A., and Mauzerall, D. C. (1984). Photochemistry of porphyrins—a model for the origin of photosynthesis, *Photochem. Photobiol.* **39**:397–405.

Mercer-Smith, J. A., Raudino, A., and Mauzerall, D. C. (1985). A model for the origin of photosynthesis. III. The ultraviolet photochemistry of uroporphyrinogen, *Photochem. Photobiol.* **42**:239–244.

Meyer-Betz, F. (1913). Untersuchungen uber die biologische (photodynamische) wirkung des hamatoporphyrins und anderen derivate des blut und gallenfarbstoffs, *Deutsch. Arch. Klin. Med.* **112**:476–503.

Mindegaard, J. (1976). Studier verrend porphyrinsynthese og porfyrinholdige biologiske pigmentinkorns oprindelse og ultrastruktur, Afdelingen for biokemi og erneering, Danmarks Tekniske Hojskole.

Möller-Sorensen, A. (1920). On haemochromatosis ossium (Ochronose) has husdyrene, Den KGL, Veterinaer-Og Landbohojskoles Aarsskrift, Copenhagen, pp. 122–139.

Moore, M. R. (1980). International review of drugs in acute porphyria, *Int. J. Biochem.* **12**:1089–1097.

Moore, M. R., Beattie, A. D., Thompson, G. G., and Goldberg, A. (1971). Depression of 5-aminolaevulinic acid dehydratase activity by ethanol in man and rat, *Clin. Sci.* **40**:81–88.

Moore, M. R. and Goldberg, A. (1985). Health implications of the hemopoietic effects of lead, *Dietary and Environmental Lead: Human Health Effects* (K. Mahaffey, Ed.), Elsevier, Amsterdam.

Moore, M. R., and McColl, K. E. L. (1987). *The Porphyrias—Drug Lists*, University of Glasgow.

Moore, M. R., McColl, K. E. L., and Goldberg, A. (1979). The porphyrias, *Diabet. Metab.* **5**:323–336.

Moore, M. R., McColl, K. E. L., and Goldberg, A. (1984). The effects of alcohol on porphyrin biosynthesis and metabolism, *Clinical Biochemistry of Alcoholism* (S. B. Rosalki, Ed.), Churchill Livingstone, pp. 161–187.

Moore, M. R., McColl, K. E. L., Rimington, C., and Goldberg, A. (1987). *Disorders of Porphyrin Metabolism*, Plenum, New York.

Moore, M. R., Thompson, G. G., Payne, A. P., and McGadey, J. (1980). Seasonal variation in 5-aminolaevulinate synthase and porphyrin content in the Harderian gland of the female golden hamster (*Mesocricetus auratus*), *Int. J. Biochem.* **12**:501–504.

Morris, C. R., and Cabral, J. R. P. (1986). *Hexachlorobenzene: Proceedings of International Symposium*, IARC Sci. Pub., IARC, Lyon.

Mosselman, D., and Hebrant, A. (1898). Coloration abnormale du squelette chez une beta de boucherie, *Ann. Med. Vet.* **47**:201–206.

Mueller, A. P., Sato, K., and Glick, B. (1971). The chicken lacrimal gland, gland of Harder, caecal tonsil and accessory spleens as sources of antibody-producing cells, *Cell Immunol.* **2**:140–152.

Muir, H. M., and Neuberger, A. (1950). The biogenesis of porphyrins. 2. The origin of the methyne carbon atoms, *Biochem. J.* **47**:97–104.

Mülder, G. H. (1844). Uber eisenfreises hamatin, *J. Prakt. Chem.* **32**:186–197.

Murphy, G. M., Hawk, J. L. M., and Magnus, I. A. (1985). Late-onset erythropoietic protoporphyria with unusual cutaneous features, *Arch. Dermatol.* **121**:1309–1312.

Murphy, G. M., Hawk, J. L. M., Magnus, I. A., Barrett, D. F., Elder, G. H., and Smith, S. G. (1986). Homozygous variegate porphyria—two similar cases in unrelated families, *J. Roy. Soc. Med.* **79**:361–363.

Mustajoki, P. (1981). Normal erythrocyte uroporphyrinogen-1 synthase in a kindred with acute intermittent porphyria, *Ann. Intern. Med.* **95**:162–166.

Mustajoki, P., Tenhunen, R. Niemi. K. M., Nordmann, Y., Kaarianen, H., and Norio, R. (1987). Homozygous variegate porphyria, *Clin. Genet.* **32**:300–305.

Nencki, M., and Sieber, N. (1888). Uber das hämatoporphyrin, *Arch. Exp. Pathol. Pharmacol.* **24**:430–446.

Neuberger, A. (1980). The regulation of chlorophyll and porphyrin biosynthesis, *Int. J. Biochem.* **12**:787–789.

Neuberger, A., and Scott, J. J. (1953). Aminolaevulinic acid and porphyrin synthesis, *Nature* **172**:1093–1094.

Noorden, G. Von (1916). Uber chronische trionalvergiftung, *Mun. Med. Wschr.* **63**:683.

Nordmann, Y., Grandchamp, B., De Verneuil, H., Phung, L., Cartigny, B., and Fontaine, G. (1983). Harderoporphyrin—a rare variant hereditary coproporphyria, *J. Clin. Invest.* **72**:1139–1149.

Offenstadt, G., Bienvenu, M. P., Hericord, P., Tawell, S., and Amstatz, P. (1980). Catatonie grave schizophrenie et coproporphyrie hereditaire, *Sem. Hop. Paris* **56**:1727–1730.

Olmstead, E. G. (1953). The neuropsychiatric aspects of abnormal porphyrin metabolism, *J. Nerv. Men. Dis.* **117**:300–311.

Orten, J. M., Doehr, S. A., Bond, C., Johnson, H., and Pappos, A. (1963). Urinary excretion of porphyrins and porphyrin intermediates in human alcoholics, *Quart. J. Studies on Alcohol* **24**:598–609.

Owen, L. N., Stevenson, D. E., and Keilin, J. (1962). Abnormal pigmentation and fluorescence in canine teeth, *Res. Vet. Sci.* **3**:139–146.

Payne, A. P., McGadey, J., Moore, M. R., and Thompson, G. G. (1977). Androgenic control of the Harderian gland in the male golden hamster, *J. Endocr.* **75**:73–82.

Payne, A. P., McGadey, J., Moore, M. R., and Thompson, G. G. (1979). Changes in Harderian gland activity in the female golden hamster during the oestrous cycle, pregnancy and lactation, *Biochem. J.* **178**:597–604.

Pepplinkhuizen, L., Bruinvels, J., Blom, W., and Moelman, P. (1980). Schizophrenia-like psychosis caused by a metabolic disorder, *Lancet* **i**:454–456.

Pinol Aguade, J., Castells, A., Indocochea, A., and Rodes, J. (1969). A case of biochemically unclassifiable hepatic porphyria, *Brit. J. Dermatol.* **81**:270–275.

Poh-Fitzpatrick, M. B. (1986). Porphyria, pseudoporphyria, pseudopseudoporphyria, *Arch. Dermatol.* **122**:403–404.

Policard, A. (1924). Etude sur les aspects offerts par des tumeurs experimentales examinees a la lumiere de Wood. *C. R. Seances Soc. Biol.* **91**:1423–1424.

Poulson, R., and Polglase, W. J. (1975). The enzymic conversion of protoporphyrinogen IX to protoporphyrin IX. Protoporphyrinogen oxidase activity in mitochondrial extracts of saccaromyces cerevisiae, *J. Biol. Chem.* **250**:1269–1274.

Poulson, V. (1910). Om ochronotiske tilstande hos mennesker og. dyr. (on ochronotic states in man and animals), Med. Diss., University of Copenhagen.

Prunty, F. T. G. (1945). Acute porphyria—some properties of porphobilinogen, *Biochem. J.* **39**:446–451.

Qadiri, M. R., Church, S. E., McColl, K. E. L., Moore, M. R., and Youngs, G. R. (1986). Chester porphyria—a clinical study of a new form of acute porphyria, *Brit. Med. J.* **292**:455–459.

Ranking, J. E., and Pardington, G. L. (1890). Two cases of haematoporphyrin in the urine, *Lancet* **ii**:607–609.

Rassmussen-Taxdal, D. S., Ward, G. E., and Figge, F. H. J. (1955). Fluorescence of human lymphatic and cancer tissues following high doses of intravenous hematoporphyrin derivative, *Cancer* **8**:78–81.

Rimington, C. (1936). Some cases of congenital porphyrinuria in cattle—chemical studies upon living animals and post-mortem material, *Onderstepoort J. Vet. Sci. Animal Ind.* **7**:567–609.

Rimington, C. (1939). A re-investigation of turacin, the copper porphyrin pigment of certain birds belonging to the musophagidae, *Proc. Roy. Soc. Lond. Ser. B.* **127**:106–120.

Rimington, C. (1955). Porphyrins, *Endeavour* **14**:126–135

Rimington, C., and Hemmings, A. W. (1939). Porphyrinuric action of drugs related to sulphonalmide, *Biochem. J.* **33**:960–968.

Rimington, C., Roets, G. C. S., and Fourier, P. J. J. (1938). Quantitative studies upon porphyrin excretion in bovine congenital porphyrinuria (Pink tooth), *Onderstepoort J. Vet. Sci. Animal Ind.* **10**:421–429.

Romeo, G., and Levin, E. Y. (1969). Uroporphyrinogen III cosynthetase in human congenital erythropoietic porphyria, *Proc. Nat. Acad. Sci. (U.S.A.)* **63**:856–863.

Ross, B. D. (1957). A suspected case of congenital porphyria (pink tooth) in a heifer, *Vet. Res.* **63**:345–346.

Roth, N. (1945). The neuropsychiatric aspects of porphyria, *Psych. Med.* **7**:291–301.

Roth, N. (1968). The psychiatric syndromes of porphyria, *Int. J. Neuropsych.* **4**:32–44.

Ruth, G. R., Schwartz, S., Stephenson, B., Bates, F., and Shave, H. (1978). A new disease of cattle—bovine protoporphyria: Clinical and diagnostic features, *Amer. Assoc. Vet. Lab. Diag. 21st Ann. Proc.* 91–96.

Sachs, P. (1931). Ein fall von akuter porphyrie mit hochgradiger muskelatrophied, *Klin. Wschr.* **10**:1123–1125.

Saillet, H. (1896). De l'urospectrine (ou urohematoporphyrine urinale normlae), *Rev. Med.* **16**:542–552.

Salkowski, E. (1891). Uber vorkommen und nachweis des hamatoporphyrins in harn, *Hoppe-Seyler's Z. Physiol. Chem.* **15**:286–309.

Scherer, J. (1841). Chemische-physiologische untersuchungen, *Ann. Chem. Pharm.* **40**:1–64.

Schmey, M. (1913). Uber ochronose bei mensch und tier, *Frankfurter Z. Pathol.* **12**:218–328.

Schmid, R., and Schwartz, S. (1952). Experimental porphyria: Hepatic type produced by sedormid, *Proc. Soc. Exp. Biol. Med.* **81**:685–689.

Schmid, R., Schwartz, S., and Sundberg, R. D. (1955). Erythropoietic (congenital) porphyria—a rare abnormality of the normoblasts, *Blood* **10**:416–428.

Schmid, R., Schwartz, S., and Watson, C. J. (1954). Porphyrin content of bone marrow and liver in the various forms of porphyria, *Arch. Intern. Med.* **93**:167–190.

Schneck, J. M. (1946). Porphyria—neuropsychiatric aspects in the case of a Negro, *J. Nerv. Men. Dis.* **104**:432–448.

Schulman, M. P., and Richert, D. A. (1957). Heme synthesis in vitamin B6 and pantothenic acid deficiencies, *J. Biol. Chem.* **226**:181–189.

Schultz, J. H. (1874). Ein fall von pemphigus leprosus, complicirt durch lepra visceralis, Inaugural Diss., Griefswald.

Schumm, O. (1924). Uber die naturlichen porphyrine, *Z. Physiol. Chem.* **126**:169–202.

Schwartz, S., Absolon, K., and Vermund, H. (1955). Some relationships of porphyrins, X-rays and tumors, *Univ. Minnesota Med. Bull.* **27**:7–13.

Seubert, A., Ippen, H., and Lang, H. (1985). Animal models for porphyria, *Models in Dermatology* (Maibach and Lowe, Eds.), Kargar, Basel, Vol. 1, pp. 296–302.

Seubert, S., Seubert, A., Rumpf, K., and Koffe, H. (1985). A porphyria cutanea tarda-like distribution pattern of porphyrins in plasma hemodialysate hemofiltrate in urine of patients on chronic hemodialysis, *J. Invest. Dermatol.* **85**:107–109.

Shemin, D., and Rittenberg, D. (1946). The biological utilisation of glycine for the synthesis of the protoporphyrin of hemoglobin, *J. Biol. Chem.* **166**:621–625.

Shemin, D., and Russell, C. S. (1953). Succinate glycine cycle, *J. Amer. Chem. Soc.* **75**:4873–4875.

Shemin, D., Russell, C. S., and Abramsky, T. (1955). The succinate glycine cycle. 1. The mechanism of pyrrole synthesis, *J. Biol. Chem.* **215**:613.

Shemin, D., and Wittenberg, J. (1951). The mechanism of porphyrin formation—the role of the tri-carboxylic acid cycle. *J. Biol. Chem.* **192**:315.

Skulj, M. (1979). A case of porphyria with psychotic symptoms, *Zdrav. Vestn.* **48**:281–282.

Smith, A. G., and De Matteis, F. (1980). Drugs and the hepatic porphyrias, *The Porphyrias: Clinics in Haematology* (A. Goldberg and M. R. Moore, Eds.), Saunders, London, Vol. 9, pp. 399–425.

Smith, K. M. (1975). *Porphyrins and Metalloporphyrins*, Elsevier, Amsterdam.

Smith, S. G. (1986) Hepatoerythropoietic porphyria, *Sem. Dermatol.* **5**:125–137.

Solomon, H. M., and Figge, F. H. J. (1959). Disturbance in porphyrin metabolism caused by feeding diethyl-1,4-dihydro-2,4,6-trimethylpyridine-3,5-dicarboxylate, *Proc. Soc. Exp. Biol. Med.* **100**:583–586.

Soret, J. L. (1883). Recherches sur l'absorption des rayons ultraviolets par diverses substances, *Arch. Sci. Phys. Nat.* **10**:430–485.

Spike, R. C., Johnston, H. S., McGadey, J., Moore, M. R., Thompson, G. G., and Payne, A. P. (1985). Quantitative studies on the effects of hormones on structure and porphyrin synthesis in the Harderian gland. 1. The effects of ovariectomy and androgen administration, *J. Anat.* **142**:59–72.

Stein, J. A., and Tschudy, D. P. (1970). Acute intermittent porphyria—a clinical and biochemical study of 46 patients, *Medicine* **49**:1–16.

Stokvis, B. J. (1889). Over twee zeldsame kleurstoffen in urine van zicken, *Ned. Tijds. Geneesk.* **13**:409–417.

Stokvis, B. J. (1895). Zur pathogenese der hamatoporphyrinurie, *Z. Klin. Med.* **28**:1–9.

Strand, L. J., Felsher, B. F., Redeker, A. G., and Marver, H. S. (1970). Heme biosynthesis in acute intermittent porphyria: decreased hepatic conversion of porphobilinogen to porphyrin and increased delta-aminolaevulinic acid synthetase activity, *Proc. Nat. Acad. Sci. (U.S.A.)* **67**:1315–1320.

Strik, J. J. T. W. A., and Koeman, J. H. (1979). *Chemical Porphyria in Man*, Elsevier North-Holland, Amsterdam.

Sutherland, D. A., and Watson, C. J. (1951). Studies of coproporphyrin. VI. The effect of alcohol on the per diem excretion and isomer distribution of the urinary coproporphyrins, *J. Lab. Clin. Med., St. Louis* **37**:29–39.

Sutka, P., and Durko, I. (1981). Bovine porphyria caused by *Candida guilliermondii* infection, *Acta Vet. Acad. Sci. Hungar.* **29**:37–43.

Sweeney, G. D. (1986). Porphyria cutanea tarda—or the uroporphyrinogen decarboxylase deficiency diseases, *Clin. Biochem.* **19**:3–15.

Tappeiner, H. (1885). Untersuchung pigmentirter knochen vom schweine, *Sitzungserber, Ges. Morph. Physiol. München* **1**:38–41.

Tephly, T. R., Coffman, B. L., Ingall, G., Zeit-Har, M. S. A., Goff, H. M., Tabba, H. D., and Smith, K. M. (1981). Identification of *N*-methylprotoporphrin IX in livers of untreated mice and mice treated with 3,5-diethoxycarbonyl-1,4-dihydrocollidine—source of the methyl group, *Arch. Biochem. Biophys.* **212**:120–126.

Tephly, T. R., Gibbs, A. H., and De Matteis, F. (1979). Studies on the mechanism of experimental porphyria produced by 3,5-diethoxycarbonyl-1,4-dihydrocollidine—role of a porphyrin-like inhibitor of protohaem ferrolyase, *Biochem. J.* **180**:241–244.

Tephly, T. R., Gibbs, A. H., Ingall, G., and De Matteis, F. (1980). Studies on the mechanism of experimental porphyria and ferrochelatase inhibition produced by 3,5-diethoxycarbonyl-1,4-dihydrocollidine, *Int. J. Biochem.* **12**:993.

Thiessen, D. D., Pendergrass, M., and Harriman, A. E. (1982). The thermoenergetics of coat colour maintenance by the Mongolian gerbil (*Meriones unguiculatus*), *J. Thermal Biol.* **7**:51–56.

Thompson, G. G., Hordovatzi, X., Moore, M. R., McGadey, J., and Payne, A. P. (1984). Sex differences in haem biosynthesis and porphyrin content in the Harderian gland of the golden hamster, *Int. J. Biochem.* **16**:849–852.

Thudichum, J. L. W. (1867). Report on researches intended to promote an improved chemical identification of disease, *10th Report of The Medical Officer, Privy Council*, H.M.S.O., London, App. 7, pp. 152–233.

Tio, T. H. (1956). Beschouwingen over de porphyria cutanea tarda, Doctoral Thesis, Amsterdam.

Tio, T. H., Leijnse, B., Jarrett, A., and Rimington, C. (1957). Acquired porphyria from a liver tomour, *Clin. Sci.* **16**:517–527.

Tishler, P. V., Woodward, B., O'Connor, J., et al. (1985). High prevalence of intermittent acute porphyria in a psychiatric in-patient population, *Amer. J. Psych.* **142**:1430–1436.

Tobias, G. (1964). Congenital porphyria in a cat, *J. Amer. Vet. Med. Assoc.* **145**:462–463.

Topi, G. C., D'Alessandro, G. L., De Costanza, F., and Cancarini, G. C. (1980). Porphyria and pseudoporphyria in hemodialized patients. *Int. J. Biochem.* **12**:963–967.

Trafford, P. A. (1976) Homicide in acute porphyria, *Forensic Sci.* **7**:113–120.

Turner, W. J. (1937). Studies on Porphyria. 1. Observations on the fox squirrel (*Sciurus niger*), *J. Biol. Chem.* **118**:519–530.

Udagawa, M., Horie, Y., and Hirayama, C. (1984). Aberrant porphyrin metabolism in hepatocellular carcinoma, *Biochem. Med.* **31**:131–139.

Urban, S. (1985). Mental disorders in acute intermittent porphyria, *Psych. Pol.* **19**:233–238.

Vaidya, M. C., and Kanan, K. (1987). Dual porphyria—an underdiagnosed entity, *Clin. Chem.* **33**:1190–1193.

Vannotti, A. (1954). *Porphyrins—Their Biological and Chemical Importance*, Hilger and Watts, London.

Vischer, J. S., and Aldrich, C. K. (1954). Acute intermittent porphyria—a case study, *Psychosomat. Med.* **16**:163.

Vollmer, E. (1903). Uber hereditare syphilis und haematoporphyrinurie, *Arch. Dematol and Syphilogy* (*Berlin*) **65**:221–234.

Waldenström, J. (1937). Studien uber porphyrie, *Acta Med. Scand. Suppl.* **82**:120.

Waldenström, J. (1956). Studies on the incidence and heredity of acute porphyria in Sweden, *Acta Genet.* **6**:122–131.

Waldenström, J. (1957). The porphyrias as inborn errors of metabolism, *Amer. J. Med.* **22**:758–773.

Waldenström, J., and Vahlquist, B. C. (1939). Studien uber die entstehung der roten harnpigmente (uroporphyrin und porphobilin) bein der akuten porphyrie aus ihrer farblosen vorstufe (porphobilinogen), *Hoppe-Seyler's Z. Physiol. Chem.* **260**:189–209.

Ware, M. (1968). *Porphyria—A Royal Malady*, British Medical Association, London.

Watson, C. J. (1960). The problem of porphyria—some facts and questions, *N. Engl. J. Med.* **263**:1205–1215.

Watson, C. J. (1965). Reminiscences of Hans Fischer and his laboratory, *Perspectives in Biol. Med.* **8**:419–435.

Watson, C. J., and Schwartz, S. (1941). Simple test for urinary porphobilinogen, *Proc. Soc. Exp. Biol. Med.* **47**:393–394.

Went, L. N., and Klasen, E. C. (1984). Genetic aspects of erythropoietic protoporphyria, *Ann. Hum. Genet.* **48**:105–117.

Westall, R. G. (1952). Isolation of porphobilinogen from the urine of a patient with acute porphyria, *Nature* **170**:614.

Wetterberg, L. (1976). Report on an International Survey of Safe and Unsafe Drugs in acute intermittent porphyria, *Porphyrins in Human Diseases* (M. Doss and P. Nawrocki, Eds.), Falk, Freiburg, pp. 191–202.

Wetterberg, L., Geller, E., and Yuwiler, A. (1970). The Harderian gland—an extraretinal photoreceptor influencing the pineal gland in neonatal rats, *Science* **167**:884–885.

Wetterberg, L., and Osterberg, E. (1970). Acute intermittent porphyria—a psychometric study of 25 patients, *J. Psychosomat. Res.* **13**:91–93.

Willstätter, R., and Mieg. W. (1906). Untersuchungen uber das chlorophyll, *Liebigs Ann. Chem.* **350**:1–47.

Willstätter, R., and Stoll, A. (1913). *Untersuchungen uber chlorophyll*, Springer, Berlin.

With, T. K. (1973). Porphyrins in egg shells, *Biochem. J.* **137**:597–598.

With, T. K. (1978). On porphyrias in the feathers of owls and bustards, *Int. J. Biochem.* **9**:893–895.

With, T. K. (1980). A short history of porphyrins and the porphyrias, *Int. J. Biochem.* **11**:189–200.

Witte, H. (1914). Ein fall von ochronose bei einem bullen und einem von ihre stammenden kalbe, *Z. Fleisch U. Milchhyg.* **24**:334.

Yeung-Laiwah, A. C., Moore, M. R., and Goldberg, A. (1987). Pathogenesis of acute porphyria, *Quart. J. Med.* **63**:377–392.

Yeung-Laiwah, A. C., Rapeport, W. G., Thompson, G. G., Macphee, G. J., Philip, M. F., Moore, M. R., Brodie, M. J., and Goldberg, A. (1983). Carbamazepine-induced nonhereditary acute porphyria, *Lancet* **i**:790–792.

Zaleski, J. (1903). Untersuchungen uber das mesoporphyrin, *Hoppe-Seyler's Z. Physiol. Chem.* **37**:54–74.

2

Biosynthesis of 5-Aminolevulinic Acid and Its Transformation into Coproporphyrinogen in Animals and Bacteria

Peter M. Jordan

I. Introduction

The biosynthesis of the tetrapyrrole ring system is a brilliant example of economy of biosynthetic effort since in only a few enzymic stages the complex tetrapyrrole structure is fashioned from simple precursor molecules. The pathway for the biosynthesis of tetrapyrroles is broadly similar in all living systems and commences with the biosynthesis of the highly reactive aminoketone 5-aminolevulinic acid. There are two distinct routes by which 5-aminolevulinic acid is produced; one in animals and some bacteria which utilize glycine and succinyl-CoA; and the other, involving the carbon skeleton of glutamate, which has been shown more recently to operate in plants and some anaerobic bacteria. Once formed, 5-aminolevulinic acid is transformed into the tetrapyrrole macrocycle in only three stages. First, two molecules of 5-aminolevulinic acid condense with one another and form the basic pyrrole building block, porphobilinogen. Second, four molecules of porphobilinogen then polymerize together in a chain to generate a highly unstable hydroxymethylbilane called preuroporphyrinogen. Last, preuroporphyrinogen is cyclized, with rearrangement of one of the pyrrole rings, the d ring, to yield the key intermediate uroporphyrinogen III. Uroporphyrinogen III is the universal precursor from which porphyrins, hemes, chlorophylls, corrins, and all other tetrapyrroles are derived. At this branch point uroporphyrinogen III may either embark upon the route to heme or chlorophyll, first by decarboxylation to coproporphyrinogen III, followed by further conversion to protoporphyrin IX or, alternatively, it may be methylated to be further transformed into siroheme, corrins, or F_{430}. A summary of these pathways is shown in Fig. 2.1.

This chapter deals with the enzymic stages up to coproporphyrinogen III. The subsequent stages from coproporphyrinogen III to protoporphyrin IX are described in Chap. 3.

A. Early investigations on the biosynthesis of the tetrapyrrole ring

The elucidation of the early stages in the tetrapyrrole biosynthesis pathway was largely complete by the end of the 1950s and all the intermediates with the exception of preuroporphyrinogen had been characterized. The major contributions stemmed from the investigations carried out by David Shemin and his co-workers in the United States and the group of Albert Neuberger in the United Kingdom. Central to their methodology was the use of isotopes in order to follow the path by which precursors were incorporated into heme. Shemin, using himself as an experimental subject, orally administered [^{15}N]glycine and established that this amino acid was the most efficient precursor of the heme nitrogen atoms (Shemin and Rittenberg, 1945). Subsequently, experiments carried out with [^{14}C]-labeled glycine, using enzyme extracts from avian erythrocytes established that the C-2 carbon atom, but not the carboxyl carbon, of glycine was incorporated into eight of the positions in the heme macrocyclic ring (Shemin et al., 1950; Muir and Neuberger, 1950). This was deduced by painstakingly degrading the labeled heme by a procedure which yielded ethylmethylmaleimide and hematinic acid. The maleimides were then further degraded by methods which permitted the isolation and positional assignment of each of the carbon atoms present in the heme macrocycle. Additional labeling experiments using 1-[^{14}C]- and 2-[^{14}C]acetate established that the remaining carbon atoms of heme were derived from an unsymmetrical 4-carbon compound arising from the tricarboxylic acid cycle (Shemin and Wittenberg, 1951) and a succinyl derivative, such as succinyl-CoA, was suggested as a possible candidate. Subsequently, experimental proof for the involvement of succinyl-CoA was obtained from in vitro experiments using avian erythrocyte preparations (Gibson et al., 1958).

From these pioneering studies the origin of all the carbon and nitrogen atoms of heme were established and the findings are summarized in Fig. 2.2.

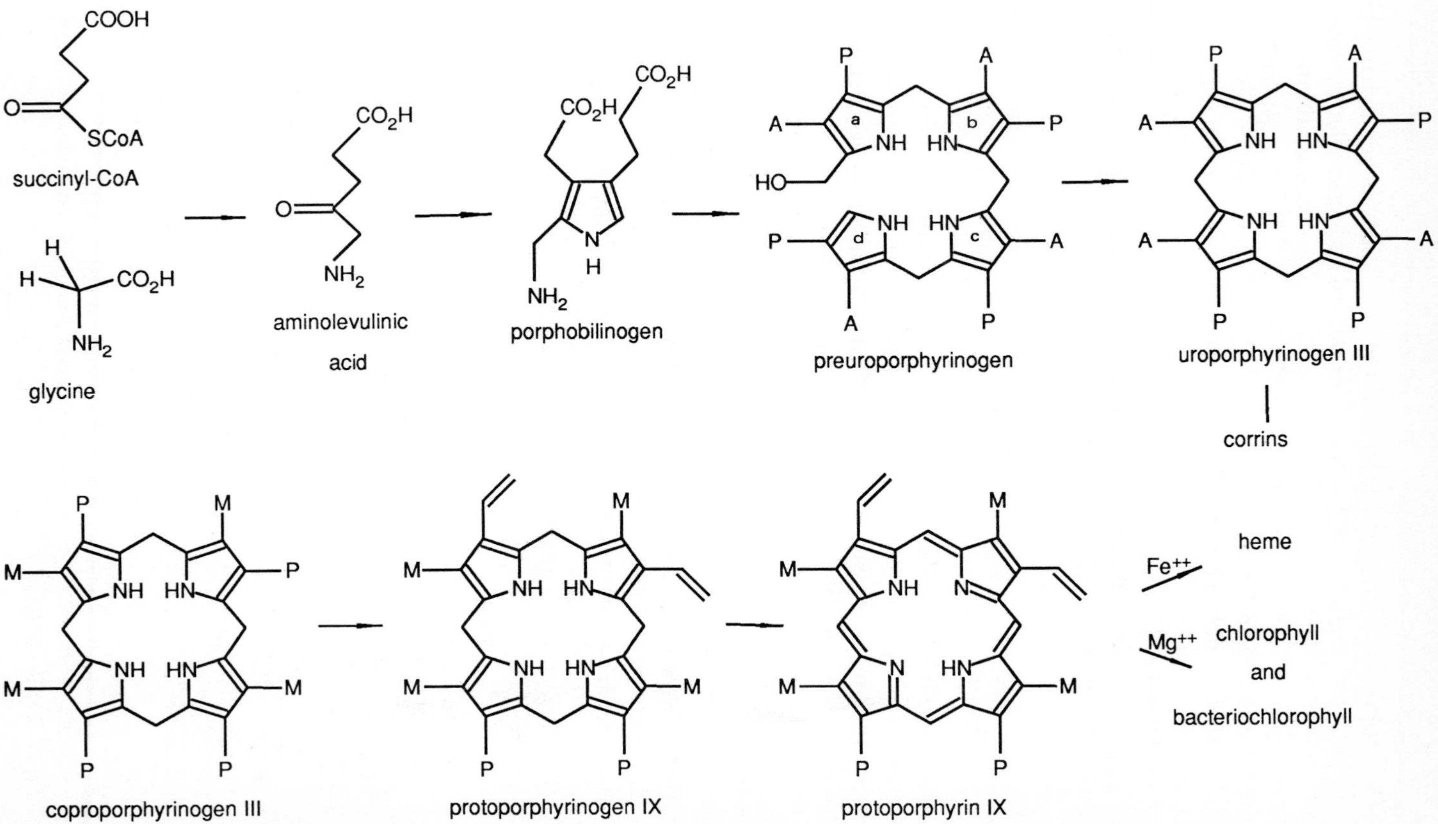

Figure 2.1 Biosynthesis of tetrapyrroles.

This applied to tetrapyrroles biosynthesized in mammalian, avian, and some bacterial systems but not to those formed in higher plants, algae, and anaerobic bacteria where glutamic acid provides the carbon and nitrogen atoms. This latter aspect is only discussed briefly below but is covered in detail in Chap. 7.

The labeling data obtained from the incorporation experiments with radioactive glycine and acetate, and especially the observation that the carboxyl-carbon atom of glycine was not incorporated into heme, led to the hypothesis that glycine and succinyl-CoA condense together to form 2-amino 3-ketoadipic acid which yields 5-aminolevulinic acid on decarboxylation (Shemin and Russell, 1953). This was confirmed when 5-amino[5-^{14}C]levulinic acid was chemically synthesized and shown to be incorporated into heme in high yield and with a labeling pattern identical to that given by [2-^{14}C]glycine (Shemin et al., 1955). The discovery of 5-aminolevulinic acid was a triumph of intuitive brilliance and decisive experimentation and ranks highly in the history of biochemical investigation. It is most educational to read first-hand accounts of this early phase in the elucidation of the tetrapyrrole pathway.

At the time that 5-aminolevulinic acid was first described, the existence of the next intermediate in the porphyrin biosynthetic pathway, porphobilinogen, had already been known for several years, having been isolated from the urine of patients suffering from acute intermittent porphyria (Westall, 1952). The implication of porphobilinogen as an intermediate in the heme biosynthetic pathway was not appreciated, however, until its structure had been elucidated by X-ray crystallography

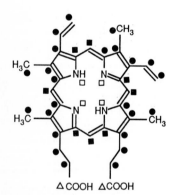

△COOH △COOH

● = CH$_3$ carbon of acetate

△ = COOH carbon of acetate

■ = CH$_2$ carbon of glycine

□ = N of glycine

Figure 2.2 Origin of carbon and nitrogen atoms in protoporphyrin IX.

(Kennard, 1953) and found to be strikingly similar to that postulated for the heme precursor pyrrole. It was then quite evident that two molecules of 5-aminolevulinic acid could account for all the carbon and nitrogen atoms of porphobilinogen. Porphobilinogen was subsequently shown to act as an excellent precursor for porphyrins (Falk et al., 1953), and its role as an intermediate was finally confirmed when it was shown to be formed enzymically from 5-aminolevulinic acid (Schmid and Shemin, 1955; Gibson et al., 1955). Three years later Bogorad (1958a, b) described enzyme systems that would transform porphobilinogen into uroporphyrinogen III and although the complexity of this latter system was not fully appreciated, the basis of the early stages of the tetrapyrrole biosynthesis pathway was largely complete. Information about porphyrin biosynthesis is available in comprehensive accounts (Dolphin, 1976; Granick and Beale, 1978; Battersby and McDonald, 1975; Akhtar and Jordan, 1979; Leeper, 1985).

II. Biosynthesis of 5-Aminolevulinic Acid

A. Occurrence and properties of 5-aminolevulinic acid synthase

The discovery of 5-aminolevulinic acid as the first committed intermediate in the tetrapyrrole biosynthesis pathway preceded by several years the identification of the enzyme which is responsible for its biosynthesis. The enzyme 5-aminolevulinic acid synthase (EC 2.3.1.37) was described simultaneously by Shemin and his co-workers (Kikuchi et al., 1958) in bacterial extracts and by Neuberger and his group in avian preparations (Gibson et al., 1958). Since that time the enzyme has been purified from many sources including *Rhodobacter spheroides* (Warnick and Burnham, 1971), rat liver (Ohashi and Kikuchi, 1979), chicken liver (Borthwick et al., 1983), *Euglena* (Dzelzkalns et al., 1982), and yeast (Volland and Felix, 1984).

All 5-aminolevulinic acid synthases catalyze the same reaction; namely, the condensation between glycine and succinyl-CoA to yield 5-aminolevulinic acid, CoA, and carbon dioxide as shown in Fig. 2.3.

In eukaryotes the enzyme is located in the mitochondria, reflecting the requirement for succinyl-CoA as one of the substrates. Although succinyl-CoA is generated by other enzyme systems such as methylmalonyl-CoA mutase, succinate thiokinase, and acetacetyl-CoA : succinate transferase, the major source of succinyl-CoA for heme synthesis is from the tricarboxylic acid cycle. It is worth mentioning that succinyl-CoA also provides the major source of energy for the entire porphyrin biosynthesis pathway, the remaining steps being energetically favorable as a result of aromatic ring formation, decarboxylations, or oxidations.

Because of the mitochondrial location of the 5-aminolevulinic acid synthase in eukaryotes a considerable amount of investigation has been focused on the mechanism by which the enzyme is first synthesized in the cytosol and then transported across the mitochondrial membrane to its ultimate location. Experiments with chick embryo liver (Borthwick et al., 1985) and yeast (Urban-Grimal et al., 1986) have established that the enzyme is first synthesized in the cytosol as a pre-enzyme which is rapidly imported into the mitochondria and processed to give the mature form. The chick embryo liver enzyme appears to be synthesized initially as a precursor molecule of molecular weight 74,000 with an amphipathic N-terminus which is recognized by the mitochondrial transport system. After its import across the mitochondrial membrane the first 56 N-terminal amino acids are removed to yield the mature enzyme with a molecular weight of 68,000. A similar situation exists in yeast where the pre-enzyme, which has a molecular weight of 59,000, is rapidly converted into the mature enzyme after import into mitochondria. The N-terminal portion of the yeast pre-enzyme is quite basic with several threonine and serine residues and represents a good recognition sequence for mitochondrial targeting. The mature yeast 5-aminolevulinic acid synthase subunit has a molecular weight of 55,000. The human liver 5-aminolevulinic acid synthase cDNA also shows the presence of an N-terminal sequence of 56 amino acids (Bawden et al., 1987).

B. Regulation of 5-aminolevulinic acid synthase

There is evidence that the enzyme from *R. spheroides* also exists in two or more forms (Tuboi et al., 1970), although it is not known whether these represent pre- and mature forms of the same enzyme or completely distinct enzymes (or both possibilities). The proportion of the enzymic

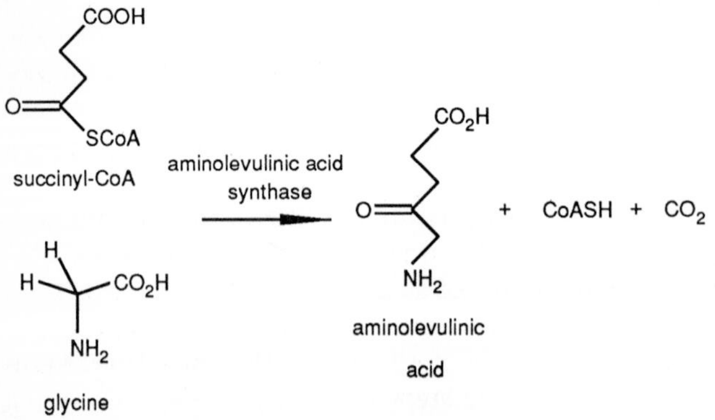

Figure 2.3   5-Aminolevulinic acid synthase reaction.

forms and the enzyme activity vary according to the conditions under which the bacteria are grown. *R. spheroides* is unusual in being able to biosynthesize heme, bacteriochlorophyll, and corrin, thus, necessitating the regulation of tetrapyrrole precursors along three branches. During adaptation from nonphotosynthetic, aerobic growth to photosynthetic anaerobic growth, a large number of proteins are induced many of which are required for the generation of the photosynthetic apparatus. The demand for bacteriochlorophyll biosynthesis may increase by as much as 100-fold (Lascelles, 1968) and 5-aminolevulinic acid synthase is therefore induced to high levels. Heme is an important regulator acting as both a feedback inhibitor of the enzyme directly and also as a regulator at the nucleic acid level. It is also tempting to speculate that two distinct 5-aminolevulinic acid synthase genes exist, one to subserve the background levels of 5-aminolevulinic acid required for heme and corrin biosynthesis and a second enzyme to cater for the 5-aminolevulinic acid required for bacteriochlorophyll biosynthesis. Evidence for the presence of "aerobic" and "anaerobic" coproporphyrinogen oxidase enzymes (Tait, 1972) has set a precedent for the existence of dual gene and enzyme systems.

Another regulatory mechanism which appears to be present in photosynthetic bacteria relates to the regulation of preexisting levels of 5-aminolevulinic acid synthase by a mechanism linked to the oxygen status of the cells. Evidence for the presence of both an inhibitor and an activator of the enzyme have been obtained which indicates that it may be regulated through sulfur-containing metabolites such as the trisulfides of cysteine and glutathione (Neuberger et al., 1973). These compounds are able to activate the 5-aminolevulinate synthase enzyme in vitro by converting a low-activity form to a high-activity form. This complex situation deserves further investigation at both the gene and protein level both in vitro and in vivo.

As the first enzyme of the tetrapyrrole biosynthetic pathway, 5-aminolevulinic acid synthase from eukaryotes has also, predictably, been the focus of attention with respect to the regulation of the flux of intermediates through the pathway (Granick et al., 1975). Regulation at the nucleic acid and at the enzyme levels have both been implicated. Heme plays a crucial role in the regulation of 5-aminolevulinic acid synthase activity, although the same feedback inhibition mechanism exhibited by the bacterial enzyme may be less significant in eukaryotes. Under conditions where the heme pool is depleted, as is the case when heme-requiring apoproteins like P450 are required for drug detoxification or when heme breakdown has been stimulated by drugs, the level of 5-aminolevulinic acid synthase may reach greatly elevated levels. Here the heme seems to act at the posttranscriptional level (Sassa and Granick, 1970). These studies suggest that the half-life of the 5-aminolevulinic acid synthase mRNA in chick embryo liver cells appears to be decreased by increases in the heme level. The 5-aminolevulinate synthase levels in erythroblasts seem to be less responsive to heme suggesting that it may be produced almost constituitively to provide the constant, high-level requirement of heme for hemoglobin synthesis.

Evidence for intrinsic instability of rat liver 5-aminolevulinate synthase indicates that this is also a most important regulatory mechanism (Hayashi et al., 1969). Similar findings have been forthcoming from studies on both mitochondrial and cytosolic forms of the enzyme from chick embryo liver cells (Ohashi and Kikuchi, 1972). Clearly, alterations in the balance between rapid synthesis and rapid breakdown of the enzyme permit a fast response to the cellular requirements for heme. Full coverage of the mechanisms involved in the regulation of heme biosynthesis is outside the scope of this chapter but may be found in Chaps. 4 and 5.

C. Substrate specificity and kinetics

All the 5-aminolevulinic acid synthase enzymes purified to date appear to exist as homodimers with subunit molecular weights varying from 40,000 to 60,000. None of the enzymes appear to accept any other amino acid substrate other than glycine. Even glycine is bound to the enzyme with a relatively low affinity and K_m values in the millimolar range are found for most of the enzymes whose kinetics have been investigated (Jordan and Shemin, 1972). Glycine analogues such as methylamine, β-alanine, and aminoethanol are only very poor inhibitors. Some amino acids such as alanine and serine also act as weak inhibitors, the L-amino acids showing preference over the D-amino acids. The most spectacular inhibition is shown by aminomalonate, with a K_i of 6 μM for the enzyme from R. *spheroides* (Matthew and Neuberger, 1963). Aminomalonate does not act as a substrate and is not, perhaps surprisingly, decarboxylated to glycine.

The rigid substrate specificity seen for glycine is not adhered to when one considers the acyl-CoA substrate. Although succinyl-CoA is by far the most favored substrate with K_m values in the low micromolar range, succinyl-CoA monomethyl ester, α-glutamyl-CoA, and acetyl-CoA are all accepted as poor substrates by the enzyme yielding the corresponding aminoketone products in yields which relate closely to their chemical reactivity (Jordan and Shemin, 1972).

The elucidation of the mechanism by which 5-aminolevulinic acid synthase catalyzes the synthesis of 5-aminolevulinic acid has been approached from several directions, including kinetic analysis, studies with exchange reactions, and the use of stereospecifically tritiated glycine. Most of the mechanistic details have been deduced from investigations with the enzyme isolated from *R. spheroides* and there is no reason to expect that other 5-aminolevulinic acid synthases follow a different mechanistic course.

Analysis of the 5-aminolevulinic acid synthase from *R. spheroides* Y using steady-state kinetics (Fanica-Gaignier and Clement-Metral, 1973) has revealed a reaction course in which there is an ordered binding of glycine followed by succinyl-CoA. The CoA is released from the enzyme before the product.

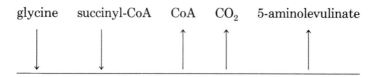

All 5-aminolevulinic acid synthases require pyridoxal 5'-phosphate for activity but unlike many other pyridoxal 5'-phosphate-dependent enzymes the cofactor is very loosely bound and may be removed by dialysis. The activity of the *R. spheroides* enzyme is maximal at 50 mM pyridoxal 5'-phosphate (Warnick and Burnham, 1971), but the nature of the interaction of the coenzyme with the enzyme is complex such that it is not possible to determine the binding constant with any precision. Spectroscopic studies (Fanica-Gaignier and Clement-Metral, 1973) have shown that the holoenzyme does not exhibit the characteristic peak of a Schiff base at 420 nm but rather indicate the presence of a carbinolamine species absorbing at about 333 nm. Treatment of the holoenzyme with sodium borohydride leads to inactivation of the enzyme but only efficiently at pHs either side of pH 7 (Jordan and Laghai, unpublished observations). At neutral pH the enzyme is not inactivated to any great extent by the reagent. This suggests that under neutral conditions the pyridoxal 5'-phosphate is bound in a less-reactive form, possibly as a carbinolamine substituted by an enzyme thiol rather than as a fully formed Schiff base as has previously been suggested (Fanica-Gaignier and Clement-Metral, 1973).

D. Mechanism of 5-aminolevulinic acid synthase

The mechanistic and steric course of the 5-aminolevulinic acid synthase reaction has received comprehensive investigation in our laboratories at Southampton in which the biosynthesis of tetrapyrroles has been investigated since 1966 by Professor Akhtar, myself, and our co-workers. Since the condensation between glycine and succinyl-CoA occurs at the α-carbon it was reasoned that a detailed study of the behavior of the α-hydrogen atoms of glycine during the transformation into 5-aminolevulinic acid would provide insight into the enzyme reaction mechanism. In common with other pyridoxal 5'-phosphate-catalyzed enzyme reactions (Snell and di Mari, 1970) the first event in the synthesis of 5-aminolevulinic acid involves the binding of glycine to the pyridoxal 5'-phosphate enzyme complex [Fig. 2.4(i)] to form an enzyme-pyridoxal 5'-phosphate-glycine Schiff-base complex [Fig. 2.4(ii)]. Further reaction of this complex requires the generation of a stabilized carbanion at the glycine-α-carbon atom which could, in principle, occur either by loss of one of the α-hydrogen atoms or by decarboxylation. When $2RS[^3H_2]$glycine was incubated with succinyl-CoA and highly purified 5-aminolevulinic acid synthase only half of the tritium label was incorporated into 5-aminolevulinic acid, suggesting that the carbanion species which reacts with succinyl-CoA is generated by the loss of a proton [Fig. 2.4(iii)] (Akhtar and Jordan, 1968). Had the alternative reaction course occurred, namely, decarboxylation followed by condensation, then all of the tritium originally present in the glycine would have been incorporated into the 5-aminolevulinic acid.

Having established the broad mechanistic features of the 5-aminolevulinic acid synthase reaction, the steric course was investigated by following the incorporation of the two tritiated enantiomers of glycine into 5-aminolevulinic acid. $2R[^3H]$Glycine and $2S[^3H]$glycine were synthesized enzymically using the enzyme serine hydroxymethyltransferase which stereospecifically exchanges the pro-S hydrogen atom of glycine (Jordan and Akhtar, 1970). Incorporation of $2R[^3H]$glycine into 5-aminolevulinic acid proceeded with loss of the tritium label, whereas the tritium from the $2S[^3H]$glycine was largely incorporated into 5-aminolevulinic acid. These experiments established that it is the pro-R hydrogen atom of glycine that is lost in the overall enzymic transformation (Zaman et al., 1973). Exchange reactions carried out with highly purified 5-aminolevulinic acid synthase from *R. spheroides* (Laghai and Jordan, 1976) confirmed these findings. In the absence of the second substrate, succinyl-CoA, the enzyme catalyzes a partial reaction in which the pro-R hydrogen atom of glycine is exchanged with the protons of the solvent. The pro-R hydrogen atom of glycine occupies the same orientation in space as the α-hydrogen atom of L-amino acids and probably accounts for the fact that L-amino acids are far better inhibitors of the enzyme than D-amino acids.

Since the reaction of succinyl-CoA with the enzyme-pyridoxal 5'-phosphate-glycine carbanion intermediate precedes decarboxylation, it follows that the condensation will yield an enzyme-pyridoxal 5'-phosphate-2-amino-3-ketoadipic acid complex [Fig. 2.4(iv)]. Further transformation of this intermediate into 5-aminolevulinic acid could, in principle, occur by one of two routes—either by hydrolysis of the Schiff base in this intermediate to yield free 2-amino-3-ketoadipic acid which could

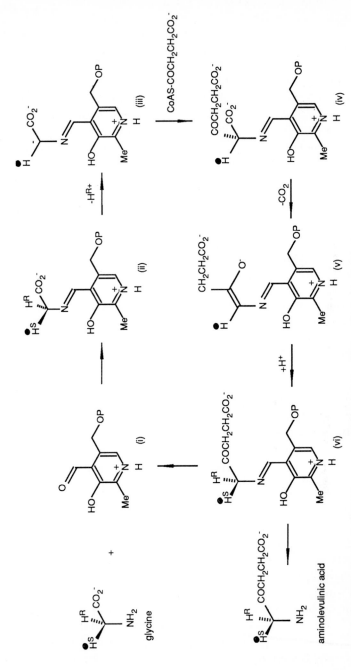

Figure 2.4 Mechanism and steric course of the 5-aminolevulinic acid synthase reaction.

decarboxylate nonenzymically to 5-aminolevulinic acid, or by an alternative mechanism in which the 5-aminolevulinic acid synthase also acts as
a decarboxylase. The latter mechanism would require that the enzyme-
bound intermediate enol [Fig. 2.4(v)] generated by the decarboxylation
would be protonated stereospecifically to generate the enzyme-pyridoxal
5'-phosphate Schiff base of 5-aminolevulinic acid [Fig. 2.4(vi)], hydrolysis
of which would yield 5-aminolevulinic acid. These two possibilities were
resolved by incorporating $2RS[^3H_2]$glycine into 5-aminolevulinic acid
and determining whether the remaining tritium is stereospecifically
located in this product. Experimental evidence (Abboud et al., 1974)
showed that the tritium originally present in the pro-S configuration is,
in fact, incorporated into the pro-S configuration at the C-5 position in
the product, thus, establishing that 5-aminolevulinic acid synthase acts
as a decarboxylase as well as a condensing enzyme. This conclusion is
strengthened by the finding that the enzyme catalyzes the stereospecific
exchange of the pro-R hydrogen atom at the C-5 position of 5-amino-
levulinic acid (Laghai and Jordan, 1977). This would not have been
expected if 2-amino-3-ketoadipic acid had been the final enzymic product.

Further powerful evidence for the enzyme-catalyzed decarboxylation
has stemmed from studies of the 5-aminolevulinic acid synthase reaction
working in reverse. Incubation of 5-aminolevulinic acid with ^{14}C carbon
dioxide in the presence of the enzyme led to the formation of radioactive
glycine, but only in the presence of 5-aminolevulinic acid and CoA
(Nandi, 1978a). This could only have occurred had the enzyme been able
to catalyze the reverse of its normal reaction.

The overall steric course of the reaction is somewhat confusing since
the reaction occurs with overall inversion yet the tritium label originally
in the pro-S configuration in the glycine is found in the pro-S configuration of the product. This cryptic stereochemistry may be explained by
the fact that the $-COCH_2CH_2COOH$ group occupies the same position
in space as the original $-COOH$ group from glycine, yet, because of the
nature of the mechanism, the $-COCH_2CH_2COOH$ replaces the proton
lost from the pro-R position of glycine and adopts its final configuration
only after the decarboxylation and reprotonation have occurred.

A survey of the literature on the mechanism of pyridoxal 5'-phos-
phate-requiring enzymes (Emery and Akhtar, 1987) reveals an almost
unerring uniformity in the steric course of substitution reactions in
which the new group occupies the same position in space as the outgoing
proton. There is, thus, a precedent for the addition of the succinyl
moiety with retention of the configuration. Decarboxylation of the
enzyme-bound 2-amino-3-ketoadipic acid would generate the enol which,
being planar, could easily be protonated from the opposite side and,
therefore, account for the inversion. This is even more attractive when

one considers that the enzymic group responsible for the original depro-tonation of the pro-R hydrogen atom of the glycine Schiff base would be in an ideal position to carry out the final reprotonation to give the desired stereochemistry in the 5-aminolevulinic acid. Consistent with this view is the observation that the enzyme catalyzes a partial reaction in which the pro-R hydrogen atom at C-5 of 5-aminolevulinic acid is stereospecifically exchanged with the protons of the medium. Thus, both the glycine and the 5-aminolevulinic acid can participate in proton exchange reactions with what is almost certainly the same catalytic group at the enzyme active site.

The effect of inhibitors of the enzyme on the exchange reactions has revealed additional information regarding the mechanism of inhibition by heme with the *R. spheroides* enzyme. The glycine exchange reaction was inhibited by 5-aminolevulinic acid and the 5-aminolevulinic acid exchange reaction was, in turn, inhibited by glycine (Laghai and Jordan, 1977). Both exchange reactions were strongly inhibited by 0.125 mM aminomalonate consistent with the inhibition of the overall reaction by this glycine analogue. Most interestingly, heme at a concentration of 2 μM inhibited the 5-aminolevulinic acid exchange reaction but had no effect on the glycine reaction. This suggests that the binding site at which heme exerts its inhibitory effect may overlap with the area of the active site required for binding the succinyl moiety ($-COCH_2CH_2COOH$). Alternatively, the interaction of the heme with the enzyme could induce a conformational change which perturbs the protein structure in the vicinity of the succinyl-CoA binding site.

E. Structure of the enzyme and molecular biology

The structure of the enzyme and the nature of the enzyme groups involved with catalysis have not yet been identified since hitherto the amounts of 5-aminolevulinic acid synthase available for study have been very limited. The enzymes from all sources are sensitive to sulfhydryl reagents such as iodoacetic acid and *p*-chloromercuribenzoate. Although cysteine is unlikely to be an important catalytic group, it has been implicated as a binding group for pyridoxal 5'-phosphate (Fanica-Gaignier and Clement-Metral, 1973).

Recently, important structural information has become available as a result of the application of molecular biology to the 5-aminolevulinic acid synthase enzyme which has led to the cloning and sequencing of the cDNA for the chick embryo liver pre-enzyme (Borthwick et al., 1985; Maguire et al., 1986), the yeast *HEM*1 gene (Urban-Grimal et al., 1986), the human liver cDNA (Bawden et al., 1987), the mouse cDNA (Schoenhaut and Curtis, 1986), and the *Bradyrhizobium japonicum* *hemA* gene (McClung et al., 1987). Partial sequence information has been obtained from *Rhizobium meliloti* (Leong et al., 1985). Yeast, chicken, and human nucleotide sequences have provided information about the primary structure of the 5-aminolevulinic acid synthase precursor and the nature of the sequences required for mitochondrial targeting and protein maturation.

The nucleotide sequence data have also revealed interesting similarities between the primary structures which are obvious targets for further investigation. For instance, the predicted protein primary structures of the 5-aminolevulinic acid synthases from *R. meliloti*, yeast, *Bradyrhizobium japonicum*, chicken embryo liver, and human liver all show highly conserved sequences. Overall, the comparison between the derived protein sequences of yeast and chick embryo liver revealed, after optimal alignment, about 41% similarity. Comparison between the sequences from *Bradyrhizobium* and chicken embryo liver showed about 49% similarity. Interestingly, comparison of the human sequence with the rat and chicken shows 83 and 78% similarity, respectively, but only 43% similarity with the mouse amino acid sequence. This suggests the existence of two distinct gene families, one representing the hepatic mitochondrial enzyme and the other perhaps from the erythroid system. Some direct evidence in support of two genes comes also from the isolation of a specific cDNA for the erythroid form (Yamamoto et al., 1985). The availability of genes for 5-aminolevulinic acid synthase opens up new and exciting possibilities for the study of both regulatory aspects and mitochondrial targeting of the enzyme.

III. Biosynthesis of 5-Aminolevulinic Acid from Glutamate

A. Discovery and occurrence of the C-5 pathway

Investigators were puzzled for many years by their inability to detect 5-aminolevulinic acid synthase in higher plants and except for a few poorly documented reports there was little evidence to suggest that glycine and succinyl-CoA were the immediate precursors of tetrapyrroles. The problem was solved by Beale and Castelfranco (1974), who made the crucial breakthrough when they demonstrated that 5-aminolevulinic acid was derived from the carbon skeleton of glutamate in greening cucumber cotyledons and the "C-5 pathway" was born (see Chap. 7). Further experiments with [^{14}C]-labeled glutamate in greening barley showed that it was incorporated into 5-aminolevulinic acid with the carbon skeleton intact, and with the C-1 of glutamate giving rise to the C-5 of 5-aminolevulinic acid (Beale et al., 1975). The existence of the C-5 pathway has been confirmed in barley (Kannangara and Gough, 1977), *Cyanidium caldarium* (Weinstein and Beale, 1984), *Chlamydomonas reinhardtii* (Wang et al., 1984), and in *Chlorella vulgaris* (Weinstein and Beale, 1985). As well as occurring in plants and algae, the C-5 pathway has been demonstrated in *Euglena gracilis* (Weinstein and Beale, 1983; Mayer et al., 1987), cyanobacteria such as *Spirulina platensis* (Einav and Avissar, 1984), archeabacteria such as *Methanobacterium thermoautotrophicum* (Freidmann et al., 1987), and in the eubacteria such as *Clostridium tetanomorphum* (Smith and Huster, 1987). Recent experimental evidence is beginning to reveal that the operation of the C-5 or glutamate pathway in the biosphere is more common than the glycine pathway.

Experiments in which $[^{13}C]$-labeled glutamate was incorporated into chlorophyll (Oh-hama et al., 1982; Porra et al., 1983) demonstrated conclusively that the glutamic acid carbon skeleton was incorporated into 5-aminolevulinic acid intact and that the C-1 of glutamate occupies those positions in the resulting chlorophyll which would have arisen from the C-5 of 5-aminolevulinic acid.

B. Enzymes of the C-5 pathway

The elucidation of the pathway by which glutamate is transformed into 5-aminolevulinic acid has been the subject of intensive research over the last decade. The enzymes have been characterized most fully in barley and it is assumed, though not proven, that similar enzymes are operative in algae and bacteria. In energetic terms the overall reaction is unfavorable since it involves the reduction of a carboxylic acid, necessitating the participation of ATP, or its equivalent. In addition, there is a requirement for a reducing agent such as NADPH. In a brilliant series of experiments the isolation and characterization of the enzymes involved in the transformation of glutamate into 5-aminolevulinic acid have been achieved by Kannangara and his colleagues in Copenhagen. Altogether, three enzymes have been detected in extracts of greening barley (Wang et al., 1981). In addition, the involvement of tRNA[glu] has also been established (Kannangara et al., 1984; Schon et al., 1986; Huang and Wang, 1986), a completely unexpected finding, but one which makes mechanistic sense since it solves the problem of activation of the α-carboxyl group of glutamate prior to reduction.

Three enzymes are thought to be involved with the transformation of glutamate into 5-aminolevulinic acid. The first enzyme, glutamate-tRNA ligase (Bruyant and Kannangara, 1987), catalyzes the coupling of glutamate to tRNA[glu], a reaction which requires ATP and magnesium ions. The glutamyl-tRNA is then reduced by a second enzyme in an

NADPH-requiring reaction to generate a new intermediate, the structure of which has not yet been unequivocally established. Kannangara and his colleagues have proposed glutamate 1-semialdehyde (Houen et al., 1984) as the structure of this intermediate, however, such α-aminoaldehydes are extremely labile compounds and rapidly polymerize to ill-defined products. The third enzyme, an aminotransferase, catalyzes the conversion of this intermediate into 5-aminolevulinic acid in a reaction which requires no transaminating amino acid donor (Hoober et al., 1988). This pathway is shown in Fig. 2.5a.

C. Alternatives to the pathway

In this pathway, glutamate 1-semialdehyde is transformed into 5-aminolevulinic acid by a single enzyme, glutamate 1-semialdehyde aminotransferase. This has been challenged by Dornemann (Breu and Dornemann, 1988; Breu et al., 1988) as a result of experiments carried out with *Scenedesmus*. In this organism 4,5-dioxovalerate appears to be a better precursor for 5-aminolevulinic acid than glutamate 1-semialdehyde. The presence of the enzyme 4,5-dioxovalerate transaminase has also been presented as evidence for a two-stage transformation of glutamate 1-semialdehyde into 5-aminolevulinic acid via 4,5-dioxovalerate. As yet these points of contention are unresolved. It is possible that variations on the pathway shown in Fig. 2.5b exist in different organisms with 4,5-dioxovalerate as an intermediate between glutamate 1-semialdehyde and 5-aminolevulinic acid in *Scenedesmus* but not in barley.

One additional question which has been of some concern relates to the remarkably stable nature of the proposed glutamate 1-semialdehyde intermediate. α-Aminoaldehydes of this type have never been successfully prepared because of their extreme reactivity. It was, therefore, quite inexplicable when it was reported that not only was glutamate 1-semialdehyde an intermediate but that it accumulated when the inhibitor gabaculine was added to etiolated barley leaves (Kannangara and Schouboe, 1985). The material extracted from the leaves had all the properties of the synthetic compound (Houen et al., 1984).

In order to resolve this paradox we prepared glutamate 1-semialdehyde by a route which involved its chemical generation from a purified, N-protected precursor (Jordan et al., 1989). Proton nmr showed, as expected, a strong aldehyde resonance. In contrast to the intermediate isolated from barley leaves, which has no free aldehyde proton, our material rapidly turned brown and the aldehyde nmr signal disappeared within a few minutes as one would have predicted. The material synthesized by Houen et al. (1984), therefore, had altogether different properties from the α-aminoaldehyde prepared in our laboratory. Most significantly, incubation of enzyme extracts from greening barley with

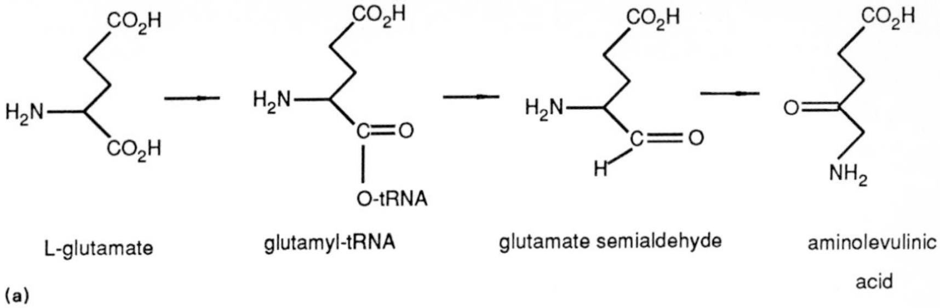

(a)

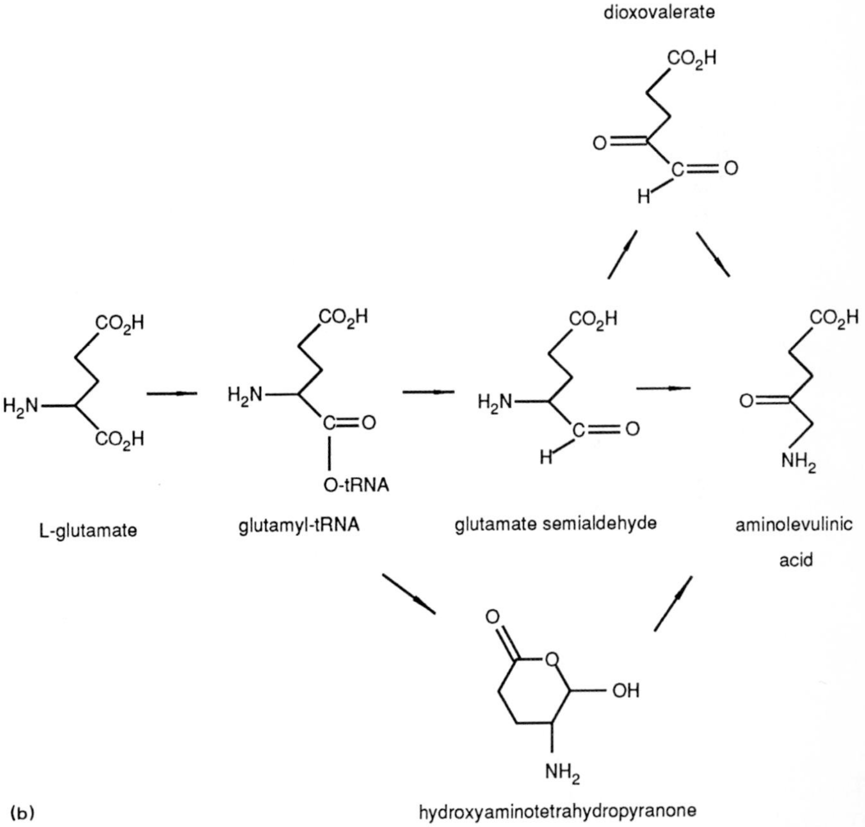

(b)

Figure 2.5 Glutamate pathway for the biosynthesis of 5-aminolevulinic acid.

our synthetic material failed to generate 5-aminolevulinic acid or porphyrins. In contrast, synthesis of the intermediate by a route related to that used by Kannangara and Gough (1978) generated a stable material which, after purification, acted as the substrate for the aminotransferase. We are, therefore, of the opinion that glutamate 1-semialdehyde with its free aldehyde group may not be involved as an intermediate. We proposed that the material generated by the synthesis of Houen et al. (1984) is not glutamate 1-semialdehyde but its cyclic form, 2-hydroxy,3-amino-tetrahydropyran-1-one (HAT) (Fig. 2.5b), and that it is this which acts as the true precursor for 5-aminolevulinic acid (Jordan et al., 1989). By analogy with the structure and properties of glucoseamine this cyclic structure should be reasonably stable in acid but highly unstable in base in which the ring would open to give the α-aminoaldehyde which would then polymerize. The observed properties of the intermediate, synthesized both chemically and enzymically, are consistent with a cyclic structure. We are of the opinion that the synthetic route used initially by Kannangara and Gough (1978) yielded the cyclic compound (HAT) and not the free α-aminoaldehyde.

The plausible mechanism for the aminotransferase reaction has been proposed by Hoober et al. (1988) in which the glutamate semialdehyde binds to the enzyme which contains a pyridoxamine phosphate cofactor at the active site. The amino group transaminates with the substrate to yield an enzyme-bound 4,5-diaminovalerate intermediate. This is now transformed into 5-aminolevulinic acid by donating the amino group in the C-4 position to the pyridoxal 5′-phosphate to regenerate the pyridoxamine 5′-phosphate-enzyme ready to receive the next substrate. This mechanism explains why an amino donor other than the substrate is required. This mechanism is also consistent with the elegant nmr experiments of Mau and Wang (1988) which showed that there was intermolecular transfer of the amino group during the reaction. The likely involvement of the cyclic intermediate (HAT) as a substrate need not affect the above mechanism since the transaminase would ring open the compound as the first step in the mechanism. Such ring opening occurs in enzyme reactions which involve transformations of hexoses such as occur in glucose metabolism.

There is a growing amount of evidence to suggest that some photosynthetic organisms as well as higher plants may operate both glycine and glutamate pathways, the former being employed for the synthesis of heme and the latter for chlorophyll production. In *Euglena gracilis* [14C]glycine is preferentially incorporated into heme, whereas radioactivity from [14C]glutamate is found predominantly in chlorophyll (Weinstein and Beale, 1983). The relative importance of the two systems may vary according to the metabolic status. For instance, during germination, it is likely that the glycine pathway would be active since respiratory activity would be high. Once photosynthetic growth was established then the glutamate pathway would assume a dominant, though not total, role. Aspects of the C-5 pathway have been reviewed elsewhere (Castelfranco and Beale, 1983; Kannangara et al., 1988) and a detailed account is presented in Chap. 7.

IV. Biosynthesis of Porphobilinogen

After the discovery of 5-aminolevulinic acid and the elucidation of the structure of porphobilinogen, the enzyme 5-aminolevulinic acid dehydratase (EC 4.2.1.24), also called porphobilinogen synthase, was initially shown to be present in ox liver (Gibson et al., 1955) and avian erythrocytes (Schmid and Shemin; 1955). The enzyme has since been shown to exist in virtually all living organisms and has been highly purified from a variety of sources including human erythrocytes (Anderson and Desnick, 1979; Gibbs et al., 1985a), bovine liver (Bevan et al., 1980; Jordan and Seehra, 1986), R. spheroides (Nandi et al., 1968), yeast (Clara de Barreiro, 1967), and spinach (Liedgens et al., 1983). The reaction catalyzed by the enzyme involves the dimerization of two molecules of 5-aminolevulinic acid in a Knorr reaction with the elimination of two molecules of water as shown in Fig. 2.6.

A. General properties of 5-aminolevulinic acid dehydratases

5-Aminolevulinic acid dehydratase enzymes have been grouped into two classes according to molecular weight, pH optimum, metal requirement, and susceptibility to inhibition with EDTA. Comprehensive reviews of the properties of the enzymes are available (Shemin, 1972; Cheh and Neilands, 1976). The mammalian and avian enzymes are zinc metalloenzymes of all which have pH optima in the range 6.3 to 7.0 and are inhibited by EDTA. During purification, a small proportion of the zinc is lost from the enzyme but full enzymic activity can be restored by adding exogeneous zinc as long as the enzyme is maintained under anaerobic

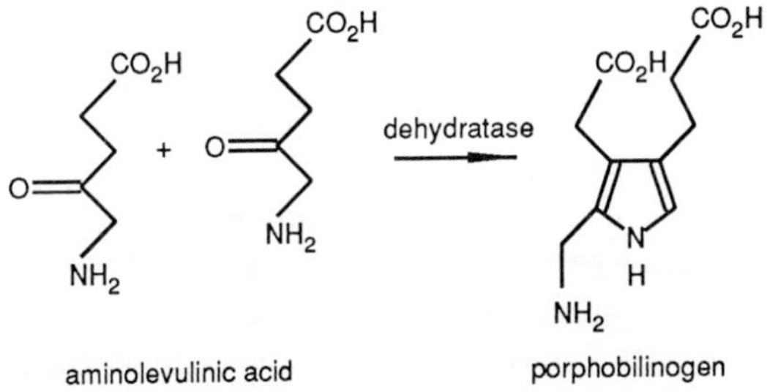

Figure 2.6 Formation of porphobilinogen from 5-aminolevulinic acid.

conditions by the presence of dithioerythritol (Cheh and Neilands, 1976; Tsukamoto et al., 1979; Gibbs et al., 1985a). Dehydratases of this class have molecular weights of about 280,000 made up of eight identical subunits of molecular weight 35,000.

The bacterial enzymes have very different properties with pH optima from 8 to 8.5 and a requirement for monovalent cations such as K^+ for maximum activity. Although the bacterial enzymes show no inhibition with EDTA and are not activated by zinc ions, this does not necessarily preclude the presence of a very tight zinc binding site. The enzyme from *R. spheroides* has a molecular weight of 240,000 and early reports suggested that it is made up of six identical subunits each of molecular weight 39,500 (van Heyningen and Shemin, 1971). More recent experiments have shown that this enzyme may, in fact, exist as an octamer (Gurne et al., 1977) like the mammalian dehydratases. In the presence of K^+ ions the *R. spheroides* enzyme aggregates to octameric dimers, trimers, and tetramers with an accompanying increase in the specific activity of the enzyme (Nandi and Shemin, 1968a). Even without activation, bacterial dehydratases have a specific activity substantially higher than that of the mammalian enzymes. Dehydratases isolated from plants (Leidgens et al., 1983) and yeast (Clara de Barreiro, 1967) seem also to be zinc metalloenzymes as judged by their susceptibility to EDTA, however, their pH optima are somewhat higher than those of the mammalian enzymes.

Electron microscopy of the bovine 5-aminolevulinic acid dehydratase has revealed that the eight subunits are arranged as if they were at the corners of a cube with dihedral symmetry (Wu et al., 1974). The way in which the subunits interact has been followed by treatment of the enzyme with urea of increasing concentrations (Jordan and Chaudhry, unpublished data). This results in the formation of a tetramer at 4 M urea and a dimer at 5.5 M urea, both of which can be separated by gel filtration. Both forms exhibit some catalytic activity, however, increasing the urea concentration further leads to the precipitation of the enzyme and complete loss of activity, as the dimeric structure collapses to give free subunits. These observations suggest that the octamer is a dimer of tetramers and that each tetramer is a dimer of dimers. The conclusions from these studies are consistent with the enzyme structure being composed of four functional dimers. In this connection there is a considerable amount of evidence to suggest that the bovine enzyme, at least, exhibits half-site reactivity (Cheh and Neilands, 1976). It has been observed that 5-aminolevulinic acid dehydratase from *R. spheroides* also dissociates into two functional tetramers in the absence of potassium ions. This has been shown by an elegant experiment (Gurne et al., 1977) in which the bacterial enzyme was first immobilized in a chromatography column. The column was subsequently treated with buffers lacking potassium ions which released half of the enzyme activity, the other half remaining bound to the column as a functional tetramer. The immobilized enzyme has also been successfully employed for the synthesis of porphobilinogen.

B. Importance of sulfhydryl groups

One common feature of all dehydratases is the remarkable sensitivity of their sulfhydryl groups to oxygen or to thiol reagents. On exposure of the native bovine enzyme to oxygen there is a rapid loss of enzyme activity which is associated with the oxidation of two highly reactive SH groups to form an S—S bond (Barnard et al., 1977; Tsukamoto et al., 1979; Seehra et al., 1981). Full catalytic activity can be restored on treatment of the enzyme with an exogenous thiol. Addition of 5,5'-dithiobis(2-nitrobenzoic acid) to the active enzyme also results in the formation of the S—S bond between these two sulfhydryl groups. Two other less-reactive sulfhydryl groups react with 5,5'-dithiobis(2-nitrobenzoic acid) (Seehra et al., 1981) and a further three or four become available when the enzyme is denatured with sodium dodecylsulfate (Tsukamoto et al., 1979). The importance of the reactive SH groups in the binding of the metal ion has been demonstrated by labeling the human 5-aminolevulinic acid dehydratase with $^{65}Zn^{2+}$ (Gibbs and Jordan, 1981). Exposure of the labeled enzyme to oxygen or treatment of the enzyme with 5,5'-dithiobis(2-nitrobenzoic acid) causes the immediate displacement of the $^{65}Zn^{2+}$ ion and a loss of enzyme activity. All these studies suggest that —SH groups are involved with the binding of the metal ion.

C. Requirement for zinc

The metal requirements for the dehydratase enzymes have been investigated largely with the mammalian enzymes especially those isolated from human erythrocytes and bovine liver. It has been established that one zinc ion is bound per subunit, eight per octamer, on the basis of experiments with both nonradioactive zinc (Tsukamoto et al., 1979) and with ^{65}Zn (Gibbs and Jordan, 1981).

Whether zinc is essential for catalytic activity is still in some doubt. Investigations by Tsukamoto et al. (1979) suggest that zinc plays only a conformational role and is not essential for activity, whereas others (Bevan et al., 1980) have suggested that only four zinc ions per octamer may be required for full catalytic activity and that only half of the subunits may be catalytically active at one time. Using $^{65}Zn^{2+}$, we have demonstrated that when only four zinc ions are bound per octamer, the enzyme is half-active and that eight zinc ions are necessary for full catalytic activity (Gibbs and Jordan, unpublished data). Zinc has also been shown to activate the enzyme in vivo in humans (Meredith and Moore, 1980) and to be essential for the de novo synthesis of the enzyme in fungi (Komai and Neilands, 1968). Cadmium displaces $^{65}Zn^{2+}$ from the enzyme more rapidly than nonlabeled zinc (Gibbs and Jordan, 1981) in keeping with the higher affinity of the enzyme for cadmium ions (Cheh and Neilands, 1976).

Evidence from x-ray absorption spectroscopy (Hasnain et al., 1985) has revealed that zinc is ligated to three sulfur atoms. The availability of the cDNA sequence from human 5-aminolevulinic acid dehydratase has provided the opportunity to examine the derived primary structure of the human enzyme and to suggest the possible location of these three sulfhydryl groups (Wetmer et al., 1986). A sequence is present which is very close to the consensus sequence of zinc binding sites as deduced from sequences described in other zinc metalloenzymes (Kozak, 1984). This sequence contains four cysteine residues, two of which are the oxygen-sensitive groups responsible for the formation of the S—S bond. In addition, there are two histidine residues, one of which is thought to interact with the zinc ion. Evidence for the involvement of histidine has been provided from inactivation studies (Tsukamoto et al., 1979), how-ever, whether the putative metal binding site comprises these histidines is not known. The proposed metal-binding-site sequence runs from residues 119 to 132 in the human enzyme with the four amino acids which are proposed as metal ligands indicated (×). This sequence is identical to that determined for the rat (Bishop et al., 1986) and is very similar to the primary protein structure derived from the *E. coli* gene sequence (Echelard et al., 1988) with all but one of the putative cysteine residues and both histidine residues conserved (*).

```
                        ×     ×               ×       ×
Human enzyme      C  D  V  C  L  C  P  Y  T  S  H  G  H  C  G
                     *     *     *     *  *  *  *  *  *  *  *
Rat enzyme        C  D  V  C  L  C  P  Y  T  S  H  G  H  C  G
                     *     *     *     *  *  *  *  *  *  *  *
E. coli enzyme    S  D  T  C  F  C  E  Y  T  S  H  G  H  C  G
```

The presence of a putative zinc binding site in the prokaryote enzyme throws some doubt on the previous attempts to classify the enzymes into metalloenzymes and Schiff-base enzymes since the *E. coli* enzyme, if it is typical of other bacterial enzymes, would also seem to have the metal binding site. The structural differences may, however, make a difference in the tightness of the metal binding which could account for the lack of EDTA inhibition seen in the bacterial enzymes.

D. Inhibition by lead

One of the most interesting properties of the mammalian 5-aminolevulinic acid dehydratases is their reaction with, and inactivation by, lead ions. The activities of human (Meredith and Moore, 1980) and rat

(Finnelli et al., 1975) erythrocyte 5-aminolevulinic acid dehydratases are inhibited by lead, both in vivo and in vitro, however, zinc is able to overcome this inhibition. Such is the sensitivity of the dehydratase to lead in vivo that its activity has been used to monitor plasma lead levels in humans with lead poisoning (Chisholm, 1971). One of the effects of lead poisoning which directly relates to the inhibition of the 5-amino-levulinic acid dehydratase enzyme is the sharp rise in 5-aminolevulinic acid in the blood and the severe accompanying neurological symptoms caused by this compound. 5-Aminolevulinic acid has been shown to act as a 4-aminobutyric acid agonist and found to inhibit the activity of mammalian spinal motor neurons probably via 4-aminobutyric acid inhibitory synapses (Bagust et al., 1985). Similar symptoms have also been observed in patients with porphyrias, one of which is the result of an inherited defect in 5-aminolevulinic acid dehydratase (Thunell et al., 1987) and the other type, acute intermittent porphyria (Kappas et al., 1963), which is caused by a defect in porphobilinogen deaminase, the next enzyme in the pathway.

The most obvious mechanism by which lead inhibits the mammalian dehydratases is thought to be by displacement of the zinc. However, our studies have shown that lead completely inactivates the $^{65}Zn^{2+}$-labeled human enzyme but that only about half the radioactivity has been displaced from the enzyme (Gibbs and Jordan, unpublished data). These findings suggest that either zinc and lead may interact with the human enzyme at more than one site (Gibbs et al., 1985b) or half-site reactivity is involved. It is also possible that the binding of lead to only half of the subunits in the octamer may cause a conformational change which accounts for the loss of all the activity.

E. Nature of the active-site groups

The first detailed studies on the mechanism of action of 5-aminolevulinic acid dehydratase were those carried out by Shemin and his colleagues using the enzyme from *R. spheroides*. These studies established several interesting features about the dehydratase, the most important being that the substrate interacts with the enzyme via a Schiff base (Nandi and Shemin, 1968b). Incubation of the substrate, 5-aminolevulinic acid, and with the enzyme in the presence of sodium borohydride led to irreversible inactivation. When 5-amino[^{14}C]levulinic acid was used, radioactive label was incorporated into the inactivated enzyme protein. Further investigations established that substrate analogues were also able to form a Schiff base with the enzyme. The structural requirement for recognition by the enzyme, therefore, appears to be a carboxylic acid with a keto-function in the 4-position. A neutral or positively charged group is thought to be required at the C-5 position since 2-ketoglutarate was found to be a very poor inhibitor. More recently, succinylacetone has been found to act as a potent inhibitor of the enzyme (Brumm and Friedmann, 1981).

The enzymic group involved with the binding of 5-aminolevulinic acid to the bacterial enzyme has been identified as a lysine residue (Nandi, 1978b). Lysine has also been shown to be involved in the human and bovine enzymes (Gibbs and Jordan, 1986). Using 5-amino[^{14}C]levulinic acid, the active-site lysine has been labeled in the human and bovine 5-aminolevulinic acid dehydratases by reduction with borohydride and the cyanogen bromide peptides from both enzymes have been sequenced (Gibbs and Jordan, 1986). The sequence of amino acids in the vicinity of the lysine appears to be highly conserved although the cyanogen bromide peptides were of different size due to the presence of a methionine in the human enzyme in place of an arginine in the bovine sequence, a change which can be accounted for by a difference of a single base in the codons—ATG for methionine to CTG for arginine. The cloning and sequencing of the full-length cDNA for the 5-aminolevulinic acid dehydratases from both human (Wetmer et al., 1986) and rat (Bishop et al., 1986) have resulted in derived protein sequences for both enzymes which also reveal a high degree (88%) of conservation. The bacterial protein sequence derived from the *hemB* gene from *E coli* (Echelard et al., 1988) also shows a substantial similarity (37%) with the human sequence. A comparison of the peptide sequences and derived sequences in the vicinity of the active-site lysine are shown below with the similarities indicated (*).

```
Peptides            *  *  *  *  *
 Human              M  V  K  P  G  M
Peptides            *  *  *  *  *      *  *  *  *      *        *
 Bovine             M  V  K  P  G  R  P  Y  L  D  L  V  R  E
          *  *  *    *  *  *  *  *  *      *  *  *  *      *        *
 Human    G  A  D  M  L  M  V  K  P  G  M  P  Y  L  D  I  V  R  E
          *  *  *    *  *  *  *  *  *      *  *  *  *      *        *
 Rat      G  A  D  I  L  M  V  K  P  G  L  P  Y  L  D  M  V  Q  E
          *  *  *    *  *  *  *  *  *      *  *  *      *        *
 E. coli  G  A  D  C  L  M  V  K  P  A  G  A  Y  L  D  I  V  R  E
```

On the basis of the active-site peptide sequences (Gibbs and Jordan, 1986), it has been possible to locate the exact position of the active-site lysine in the derived protein sequences which is at position 252 in human, position 252 in rat, and position 247 in *E. coli* dehydratases. The polar active-site lysine is flanked by hydrophobic groups which may increase its reactivity. The highly significant similarity between the prokaryote enzyme and the mammalian enzymes, especially in the vicinity of the active-site lysine and the putative metal binding site, suggest they may have very similar three-dimensional structures.

F. Order of binding the two substrates

5-Aminolevulinic acid dehydratase uses two molecules of the same substrate and, therefore, the order of substrate binding in relation to their final position in the product cannot be determined by a kinetic approach. 5-Aminolevulinic acid dehydratase is very specific for its substrate 5-aminolevulinic acid and only the bacterial enzymes will accept alternative substrates. The use of the substrate analogue levulinic acid, together with 5-aminolevulinic acid, leads to the formation of a "mixed" pyrrole (Fig. 2.7) in which the acetic acid (A) side is composed of levulinic acid and the propionic acid side (P) of 5-aminolevulinic acid (Nandi and Shemin, 1968b).

The fact that levulinic acid also acts as a competitive inhibitor and forms a covalent link with the enzyme suggested a mechanism in which the substrate binding as a Schiff base gives rise to the A side of the product porphobilinogen (Nandi and Shemin, 1968b). This mechanism was accepted until recently when single-turnover experiments were designed to investigate the precise order of binding of the two substrates (without using substrate analogues) in the bovine and bacterial dehydratases (Jordan and Seehra, 1980a, b) and in the human enzyme (Jordan and Gibbs, 1985). In these experiments stoichiometric amounts of either ^{13}C or ^{14}C substrate were reacted rapidly with the enzyme to occupy one of the substrate-binding sites. Nonlabeled substrate was then added to complete the turnover of the bound labeled substrate. It was hoped that the labeled 5-aminolevulinic acid, initially bound to the enzyme, would occupy only one side of the porphobilinogen and that this would reveal which of the two substrate molecules had originally bound to the enzyme. The position of the label in the porphobilinogen was determined either by nmr or by chemical degradation. The results showed clearly that the 5-aminolevulinic acid molecule initially bound to the enzyme gives rise to the P side of the substrate and not the A side as had been suggested previously (Nandi and Shemin, 1968b). These workers had assumed incorrectly that levulinic acid was acting as a substrate

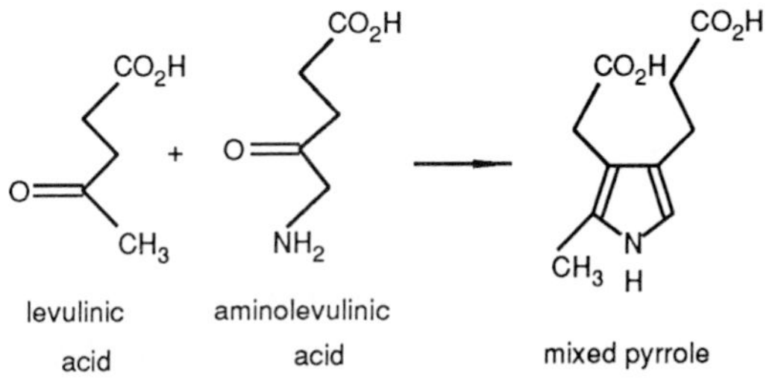

Figure 2.7 Formation of a mixed pyrrole between 5-aminolevulinic acid and levulinic acid.

and an inhibitor at the same site—the A site. However, levulinic acid is clearly acting as a substrate at the A site but acting only as an inhibitor at the P site (since levulinic acid has no NH_2 it cannot supply the nitrogen necessary for the pyrrole ring and cannot act as a substrate at the P site). Hence, the reaction to form a Schiff base must have occurred at the P site. It, thus, appears that the mechanism of the human, bovine, and bacterial enzymes all proceed with the initial binding of a molecule of 5-aminolevulinic acid to form a Schiff base and that this substrate gives rise to the P side of the porphobilinogen.

G. Mechanism of the 5-aminolevulinic acid dehydratase reaction

On the basis of the order in which the two substrates bind a new mechanism may be written (Fig. 2.8). The formation of porphobilinogen from two molecules of 5-aminolevulinic acid requires an aldol condensation, the formation of a C—N bond, the loss of two molecules of water, and a tautomeric shift. It is proposed that the initial event is the binding of the first substrate molecule to the P site in the form of a Schiff base. The 5-aminolevulinic acid Schiff base provides a good electrophile for reaction with the second substrate molecule. Dehydration would proceed followed by Schiff-base formation to form the five-membered ring. The bond formations between the two substrate molecules could occur in the converse fashion (aldol reaction second) as shown in Fig. 2.8. The final tautomerization is not left to chance and is catalyzed by the enzyme. Evidence for this has come from the use of 5-aminolevulinic acid tritiated in the 5-position (Abboud and Akhtar, 1976; Chaudhry and Jordan, 1976). Incubation of 5-amino[$5RS$-$^3H_2$]levulinic acid with dehydratases from bacterial or mammalian sources leads to the removal of half the label from the 2 position of porphobilinogen. The use of substrate, stereospecifically tritiated in the pro-S position, gives rise to porphobilinogen with no loss of label. These observations, therefore, establish that in this last stage, the pro-R hydrogen atom is stereoselectively removed and must, therefore, occur while the intermediate is bound to the active site. These mechanistic details are included in Fig. 2.8.

H. Half-site reactivity and the role of zinc in binding substrate

Several additional questions still need to be answered before the mechanistic course can be fully understood. First, is the role of zinc a structural or a mechanistic one (or both)? Second, how many active sites are present? Third, what are the main catalytic groups involved? Although the weight of evidence points to zinc being essential for activity, several pieces of information point to its noninvolvement directly with the catalytic events. Substitution by [113]Cd ions at the zinc binding site yields an active enzyme with a single [113]Cd nmr resonance at $\delta = 79$ ppm. This signal is not affected by the addition of 5-aminolevulinic acid, suggesting that the substrate is not interacting directly with the metal ion (Sommer and Beyersmann, 1984).

Experiments by Jordan et al. (1976) established that the removal of zinc by alkylation of the essential SH group with iodoacetic acid did not affect the ability of the bovine enzyme to form a Schiff base with the substrate. In fact when 5-amino[14C]levulinic acid and borohydride were used, twice the amount of radioactivity was incorporated into the alkylated protein compared with the native enzyme. These findings have

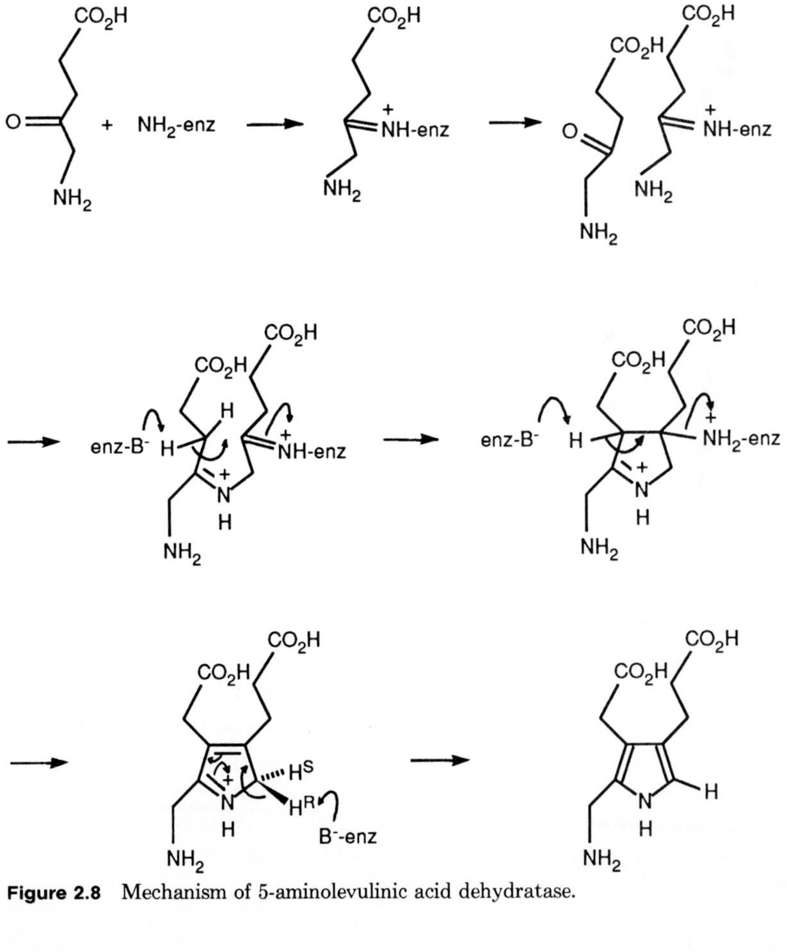

Figure 2.8 Mechanism of 5-aminolevulinic acid dehydratase.

been confirmed and extended (Jaffe and Hanes, 1986) by observations on the enzyme alkylated with methylmethanethiosulfonate, a reagent which reacts reversibly with SH groups. It, therefore, appears that the metal binding site is not essential for the initial formation of the Schiff-base intermediate but is involved in some way with the ability of the enzyme to accept the second molecule of substrate. It is interesting to note that the enzyme, temporarily incapacitated by the methylmethanethiosulfonate reagent, is twice as sensitive to inactivation with borohydride in the presence of the substrate and loses almost all its activity, whereas native enzyme loses only half of its activity under similar conditions. Related observations have been made by Nandi and Shemin (1968b) in that the enzyme treated with levulinic acid and borohydride is totally inactivated, whereas only 55 to 65% of the activity is lost in equivalent reactions with the substrate. It must be concluded that if turnover is prevented the enzyme may bind efficiently to either the substrate or an analogue such as levulinic acid in the form of a reducible Schiff-base intermediate. In the native enzyme where turnover occurs, catalytic intermediates and products occupy the active site at the expense of the Schiff-base intermediate with an accompanying protection against inactivation. Porphobilinogen, the product is in fact a respectable competitive inhibitor inhibiting the bacterial enzyme 50% at a concentration of $2mM$ (Jordan, unpublished data).

The numerous reports on half-site reactivity need to be further studied. Half the subunits of the bovine dehydratase (Shemin, 1976; Jaffe and Hanes, 1986) are modified on reduction with borohydride in the presence of [14]C 5-aminolevulinic acid, suggesting that half-site reactivity may be operative. Studies with the active-site-directed reagent, chlorolevulinic acid, have also revealed an element of half-site reactivity (Seehra and Jordan, 1981). Aspects of half-site reactivity of 5-aminolevulinic acid dehydratases have been discussed in detail elsewhere (Cheh and Neilands, 1976).

The enzyme groups responsible for catalysis have not been identified with any certainty with the exception of the active-site lysine (Gibbs and Jordan, 1986) (K252 in the human and rat enzymes and K247 in the *E. coli* enzyme). Two histidines have also been implicated from photoinactivation studies (Tsukamoto et al., 1979). Interestingly, there are two conserved histidines at the proposed zinc binding site as predicted from this work and one seems to be particularly important and may be involved as a catalytic group (Tsukamoto et al., 1980). A close study of the gene and cDNA-derived protein sequences reveal several potential catalytic residues in areas of high conservation. The wealth of knowledge emanating from the molecular biology studies suggests that many of the above questions will soon be answered.

V. Biosynthesis of Uroporphyrinogen III

A. Introduction

The transformation of four molecules of porphobilinogen into uroporphyrinogen III requires the participation of two enzymes. The first of these enzymes is called porphobilinogen deaminase (EC 4.3.1.8). The enzyme was originally known as uroporphyrinogen I synthase, a name still used in the medical sphere. More recently, the use of a third name, hydroxymethylbilane synthase, has made matters even more confusing. The most widely used name, porphobilinogen deaminase, is the least ambiguous and will be used throughout this section. The second enzyme required for the biosynthesis of uroporphyrinogen III is called uroporphyrinogen III synthase (EC 4.2.1.75). This enzyme was first called uroporphyrinogen III cosynthase since it was thought to function together with the deaminase rather than to catalyze its own individual reaction. This enzyme has also been referred to as uroporphyrinogen III isomerase in some early literature.

The role of porphobilinogen deaminase is to tetrapolymerize the pyrrole porphobilinogen into preuroporphyrinogen, a highly labile 1-hydroxymethylbilane. This involves the stepwise addition of four porphobilinogen molecules to the enzyme with loss of each amino group as ammonia. The enzyme-bound linear tetrapyrrole is then released into solution as preuroporphyrinogen which acts as the substrate for uroporphyrinogen III synthase. The uroporphyrinogen III synthase carries out an amazing reaction in which the fourth ring (ring d) of preuroporphyrinogen is rearranged and the molecule is cyclized to give the uroporphyrinogen III isomer. The order of these two events is not yet known. In the absence of uroporphyrinogen III synthase, the highly reactive preuroporphyrinogen cyclizes without rearrangement in a nonenzymic reaction, to give uroporphyrinogen I. Since many of the studies on the deaminase and synthase have been closely interwoven, the two enzymes will be considered in this section together. Their combined reactions are shown in Fig. 2.9.

The enzymic production of uroporphyrinogen III from porphobilinogen was first demonstrated by Bogorad and Granick (1953) using enzyme extracts from spinach. On heating the extracts prior to incubation with porphobilinogen, the uroporphyrinogen I isomer was formed providing the first indication that a labile protein was responsible for the isomerization reaction. Porphobilinogen deaminase and uroporphyrinogen III synthase were subsequently isolated by Bogorad (1958a, b), although at that time the uroporphyrinogen III synthase was termed uroporphyrinogen isomerase. Bogorad found that extracts of acetone powder from

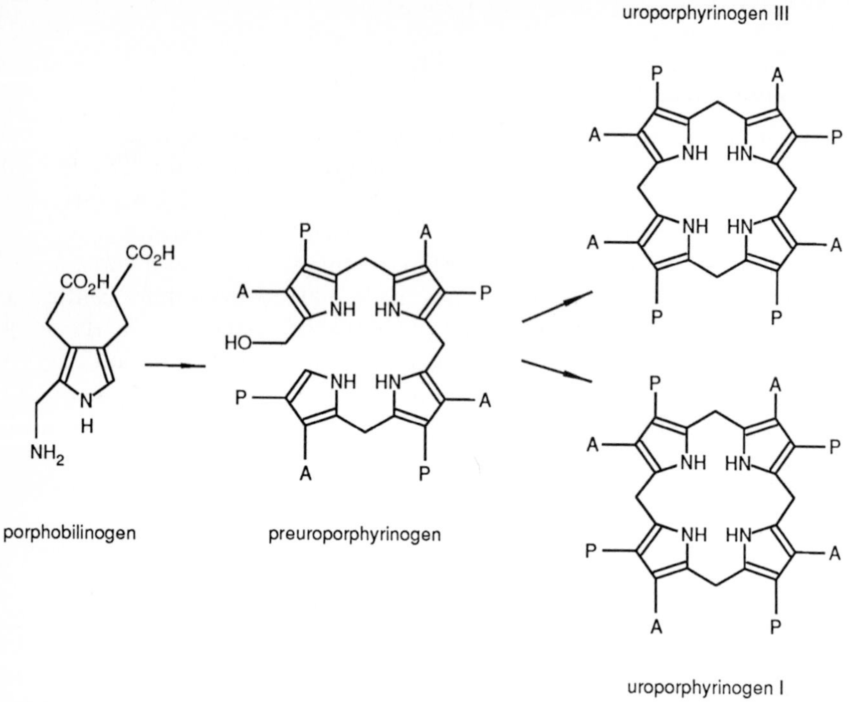

uroporphyrinogen III

porphobilinogen   preuroporphyrinogen

uroporphyrinogen I

Figure 2.9 Biosynthesis of uroporphyrinogens from porphobilinogen.

spinach leaves catalyzed the formation of uroporphyrinogen I from four molecules of porphobilinogen with the liberation of four molecules of ammonia. When the semipurified "isomerase" from wheat germ was added to the spinach enzyme, uroporphyrinogen III was produced. Bogorad concluded that the role of the first enzyme was to catalyze the formation of a polypyrromethane intermediate and that the "isomerase" acted on this intermediate, in the presence of porphobilinogen, to produce the uroporphyrinogen III isomer. Most importantly, it was established that the "isomerase" alone did not catalyze the isomerization of uroporphyrinogen I into uroporphyrinogen III neither would it act on porphobilinogen alone as a substrate.

B. Properties of porphobilinogen and uroporphyrinogens

Since these original experiments the pursuance of the mechanism by which the two enzymes catalyze the biosynthesis of uroporphyrinogen III has, until relatively recently, consistently baffled all investigators and has left a trail of incorrect theories and erroneous conclusions. Of all the problems in the tetrapyrrole field it is still one of the most fascinat-

uroporphyrinogen I

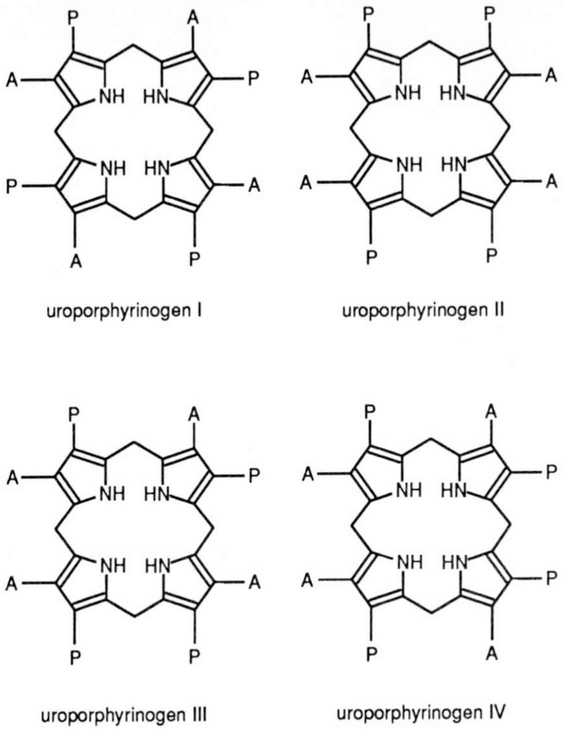

uroporphyrinogen II

uroporphyrinogen III

uroporphyrinogen IV

Figure 2.10   Structure of uroporphyrinogen isomers.

ing, the most enigmatic aspect being the mechanism by which the d ring in uroporphyrinogen III becomes switched during the overall transformation. Interestingly, the intrinsic chemistry of porphobilinogen and its polymerization products appear to favor the uroporphyrinogen III isomer since investigations into the nonenzymic polymerization of porphobilinogen have revealed that in acid uroporphyrinogen III is the major product. Analysis of the uroporphyrinogen isomers produced showed a statistical distribution of uroporphyrinogens III : IV : II : I (Fig. 2.10) in a ratio of 4 : 2 : 1 : 1 (Mauzerall, 1960a, b).

This established that, in chemical terms at least, it was possible for the CH_2NH_2 side chain of porphobilinogen to react, after elimination of ammonia, with either a free or a substituted α-position of another porphobilinogen unit. The involvement of hydroxymethyl intermediates was suggested to explain the mechanism by which any one of the uroporphyrinogen isomers could interconvert to the same equilibrium mixture of all the four isomers. Subsequent chemical studies showed that porphobilinogen is unique among substituted pyrroles since it actually prefers to react at the substituted α-position of another molecule of porphobilinogen. Furthermore, the "polypyrroles" formed on self-condensation of porphobilinogen were unusually stable in solution (Frydman et al., 1971). Nature has, thus, accepted that uroporphyrinogen III is the chemically favored product and has exploited the asymmetry of this isomer in the pathway. For instance, coproporphyrinogen oxidase only accepts the type III isomer and hence the final product of the pathway, heme, is also asymmetric. This asymmetry or "sidedness" of heme is perfectly suited to its role as a prosthetic group in proteins since the hydrophobic portion interacts with the nonpolar amino acid side chains in the protein interior, while the paired, adjacent propionic acid side chains occupy positions near the more polar surface of the proteins.

C. Porphobilinogen deaminase

The isolation of porphobilinogen deaminase and uroporphyrinogen synthase has been accomplished from a wide variety of sources. The two enzymes have been isolated either together as "porphobilinogenase" (Sancovich et al., 1969; Llambias and Batlle, 1971; Frydman and Feinstein, 1974) or as separate enzymes. Porphobilinogen deaminases have been isolated in homogeneous form from *R. spheroides* (Jordan and Shemin, 1973; Davies and Neuberger, 1973), spinach (Higuchi and Bogorad, 1975), human erythrocytes (Anderson and Desnick, 1980), *Euglena gracilis* (Williams et al., 1981), and *E. coli* (Hart et al., 1986). The *E. coli* enzyme, isolated from a genetically engineered strain has been crystallized (Jordan et al., 1988b). All the porphobilinogen deaminases exist as monomeric proteins with molecular weights ranging from 34,000 to 44,000 and most have similar properties with optimal activities at pH 8.0 to 8.5 and isoelectric points between pH 4 and 5. The K_m values for porphobilinogen are all in the low micromolar range. One unifying property of the deaminases is their remarkable heat stability which contrasts sharply with the uroporphyrinogen III synthases which are, in general, extremely heat-labile. Porphobilinogen deaminases are rather slow enzymes and take about 2 s to catalyze the tetrapolymerization of porphobilinogen at 20°C.

D. Uroporphyrinogen III synthase (cosynthase)

Far fewer uroporphyrinogen III synthases have been isolated in homogeneous form due to their extreme instability and the lack of a convenient assay method. These problems have largely been overcome by the advent of fast protein liquid chromatography purification methods and the development of a rapid assay method for the enzyme (Jordan, 1982). The uroporphyrinogen synthases have been isolated in homogeneous form from human erythrocytes (Tsai et al., 1987) and from a genetically engineered strain of *E. coli* (Alwan and Jordan, 1988; Jordan et al., 1988a). The enzyme has also been obtained in high purity from spinach (Higuchi and Bogorad, 1975), rat liver (Kohashi et al., 1984; Smythe and Williams, 1988), and *Euglena gracilis* (Hart and Battersby, 1985). The synthases are generally smaller enzymes than the deaminases, the molecular weights of the human and *E. coli* enzymes being 29,500 and 28,000, respectively. The *Euglena* enzyme is slightly larger (molecular weight 31,000). All the synthases, like the deaminases, appear to be monomeric enzymes with isoelectric points around pH 5. These enzymes are much faster than deaminases catalyzing at least 200 turnovers/s. The K_m for preuroporphyrinogen varies according to source but ranges from 10 to 25 μM.

E. Early investigations on the mechanism
of uroporphyrinogen biosynthesis

The mechanism by which the porphobilinogen deaminase and uroporphyrinogen III synthase catalyze the transformation of four porphobilinogen molecules into the tetrapyrrole uroporphyrinogen III has attracted the attention of numerous researchers over a period of a quarter of a century and many mechanisms have been proposed. Several of these have been covered in reviews which were published in the 1970s (Battersby and McDonald, 1975; Batlle and Rossetti, 1977; Akhtar and Jordan, 1979). The elucidation of the mechanism by which the deaminase and synthase catalyze the transformation of porphobilinogen into uroporphyrinogen III has tantalized even the finest minds and the deaminase enzyme, in particular, is only now beginning to reveal the secrets of its reaction mechanism. Few workers in this field have escaped without making incorrect conclusions at some point. Included in the catalog of errors is the early rearrangement mechanism (Frydman et al., 1976), the headless dipyrrole (Scott et al., 1976), the aminomethylbilane (Battersby et al., 1978a, b; Battersby and McDonald, 1979), and the N-alkylporphyrinogen (Burton et al., 1979b), to name but four.

The first significant pointer to the mechanism by which porphobilinogen deaminase catalyzes its reaction came from observations made in the laboratories of Bogorad (Pluscec and Bogorad, 1970) and Neuberger (Davies and Neuberger, 1973), who found that incubation of the deaminase with porphobilinogen in the presence of the bases NH_3, NH_2OH, or NH_2OCH_3 led to the interception of enzyme-bound species which were liberated into the medium in the form of pyrromethanes linked to the inhibitory base. Pyrromethanes with two, three, and four rings could be detected by electrophoresis (Pluscec and Bogorad, 1970). Incubation of the deaminase with porphobilinogen in the presence of tritiated methoxyamine ($NH_2OC^3H_2$) led to the formation of a tritiated tetrapyrromethane (Davies and Neuberger, 1973). These observations pointed to a mechanism in which the four porphobilinogen molecules are incorporated into the tetrapyrrole in a stepwise fashion. The results also suggested that a covalent linkage existed between the enzyme and the bound substrates.

F. Experiments with aminomethyldipyrromethanes, aminomethyltripyrranes, and aminomethylbilanes

A period of investigation followed in which various synthetic aminomethyldipyrromethanes and aminomethyltripyrranes were prepared chemically to determine whether they were able to act as tetrapyrrole precursors. However, when these compounds were incubated with either deaminase or with the combined deaminase/synthase system in the presence of porphobilinogen, the results were disappointing since the deaminase preferred to use porphobilinogen rather than the di- and tripyrroles which acted as inhibitors (Frydman et al., 1976, 1978; Battersby and McDonald, 1976).

An important breakthrough was made, however, when it was found that two polypyrroles D and P accumulated in solution when extracts of *Euglena* were incubated with porphobilinogen in the presence of porphobilinogen deaminase or the combined deaminase/synthase system, respectively, and it was suggested that these compounds were natural intermediates in the biosynthesis of uroporphyrinogens. The structure of polypyrrole D was proposed as NH_2CH_2-AP-AP-AP-AP and polypyrrole P as NH_2CH_2-PA-PA-PA-AP (Rossetti et al., 1977) (Fig. 2.11). When polypyrrole D was incubated with the deaminase/synthase enzymes some uroporphyrinogen III was formed, whereas with the deaminase alone uroporphyrinogen I was the major product. In the case of the compound P, deaminase alone yielded equal amounts of the two uroporphyrinogen isomers, whereas incubation with the two enzymes resulted in the exclusive production of uroporphyrinogen III. Although there was insufficient definitive structural information about the nature of P and D, their possible involvement in the biosynthetic mechanism was a great stimulus to further studies on aminomethylbilanes. Chemical synthesis of the aminomethylbilane NH_2CH_2-AP-AP-AP-AP (Battersby et al., 1977) and its incubation with the combined deaminase/synthase system produced good yields of uroporphyrinogen III.

Although it has been well-established by early investigators that the d ring is inverted during the biosynthesis of uroporphyrinogen III, elegant ^{13}C nmr studies using [2,11-$^{13}C_2$]porphobilinogen, which was diluted with nonlabeled porphobilinogen, left no doubt that a single intramolecular rearrangement occurred (Battersby and McDonald, 1976). This was further confirmed at the tetrapyrrole level by synthesizing the aminomethylbilane NH_2CH_2-AP-AP-AP-AP, labeled with ^{13}C in either positions 16 and 20 (■) or at positions 15 and 19 (●) (Battersby et al., 1978b). The uroporphyrinogen III biosynthesized from either of these labeled materials showed direct ^{13}C–^{13}C coupling since the label originally at position 16 now occupied the adjacent position 19, and, in the other case, the label once at position 19 now coupled to C-15 as a result of its new location at position 16 (Fig. 2.12).

These experiments also established that the terminal pyrrole ring having the aminomethyl group in the aminomethyl bilane NH_2CH_2-AP-AP-AP-AP gave rise to the a ring in uroporphyrinogen III. On the basis of these observations it was also proposed that the aminomethylbilane NH_2-AP-AP-AP-AP was the key intermediate which was produced by the deaminase and which subsequently acted as the substrate for the synthase (Battersby et al., 1978a, b; Battersby and McDonald, 1979).

In order to explore further the role of aminomethylbilanes in the enzymic formation of uroporphyrinogens, a range of aminomethylbilanes was chemically synthesized, each of which had a single ring rearranged,

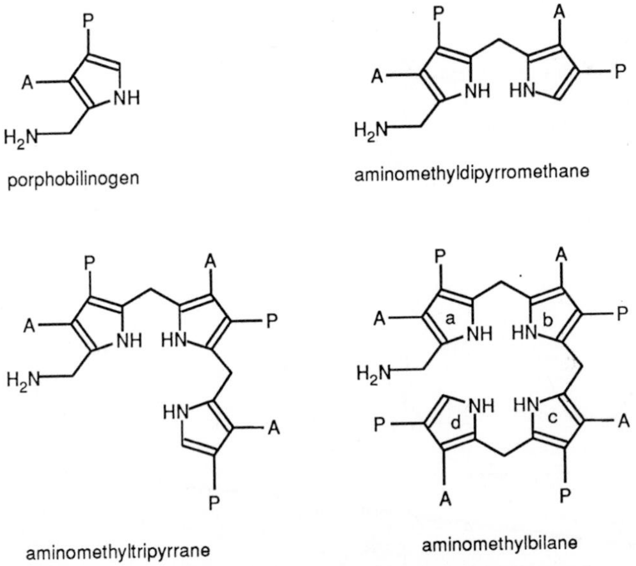

porphobilinogen

aminomethyldipyrromethane

aminomethyltripyrrane

aminomethylbilane

Figure 2.11 Structure of the aminomethyldipyrromethane, aminomethyltripyranne, and aminomethylbilane related to porphobilinogen.

and their ability to act as substrates with the combined deaminase/synthase system from *Euglena* was investigated (Battersby et al., 1978a).

Aminomethylbilane	Rate
NH_2CH_2-AP-AP-AP-AP	+ + + + + + +
NH_2CH_2-PA-AP-AP-AP	−
NH_2CH_2-AP-PA-AP-AP	+ + + +
NH_2CH_2-AP-AP-PA-AP	+
NH_2CH_2-AP-AP-AP-PA	+ +
NH_2CH_2-PA-PA-PA-AP	−

The compounds which contained the A and P substituents reversed in the a ring (i.e., the ring with the aminomethyl substituent) were not utilized by the enzymes, although, as will be seen later, this was almost certainly a reflection of the inability of the porphobilinogen deaminase to accept these two aminomethylbilanes. Since purified uroporphyrinogen III synthase was not available these workers were not aware that this enzyme could not accept an aminomethylbilane since these compounds are not physiological intermediates. It was noticed, however, that deaminase alone accelerated the formation of uroporphyrinogen I from the aminomethylbilane NH_2-AP-AP-AP-AP but the significance of this was yet to be appreciated. Related studies were also carried out by Sburlati et al. (1983) using the enzyme from *R. spheroides*.

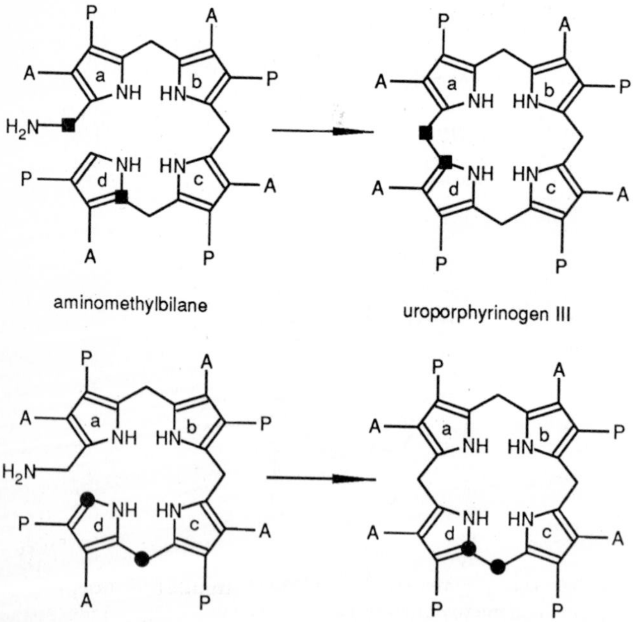

aminomethylbilane   uroporphyrinogen III

Figure 2.12 Intramolecular rearrangement of the aminomethylbilane NH_2CH_2-AP-AP-AP-AP using ^{13}C nmr.

G. Discovery of preuroporphyrinogen, the substrate for uroporphyrinogen III synthase

The discovery of preuroporphyrinogen, the last remaining tetrapyrrole pathway intermediate to be described, deserves special coverage. In 1978, while on sabbatical with Ian Scott at Texas A & M University, the major breakthrough was made toward our understanding of the mechanism by which porphobilinogen deaminase and uroporphyrinogen III synthase participate together in the biosynthesis of uroporphyrinogen III. While incubating porphobilinogen deaminase with 11-^{13}C-porphobilinogen in the nmr tube in an attempt to observe enzyme-bound intermediate complexes, in addition to the nmr signal forming at $\delta = 22$ ppm due to the formation of uroporphyrinogen I, we observed an additional complex signal at about $\delta = 23$ ppm which appeared transiently. Since there was insufficient enzyme to identify any enzyme-bound species, it was immediately obvious that we were observing an unstable enzyme-free intermediate, which, on prolonged incubation, finally produced uroporphyrinogen I. Further investigation with larger amounts of enzyme revealed that in addition to a complex signal at $\delta = 23$ ppm there was a further resonance at $\delta = 57$ ppm, approximately 20 ppm from the aminomethyl resonance of the substrate ($\delta = 36$ ppm). Most importantly, the integration of the signals showed an almost perfect $3:1$ distribution for the resonance at $\delta = 23$ ppm and $\delta = 57$ ppm, respectively (Burton et al., 1979a). Clearly, this was not a spectrum due to uroporphyrinogen I but to some tetrapyrrole which contained three similar, though not identical, labeled carbon atoms together with a fourth carbon in a very different environment. The aminomethylbilane previously proposed (Battersby and McDonald, 1979) would have given signals at 23 and 36 ppm so this was eliminated as a candidate immediately. We considered a hydroxymethylbilane structure as one of the main candidates for the structure of the intermediate (Burton et al., 1979a) since substitution of $-OH$ for $-NH_2$ characteristically produces a shift of about 20 ppm, similar to that observed. In the absence of an authentic standard it was not possible to be certain, however, and several other possibilities were also considered. The most important question, however, still needed to be answered, namely, what was the significance of the transient species and had we discovered the elusive substrate for the uroporphyrinogen III synthase enzyme. When the same nmr experiment was performed but in the presence of both enzymes there was no appearance of the transient nmr signals and uroporphyrinogen III was formed.

In a series of enzymic experiments Burton and I incubated porphobilinogen with a large amount of deaminase enzyme so that the consumption of porphobilinogen was complete in about 10 min. The solution was cooled to 0°C to stabilize the intermediate which was totally separated from the deaminase by ultrafiltration. The next stage was to incubate the intermediate with highly purified uroporphyrinogen III synthase, which had been isolated by other members of the group, and to determine if any uroporphyrinogen III was produced. As we had predicted, the intermediate was transformed quantitatively into uroporphyrinogen III. Interestingly, when the intermediate was incubated with buffer alone uroporphyrinogen I was generated with a half-life of 4.5 min at 37°C. These enzymic experiments, thus, firmly established the transiently formed compound as the substrate for the uroporphyrinogen III synthase (Jordan et al., 1979) and at a stroke eliminated virtually all previous mechanistic postulates. The overall conclusions from these experiments are as follows.

1. The deaminase is responsible for assembling a tetrapyrrole intermediate from four molecules of porphobilinogen in the absence of uroporphyrinogen III synthase.

2. The intermediate is not an aminomethylbilane of the type previously proposed (Battersby and McDonald, 1979).

3. The intermediate is highly unstable with a half-life of only 4.5 min at pH 8.5 and is converted into uroporphyrinogen I in a nonenzymic reaction.

4. The intermediate acts as the substrate for the uroporphyrinogen III synthase enzyme and is rapidly and quantitatively transformed into uroporphyrinogen III.

5. The transformation of the intermediate into uroporphyrinogen III does not require the participation of porphobilinogen deaminase or additional porphobilinogen units.

6. The two enzymes function independently and sequentially in the overall transformation of porphobilinogen into uroporphyrinogen III.

7. The aminomethylbilane NH_2CH_2-AP-AP-AP-AP is accepted as a poor substrate for deaminase and is transformed into the new intermediate which only then can act as the substrate for uroporphyrinogen III synthase (this point explained why the aminomethylbilane had mistakenly been identified as an important physiological intermediate).

Since the intermediate was the enzymic precursor for uroporphyrinogen III and the nonenzymic precursor for uroporphyrinogen I, it was named preuroporphyrinogen. Further investigations with uroporphyrinogen III synthases from several sources firmly established that preuroporphyrinogen was a universal substrate in all living organisms (Jordan

and Berry, 1980). Furthermore, the fact that preuroporphyrinogen generated by *R. spheriodes* was consumed by uroporphyrinogen III synthases
from different sources suggested that the two enzymes were working
independently and not in a functional complex as had previously been
suggested (Higuchi and Bogorad, 1975). The conclusions from these
investigations are summarized in Fig. 2.13.

The publications concerning the discovery and structure of preuroporphyrinogen are extremely confusing to the nonspecialist in this field and
deserve a brief explanation. The original ^{13}C nmr spectral data (Burton
et al., 1979a) were entirely consistent with the intermediate, preuroporphyrinogen, having a hydroxymethyl rather than an aminomethyl side
chain, and this was confirmed subsequently by Battersby et al. (1979a)
who repeated the original ^{13}C nmr experiments with essentially similar
results. Most significantly, the hydroxymethylbilane HOCH$_2$-AP-AP-
AP-AP, although a most challenging compound to prepare, had been
quickly synthesized by Battersby et al. (1979a) and was shown to have
identical chemical and enzymic properties to the intermediate, preuroporphyrinogen, which had been described earlier (Burton et al., 1979a;
Jordan et al., 1979).

The reader of these papers may get the impression that the intermediate obtained by Burton et al. (1979a) was different from that subsequently described by Battersby et al. (1979a). This was not so. It was
unfortunate that further experiments in which porphobilinogen deaminase was incubated with [1-^{15}N,11-^{13}C]porphobilinogen yielded an nmr
spectrum which appeared to exhibit ^{13}C–^{15}N single-bond coupling. This
was interpreted at the time as evidence for an *N*-alkylporphyrinogen
type of compound as being the structure of preuroporphyrinogen
(Burton et al., 1979b). The signals observed were in fact due to a
three-bond coupling between the ^{15}N in ring a with the ^{13}C atom of the
hydroxymethyl side chain which gave rise to the splitting of the signal at
$\delta = 57$ ppm.

Now that we had solved the essential features of the deaminase/syn-
thase reaction we were able, for the first time, to design a rapid assay
method for the synthase enzyme (Jordan, 1982). Previously, this had
involved laborious analyses of the uroporphyrinogen isomers by decarboxylation to the corresponding coproporphyrins and identification of
the esters by TLC. The assay principle was based on the fact that
uroporphyrinogen is formed more slowly from porphobilinogen with
deaminase alone than when the deaminase and synthase enzymes are
present together. It is, thus, possible to assay the uroporphyrinogen III
synthase directly by simply subtracting the amount of uroporphyrinogens formed in a blank containing deaminase alone from the uroporphyrinogens formed in the presence of the two enzymes. This gives, with
minor corrections, the amount of uroporphyrinogen III produced. The

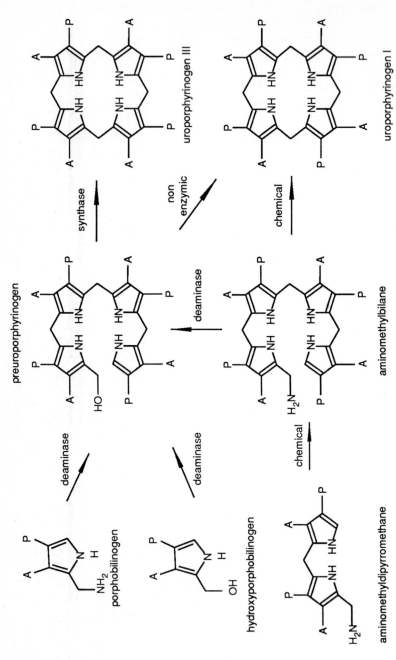

Figure 2.13 Formation of preuroporphyrinogen and its conversion to uroporphyrinogen.

ability to be able to assay the synthase in minutes rather than hours has enabled what is a very unstable enzyme to be isolated far more rapidly than had been possible previously.

H. Order of assembly of the four pyrrole rings of the tetrapyrrole

The recognition that the role of the deaminase was to construct a linear tetrapyrrole prompted us to investigate the order in which the four pyrrole rings are incorporated into preuroporphyrinogen by the deaminase enzyme. Two realistic possibilities existed—either the four porphobilinogen units could be assembled by the deaminase in the order a, b, c, and d or, alternatively, in the order d, c, b, and a. The problem was solved by two different approaches from two independent groups.

Using a radiochemical approach (Jordan and Seehra, 1979; Seehra and Jordan, 1980), purified deaminase enzyme was exposed to a limiting amount of $[3,5^{14}C_2]$porphobilinogen with the aim of labeling specifically the sites which first bind the substrate. Addition of nonlabeled porphobilinogen to complete the turnover of the enzyme-bounded label was followed by conversion of the resulting preuroporphyrinogen into protoporphyrin by enzymes from *R. spheroides*. Chemical degradation of the tetrapyrrole gave ethylmethylmaleimide from rings a and b and hematinic acid from rings c and d. Analysis showed that all the label was present in the ethylmethylmaleimide and almost none in the hematinic acid.

Using a most elegant ^{13}C nmr method, Battersby et al. (1979b) exposed the deaminase enzyme first to a limiting amount of unlabeled porphobilinogen in order to fill the active sites which first bind the substrate. This was then followed by $[11-^{13}C]$porphobilinogen to occupy the remaining binding sites. The resulting tetrapyrrole product was transformed into uroporphyrinogen III and thence to coproporphyrin which was analyzed by proton nmr as the tetramethyl ester. The spectra showed clearly that the ^{12}C content of the meso-bridge atoms decreased in the order C-20, C-5, C-10, and C-15.

The conclusions from these two independent approaches were the same, namely, that the tetrapyrrole ring is built up by the deaminase with ring a first binding to the enzyme, followed by rings b, c, and finally d.

I. Enzyme intermediate complexes

Shortly after these studies, Anderson and Desnick (1980) made the important observation that incubation of porphobilinogen deaminase with porphobilinogen led to the formation of several enzyme species which had a higher negative charge than the native enzyme and which could be separated either by ion exchange chromatography or by electrophoresis. Using tritiated porphobilinogen, the enzyme species were shown to be enzyme-intermediate complexes with one, two, three, and four pyrrole units linked to the enzyme. These will be referred to as ES, ES_2, ES_3, and ES_4, respectively. Similar behavior has been observed on adding a substrate to the purified deaminases isolated from *R. spheroides* (Berry et al., 1981) and *E. coli* (Jordan et al., 1988b), and the enzyme-intermediate complexes have each been characterized by chemical and radiochemical techniques. The ES, ES_2, and ES_3 complexes can be isolated using either of the bacterial enzymes, but the ES_4 complex is too unstable to be recovered and has not been observed except with eukaryotic enzymes. Treatment of the enzyme-intermediate complexes with sodium dodecyl sulfate was not able to release the bound substrate, thus, providing strong evidence for the existence of a covalent link between the enzyme and its substrates (Jordan and Berry, 1981). Such a link had been inferred from the experiments of Pluscec and Bogorad (1970) and Davies and Neuberger (1973). The enzyme therefore catalyzes the synthesis of the tetrapyrrole in a stepwise order with stable intermediate complexes all of which may be isolated and characterized (Fig. 2.14).

J. Nature of the enzymic group involved in substrate covalent binding

The nature of the enzymic group which is responsible for the binding of the substrate has been of considerable interest to several research groups. On the basis of ^{13}C nmr evidence, a covalent link between the substrate and a lysine residue had been proposed in the *Euglena* enzyme (Battersby et al., 1983). Inhibition studies with pyridoxal 5′-phosphate

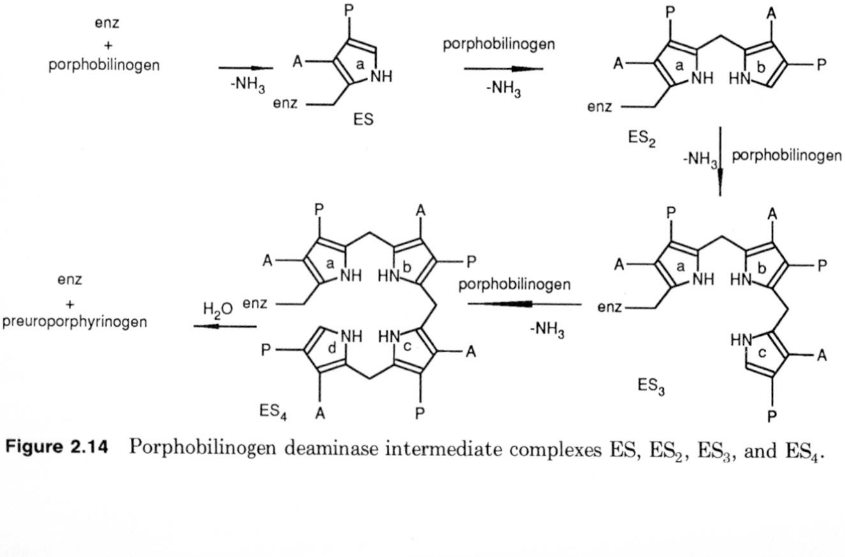

Figure 2.14 Porphobilinogen deaminase intermediate complexes ES, ES_2, ES_3, and ES_4.

consolidated the case for lysine (Hart et al., 1984) since the *Euglena* enzyme is inactivated by pyridoxal 5'-phosphate and borohydride, but only in the absence of porphobilinogen. A reduced pyridoxal-lysine adduct has been isolated from the inactivated enzyme. On the other hand, studies using ^{3}H nmr with the *R. spheroides* enzyme have pointed to the involvement of a cysteine residue as the amino acid responsible for the covalent link with the substrate (Evans et al., 1986). Arginine has been implicated at the active site as a result of inactivation experiments with butanedione (Russell et al., 1984). In fact, none of these amino acids are involved in the *covalent* linkage with the substrate in view of the conclusions from the following section.

Mechanistic studies on the deaminase seem to have switched to the *E. coli* enzyme since the identification, cloning, and sequencing of the *hemC* gene (Thomas and Jordan, 1986). This has already resulted in the isolation of the *E. coli* enzyme (Hart et al., 1986). The application of molecular biology has permitted the construction of strains which over-produce the deaminase enzyme (Jordan et al., 1988b), permitting the isolation of milligram quantities of the enzyme and its crystallization. As a result, it has been possible to explore the structure of the *E. coli* enzyme with classical protein chemistry techniques.

K. Discovery of a cofactor in all porphobilinogen deaminases: the dipyrromethane cofactor

Initial attempts, using the *R. spheroides* deaminase, to isolate a peptide to which the substrate is attached met with little success since the link between the enzyme and bound substrates was found to be rather labile. However, while purifying peptides from a proteolytic digest of native *R. spheroides* deaminase (Jordan and Berry, unpublished data), a pink material was observed which had properties remarkably similar to those of an oxidized dipyrromethane. After switching to the more abundant *E. coli* enzyme, peptide mapping (Thomas and Jordan, 1986) resulted in the appearance of a red fluorescent material which was quickly identified as uroporphyrin I. Since this work had been carried out on the native enzyme rather than an enzyme-intermediate complex we concluded that the *E. coli* deaminase contained resident porphobilinogen-like pyrroles which, on acid treatment, give rise to uroporphyrinogen. The treatment of the deaminase with Ehrlich's reagent confirmed our suspicions (Jordan and Warren, 1987) and showed a reaction typical of a dipyrromethane (Pluscec and Bogorad, 1970), thus, corroborating our earlier observations with the *R. spheroides* enzyme.

The next task was to determine the role of the dipyrromethane. When the enzyme was treated with substrate to give ES_2 and this complex was reacted with Ehrlich's reagent, a very rapid color reaction occurred which was now indicative of the reaction of a tetrapyrromethane (Radmer and Bogorad, 1972). It, thus, appeared that the two substrate molecules were interacting directly with the enzyme-bound dipyrromethane to form an enzyme-bound tetrapyrrole (bilane). Treatment of the ES_2 complex with formic acid yielded twice as much uroporphyrin compared to the reaction with the native enzyme. These results pointed to a most important conclusion, namely, the existence of a dipyrromethane which was resident at the active site of the enzyme and which provided the attachment site for the covalent binding of the substrate (Jordan and Warren, 1987).

Further evidence for this proposal was obtained when α-bromoporphobilinogen (an analogue of porphobilinogen with the reactive α-position blocked with a bromine atom) was incubated with the native deaminase. Not only was the dipyrromethane Ehrlich reaction inhibited, showing that the inhibitor had reacted directly with the dipyrromethane, but the enzyme was completely inactivated. Clearly, the inhibitor was recognized by the deaminase, it was deaminated like a substrate and covalently linked to the dipyrromethane. However, the presence of the bromine atom blocked further reaction of the substrate, resulting in loss of enzymic activity (Warren and Jordan, 1986b).

One crucial experiment needed to be carried out to prove that the dipyrromethane was not merely substrate-bound tightly to the enzyme. Since the dipyrromethane was able to generate uroporphyrin in acid, it followed that it must be made up of pyrrole units similar to the substrate porphobilinogen. It would, therefore, be possible to label the dipyrromethane specifically with ^{14}C radioactivity by growing a deaminase overproducing strain of *E. coli* in the presence of 5-amino[^{14}C]levulinic acid. When the deaminase containing ^{14}C-labeled dipyrromethane was isolated and incubated with nonradioactive porphobilinogen no radioactivity was incorporated into the enzymic product, and most significantly the enzyme retained all the original label (Jordan and Warren, 1987; Warren and Jordan, 1988b). Only formic acid treatment released the radioactivity which was then found in uroporphyrin. These investigations proved that the deaminase from *E. coli* contains a resident dipyrromethane which is *not* subject to catalytic turnover and which is responsible for the covalent binding of the substrate molecules during the assembly of the tetrapyrrole. It was, therefore, named the *dipyrromethane cofactor* (Jordan and Warren, 1987).

The Ehrlich positive group has also been identified by Hart et al. (1987), also in the *E. coli* enzyme, and ^{13}C nmr experiments in which the deaminase has been incubated with the [11-^{13}C]porphobilinogen have revealed a resonance at $\delta = 24.6$ ppm. This is also presented as evidence for a pyrromethane group as the substrate binding site.

Further investigations have revealed that the dipyrromethane cofactor is present in animals, dicotyledonous, and monocotyledonous plants as well as in bacteria. Purified deaminases which have been investigated in addition to the *R. spheroides* and *E. coli* enzymes include those from human erythrocytes, spinach, and barley (Warren and Jordan, 1988a). In view of these findings it is most unlikely that lysine, arginine, or cysteine is involved in the covalent binding with the substrate although these amino acids may be important for noncovalent interaction.

L. Attachment site and assembly of the dipyrromethane cofactor

The discovery that the substrate binding site of porphobilinogen deaminase contains a covalently bound dipyrromethane cofactor (Jordan and Warren, 1987) posed new questions, namely, how is the cofactor attached to the deaminase and what is the mechanism of its assembly. The answer to the former question has come from ^{13}C nmr studies in which a recombinant strain of *E. coli* was grown in the presence of 5-amino[^{13}C]levulinic acid to generate deaminase containing the ^{13}C-labeled cofactor. The spectrum of the purified enzyme, which was obtained by Scott's group in Texas (Jordan et al., 1988c), revealed four resonances, two from the aromatic carbon atoms, one from the meso position, and a fourth with a chemical shift which indicates that the cofactor is attached to a cysteine residue. The structure of the cofactor and its binding site are shown in Fig. 2.15.

Protein chemistry and site-directed mutagenesis have shown that, of the four cysteine residues in the *E. coli* deaminase, it is cysteine-242 which binds the cofactor (Jordan et al., 1988c). From a comparison of the *E. coli* gene-derived deaminase protein sequence (Thomas and Jordan, 1986) with that of human deaminase (Raich et al., 1986) the cofactor binding site is found in the human enzyme at cysteine-247 in the center of a highly conserved sequence shown below.

    E. coli   M N T R L E G G C Q V P I G S Y A E L
                      * * * * *   * *
    Human   F L R H L E G G C S V P V A V H T A M

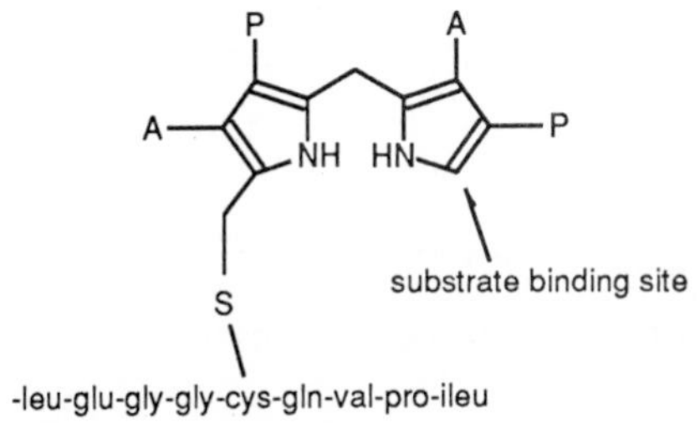

Figure 2.15 Structure of the dipyrromethane cofactor and its enzymic attachment site.

The question of how the cofactor is assembled has also been addressed (Hart et al., 1988). Using hydrochloric acid, the cofactor was removed from the denatured enzyme and the resulting apoenyzme was treated with ^{13}C-porphobilinogen in the presence of a reducing agent. This led to the recovery of part of the enzymic activity, suggesting, as expected, that the deaminase can also catalyze the self-assembly of its own cofactor. This reaction is merely the same generic reaction as the normal deamination of porphobilinogen which occurs during the construction of the tetrapyrrole product. The nmr resonance obtained showed that the porphobilinogen units had linked to a cysteine residue.

M. Mechanism of action of porphobilinogen deaminase

The mechanism by which porphobilinogen deaminase catalyzes the remarkable tetrapolymerization reaction can now be deduced from the wealth of experiments described above. The evidence points to the presence of a single catalytic site which is able to catalyze two basic reactions: first, the deamination of the substrate and the condensation of the deaminated substrate either with the dipyrromethane cofactor or an enzyme-intermediate complex; second, the hydrolytic cleavage to yield a hydroxymethyl product. The latter activity is normally confined to the release of the tetrapyrrole product, preuroporphyrinogen, but in the absence of sufficient substrate, any of the enzyme-intermediate complexes can be similarly cleaved. Both reactions can occur in reverse so that ammonia is able to release bound intermediates (Pluscec and Bogorad, 1970) and the enzyme can accept a hydroxymethyl substrate.

The topography of the catalytic center may be envisaged as having two pyrrole recognition sites, one for the incoming substrate, *site S*, and a second, *site C* (C for cofactor), which can accommodate a pyrrole ring with a free α position in readiness for the reaction with the substrate bound at site S. In the free holoenzyme this second site is occupied by the dipyrromethane cofactor, hence the designation *site C*. In the case of the apoenzyme the cofactor is first assembled (Fig. 2.16) by the deamination of one porphobilinogen molecule at site S, followed by reaction with cysteine-242 (cys). The second porphobilinogen unit of the dipyrromethane cofactor is inserted similarly, and the deaminase assumes the conformation of the holoenzyme in which the cofactor is permanently bound to the deaminase. Evidence for a conformational change comes from the fact that the apoenzyme is heat-labile unlike the holoenzyme (Warren and Jordan, 1988b).

The subsequent stages in Fig. 2.16 outline the stepwise addition of the four substrates in the assembly of the tetrapyrrole, preuroporphyrinogen. The first substrate occupies site S and reacts with the

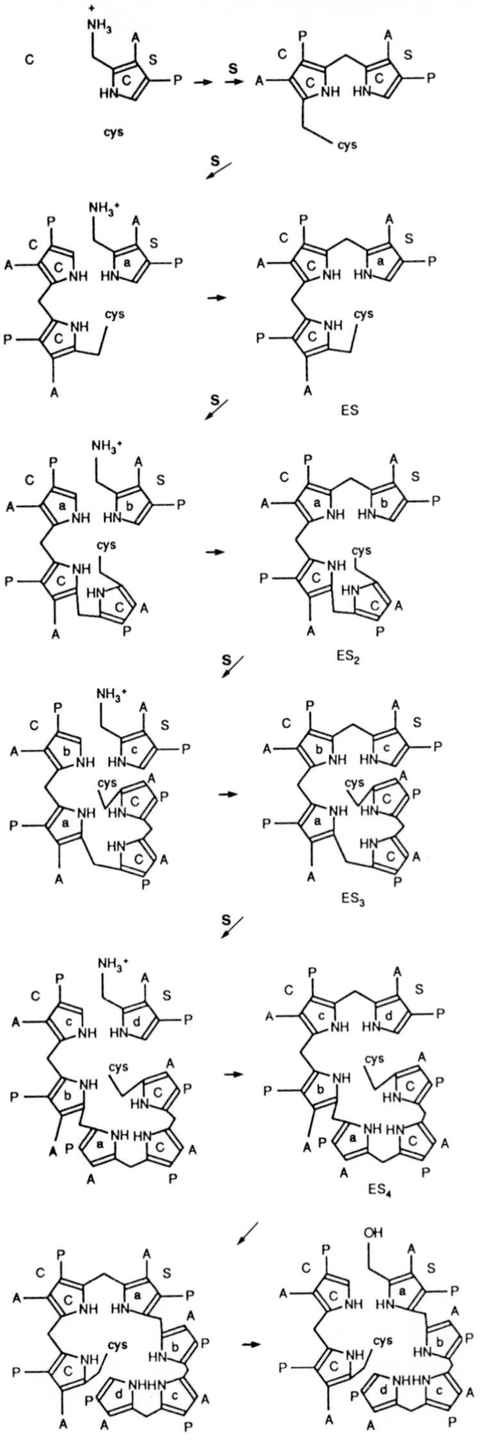

Figure 2.16 Mechanism of assembly of the dipyrromethane cofactor and its role in substrate binding and pyrrole chain extension.

dipyrromethane cofactor, which acts as a "primer" for the reaction. The resulting cofactor enzyme-intermediate complex is then translocated at the active site so that the newly incorporated pyrrole unit occupies site C. The translocation occurs as a result of the binding of porphobilinogen which has a higher affinity for site S than the newly incorporated pyrrole unit. In the absence of a substrate the pyrrole ring bound in this ES complex remains in the S site and can be released by hydrolytic cleavage to yield hydroxyporphobilinogen. In the presence of an additional substrate, sequential deamination occurs at site S, followed by translocation, resulting in the formation of ES_2, followed by ES_3 and finally ES_4. At this stage it is envisaged that steric considerations, caused by the fact that the cofactor is bound both to the enzyme and to the tetrapyrrole, prevent the binding of a "fifth" substrate and that hydrolytic cleavage, which is normally far slower than the condensation reaction, becomes significant and results in the liberation of the hydroxymethylbilane product, preuroporphyrinogen. This would require that the a ring of ES_4 occupies site S. It is well-established that an enzyme-bound tetrapyrrole can exist in this form since incubation of deaminase with a substrate in the presence of ammonia leads to the production of aminomethylbilanes of the type NH_2CH_2-AP-AP-AP-AP (Radmer and Bogorad, 1972). Furthermore, the enzyme is also able to deaminate the synthetic aminomethylbilane NH_2CH_2-AP-AP-AP-AP to the hydroxymethyl equivalent. The function of the cofactor is thus two-fold—first, to act as a primer on which to assemble the tetrapyrrole chain and, second, to impose a steric restriction on the number of pyrrole rings which can be incorporated to four. This latter property is due to the fact that the cofactor is permanently linked to the deminase protein. This mechanism is discussed in detail elsewhere (Warren and Jordan, 1988b).

Porphobilinogen deaminase has a high substrate specificity and recognizes pseudosubstrates where the a ring resembles porphobilinogen. Thus, the enzyme can recognize the aminomethyldipyrromethane NH_2CH_2-AP-AP, the aminomethyltripyrrane NH_2CH_2-AP-AP-AP, and the aminomethylbilane NH_2CH_2-AP-AP-AP-AP (see Fig. 2.11). The enzyme is unable to use the di- and tripyrroles as substrates because they cannot be translocated and, thus, they act as inhibitors. The aminomethylbilane, however, can act as pseudosubstrate and is deaminated and released as the equivalent hydroxymethylbilane, preuroporphyrinogen. This accounts for the observation that in the presence of deaminase and synthase, uroporphyrinogen III is formed (see Fig. 2.13). It should be pointed out, however, that this aminomethylbilane is not a physiological intermediate as had been suggested on numerous occasions (Battersby and McDonald, 1979) and plays no part in the natural biosynthesis of porphyrinogens. The isomeric aminomethylbilane NH_2CH_2-PA-AP-AP-AP (Battersby et al., 1978a) cannot act as a substrate because the a ring is not recognized by the enzyme. The inhibition caused by the aminomethylbilane NH_2CH_2-PA-PA-PA-AP is the most interesting. This compound may interact with the synthase as an intermediate analogue resembling the structure prior to final ring closure to uroporphyrinogen III (see Fig. 2.18).

N. Steric course of porphobilinogen deaminase and uroporphyrinogen III synthase reaction

One of the most challenging stereochemical problems in bioorganic chemistry is the determination of the absolute configuration of each meso position in uroporphyrinogen III and to relate it to the configuration of the paired hydrogen atoms at position 11 of the precursor porphobilinogen. Although the ultimate experiments have not been accomplished, important advances have been made in the understanding of the problem. For instance, it has been shown that, using avian erythrocyte enzymes, the incorporation of $[11RS-^3H_2;2,11-^{14}C_2]$- and $[11S-^3H;2,11-^{14}C_2]$porphobilinogen into porphyrinogens proceeds by a mechanism in which all four methylenes of porphyrinogens and, therefore, of preuroporphyrinogen, are formed by stereospecific processes (Jones et al., 1984). This observation establishes unambiguously that the hydroxyl group of the hydroxymethylbilane, preuroporphyrinogen, must have arisen by an enzymic process at the active site of the deaminase and not by the nonenzymic hydration of an azafulvene-type intermediate favored by some workers (Fig. 2.17).

The complete retention of tritium in the uroporphyrinogen synthesized from $[11RS-^3H_2]$porphobilinogen at positions C-5, C-10, C-15, and C-20 of the porphyrinogens is powerful evidence for the participation of a mechanism involving a retention mode at all bond-forming and breaking events which occur at the active site of *both* enzymes. Had an inversion of configuration occurred, then a considerable amount of tritium loss would have ensued, particularly at the C-20 position, as a result of the ability of the preuroporphyrinogen intermediate to bind

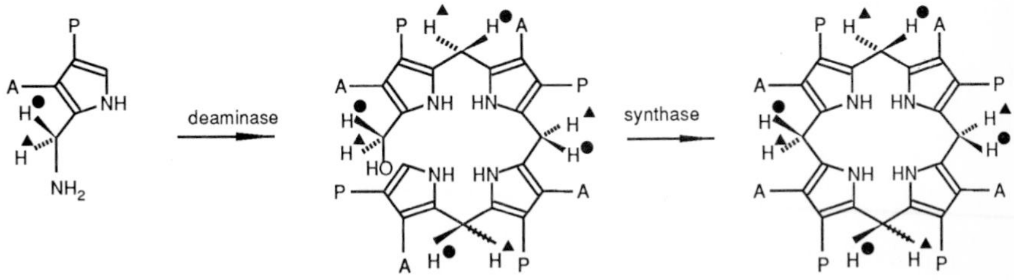

Figure 2.17 Steric course of the deaminase reaction.

reversibly to the deaminase enzyme (Battersby et al., 1985). Indirect evidence for a retention mode comes from the many experiments carried out on Mannich systems such as those found in porphobilinogen which indicate that such substitutions follow a strict retention mode.

Confirmation of our thesis has come from recent experiments in which porphobilinogen, also stereospecifically tritiated at C-11, was transformed with deaminase into the hydroxymethylbilane, preuroporphyrinogen (Schauder et al., 1987). Chiral analysis of the product indicated that the overall steric course is one of retention, allowing the same conclusion as Jones et al. (1984), namely, that the hydroxy group is added to the tetrapyrrole while it is bound within the confines of the deaminase catalytic site.

O. Use of synthetic analogues to investigate the uroporphyrinogen III synthase reaction

Few experiments have been carried out on the uroporphyrinogen III synthase (Fig. 2.18) in isolation because of the difficulties in purifying the enzyme and preparing the unstable substrate. However, several analogues of preuroporphyrinogen (hydroxymethylbilanes) have been synthesized and their effectiveness as substrates has been assessed (Battersby et al., 1983).

Hydroxymethylbilane	Percentage enzymic inversion
HOCH$_2$-AP-AP-AP-AP	100 (natural substrate)
HOCH$_2$-AP-PA-AP-AP	0
HOCH$_2$-AP-AP-PA-AP	95
HOCH$_2$-AP-AP-AP-PA	45
HOCH$_2$-PA-PA-PA-AP	0

The results of this study highlight the importance of the a and b rings for the recognition of the catalytic site. The most remarkable

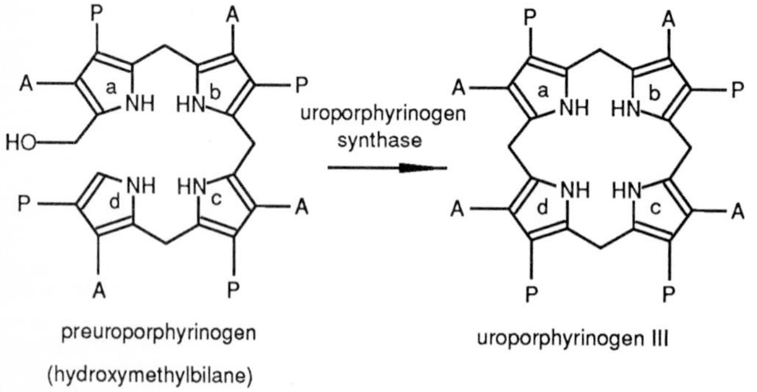

Figure 2.18 Reaction of uroporphyrinogen III synthase.

finding, however, was that the analogue with the d ring inverted acted as a reasonable substrate and that the product was uroporphyrinogen I! These results point to a mechanism in which the cyclization and inversion reactions are inexorably linked. This is simply explained by the fact that the enzyme-substrate complex has a single conformation and, thus, can only react in a single unidirectional fashion. Poor substrates would bind more loosely and the specificity would not be so high. This is exactly what appears to occur.

P. Mechanisms of action of uroporphyrinogen III synthase

The most-favored mechanism by which the enzyme catalyzes this gymnastic feat was proposed by Mathewson and Corwin (1963) and is one of a few early postulates that have not yet been disproved by subsequent experimental investigations (Fig. 2.19). A key feature of this mechanism is the formation of a spiro intermediate. Ring opening by scission of the opposite bond, followed by final ring closure, would yield uroporphyrinogen III. Attempts to synthesize the challenging spiro intermediate are

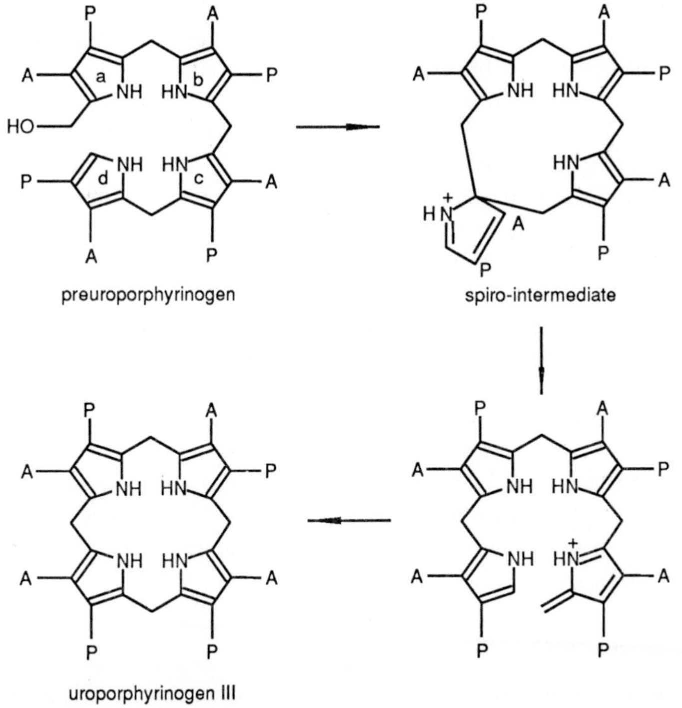

Figure 2.19 Mechanism for the biosynthesis of uroporphyrinogen III from preuroporphyrinogen.

under way (Stark et al., 1986) and one analogue has been shown to act as a good competitive inhibitor (K_i 1 μM). Only one of the two possible isomers acts as an inhibitor as predicted for a unidirectional sequence.

The steric course of the reaction of the porphobilinogen deaminase/uroporphyrinogen III synthase system has been discussed above. The experiments revealed that all four methylene positions of uroporphyrinogen III, and hence of preuroporphyrinogen, are produced through stereospecific processes. It follows that the cyclization and rearrangement of preuroporphyrinogen to uroporphyrinogen III must all occur at enzyme active sites (Jones et al., 1984).

Q. Molecular biology and protein structure of deaminase and synthase

The availability of the nucleotide sequences for the *E. coli* genes of porphobilinogen deaminase (*hemC*) (Thomas and Jordan, 1986) and the uroporphyrinogen III synthase (*hemD*) (Sasarman et al., 1987; Jordan et al., 1987), together with the human cDNA (Raich et al., 1986), has allowed direct comparisons to be made between the derived protein structures. There is a considerable similarity between the *E. coli* and human deaminases with highly conserved areas -V-G-T-S-S-L-R-R- and the cofactor binding site (see above). Several conserved arginine and lysine residues are apparent and it is tempting to suggest that they too may be involved in substrate binding. An interesting situation exists in the case of the human deaminase since the erythroid and nonerythroid isoenzymes both arise from the same gene (Grandchamp et al., 1987).

The sequence of the *E. coli hemD* was determined in two laboratories (Sarsaman et al., 1987; Jordan et al., 1987). The *hemD* gene is immediately adjacent to the *hemC* gene and under the control of the *hemC* promoter. There may be several *hem* genes in this operon under control of the *hemC* promoter. The *E. coli* synthase has been isolated from an overproducing strain and shown to have a molecular weight of about 29,000 (Jordan et al., 1988a). The N terminus of the *E. coli* enzyme has been sequenced, NH_2-S-I-L-V-T-R- and has lost the terminal methionine predicted from the gene sequence. The N terminus of the human enzyme NH_2-M-L-V-L-L-L-, however, appears to be intact. The human uroporphyrinogen III synthase cDNA has now been sequenced and comparison of the *E. coli* and human-derived protein sequences show very little homology, a surprising fact considering the high degree of similarity with the deaminases (Tsai et al., 1988).

VI. Biosynthesis of Coproporphyrinogen III

The oxidized form of coproporphyrinogen III, coproporphyrin III, had been known for many years from studies with porphyric patients but in early in vitro experiments it was not found to act as a substrate for protoporphyrin IX biosynthesis. It was also observed that when ^{14}C-glycine was incorporated into protoporphyrin, neither uroporphyrin III nor coproporphyrin III were able to dilute the label when added to incubations, pointing to the fact that porphyins were not the true intermediates (Shemin et al., 1955). The first experimental evidence that reduced porphyrins were involved came from studies by Bogorad (1955), who was able to demonstrate the formation of coproporphyrin from a colorless precursor in extracts from *Chlorella*. The major breakthrough was made when chemically reduced uroporphyrin III, uroporphyrinogen III, was shown to stimulate the incorporation of ^{59}Fe into heme whereas the nonreduced porphyrin was ineffective (Neve et al., 1956).

A. Intermediates in the decarboxylation and substrate specificity

The appearance of porphyrins with seven, six, and five carboxyl groups had been observed on numerous occasions by investigators in the field and a stepwise decarboxylation had always seemed likely. However, the first experimental evidence for such a pathway was obtained by Batlle and Grinstein (1964a, b), who demonstrated that uroporphyrinogen III could be decarboxylated to 7-COOH porphyrinogen as part of the natural heme pathway. The 6-COOH and 5-COOH porphyrinogens were soon described as later intermediates using elegant isotope dilution experiments (San Martin de Vaile and Grinstein, 1968), and a stepwise decarboxylation mechanism was firmly established. Responsible for all these reactions is a single enzyme named uroporphyrinogen decarboxylase (EC 4.1.1.37), also known as uroporphyrinogen carboxy-lyase. The enzyme catalyzes the decarboxylation of all four acetic acid side chains of uroporphyrinogen III to methyl groups yielding coproporphyrinogen III by the following sequence.

uroporphyrinogen III → 7-COOH → 6-COOH

→ 5-COOH → coproporphyrinogen III

The enzyme is able to carry out the decarboxylation of uroporphyrinogen I as well as the nonphysiological II and IV isomers (Mauzerall and Granick, 1958) and, thus, there are potentially 39 substates for the enzyme. Of the naturally occurring isomers, uroporphyrinogen III is decarboxylated at a preferential rate to the uroporphyrinogen I isomer, however, the selectivity varies between sources of the enzyme and conditions of the assay. Although it was always likely that a single enzyme was involved in catalyzing the decarboxylation of all four acetic acid side chains of uroporphyrinogen III, it was not possible to be certain of this until the homogeneous enzyme had been purified. The isolation of a single-enzyme protein capable of catalyzing all four decarboxylations from human erythrocytes (Elder et al., 1983; de Verneuil et al., 1983; Kawanishi et al., 1983; Straka and Kushner, 1983) has confirmed that the uroporphyrinogen decarboxylase is indeed endowed with a very broad substrate specificity.

It has been suggested that the enzyme has two catalytic sites in order to cater to the differences in the structure of the substrates. This has stemmed from the observation that uroporphyrinogen I inhibits the decarboxylation of uroporphyrinogen III but has little effect on the decarboxylation of the 7-COOH, 6-COOH, and 5-COOH intermediates (de Verneuil et al., 1980). This may simply reflect the higher affinity of uroporphyrinogen III for the active site when compared to the other intermediates. What is generally accepted by most workers is that the decarboxylation of uroporphyrinogen III is the fastest reaction and that the subsequent decarboxylations occur at a somewhat slower rate. A comparison between the isomers is shown below, although there seems to be considerable variation in the enzyme source and the investigators.

$$\text{III series } 8 > > > > > 7 > > 6 > > 5 > > > 4$$
$$\text{I series } 8 > > 7 > > 6 > > 5 > 4$$

Since uroporphyrinogen III is the best substrate it tends to compete for the first decarboxylation product, the 7-COOH intermediate, which in high concentrations of uroporphyrinogen III accumulates until the uroporphyrinogen III level has decreased. This has the effect of delaying the formation of the final product, coproporphyrinogen III (Smith and Francis, 1981).

B. Order of the decarboxylation reactions

The order of decarboxylation of the four acetic acid side chains of uroporphyrinogen III has been studied comprehensively by Jackson and his colleagues and is reviewed (Jackson et al., 1976). Theoretically, there are 14 possible intermediates between uroporphyrinogen III and coproporphyrinogen III made up of partially decarboxylated porphyrinogens containing 7, 6, or 5 carboxyl groups. Several of these intermediates, in the oxidized porphyrin form, have been isolated from patients suffering from the disease porphyria cutanea tarda, PCT (San Martin de Viale and Grinstein, 1968) or from laboratory animals that have been treated with chlorinated hydrocarbons (Sinclair et al., 1984). These partially decarboxylated porphyrins are all of the type III series since they yield coproporphyrinogen III on chemical decarboxylation. The heptacarboxylic acid isomer which accumulates, phriaporphyrin, has been identified by unambiguous chemical synthesis as the d ring decarboxylation product. Similarly, the hexacarboxylic acid porphyrin, of which there are six type III isomers, has been identified as arising from the decarboxylation of rings d and a with only small amounts of other isomers. Out of the four pentacarboxylic acid porphyrins, clearly, only two isomers were candidates, namely, the one with the d, a, and b rings decarboxylated or alternatively the isomer with d, a, and c rings decarboxylated. The naturally occurring intermediate was identical to the isomer chemically synthesized with methyl groups in the d, a, and b rings. In these experiments the isomers were characterized by proton nmr using shift reagents to maximize the difference between the relevant meso protons (Jackson et al., 1976). From this arduous series of determinations it was, therefore, established that a preferred decarboxylation route occurs (Fig. 2.20) commencing with ring d, with ring a and b next in sequence, and finally ending with ring c (Jackson et al., 1980). It is surprising that the complete series of decarboxylations is carried out by one enzyme since the substrates are really quite different and, as the intermediates form, the differences become even more acute. However, a consideration of the structure of each intermediate does allow one to make guarded suggestions about the number of pyrrole binding sites and their possible properties.

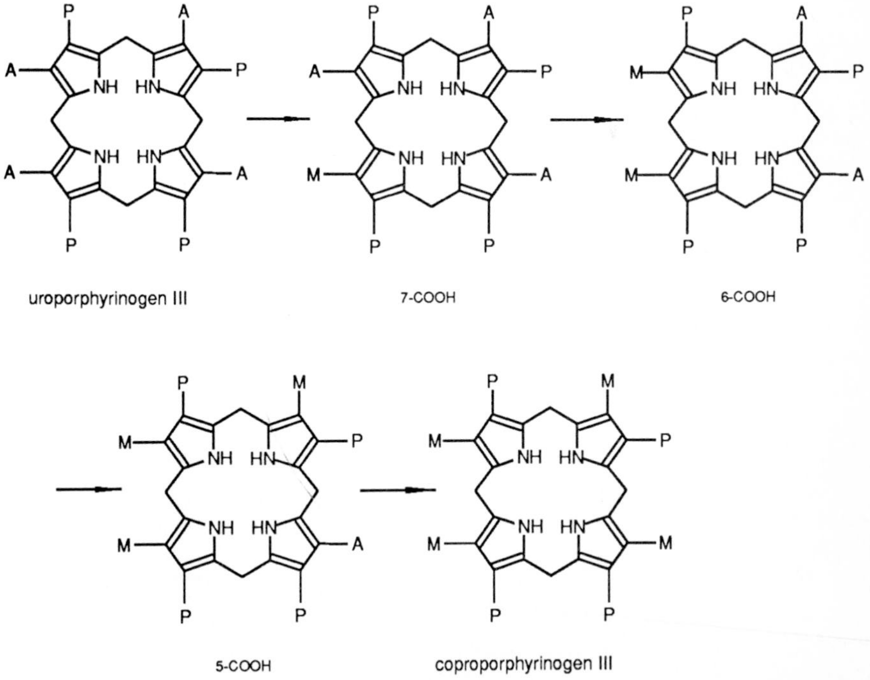

uroporphyrinogen III   7-COOH   6-COOH

5-COOH   coproporphyrinogen III

Figure 2.20 Stepwise decarboxylation of uroporphyrinogen III to coproporphyrinogen III.

In order to accommodate each of the four rings, the catalytic site will clearly have amino acid residues which can bind the acetic acid and propionic acid side chains of the ring which is to be decarboxylated. Any major change to this catalytic site would cause a complete loss of activity for all uroporphyrinogen substrates. The more interesting aspect of the enzyme function relates to structural abnormalities in which the catalytic site of the decarboxylase is functional, but where the peripheral binding sites appear to be affected. This may be seen in the case of hexachlorobenzene-poisoned rats and in patients with porphyria cutanea tarda and hepatoerythroporphyria, a homozygous form of porphyria cutanea tarda (Elder, 1983), in which the decarboxylase appears to carry out only a single decarboxylation with any efficiency. This leads to the accumulation of heptacarboxylic acid porphyrin and uroporphyrin III in the skin. In all these cases the enzyme appears catalytically active but its ability to recognize the substrates following the heptacarboxylic acid porphyrinogen is severely impaired. In order to decarboxylate the second ring, ring a, the heptacarboxylic acid porphyrinogen intermediate has to vacate the active site completely and the whole macrocyclic ring has to turn over before it can bind for the subsequent decarboxylations. It may well be that this subsequent rebinding is impaired due either to structural changes caused by chemical modification or to an amino acid substitution. Alternatively, the accumulation of uroporphyrinogen III may decrease the rate of decarboxylation of the hepta intermediate by competing for the decarboxylation site. One of the most important factors which has emerged is that the ratio of the substrate uroporphyrinogen III to enzyme should be low to avoid the buildup of intermediates.

C. Structure of the enzyme

The cDNAs for the rat and human decarboxylase enzymes have been cloned and both have been sequenced (Romana et al., 1987; Romeo et al., 1986). The derived protein sequences show striking similarities at both the DNA and protein levels with 85 and 90% homology, respectively. The main features are the occurrence of a group of three cysteine residues which may account for the fact that the enzyme is susceptible to reagents which interact with cysteine residues (de Verneuil et al., 1983; Straka and Kushner, 1983). There are a large number of aromatic residues, an emerging feature of enzymes that interact with porphyrinogens.

Elegant studies by de Verneuil et al., (1986) have shown that there is a mutation of glycine-281 to a glutamate in the human decarboxylase which causes an inherent susceptibility of the enzyme to proteolytic degradation. The lowered level of the decarboxylase causes the porphyria.

D. Mechanism of uroporphyrinogen decarboxylase

The mechanism by which the uroporphyrinogen decarboxylase catalyzes the reaction has been investigated by Barnard and Akhtar (1975). Succinate, stereospecifically tritiated and deuterated at the C-2 position, was incorporated into heme with an enzyme preparation from hemolyzed chicken erythrocytes. The C-2 position of succinate is incorporated into the methyl groups of coproporphyrinogen and, thence, to heme. Degradation of the heme to ethylmethylmaleimide and hematinic acid, followed by further degradation of the rings, yielded chiral acetic acid containing protium, deuterium, and tritium in the same molecule. Determination of the chirality revealed that the acetic acid was of the S configuration. Consideration of the original configuration of the succi-

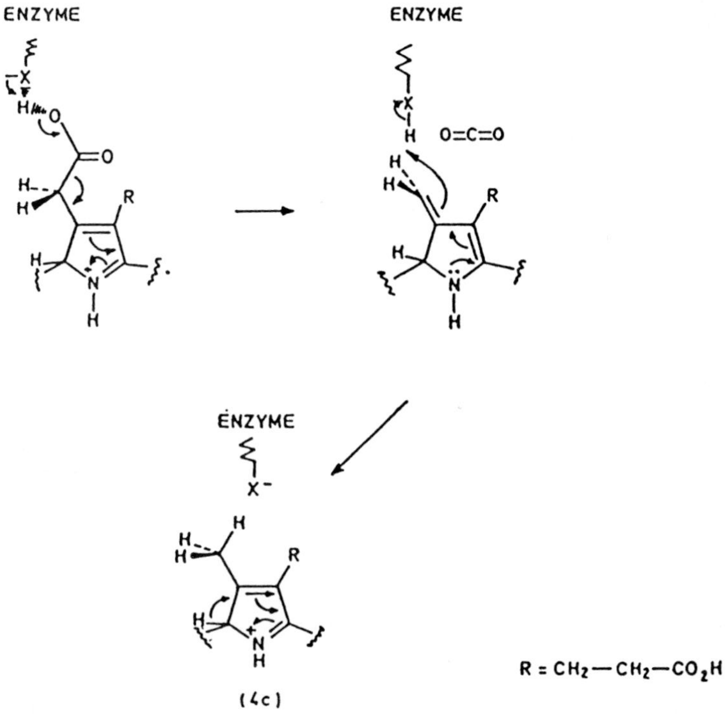

Figure 2.21   Mechanism of steric course of the uroporphyrinogen decarboxylase reaction.

nate in comparison to the S-acetic acid allowed the conclusion that the decarboxylation of the acetic acid chains to methyl groups occurs with retention of configuration. This is shown in Fig. 2.21.

In the proposed mechanism, the protonated pyrrole ring of the porphyrinogen functions in a similar capacity to the pyridine ring of pyridoxal phosphate in order to promote electron withdrawal. The reason for the porphyrinogen, rather than the porphyrin, oxidation state, not only for this reaction, but also for the coproporphyrinogen oxidase stage, is, therefore, easier to appreciate. A similar steric course has been shown to occur in $R.$ spheroides (Battersby et al., 1981).

REFERENCES

Abboud, M. M., and Akhtar, M. (1976). Stereochemistry of hydrogen elimination of the enzymic formation of the C-2–C-3 double bond of porphobilinogen, *J. Chem. Soc. Chem. Comm.* 1007–1008.

Abboud, M. M., Jordan, P. M., and Akhtar, M. (1974). Biosynthesis of 5-aminolevulinic acid. Involvement of a retention/inversion mechanism, *J. Chem. Soc. Chem. Comm.* 643–644.

Akhtar, M., and Jordan, P. M. (1968). Mechanism of action of 5-aminolevulinic acid synthase and the synthesis of stereospecifically tritiated glycine, *J. Chem. Soc. Chem. Comm.* 1691–1692.

Akhtar, M., and Jordan, P. M. (1979). Porphyrin, chlorophyll and corrin biosynthesis, *Comprehensive Organic Chemistry* (D. H. R. Barton, and W. D. Ollis, Eds.), Pergamon, pp. 1121–1166.

Alwan, A. F., and Jordan, P. M. (1988). Isolation of uroporphyrinogen III synthase from *E. coli*, *Biochem. Soc. Trans.* **16**:965–966.

Anderson, P. M., and Desnick, R. J. (1979). Purification and properties of 5-aminolevulinic acid dehydratase from human erythrocytes, *J. Biol. Chem.* **254**:6924–6930.

Anderson, P. M., and Desnick, R. J. (1980). Purification and properties of uroporphyrinogen I synthase from human erythrocytes, *J. Biol. Chem.* **255**:1993–1999.

Bagust, J., Jordan, P. M., Kelley, M. E. M., and Kerkut, G. A. (1985). Effect of 5-aminolevulinic acid on the activity in the isolated, hemisected mammalian spinal cord; *Neurosci. Lett.* **21**:S84.

Barnard, G. F., and Akhtar, M. (1975). Stereochemistry of porphyrinogen carboxylase reaction in heme biosynthesis, *J. Chem. Soc. Chem. Comm.* 494–496.

Barnard, G. F., Itoh, R., Hohberger, L. H., and Shemin, D. (1977). Mechanism of porphobilinogen synthase. Possible role of essential thiol groups, *J. Biol. Chem.* **252**:8965–8974.

Batlle, A. M. C., and Grinstein, M. (1964a). Porphyrin biosynthesis. I. Studies on erythrocyte preparations. *Biochim. Biophys. Acta* **82**:1–12.

Batlle, A. M. C., and Grinstein, M. (1964b). Porphyrin biosynthesis. II. A normal intermediate in heme biosynthesis; *Biochim. Biophys. Acta* **82**:13–20.

Batlle, A. M. C., and Rossetti, M. V. (1977). Review. Enzymic polymerization of porphobilinogen into uroporphyrinogens, *Int. J. Biochem.* **8**:251–267.

Battersby, A. R., Fookes, C. J. R., Gustafson-Potter, K. E., Matcham, G. W. J., and McDonald, E. (1979a). Proof by synthesis that unrearranged hydroxymethylbilane is the product from deaminase and the substrate for cosynthetase in the biosynthesis of uroporphyrinogen III, *J. Chem. Soc. Chem. Comm.* 1155–1158.

Battersby, A. R., Fookes, C. J. R., Matcham, G. W. J., and McDonald, E. (1978a). Biosynthesis of natural porphyrins: Enzymic experiments on isomeric bilanes, *J. Chem. Soc. Chem. Comm.* 1064–1066.

Battersby, A. R., Fookes, C. J. R., Matcham, G. W. J., and McDonald, E. (1979b). Order of assembly of the four pyrrole rings during the biosynthesis of natural porphyrins, *J. Chem. Soc. Chem. Comm.* 539–541.

Battersby, A. R., Fookes, C. J. R., McDonald, E., and Meegan, M. (1978b). Biosynthesis of type-III porphyrins. Proof of intact enzymic conversion of head-to-tail bilane into uroporphyrinogen III by intramolecular rearrangement, *J. Chem. Soc. Chem. Comm.* 185–186.

Battersby, A. R., Fookes, C. J. R., and Pandey, P. S. (1983). Linear tetrapyrrolic intermediates for biosynthesis of the natural porphyrins. Experiments with modified substrates, *Tetrahedron* **39**:1919–1926.

Battersby, A. R., Gutmann, A. L. Fookes, C. J. R., Gunther, H., and Simon, H. (1981). Stereochemistry of formation of methyl and ethyl groups in bacteriochlorophyll a, *J. Chem. Soc. Chem. Comm.* 645–647.

Battersby, A. R., and McDonald, E. (1975). Biosynthesis of porphyrins, chlorins and corrins, *Porphyrins and Metalloporphyrins* (K. M. Smith, Ed.), Elsevier, New York, pp. 61–122.

Battersby, A. R., and McDonald, E. (1976). Biosynthesis of porphyrins and corrins, *Philos. Trans. Roy. Soc. Lond. Ser. B* **273**:161–180.

Battersby, A. R., and McDonald, E. (1979). Origin of the pigments of life: The type-III problem in porphyrin biosynthesis, *Acc. Chem. Res.* **12**:14–22.

Battersby, A. R., McDonald, E., William, D. C., and Wurziger, H. K. W. (1977). Biosynthesis of the natural (type-III) porphyrins. Proof that rearrangement occurs after head-to-tail bilane formation, *J. Chem. Soc. Chem. Comm.* 113–115.

Bawden, M. J., Borthwick, I. A., Healy, H. M., Morris, C. P., May, B. K., and Elliott, W. H. (1987). Sequence of human 5-aminolevulinic acid cDNA, *Nucl. Acids Res.* **15**:8563.

Beale, S. I., and Castelfranco, P. A. (1974). The biosynthesis of 5-aminolevulinic acid in higher plants. II. Formation of 5-amino[^{14}C]levulinic acid for labelled precursors in greening plant tissues, *Plant Physiol.* **53**:291–296, 297–303.

Beale, S. I., Gough, S. P., and Granick, S. (1975). The biosynthesis of 5-aminolevulinic acid from the intact carbon skeleton of glutamic acid in greening barley, *Proc. Nat. Acad. Sci. (U.S.A)* **72**:2717–2723.

Berry, A., Jordan, P. M., and Seehra, J. S. (1981). The isolation and characterization of catalytically competent porphobilinogen deaminase-intermediate complexes, *FEBS Lett.* **129**:220–224.

Bevan, D. R., Bodlaender, P., and Shemin, D. (1980). Mechanism of porphobilinogen synthase. Requirement of zinc for enzyme activity, *J. Biol. Chem.* **255**:2030–2035.

Bishop, T. R., Frelin, L. P., and Boyer, S. H. (1986). Nucleotide sequence of rat liver 5-aminolevulinic acid dehydratase cDNA, *Nucl. Acids Res.* **14**:10115.

Bogorad, L. (1955). Intermediates in the biosynthesis of porphyrins from porphyrinogen, *Science* **121**:878–879.

Bogorad, L. (1958a). The enzymic synthesis of porphyrins from porphobilinogen. I. Uroporphyrin I, *J. Biol. Chem.* **233**:501–509.

Bogorad, L. (1958b). The enzymic synthesis of porphyrins from porphobilinogen. II. Uroporphyrin III, *J. Biol. Chem.* **233**:510–515.

Bogorad, L., and Granick, S. (1953). The enzymic synthesis of porphyrins from porphobilinogen, *Proc. Nat. Acad. Sci. (U.S.A.)* **39**:1176–1188.

Borthwick, I. A., Srivastava, G., Brooker, J. D., May, B. K., and Elliott, W. H. (1983). Purification of 5-aminolevulinic acid synthase from liver mitochondria of chick embryo, *Eur. J. Biochem.* **129**:615–620.

Borthwick, I.A., Srivastava, G., Day, A. R., Pirola, B. A., Snoswell, M. A., May, B. K., and Elliot, W. H. (1985). Complete nucleotide sequence of hepatic 5-aminolevulinic acid synthase precursor, *Eur. J. Biochem.* **150**:481–484.

Breu, V., and Dornemann, D. (1988). Formation of 5-aminolevulinic acid via glutamate 1-semialdehyde and 4,5-dioxovalerate with participation of a RNA component in *Scenedesmus obliquus* mutant C-2A, *Biochem. Biophys. Acta,* **967**:135–140.

Breu, V., Kah, A., and Dornemann, D. (1988). Quantative determination of 4,5-dioxovaleric acid as a metabolite in *Scenedesmus obliquus* after complete separation from 5-aminolevulinic acid, *Biochim. Biophys. Acta* **964**:61–68.

Brumm, P. J., and Friedmann, H. C. (1981). Succinylacetone pyrrole, a powerful inhibitor of vitamin B_{12} biosynthesis. Effect on 5-aminolevulinic acid dehydratase, *Biochem. Biophys. Res. Comm.* **102**:854–859.

Bruyant, P., and Kannangara, C. G. (1987). Biosynthesis of 5-aminolevulinic acid in greening barley leaves. VIII. Purification and characterization of the glutamate-tRNA ligase, *Carlsberg Res. Comm.* **52**:99–109.

Burton, G., Fagerness, P. E., Hosozawa, S., Jordan, P. M., and Scott, A. I. (1979a). ^{13}C nmr evidence of a new intermediate, preuroporphyrinogen, in the enzymic transformation of porphobilinogen into uroporphyrinogen III, *J. Chem. Soc. Chem. Comm.* 202–204.

Burton, G., Nordlov, H., Hosozawa, S., Matsumoto, H., Jordan, P. M., Fagerness, P. E., Pryde, L. M., and Scott, A. I. (1979b). Structure of preuroporphyrinogen. Exploration of an enzyme mechanism by ^{13}C and ^{15}N nmr spectroscopy. *J. Amer. Chem. Soc.* **101**:3114–3116.

Castelfranco, P., and Beale, S. I. (1983). Chlorophyll biosynthesis. Recent advances and areas of current interest, *Ann. Rev. Plant Physiol.* **34**:241–278.

Chaudhry, A. G., and Jordan, P. M. (1976). Stereochemical studies on the formation of porphobilinogen, *Biochem. Soc. Trans.* **4**:760–761.

Cheh, A. M. and Neilands, J. B. (1976). 5-Aminolevulinic acid dehydratase, *Struct. Bonding* **29**:123–170.

Chisholm, J. J. (1971). Lead poisoning. *Sci. Amer.* **224**:15–23.

Clara de Barreiro, O. L. (1967). 5-Aminolevulinic acid hydro-lyase from yeast. Isolation and purification, *Biochim. Biophys. Acta* **139**:479–486.

Davies, R. C., and Neuberger, A. (1973). Polypyrroles formed from porphobilinogen and amines by uroporphyrinogen synthase of *Rhodobacter spheroides*, *Biochem. J.*, **133**:471–492.

de Verneuil, H., Grandchamp, B., Beaumont, C., Picat, C., and Nordmann, Y. (1986). Uroporphyrinogen decarboxylase structural mutant (gly^{281}-glu) in a case of porphyria, *Science* **234**:732–734.

de Verneuil, H., Grandchamp, B., and Nordmann, Y. (1980). Some kinetic properties of human red cell uroporphyrinogen decarboxylase, *Biochim. Biophys. Acta* **611**:174–186.

de Verneuil, H., Sassa, S., and Kappas, A. (1983). Purification and properties of uroporphyrinogen decarboxylase from human erythrocytes, *J. Biol. Chem.* **258**:2454–2460.

Dolphin, D. (Ed.) (1976). *The Porphyrins*, Academic, New York, Vol. 6, Chaps. 1–4.

Dzelzkalns, V., Foley, T., and Beale, S. I. (1982). 5-Aminolevulinic acid synthase of *Euglena gracilis*. Physical and kinetic properties. *Arch. Biochem. Biophys.* **216**:196–203.

Echelard, Y., Dymetryszyn, J., Drolet, M., and Sasarman, A. (1988). Nucleotide sequence of the *hemB* gene of *Escherichia coli* K-12, *Mol. Gen. Genet.*, **214**:503–508.

Einav, M., and Avissar, Y. J. (1984). Biosynthesis of 5-aminolevulinic acid from glutamate in the blue green alga *Spirulina platensis*, *Plant Sci. Lett.* **35**:51–54.

Elder, G. H. (1983). Recent advances in the identification of enzyme deficiencies in the porphyrias, *Brit. J. Dermatol.* **108**:729–734.

Elder, G. H., Tovey, J. A., and Sheppard, D. M. (1983). Purification of uroporphyrinogen decarboxylase from human erythrocytes, *Biochem. J.* **215**:45–55.

Emery, V. and Akhtar, M. (1987). Pyridoxal phosphate dependent enzymes, *Enzyme Mechanisms* (M. I. Page and A. Williams, Eds.) The Royal Society of Chemistry, pp. 345–389.

Evans, J. N. S., Burton, G., Fagerness, P. E., Mackenzie, N. E., and Scott, A. I. (1986). Biosynthesis of porphyrins and corrins. 2. Isolation, purification, and nmr investigations of the porphobilinogen-deaminase covalent complex, *Biochemistry* **25**:905–912.

Falk, J. E., Dresel, E. I. B., and Rimington, C. (1953). Porphobilinogen as a porphyrin precursor and interconversion of porphyrins in a tissue system, *Nature* **172**:292–294.

Fanica-Gaignier, M., and Clement-Metral, J. (1973). 5-Aminolevulinic acid synthase from *Rhodobacter Spheroides* Y. Kinetic mechanism and inhibition by ATP, *Eur. J. Biochem.* **40**:19–24.

Finelli, V. N., Klauder, D. S., Karaffa, M. A., and Petering, H. G. (1975). Interaction of zinc and lead on 5-aminolevulinic acid dehydratase, *Biochem. Biophys. Res. Comm.* **65**:303–312.

Francis, J. E., and Smith, A. G. (1984). Assay of mouse liver, uroporphyrinogen decarboxylase by reverse phase h.p.l.c., *Anal. Biochem.* **138**:404–410.

Friedmann, H. C., Thauer, R. K., Gough, S. P., and Kannangara, C. G. (1987). 5-Amino-levulinic acid formation in the archebacterium *Methanobacterium thermoautotroph-icum* requires tRNA, *Carlsberg Res. Comm.* **52**:363–371.

Frydman, R. B., and Feinstein, G. (1974). Studies on porphobilinogen deaminawse and uroporphyrinogen III cosynthase from human erythrocytes, *Biochim. Biophys. Acta* **350**:358–373.

Frydman, B., Frydman, R. B., Valasinas, A., Levy, E. S., and Feinstein, G. (1976). Biosynthesis of uroporphyrinogen from porphobilinogen: Mechanism and the nature of the process, *Philos. Trans. Roy. Soc. Lond. Ser. B* **273**:137–160.

Frydman, R. B., Levy, E. S., Valasinas, A., and Frydman, B. (1978). Biosynthesis of uroporphyrinogens. Interaction among 2-aminomethyldipyrrylmethanes and the en-zymic systems, *Biochemistry* **17**:110–120.

Frydman, R. B., Reil, S., and Frydman, B. (1971). Relation between structure and reactivity in porphobilinogen and related pyrroles, *Biochemistry* **10**:1154–1160.

Gibbs, P. N. B., Chaudhry, A. G., and Jordan, P. M. (1985a). Purification and properties of 5-aminolevulinic acid dehydratase from human erythrocytes, *Biochem. J.* **230**:25–34.

Gibbs, P. N. B., Gore, M. G. G., and Jordan, P. M. (1985b). Investigation of the effect of metal ions on the reactivity of thiol groups in human 5-aminolevulinic acid dehydratase, *Biochem. J.* **225**:573–580.

Gibbs, P. N. B., and Jordan, P. M. (1981). 5-Aminolevulinic acid dehydratase. [65]Zinc binding and exchange with enzyme from human erythrocytes, *Biochem. Soc. Trans.* **9**:232–233.

Gibbs, P. N. B., and Jordan, P. M. (1986). Identification of lysine at the active site of human 5-aminolevulinic acid dehydratase, *Biochem. J.* **236**:447–451.

Gibson, K. D., Laver, W. G., and Neuberger, A. (1958). Initial stages in the biosynthesis of porphyrins. II. The formation of 5-aminolevulinic acid from glycine and succinyl-CoA by particles from chicken erythrocytes, *Biochem. J.* **70**:71–81.

Gibson, K. D., Neuberger, A., and Scott, J. J. (1955). The purification and properties of 5-aminolevulinic acid dehydratase, *Biochem. J.* **61**:618–629.

Grandchamp, B., de Verneuil, H., Beaumont, C., Chretien, S., Walter, O., and Nordmann, Y. (1987). Tissue specific expression of porphobilinogen deaminwase. Two isoenzymes from a single gene, *Eur. J. Biochem.* **162**:105–110.

Granick, S., and Beale, S. I. (1978). Heme, chlorophylls and related compounds. Biosynthe-sis and metabolic regulation, *Adv. Enzymol.* **46**:33–203.

Granick, S., Sinclair, P., Sassa, S., and Grieninger, G. (1975). Effects of heme, insuli and serum albumin on heme and protein synthesis in chick embryo liver cells cultured in a chemically defined medium and a spectrofluorometric assay for porphyrin composition, *J. Biol. Chem.* **250**:9215–9225.

Gurne, D., Chen, J., and Shemin, D. (1977). Dissociation and reassociation of immobilized porphobilinogen synthase: Use of immobilized subunits of enzyme isolation, *Proc. Nat. Acad. Sci. (U.S.A.)* **74**:1383–1387.

Hart, G. J., Abell, C., and Battersby, A. R. (1986). Purification, N-terminal amino acid sequence and properties of hydroxymethylbilane synthase (porphobilinogen deaminase) from *Escherichia coli*, *Biochem. J.* **240**:273–276.

Hart, G. J., and Battersby, A. R. (1985). Purification and properties of uroporphyrinogen III synthase (cosynthase) from *Euglena gracilis*. *Biochem. J.* **232**:151–160.

Hart, G. J., Leeper, F. J., and Battersby, A. R. (1984). Modification of hydroxymethylbi-lane synthase (porphobilinogen deaminase) by pyridoxal phosphate. Demonstration of an essential lysine residue, *Biochem. J.* **222**:93–102.

Hart, G. J., Miller, A. D., and Battersby, A. R. (1988). Evidence that the pyrromethane cofactor of hydroxymethylbilane synthase (porphobilinogen synthase) is bound through the sulfur atom of a cysteine residue, *Biochem. J.* **252**:909–912.

Hart, G. H., Miller A. D., Leeper, F. J., and Battersby, A. R. (1987). Biosynthesis of the natural porphyrins: Proof that hydroxymethylbilane synthase (porphobilinogen deami-nase) uses a novel binding group in its catalytic action, *J. Chem. Soc. Chem. Comm.* 1762–1765.

Hasnain, S. S., Wardell, E. M., Garner, C. D. Schlosser, M., and Beyersmann, D. (1985). Extended-x-ray absorbtion-fine-structure investigations of zinc in 5-aminolevulinic acid dehydratase, *Biochem. J.* **230**:625–633.

Hayashi, N., Yoda, B., and Kikuchi, G. (1969). Mechanism of allylisopropylacetamide-induced increase of 5-aminolevulinic acid synthase in liver mitochondria. IV. Accumulation of the enzyme in the soluble fraction of rat liver, *Arch. Biochem. Biophys.* **131**:83–91.

Higuchi, M., and Bogorad, L. (1975). Purification and properties of uroporphyrinogen I synthase and uroporphyrinogen III cosynthetase. Interaction between the enzymes, *Ann. N.Y. Acad. Sci.* **244**:401–418.

Hoober, J. K., Kahn, A., Ash, D. E., Gough, S. P., and Kannangara, C. G. (1988). Biosynthesis of 5-aminolevulinic acid in greening barley leaves. IX. Structure of the substrate, mode of gabaculine inhibition, and the catalytic mechanism of glutamate 1-semialdehyde aminotransferase, *Carlsberg Res. Comm.* **53**:11–25.

Houen, G., Gough, S. P., and Kannangara, C. G. (1984). 5-Aminolevulinic acid synthesis in greening barley. V. The structure of gluamate 1-semialdehyde, *Carlsberg Res. Comm.* **48**:567–572.

Huang, D.-D. and Wang, W.-Y. (1986). Chlorophyll biosynthesis in *Chlamydomonas* starts with the formation of glutamyl-tRNA, *J. Biol. Chem.* **261**:13451–13455.

Jackson, A. H., Sancovich, H. A., and Ferramola, A. M. (1980). Synthetic and biosynthetic studies of porphyrins. III. Structures of the intermediates between uroporphyrinogen III and coproporphyrinogen III: Synthesis of fourteen heptacarboxylic, hexacarboxylic, and pentacarboxylic porphyrins related to uroporphyrin III. *Bioorg. Chem.* **9**:71–120.

Jackson, A. H., Sancovich, H. A., Ferramola, A. M., Evans, N., Games, D. E., and Matlin, S. A. (1976). Macrocyclic intermediates in the biosynthesis of porphyrins, *Philos. Trans. Roy. Soc. Lond. Ser. B* **273**:191–206.

Jaffe, E. K., and Hanes, D. (1986). Dissection of the early steps in the porphobilinogen synthase catalysed reaction. Requirements for Schiff base formation, *J. Biol. Chem.* **261**:9348–9353.

Jones, C., Jordan, P. M., and Akhtar, M. A. (1984). Mechanism and stereochemistry of the porphobilinogen deaminase and protoporphyrinogen IX oxidase reactions: Stereospecific manipulation of hydrogen atoms at the four methylene bridges during the biosynthesis of heme, *J. Chem. Soc. Perkin Trans. I* 2625–2633.

Jordan, P. M. (1982). Uroporphyrinogen III cosynthase: A direct assay method, *Enzyme* **28**:158–169.

Jordan, P. M., and Akhtar, M. (1970). The mechanism of action of serine transhydroxymethylase, *Biochem. J.* **116**:227–286.

Jordan, P. M., and Berry A. (1980). Preuroporphyrinogen, a universal intermediate in the biosynthesis of uroporphyrinogen III, *FEBS Lett.* **112**:86–88.

Jordan, P. M., and Berry, A. (1981). Mechanism of action of porphobilinogen deaminase. The participation of stable enzyme substrate covalent intermediates between porphobilinogen and the porphobilinogen deaminase from *Rhodobacter spheroides*, *Biochem. J.* **195**:177–181.

Jordan, P. M., Burton, G., Nordlov, H., Schneider, M., Pryde, L., and Scott, A. I. (1979). Preuroporphyrinogen, a substrate for uroporphyrinogen III cosynthase, *J. Chem. Soc. Chem. Comm.* 204–205.

Jordan, P. M., Chaudhry, A. G., and Gore, M. G. (1976). Studies on the inactivation of 5-aminolevulinic acid dehydratase by alkylation, *Biochem. Soc. Trans.* **4**:301–303.

Jordan, P. M., and Gibbs, P. N. B. (1985). Mechanism of action of 5-aminolevulinic acid dehydratase from human erythrocytes, *Biochem. J.* **227**:1015–1020.

Jordan, P. M., Mgbeje, I. A. B., Alwan, A. F., and Thomas, S. D. (1987). Nucleotide sequence of *hemD* the second gene in the *hem* operon of *Escherichia coli* K-12, *Nucl. Acids Res.* **15**:10583.

Jordan, P. M., Mgbeje, I. A., Thomas, S. D., and Alwan, A. F. (1988a). Nucleotide sequence of the *hemD* gene of *Escherichia coli* encoding uroporphyrinogen III synthase and initial evidence for a *hem* operon, *Biochem. J.* **249**:613–616.

Jordan, P. M., and Seehra, J. S. (1979). The biosynthesis of uroporphyrinogen III. Order of assembly of the four porphobilinogen molecules in the formation of the tetrapyrrole ring, *FEBS Lett.* **104**:364–366.

Jordan, P. M., and Seehra, J. S. (1980a). ^{13}C nmr as probe for the study of enzyme catalysed reactions; mechanism of action of 5-aminolevulinic acid dehydratase, *FEBS Lett.* **114**:283–286.

Jordan, P. M., and Seehra, J. S. (1980b). Mechanism of action of 5-aminolevulinic acid dehydratase: stepwise order of addition of the two molecules of 5-aminolevulinic acid in the enzymic synthesis of porphobilinogen, *J. Chem. Soc. Chem. Comm.* 240–242.

Jordan, P. M., and Seehra, J. S. (1986). Purification of porphobilinogen synthase from bovine liver, *Methods Enzymol.* **123**:427–434.

Jordan, P. M., Sharma, R. P., and Warren, M. J. (1989). A cyclic intermediate, 2-hydroxy-3-aminotetrahydropyran-1-one (HAT) as a precursor for 5-aminolevulinic acid in greening barley, *Tet. Lett.*, to appear.

Jordan, P. M., and Shemin, D. (1972). 5-Aminolevulinic acid synthase, *The Enzymes* (P. D. Boyer, Ed.), 3rd ed., Academic, New York, Vol. 5, pp. 323–356.

Jordan, P. M., and Shemin, D. (1973). Purification and properties of uroporphyrinogen I synthase from *Rhodobacter spheroides*, *J. Biol. Chem.* **248**:1019–1024.

Jordan, P. M., Thomas, S. D., and Warren, M. J. (1988b). Purification, crystallization and properties of porphobilinogen deaminase from a recombinant strain of *Escherichia coli* K12, *Biochem. J.*, **254**:427–435.

Jordan, P. M., and Warren, M. J. (1987). Evidence for a dipyrromethane cofactor at the catalytic site of *E. coli* porphobilinogen deaminase, *FEBS Lett.* **225**:87–92.

Jordan, P. M., Warren, M. J., Williams, H. J., Stolowich, N. J., Roessner, C. A., Grant, S. K., and Scott, A. I. (1988c). Identification of a cysteine-242 residue as the binding site for the dipyrromethane cofactor at the active site of *Escherichia coli* porphobilinogen deaminase, *FEBS Lett.* **235**:189–193.

Kannangara, C. G., and Gough, S. P. (1977). Synthesis of 5-aminolevulinic acid and chlorophyll by isolated chloroplasts, *Carlsberg Res. Comm.* **42**:441–457.

Kannangara, G. C., and Gough, S. P. (1978). Biosynthesis of 5-aminolevulinic acid in greening barley leaves: Glutamate 1-semialdehyde aminotransferase, *Carlsberg Res. Comm.* **43**:185–194.

Kannangara, C. G., Gough, S. P., Bruyant, P., Hoober, J. K., Kahn, A., and von Wettstein, D. (1988). tRNA^{glu} as a cofactor in 5-aminolevulinic acid synthesis. Steps that regulate chlorophyll synthesis, *TIBS* **13**:139–143.

Kannangara, C. G., Gough, S. P., Oliver, R. P., and Rasmussen, S. K. (1984). Biosynthesis of 5-aminolevulinic acid in greening barley leaves. VI. Activation of glutamate by ligation to RNA, *Carlsberg Res. Comm.* **49**:417–437.

Kannangara, C. G., and Schouboe, A. (1985). Biosynthesis of 5-aminolevulinic acid in greening barley leaves. VII. Glutamate 1-semialdehyde accumulation in gabaculine treated leaves, *Carlsberg Res. Comm.* **50**:179–191.

Kappas, A., Sassa, S., and Anderson, K. E. (1963). The porphyrias, *The Metabolic Basis of Inherited Disease* (J. B. Stanbury, J. B. Wyngaarden, D. S. Fredrickson, J. J. Goldstein and M. S. Brown, Eds.), 5th ed., McGraw-Hill, New York.

Kawanishi, S., Seki, Y., and Sano, S. (1983). Uroporphyrinogen decarboxylase. Purification, properties of inhibition by polychlorinated biphenyls, *J. Biol. Chem.* **258**:4285–4292.

Kennard, O. (1953). Porphobilinogen. X-Ray crystallographic determination and molecular weight, *Nature* **171**:876–877.

Kikuchi, G., Kumar, A., Talmage, P., and Shemin, D. (1958). The enzymic synthesis of 5-aminolevulinic acid, *J. Biol. Chem.* **233**:1214–1219.

Kohashi, M., Clement, R. P., Tse, J., and Piper, W. N. (1984). Rat hepatic uroporphyrinogen III cosynthase. Purification and evidence for a bound folate coenzyme participating in the biosynthesis of uroporphyrinogen III, *Biochem. J.* **220**:755–765.

Komai, H., and Neilands, J. B. (1968). Effect of zinc ions on 5-aminolevulinic acid dehydratase in *Usilago spherogena*, *Arch. Biochem. Biophys.* **124**:456–461.

Kozak, M. (1984). Compilation and analysis of sequences upstream from the translation start site in eukaryote mRNAs, *Nucl. Acids Res.* **12**:857–872.

Laghai, A., and Jordan, P. M. (1976). A partial reaction of 5-aminolevulinic acid synthase from *Rhodobacter spheroides*, *Biochem. Soc. Trans.* 4:52–53.

Laghai, A. and Jordan, P. (1977). An exchange reaction catalysed by 5-aminolevulinic acid synthase from *Rhodobacter spheroides*, *Biochem. Soc. Trans.* 5:299–301.

Lascelles, J. (1968). The regulation of heme and chlorophyll synthesis, *Biochem. Soc. Symp.* 28:49–59.

Leeper, F. J. (1985). Biosynthesis of porphyrins, chlorophylls and vitamin B_{12}, *Natural Product Reports* 2:19–47.

Leong, S. A., Williams, P. H. and Ditta, G. S. (1985). Analysis of the 5′ regulatory region of the gene for 5-aminolevulinic acid synthase from *Rhizobium meliloti*, *Nucl. Acids Res.* 13:5965–5976.

Liedgens, W., Lutz, C., and Schneider, H. A. W. (1983). Molecular properties of 5-aminolevulinic acid dehydratase from *Spinacia olereiea*, *Eur. J. Biochem.* 135:75–79.

Llambias, E. B. C., and Batlle, A. M. C. (1971). Porphyrin biosynthesis. VIII. Avian erythrocyte porphobilinogen deaminase-uroporphyrinogen III cosynthetase, its purification, properties and separation of its components, *Biochim. Biophys. Acta* 227:180–191.

Maguire, D. J., Day, A. R., Borthwick, I. A., Srivastava, G., Wigley, P. L., May, B. K., and Elliott, W. H. (1986). Nucleotide sequence of the chicken 5-aminolevulinic acid synthase gene, *Nucl. Acids Res.* 14:1379–1391.

Matthew, M., and Neuberger, A. (1963). Aminomalonate as an enzyme inhibitor, *Biochem. J.* 87:601–612.

Mathewson, J. H., and Corwin, A. H. (1963). Biosynthesis of pyrrole pigments. A mechanism for porphobilinogen polymerization, *J. Amer. Chem. Soc.* 83:135–137.

Mau, Y.-H. L., and Wang, W.-Y. (1988). Biosynthesis of 5-aminolevulinic acid in *Chlamydomonas reinhardtii*. Study of the transamination mechanism using specifically labelled glutamate, *Plant Physiol.* 86:793–797.

Mauzerall, D. (1960a). The thermodynamic stability of uroporphyrinogens, *J. Amer. Chem. Soc.* 82:2601–2605.

Mauzerall, D. (1960b). The condensation of porphobilinogen to uroporphyrinogens, *J. Amer. Chem. Soc.*, 82:2605–2609.

Mauzerall, D., and Granick, S. (1958). Porphyrin biosynthesis of erythrocytes. III. Uroporphyrinogen and its decarboxylase, *J. Biol. Chem.* 232:1141–1162.

Mayer, S. M., Beale, S. I., and Weinstein, J. D. (1987). Enzymic conversion of glutamate to 5-aminolevulinic acid in soluble extracts of *Euglena gracilis*, *J. Biol. Chem.*, 262:12547–12549.

McClung, C. R., Somerville, J. E., Guerinot, M. L., and Chelm, B. K. (1987). Structure of the *Bradyrhizobium japonicum* gene *hemA* encoding 5-aminolevulinic acid synthase, *Gene* 54:133–139.

Meredith, P. A., and Moore, M. R. (1980). Effects of zinc and lead on 5-aminolevulinic acid dehydratase, *Biochem. Soc. Trans.* 6:760–762.

Muir, H. M., and Neuberger, A. (1950). The biogenesis of porphyrins. 2. The origin of the methyne carbon atoms, *Biochem. J.* 47:97–104.

Nandi, D. L. (1978a). Studies of 5-aminolevulinic acid synthase from *Rhodobacter spheroides*. Reversibility of the reaction, kinetic, spectral and other studies relating to the mechanism of action, *J. Biol. Chem.* 253:8872–8877.

Nandi, D. L. (1978b). Lysine as the substrate binding site of porphobilinogen synthase of *Rhodobacter spheroides*. *Z. Naturforsch. C. Biosci.* 33:799–800.

Nandi, D. L., Baker-Cohen, K. F., and Shemin, D. (1968). 5-Aminolevulinic acid dehydratase of *Rhodobacter spheroides*. I. Isolation and properties, *J. Biol. Chem.* 243:1224–1230.

Nandi, D. L., and Shemin, D. (1968a). 5-Aminolevulinic acid dehydratase of *Rhodobacter spheroides*. II. Association to polymers and dissociation to subunits, *J. Biol. Chem.* 243:1231–1235.

Nandi, D. L., and Shemin, D. (1968b). 5-Aminolevulinic acid dehydratase of *Rhodobacter spheroides*. III. Mechanism of porphobilinogen synthesis, *J. Biol. Chem.* 243:1236–1242.

Neuberger, A., Sandy, J. D., and Tait, G. H. (1973). Control of 5-aminolevulinate synthetase activity in *Rhodobacter spheroides*. The involvement of sulfur metabolism, *Biochem. J.* **136**:477–490.

Neve, R. A., Labbe, R. F., and Aldrich, R. A. (1956). Reduced uroporphyrinogen III in the biosynthesis of heme, *J. Amer. Chem. Soc.* **78**:691–692.

Ohashi, A., and Kikuchi, G. (1972). Mechanism of allylisopropylacetamide-induced increase of 5-aminolevulinic acid synthase in liver mitochondria. VI. Multiple forms of 5-aminolevulinic acid synthase in cytosol, *Arch. Biochem. Biophys.* **153**:34–46.

Ohashi, A., and Kikuchi, G. (1979). Purification and some properties of two forms of 5-aminolevulinic acid synthase from rat liver cytosol, *J. Biochem.* **85**:239–247.

Oh-hama, T., Seto, H., Otake, N. and Miyachi, S. (1982). ^{13}C nmr evidence for the pathway of chlorophyll synthesis in green algae, *Biochem. Biophys. Res. Comm.* **105**:647–652.

Pluscec, J., and Bogorad, L. (1970). A dipyrrylmethane intermediate in the enzymic synthesis of uroporphyrinogen, *Biochemistry* **9**:4736–4743.

Porra, R. J., Klein, D., and Wright, P. E. (1983). The proof by ^{13}C nmr spectroscopy of the predominance of the C-5 pathway over the Shemin pathway in chlorophyll biosynthesis in higher plants and of the formation of the methyl ester group of chlorophyll from glycine, *Eur. J. Biochem.* **130**:509–516.

Radmer, R., and Bogorad, L. (1972). A tetrapyrrole intermediate in the enzymic synthesis of uroporphyrinogen, *Biochemistry* **11**:904–910.

Raich, N., Romeo, P. H., Dubart, A., Beaupain, D., Cohen-Sohal, M., and Goossens, M. (1986). Molecular cloning and complete primary sequence of human erythrocyte porphobilinogen deaminase, *Nucl. Acids Res.* **14**:5955–5968.

Romana, M., le Boulch, P., and Romeo, P.-H. (1987). Rat uroporphyrinogen decarboxylase cDNA: Nucleotide sequence and comparison to human uroporphyrinogen decarboxylase, *Nucl. Acids Res.* **15**:7211.

Romeo, P.-H., Raich, N., Dubart, A., Beaupain, D., Pryor, M., Kushner, J. P., Cohen-Solal, M., and Goossens, M. (1986). Molecular cloning and nucleotide sequence of a complete human uroporphyrinogen decarboxylase cDNA, *J. Biol. Chem.* **261**:9825–9831.

Rossetti, M. V., Juknat de Geralnik, A. A., and Batlle, A. M. C. (1977). Porphyrin biosynthesis in *Euglena gracilis*. II. Pyrrylmethane intermediate in the enzymic cyclotetramerization of porphobilinogen, *Int. J. Biochem.* **8**:781–87.

Russell, C. S., Polack, S., and James, J. (1984). Studies on the active site of wheat germ porphobilinogen deaminase, *Ann. N.Y. Acad. Sci.* **435**:202–204.

Sancovich, H. A., Batlle, A. M. C., and Grinstein, M. (1969). Porphyrin biosynthesis. VI. Separation and purification of porphobilinogen deaminase and uroporphyrinogen isomerase from cow liver. Porphobilinogenase an allosteric enzyme, *Biochim. Biophys. Acta* **191**:130–143.

San Martin De Vaile, L. C., and Grinstein, M. (1968). Porphyrin biosynthesis. IV. 5- and 6-COOH porphyrinogens (type-III) as normal intermediates in heme biosynthesis, *Biochim. Biophys. Acta* **158**:79–91.

Sasarman, A., Nepveu, A., Echelard, Y., Dymetryszyn, J., Drolet, M., and Goyer, C. (1987). Molecular cloning and sequencing of the *hemD* gene of *Escherichia coli* and preliminary data on the *uro* operon, *J. Bacteriol.* **169**:4257–4262.

Sassa, S., and Granick, S. (1970). Induction of 5-aminolevulinic acid synthase in chick embryo liver cells in culture, *Proc. Nat. Acad. Sci. (U.S.A.)* **67**:517–522.

Sburlati, A., Frydman, R. B., Valasinas, A., Rose, S., Priestap, H. A., and Frydman, B. (1983). Biosynthesis of uroporphyrinogens. Interaction among 2-(aminomethyl)bilanes and the enzymatic system, *Biochemistry* **22**:4006–4013.

Schauder, J. R., Jendrezejewski, S., Abell, A., Hart, G. J., and Battersby, A. R. (1987). Stereochemistry of formation of the hydroxymethyl group of hydroxymethylbilane the precursor for uroporphyrinogen III, *J. Chem. Soc. Chem. Comm.* 436–439.

Schimd, R., and Shemin, D. (1955). The enzymic formation of porphobilinogen from 5-aminolevulinic acid and its conversion to protoporphyrin, *J. Amer. Chem. Soc.* **77**:506–508.

Schoenhaut, D. S., and Curtis, P. J. (1986). Nucleotide sequence of mouse 5-aminolevulinic acid synthase cDNA and expression of its gene in hepatic and erythroid tissues, *Gene* **48**:55–63.

Schon, A., Krupp, G., Gough, S. P., Berry-Lowe, S., Kannangara, C. G., and Soll, D. (1986). The RNA required in the first step of chlorophyll biosynthesis is a chloroplast glutamate-tRNA, *Nature* **322**:281–284.

Scott, A. I., Ho, K. S., Kajiwara, M., and Takahashi, T. (1976). Biosynthesis of uroporphyrinogen III from porphobilinogen. Resolution of the enigmatic switch mechanism, *J. Amer. Chem. Soc.* **98**:1589–1591.

Seehra, J. S., Gore, M. G., Chaudhry, A. G., and Jordan, P. M. (1981). 5-Aminolevulinic acid dehydratase. The role of sulfhydryl groups in 5-aminolevulinic acid dehydratase from bovine liver, *Eur. J. Biochem.* **114**:263–269.

Seehra, J. S., and Jordan, P. M. (1980). Mechanisms of action of porphobilinogen deaminase: Ordered addition of the four porphobilinogen molecules in the formation of preuroporphyrinogen, *J. Amer. Chem. Soc.* **102**:6841–6846.

Seehra, J. S., and Jordan, P. M. (1981). 5-Aminolevulinic acid dehydratase. Alkylation of an essential thiol in the bovine liver enzyme by active site directed reagents, *Eur. J. Biochem.* **113**:435–446.

Shemin, D. (1972). 5-Aminolevulinic acid dehydratase, The Enzymes (P. D. Boyer, Ed.), 3rd ed., Academic, New York, Vol. 7, pp. 323–337.

Shemin, D. (1976). 5-Aminolevulinic acid dehydratase; structure, function and mechanism, *Philos. Trans. Roy. Soc. Lond. Ser. B* **273**:109–115.

Shemin, D., London, I. M., and Rittenberg, D. (1950). Synthesis of protoporphyrin in vitro by red blood cells of the duck, *J. Biol. Chem.* **183**:757–765.

Shemin, D., and Rittenberg, D. (1945). The utilisation of glycine for the synthesis of a porphyrin, *J. Biol. Chem.* **159**:567–568.

Shemin, D., and Russell, C. S. (1953). 5-Aminolevulinic acid, its role in the biosynthesis of porphyrins and purines, *J. Amer. Chem. Soc.* **75**:4873–4875.

Shemin, D., Russell, C. S., and Abramsky, T. (1955). The succinate glycine cycle. The mechanism of pyrrole synthesis, *J. Biol. Chem.* **215**:613–626.

Shemin, D., and Wittenberg, J. (1951). THe mechanism of porphyrin formation. The role of the tricarboxylic acid cycle, *J. Biol. Chem.* **192**:315–334.

Sinclair, P. R., Bement, W. J., Bonkovsky, H. L., and Sinclair, J. F. (1984). Inhibition of uroporphyrinogen decarboxylase by halogenated biphenyls in chick hepatic cultures. Essential role for induction of cytochrome P-450, *Biochem. J.* **222**:737–748.

Smith, A. G., and Francis, J. E. (1981). Investigations with rat liver uroporphyrinogen decarboxylase. Comparison of porphyrinogens I and III as substrates and the inhibition by porphyrins, *Biochem. J.* **195**:241–250.

Smith, K. M., and Huster, M. S. (1987). Bacteriochlorophyll-c formation via the glutamate C-5 pathway in *Chlorobium* bacteria, *J. Chem. Soc. Chem. Comm.* 14–16.

Smythe, E., and Williams, D. C. (1988). Rat liver uroporphyrinogen III synthase has similar properties to the enzyme from *Euglena gracilis* including the absence of a requirement for a reversibly bound cofactor for activity, *Biochem. J.* **253**:275–279.

Snell, E. E., and di Mari, S. (1970). Schiff base intermediates in enzyme catalysis, The Enzymes (P. D. Boyer, Ed.), 3rd ed., Academic, New York, vol. 2, pp. 335–370.

Sommer and Beyersmann (1984). Zinc and cadmium in 5-aminolevulinic acid dehydratase. Equilibrium, kinitic, and [113]Cd-nmr-studies, *J. Inorg. Biochem.* **20**:131–145.

Stark, W. M., Hart, G. J., and Battersby, A. R. (1986). Synthetic studies on the proposed spiro-intermediate for the biosynthesis of the natural porphyrins: Inhibition of cosynthase, *J. Chem. Soc. Chem. Comm.* 465–467.

Straka, J. G., and Kushner, J. P. (1983). Purification and characteristics of bovine hepatic uroporphyrinogen decarboxylase, *Biochemistry* **22**:4664–4672.

Tait, G. H. (1972). Coproporphyrinogenase activity in extracts of *Rhodobacter spheroides* and *Chromatium D*, *Biochem. J.* **128**:1159–1169.

Thomas, S. D., and Jordan, P. M. (1986). Nucleotide sequence of the *hemC* locus encoding porphobilinogen deaminase of *Escherichia coli* K12, *Nucl. Acids Res.* **14**, 6215–6226.

Thunell, S., Holmberg, L., and Lundgren, J. (1987). 5-Aminolevulinic acid dehydratase porphyria in infancy. A clinical and biochemical study, *J. Clin. Chem. Clin. Biochem.* **25**:5–14.

Tsai, S. F., Bishop, D. F., and Desnick, R. J. (1987). Purification and properties of uroporphyrinogen III synthase from human erythrocytes, *J. Biol. Chem.* **262**:1268–1273.

Tsai, S.-F. Bishop, D. F., and Desnick, R. J. (1988). Human uroporphyrinogen III synthase. Molecular cloning, nucleotide sequence and expression of full length cDNA; *Proc. Nat. Acad. Sci. (U.S.A.)* to appear.

Tsukamoto, I., Yoshinaga, T., and Sano, S. (1979). The role of zinc with special reference to the essential thiol groups in 5-aminolevulinic acid dehydratase of bovine liver, *Biochim. Biophys. Acta* **570**:167–178.

Tsukamoto, I., Yoshinaga, T., and Sano, S. (1980). Zinc and cysteine residues in the active site of bovine 5-aminolevulinic acid dehydratase, *Int. J. Biochem.* **12**:751–756.

Tuboi, S. Kim, H. J., and Kikuchi, G. (1970). Occurrence and properties of two types of 5-aminolevulinic acid synthase in *Rhodobacter spheroides*, *Arch. Biochem. Biophys.* **138**:147–154.

Urban-Grimal, D., Volland, C., Garnier, T., Dehoux, P., and Labbe-Bois, R. (1986). The nucleotide sequence of the *hem*1 gene and evidence for a precursor form of the mitochondrial 5-aminolevulinate synthase in *Saccharomyces cerevisae*, *Eur. J. Biochem.* **156**:511–519.

van Heyningen, S., and Shemin, S. (1971). Quarternary structure of 5-aminolevulinic acid dehydratase from *Rhodobacter spheroides*, *Biochemistry* **10**:4676–4682.

Volland, C., and Felix, F. (1984). Isolation and properties of 5-aminolevulinic acid synthase from the yeast *Saccharomyces cerevisae*, *Eur. J. Biochem.* **142**:551–557.

Wang, W.-Y. Gough, S. P., and Kannangara, C. G. (1981). Isolation of three soluble enzymes required for the conversion of glutamate into 5-aminolevulinate, *Carlsberg Res. Comm.* **46**:243–257.

Wang, W. Y., Huang, D. D., Stachon, D., Gough, S. P., and Kannangara, C. G. (1984). Purification, characterization and fractionation of the 5-aminolevulinic acid synthesizing enzymes from light-grown *Chlamydomonas reinhardtii*, *Plant Physiol.* **74**, 569–575.

Warnick, G. R., and Burnham, B. F. (1971). Purification and characterization of 5-aminolevulinic acid synthase, *J. Biol. Chem.* **246**:6880–6885.

Warren, M. J., and Jordan, P. M. (1988a). Further evidence for the involvement of a dipyrromethane cofactor at the active site of porphobilinogen deaminases, *Biochem. Soc. Trans.* **16**:963–965.

Warren, M. J., and Jordan, P. M. (1988b). Investigation into the nature of substrate binding to the dipyrromethane cofactor of *Escherichia coli* porphobilinogen deaminase, *Biochemistry* **27**:9020–9030.

Weinstein, J. D., and Beale, S. I. (1983). Separate physiological roles and subcellular compartments for two tetrapyrrole biosynthetic pathways in *Euglena gracilis*, *J. Biol. Chem.* **258**:6799–6807.

Weinstein, J. D., and Beale, S. I. (1984). Biosynthesis of protoheme and heme a precursors solely from glutamate in the unicellular red alga *Cyanidium caldarium*, *Plant Physiol.* **74**:146–151.

Weinstein, J. D., and Beale, S. I. (1985). RNA is required for enzymic conversion of glutamate into 5-aminolevulinic acid by extracts of *Chlorella vulgaris*, *Arch. Biochem. Biophys.* **239**:87–93.

Westall, R. G. (1952). The isolation of porphobilinogen from a patient with acute porphyria, *Nature* **170**:614–616.

Wetmer, J. G., Bishop, D. F., Cantelmo, C., and Desnick, R. J. (1986). Human 5-aminolevulinic acid dehydratase: Nucleotide sequence of a full-length cDNA clone, *Proc. Nat. Acad. Sci. (U.S.A)* **83**:7703–7707.

Williams, D. C., Morgan, G. S., McDonald, E., and Battersby, A. R. (1981). Purification of porphobilinogen deaminase from *Euglena gracilis* and studies of its kinetics, *Biochem. J.* **193**:301–310.

Wu, W., Shemin, D., Richards, K. E., and Williams, R. C. (1974). The quarternary structure of 5-aminolevulinic acid dehydratase from bovine liver, *Proc. Nat. Acad. Sci. (U.S.A)* **69**:2585–2588.

Yamamoto, M., Yew, N. S., Federspeil, M., Dodgson, J. B., Hayashi, N., and Engel, J. D. (1985). Isolation of recombinant cDNAs encoding chicken, erythroid 5-aminolevulinic acid synthase, *Proc. Nat. Acad. Sci. (U.S.A.)* **82**:3702–3706.

Zaman, Z., Jordan, P. M., and Akhtar, M. (1973). Mechanism and stereochemistry of the 5-aminolevulinic acid synthase reaction, *Biochem. J.* **135**:257–263.

Conversion of Coproporphyrinogen to Protoheme in Higher Eukaryotes and Bacteria: Terminal Three Enzymes

Harry A. Dailey

I. Introduction

The terminal three steps of the heme biosynthetic pathway catalyze the conversion of coproporphyrinogen III to protoheme IX. This involves the oxidative decarboxylation of two propionate groups on the A and B rings to vinyl groups, the six-electron oxidation of the porphyrinogen to porphyrin, and the insertion of iron (Fig. 3.1). The three enzymes involved are coproporphyrinogen oxidase, protoporphyrinogen oxidase, and ferrochelatase. In eukaryotic cells these three enzymes are all located in the mitochondria in contrast to the preceding four enzymes which are cytosolic. In prokaryotes the terminal two enzymes appear to be integral membrane proteins that are associated with the cytoplasmic membrane while coproporphyrinogen oxidase may be soluble.

All three of these steps present interesting mechanistic problems. In eukaryotes oxygen is the electron acceptor for both enzymes, while in prokaryotes there appears to be a necessary coupling with the cell respiratory chain by protoporphyrinogen oxidase and a requirement for several cofactors for coproporphyrinogen oxidase. In all cell types ferrochelatase utilizes only ferrous iron and protoporphyrin IX. Thus, a source of reduced iron is necessary. The requirement for heme other than protoheme IX must apparently be met by modification of the macrocycle after iron insertion since ferrochelatase does not utilize protein-bound porphyrins or modified porphyrins such as "heme a" porphyrin.

Since the heme biosynthetic pathway in yeast and photosynthetic organisms is covered in detail in separate chapters, only higher eukaryotic and prokaryotic systems are reviewed in this chapter. Furthermore, since regulation and porphyrias are reviewed elsewhere, they are also not covered here.

II. Eukaryotic Coproporphyrinogen Oxidase

The antepenultimate step in heme biosynthesis is the oxidative decarboxylation of coproporphyrinogen III to protoporphyrinogen IX which is carried out by coproporphyrinogen oxidase (EC 1.3.3.3). This enzyme, which had also been called coproporphyrinogenase, catalyzes the conversion of two propionate groups at positions 2 and 4 to vinyl groups. Two molecules of CO_2 are eliminated and for the eukaryotic enzyme molecular oxygen is required as an electron acceptor.

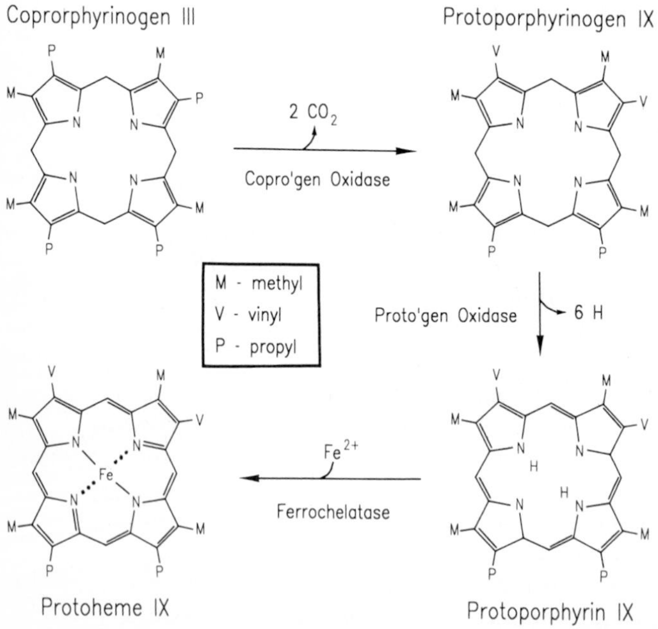

Figure 3.1 Terminal three steps of the heme biosynthetic pathway. The reactions catalyzed in these steps are identical in all organisms examined to date, but the characteristics of the individual enzymes and the specific enzymatic mechanism may vary.

This enzymatic step was identified over 35 years ago, but until Porra and Falk (1984) demonstrated the accumulation of protoporphyrinogen it was proposed that this step involved both vinyl group formation and the subsequent oxidation of the porphyrinogen to protoporphyrin IX.

A. Properties

Early attempts at the purification of coproporphyrinogen oxidase were described by Sano and Granick (1961) for the enzyme from bovine liver and later by Batlle et al. (1965) for the rat liver enzyme. While neither succeeded in preparing a homogeneous preparation, both were able to provide new information about substrate specificity and catalytic properties. The rat liver enzyme was reported to have a molecular weight of $80,000 \pm 8000$. There was no evidence for any chromophoric or dialyzable cofactors and the addition of a variety of potential electron acceptors had no effect on enzyme activity. Oxygen was found to be the obligate electron acceptor in the reaction. Sulfhydryl reagents reportedly inhibited activity and Cd^{2+} and Pb^{2+} were inhibitory.

Purification to homogeneity from bovine liver was achieved by Yoshinaga and Sano in 1980. This enzyme is a single polypeptide chain with a molecular weight of 71,600. Its amino acid composition revealed that it has a relatively high number of aromatic amino acids (12%). As was reported for the rat enzyme there is no evidence for any chromophoric cofactors, and metal analysis gave negative results. Added electron acceptors, metal ions, and sulfhydryl reagents had no effect upon coproporphyrinogen oxidase activity. One interesting feature that was reported was the stimulation of activity by some detergents and phospholipids. This will be discussed in more detail below. The pH optimum is 7.4 and the reported apparent K_m of the purified enzyme for coproporphyrinogen is 48 μM. A K_m for oxygen was not reported.

Unlike crude preparations of the enzyme, the purified bovine enzyme was reported to be unaffected by metal ions and was similarly unaffected by metal chelators. There are three free sulfhydryl groups in the protein, but modification of these did not result in the loss of activity. However, modification of two or more tyrosyl residues with tetranitromethane did result in the loss of coproporphyrinogen oxidase activity. Kinetic studies on the modified enzyme suggested that at least one tyrosyl residue was required for normal catalysis.

B. Catalytic mechanism

A number of investigators have studied the manner in which the two propionate side chains are enzymatically converted to two vinyl groups. The conversion proceeds via a tripropionate monovinyl porphyrinogen

(Sano and Granick, 1961). Two isomers are possible: harderoporphyrinogen, a 2-vinyl, 4-propionate porphyrinogen; and isoharderoporphyrinogen, a 4-vinyl, 2-propionate porphyrinogen. Harderoporphyrin is found in small amounts in many tissues and in high concentrations in the harderian gland of the rat (Kennedy, 1970; Smith and Belcher, 1974). Likewise in in vitro assays harderoporphyrin, but not isoharderoporphyrin, is found.

In elegant studies by the Elder and Jackson groups (Jackson et al., 1974, 1978, 1980; Elder et al., 1978), it had been clearly demonstrated that the enzymatic reaction proceeds in a stepwise fashion first decarboxylating the 2-position propionate and then the 4 position. Under normal conditions free harderoporphyrinogen is not released from the enzyme and exogenously supplied harderoporphyrinogen is not further decarboxylated since it does not equilibrate with enzyme-bound harderoporphyrinogen so that coproporphyrinogen is preferentially converted to protoporphyrinogen. The decarboxylation of the 2-position propionate proceeds at a faster rate than the subsequent decarboxylation of the 4 position.

Coproporphyrinogen oxidase, which utilizes the naturally occurring III isomer most rapidly, will also decarboxylate the IV but not the I or II isomers (Fig. 3.2). It has been postulated, based upon experimental data, that the enzyme recognizes the side-chain sequence of methyl(vinyl)-methyl-propionate-methyl, and will only decarboxylate a propionate that is flanked by methyl groups. These requirements are not satisfied by the 4-propionate group of coproporphyrinogen III, but they are satisfied by the 2-propionate group. Thus, the enzymatic decarboxylation proceeds with the 2 propionate first, followed by the 4 propionate, without the release of an intermediate. These studies have been extended with the examination of purified enzyme (Yoshinaga and Sano, 1980b). Yoshinaga and Sano (1980b) found that isoharderoporphyrinogen is converted at a slower rate than harderoporphyrinogen and coproporphyrinogen III, and, thus, proposed that the enzyme initially recognizes a side-chain sequence of methyl-methyl-propionate-methyl-propionate.

The manner in which the propionates are oxidized and decarboxylated to vinyl groups has attracted considerable attention. One early model suggested that the process proceeded via an acrylic acid side chain (Batlle et al., 1965). This proposal has generally been dismissed since labeling studies show that the hydrogen atoms of the methylene groups near the propionate carboxyl groups are retained (Battersby et al., 1972; Zamen et al., 1972). Currently, two models exist that are consistent with the available data. The first of these suggests a β-hydroxypropionate as an intermediate (Sano, 1966), whereas the second proposes that a hydroxyl group is not involved but that the reaction proceeds via hydride ion removal with simultaneous decarboxylation (Seehra et al., 1983) (Fig. 3.3).

In support of the hydroxypropionate model Yoshinaga and Sano (1980b) demonstrated that for the purified enzyme the 2-β-hydroxypropionate derivative is an effective substrate. Indeed, it was shown that 2-β-hydroxypropionate-4-propionate-, 2,4-bis(β-hydroxypropionate)-, and 2-propionate-4-β-hydroxypropionate deuteroporphyrinogen IX were all effectively converted to protoporphyrinogen IX by coproporphyrinogen oxidase. These studies appear to confirm the earlier hypothesis (Sano, 1966; Chaudhry et al., 1977; Jackson et al., 1978) that the enzymatic reaction proceeds via hydroxypropionate intermediates prior to decarboxylation. Inactivation studies with tetranitromethane on the purified enzyme also revealed some interesting catalytic features which are consistent with this model (Yoshinaga and Sano, 1980b). The enzyme

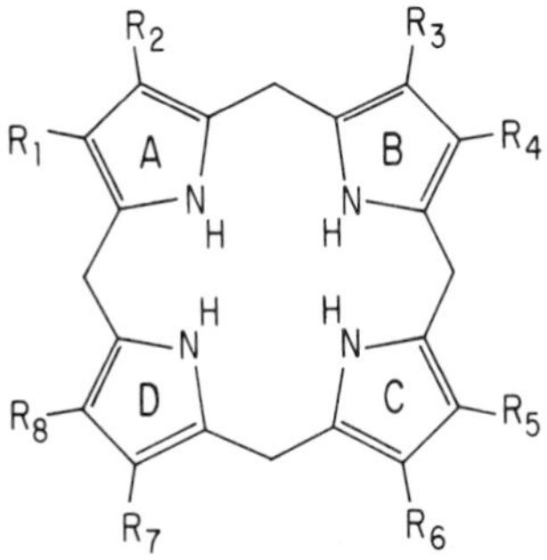

Porphyrinogen	R_1	R_2	R_3	R_4	R_5	R_6	R_7	R_8
Copro - I	M	P	M	P	M	P	M	P
Copro - II	M	P	P	M	M	P	P	M
Copro - III	M	P	M	P	M	P	P	M
Copro - IV	P	M	M	P	M	P	P	M
Hardero -	M	V	M	P	M	P	P	M
Isohardero -	M	P	M	V	M	P	P	M
Proto - IX	M	V	M	V	M	P	P	M
Proto - XIII	V	M	M	V	M	P	P	M
Meso - IX	M	E	M	E	M	P	P	M

M - methyl   P - propyl

V - vinyl   E - ethyl

Figure 3.2 Structural isomers of some common porphyrinogens.

will convert 2,4-bis(β-hydroxypropionate) deuteroporphyrinogen into protoporphyrinogen. Modification of 2.8 tyrosyl residues inactivated enzyme activity with coproporphyrinogen, but not when 2,4-bis(β-hydroxypropionate) deuteroporphyrinogen was a substrate. These data suggest that protein tyrosyl residues are involved in β-hydroxypropionate formation, but not in the subsequent dehydration and decarboxylation.

As proponents of the hydride model, Seehra et al. (1983) suggest that the enzyme does not possess the characteristics generally associated with a hydroxylation reaction, other than the requirement for oxygen. Also the ability of an anaerobic organism (see below) to catalyze this reaction in the absence of molecular oxygen does not favor a hydroxyl intermediate. In the hydride model it is suggested that the driving force of the reaction may be the pyrrolic nitrogen electrons.

Since so little is known of the anaerobic coproporphyrinogen oxidase enzyme other than the fact that it does not use oxygen and requires a variety of cofactors, it may be reasonable to suggest that nature has selectively incorporated both of the proposed schemes to catalyze this one step depending upon the nature of the organism involved.

C. Cellular location and lipid stimulation

In eukaryotic cells coproporphyrinogen oxidase is associated with the mitochondrion. Studies by Elder and Evans (1978) and Grandchamp et al. (1978) clearly demonstrate that the enzyme is located in the intermembrane space between the outer and inner mitochondrial membranes. The data suggest that the enzyme, while soluble, is associated with the outer surface of the inner membrane, thus, making it a peripherial membrane protein. This would physically position it near the next pathway enzyme, protoporphyrinogen oxidase. The stimulation of puri-

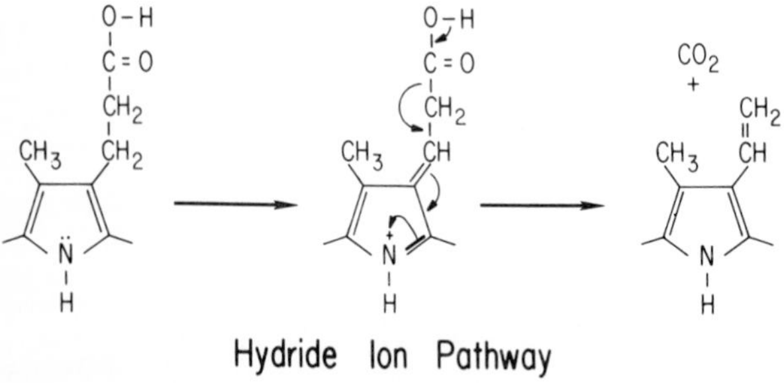

Hydride Ion Pathway

Figure 3.3 Two possible catalytic mechanisms for coproporphyrinogen oxidase. The specifics for each proposal are given in the text [adopted from Seehra et al. (1983)].

fied enzyme activity by detergents and phospholipids is then a reasonable and not unexpected finding (Yoshinaga and Sano, 1980a).

A purified, but not crude, enzyme was stimulated 3.6-fold by a crude phospholipid extract and, to a lesser extent, by neutral or choline-containing lipids. Maximal stimulation was found with phospholipids and lysophospholipids. Triglycerides and free fatty acids did not stimulate activity. The activation by phospholipids was manifested as both an increase in V_{max} as well as a decrease in K_m (apparent) from 48 to 18 μM. Nonionic detergents such as Tweens and Triton X100 also stimulated activity about twofold.

III. Eukaryotic Protoporphyrinogen Oxidase

The penultimate step in the heme biosynthetic pathway is the six-electron oxidation of protoporphyrinogen IX into protoporphyrin IX. This is catalyzed by the enzyme protoporphyrinogen oxidase (EC 1.3.3.4) in a step that requires molecular oxygen in eukaryotic cells. While chemical oxidation of protoporphyrinogen to protoporphyrin is known to occur rapidly at neutral pH, this appears not to happen normally in cells. Porra and Falk (1964) proposed the existence of an enzyme to catalyze this biological oxidation based upon the observed accumulation of protoporphyrinogen by ox liver extracts. Oxygen was required for this conversion. The existence of this enzyme was proposed by a number of investigators, based upon indirect observations, but it was the partial purification of this enzyme by Poulson and Polglase in 1975 that confirmed its existence.

A. Properties

Protoporphyrinogen oxidase was partially purified from yeast (Poulson and Polglase, 1975) and rat liver mitochondria (Poulson, 1976) during the 1970s. Both enzymes were bound to the mitochondrial membrane fraction and required detergents to solubilize them prior to purification. The solubilized rat liver enzyme was reported to have a molecular weight of 35,000. The apparent K_m for protoporphyrinogen was 11 μM, and, while there was a reported requirement for molecular oxygen as the electron acceptor, no K_m for O_2 was determined. There was no stimulation by cations or electron acceptors although thiol reagents inhibited activity. Human protoporphyrinogen oxidase has also recently been solubilized and reported to have a molecular weight of about 32,000 and an apparent K_m of 0.16 μM for protoporphyrinogen at pH 7.2 (Camadro et al., 1985). Once again, however, no K_m for oxygen was reported. Substrate inhibition by concentrations of protoporphyrinogen above 5 μM was also reported. Cobalt protoporphyrin was reported to be a noncompetitive inhibitor with a K_i of 0.8 μM.

Recently, protoporphyrinogen oxidase has been purified to apparent homogeneity from bovine liver (Siepker et al., 1987) and mouse liver (Dailey and Karr, 1987). The enzyme from these sources is a monomer with a molecular weight of approximately 65,000 in detergent solution. For the bovine enzyme Siepker et al. (1987) suggest that there is a tightly bound molecule of FAD, while Dailey and Karr reported finding no chromophoric cofactors for the mouse enzyme recent reexamination has shown the presence of one molecule of FMN (Proulx and Dailey, unpublished data). Examination of a variety of putative electron acceptors with the mouse enzyme (Dailey and Karr, 1987; Ferreira and Dailey, 1988) revealed no significant stimulation. Quinones at low concentration had a stimulatory effect, while at concentrations above 30 μM all tested quinones were inhibitory. Dicumarol, an inhibitor of quinone-utilizing enzymes, gave the same stimulation/inhibition pattern suggesting that the stimulation by low concentrations of quinones was not attributable to specific interactions but rather due to some system artifact.

Oleic acid stimulated the purified bovine enzyme 66% (Siepker et al., 1987) and mouse protoporphyrinogen oxidase was also affected by phospholipids (Ferreira and Dailey, 1987). For the mouse enzyme the apparent K_m for protoporphyrinogen was 5.6 μM when the enzyme was soluble in detergent solution, but upon incorporation into a phospholipid membrane (egg phosphatidylcholine) the apparent K_m decreased to 0.6 μM, and if cardiolipin, a mitochondrial phospholipid, was present the apparent K_m decreased to 0.2 μM. More extensive kinetic analysis with the soluble mouse enzyme yielded a K_m of 6.6 μM for protoporphyrinogen and a K_m of 125 μM for oxygen (Ferreira and Dailey, 1988). The enzyme utilizes protoporphyrinogen IX and at lower activity mesoporphyrinogen IX, but no other tested porphyrinogen. The pH optimum is 7.1. The purified bovine enzyme has a reported K_m of 16.6 μM for protoporphyrinogen and a K_m for oxygen was not reported.

B. Catalytic mechanism

In the conversion of protoporphyrinogen to protoporphyrin six electrons are removed with molecular oxygen as the electron acceptor in higher eukaryotes. Early work on the enzyme demonstrated that it exhibits relatively high substrate specificity since it will use only mesoporphyrinogen IX, protoporphyrinogen XIII, and 2(4)vinyl-4(2)hydroxyethyl deuteroporphyrinogen, although all of these are used at much lower rates than protoporphyrinogen IX (Jackson et al., 1978; Poulson and Polglase, 1975). Coproporphyrinogen I and III and uroporphyrinogen I and III are not substrates.

Two lines of evidence are available to suggest the presence of an enzymatically, rather than chemically, catalyzed oxidation of protoporphyrinogen. In the six-electron transformation, two possible intermediates exist, didehydro and tetradehydro compounds. Poulson and Polglase (1975) identified nonenzymatically oxidized prototetrahydroporphyrin in their studies, but found no evidence for the accumulation of any intermediates in the enzymatic reactions. Jackson et al. (1974) also demonstrated that meso-tritium-labeled protoporphyrinogen lost only 50% of its label in chicken hemolysate extracts rather than the 95% that would be expected from chemical oxidation.

Since the initial reports on the enzyme, it has been accepted that oxygen is the electron acceptor. This hypothesis has remained intact inspite of the examination of numerous flavin- and quinone-type compounds with the purified enzyme (Ferreira and Dailey, 1988). The data from the mouse enzyme show that oxygen serves as the electron acceptor with a K_m of 125 μM. Furthermore, the stoichiometry of the reaction demonstrates that 3 mol of O_2 is consumed per mole of protoporphyrinogen oxidized. These data, along with unpublished results, led these same investigators to propose that H_2O_2 rather than H_2O was one of the reaction products. Since the peroxide produced was not quantitatively determined, the possibility exists that additional products may be produced. Well-characterized examples of enzymes catalyzing six-electron oxidations, such as xanthine oxidase, exist in which some, but not all, of the electrons go to produce H_2O_2 (Malmstrom, 1982).

The kinetic data, when analyzed by Michaelis Menton approaches, are inconsistent with a ping-pong mechanism that one would anticipate with three molecules of O_2 per one molecule of porphyrinogen (Ferreira, 1986). These data may be explained by a penta complex, which is unlikely, or by the fact that the rate constant for the addition of the first O_2 molecule is rate-limiting and much slower than for the other two O_2 molecules.

It has been shown that the rat and bovine protoporphyrinogen oxidases are inhibited by some sulfhydryl reagents such as N-ethylmaleimide and iodoacetamide (Poulson, 1976; Siepker et al., 1987). It was proposed that enzyme sulfhydryl groups might function in binding substrates via the macrocycle vinyl groups (Poulson and Polglase, 1975). However, the lack of inhibition of the mouse enzyme by these same reagents suggests that explanations involving factors other than substrate binding or specific catalytic interactions need to be invoked to explain inhibition in the rat and bovine enzymes.

At the present time there are no sufficient data to postulate a model for catalysis or even substrate binding. Since the enzyme uses only protoporphyrinogen and mesoporphyrinogen IX, it is obvious that the enzyme binding site for porphyrinogen recognizes not only the vinyl groups at positions 2 and 4 on the A and B ring, but also the propionates at positions 6 and 7 on the C and D ring. While there is substrate inhibition at high concentrations, N-methylprotoporphyrin, a strong inhibitor of ferrochelatase, has no inhibitory effect on the oxidase (Dailey and Karr, 1987). These data support a model of relatively high specificity for substrate binding, although the critical protein features involved in binding or orientation are currently unidentified. In light of the high specificity for porphyrinogen, it is of interest to note that bilirubin, as well as its ditaurine conjugate, has been found to be a competitive inhibitor of mouse protoporphyrinogen oxidase (Ferreira and Dailey, 1988; Ferreira et al., 1988). A possible physiological consequence of inhibition may be seen in Gilbert's syndrome where bilirubin is known to accumulate and the levels of protoporphyrinogen oxidase in circulating lymphocytes are lower than normal (McColl et al., 1987).

Likewise, those features involved in actual catalysis are a mystery at present. An interesting feature of the bovine FAD is that it is only oxidized with difficulty, that is, it is present in a reduced form in the active enzyme (Siepker et al., 1987). This is unusual since one would expect that the bound FAD would normally be oxidized and would only be reduced in the presence of porphyrinogen. The mouse FMN, however, is present in the oxidized state in the isolated protein (Proulx and Dailey, unpublished data). An additional feature not yet examined is the possibility of protein tyrosyl residue involvement as has been proposed for coproporphyrinogen oxidase (Yoshinaga and Sano, 1980b).

C. Cellular location and lipid effect

Poulson demonstrated in 1976 that in rat liver and human fibroblasts a majority of protoporphyrinogen oxidase activity is associated with the mitochondrial fraction and that detergents are necessary to solubilize the activity from the membrane fraction. Deybach et al. (1985) fractionated rat liver mitochondria and found that enzyme activity is associated with the inner mitochondrial membrane. The question concerning the orientation of the enzyme on the inner mitochondrial membrane was approached by these same investigators. They suggested, based upon proteolytic digestion, chemical modification with diazobenzene sulfonate, and porphyrinogen accessibility of sonicated and intact mitoplasts, that the enzyme was accessible from both sides of the membrane. Ferreira et al. (1988) examined this question by using a membrane-impermeable inhibitor of protoporphyrinogen oxidase. They reported that the water-soluble, ditaurine conjugate of bilirubin, which is an inhibitor of purified protoporphyrinogen oxidase, inhibited enzyme activity in intact mitochondria as well as mitoplasts and sonicated mitochondria. Since this charged conjugate cannot cross biological membranes, it was concluded that the oxidase must have its active site facing the cytoplasmic side of the inner mitochondrial membrane.

The effects of lipids on protoporphyrinogen oxidase activity have not been studied in as much detail as have the effects of lipids on ferrochelatase or coproporphyrinogen oxidase, but the available reports suggest that this enzyme activity is stimulated by some lipids. The bovine enzyme is reported to be stimulated by oleic acid (Siepker et al., 1987), although additional fatty acids or phospholipids were not tested. The mouse enzyme was reconstituted into phospholipid vesicles composed of egg phosphatidylcholine with or without cardiolipin. As detailed above, the K_m for porphyrinogen decreased over 10-fold under these conditions. It was also reported that the activation energy of protoporphyrinogen oxidase was decreased from 5.7 to 4.5 kcal $\cdot$ mol^{-1} upon incorporation of the purified enzyme into dimyristoylphosphatidylcholine vesicles (Ferreira and Dailey, 1988). This compares with reported activation energies of 9.1 and 11.4 kcal $\cdot$ mol^{-1} for the partially purified rat liver and yeast enzymes, respectively (Poulson, 1976). No added phospholipids were reported to be present in the assays of these preparations.

IV. Eukaryotic Ferrochelatase

The terminal step in the heme biosynthetic pathway is the insertion of iron into protoporphyrin IX to give the final product, protoheme IX. This step is catalyzed by the enzyme called ferochelatase (occasionally heme synthase) although the proper name is protoheme ferrolyase (EC 4.9.9.1.1). Ferrochelatase activity was reported in cell extracts in 1956 by Goldberg's group and has since been found in a wide variety of tissue and cell types (Yoneyama et al., 1962, 1965; Porra and Jones, 1963; Porra and Lascelles, 1965; Labbe and Hubbard, 1960). While it is recognized that nonenzymatic insertion of iron may occur (Tokunaga and Sano, 1972; Kassner and Walchak, 1973), the description of a bacterial heme auxotroph which lacked ferrochelatase activity and exhibited an absolute requirement for protoheme established the biological role for this enzyme (Dailey and Lascelles, 1974).

A. Properties

Ferrochelatase activity was described in 1956, but the first successful purification procedure was not published until 1981. Numerous attempts were made in the 25-year interim, but difficulties in the detergent fractionation of the solubilized, low-abundance protein created major roadblocks for the purification techniques available during that period.

Although Mailer et al. (1980) reported the purification of rat liver ferrochelatase using a heme affinity column, the first bonafide purification of ferrochelatase was reported in 1981 by Taketani and Tokunaga from rat liver. The major innovation of this scheme was the use of a reactive blue-dye column in the presence of first nonionic and then anionic detergents. Using minor modifications of this procedure, ferrochelatase has now been purified from bovine liver (Dailey and Fleming, 1983; Taketani and Tokunaga, 1982), chicken erythrocytes (Hanson and Dailey, 1984), mouse liver (Dailey et al., 1986a), and human liver (Mathews-Roth et al., 1987). The enzymes from all of these sources are similar in their physical properties, although differences do exist in their kinetic parameters.

Mammalian ferrochelatases that have been purified all have a reported molecular weight of 40,000. Chicken erythrocytes possess an enzyme with a slightly higher reported molecular weight of 42,000. However, immunological cross reactivity of bovine, murine, and chicken ferrochelatases suggests a high degree of structural homology. The amino acid composition has been reported for the rat, bovine, and human enzymes and, although there are differences, none of the enzymes appear to have an unusually large number of hydrophobic residues. No amino acid sequence data are presently available.

The natural porphyrin substrate for ferrochelatase is protoporphyrin IX, but it will utilize a variety of IX isomer porphyrins with substituents at the 2,4 positions of the A and B rings that are hydroxyethyl or smaller in size and uncharged (Fig. 3.4). Only free dicarboxylate prophyrins are substrates and esterified porphyrins or protein-bound porphyrins are not used. The porphyrin specificity for a variety of tissues and animal species has been examined in a number of laboratories. In general, what is found are large quantitative variations in the data, but similar qualitative features. That is, one finds a similar porphyrin (and metal) usage profile (e.g., proto-, hemato-, meso-, and deuteroporphyrin), but with significant quantitative differences in the calculated K_m's for a given substrate.

Two possible explanations may account for the differences in these data: (1) The values actually do differ substantially in quantitative terms from animal to animal; or (2) the difference in values reflects, in part, differences in the techniques used by various laboratories in porphyrin preparation and assay procedures. In support of this second proposal, one need only look at the data published for bovine ferrochelatase to find apparent K_m's for protoporphyrin varying from 11 to 54 μM and the rat enzyme with reported K_m's for mesoporphyrin of 5 to 27 μM (see the references in Table 3.1). Thus, the results from two different laboratories should be carefully compared. Perhaps the most reliable comparisons are either of a qualitative nature or a quantitative nature from a single laboratory.

Other factors that need to be considered are the purity of porphyrins used, the manner in which porphyrin solutions were prepared, and the nature of the enzyme (i.e., membrane-bound vs. solubilized and purified). Recent enzymatic studies have generally made use of high-purity porphyrins, whereas researchers in the 1970s only had much cruder porphyrins available. This may be most critical for protoporphyrin because of the propensity of the vinyl groups to hydrate, thus, forming hematoporphyrin and mixtures of monovinyl, monohydroxyethyl porphyrin.

The manner in which porphyrin solutions are made and stored is also important because of the facility with which aqueous porphyrin solutions form aggregates. One result of this was the early "observation" that ferrochelatase had a biphasic pH optima curve which, in fact, was an artifact attributable to using stored porphyrin solutions since freshly prepared porphyrin solutions yield a single optimum (Dailey and Lascelles, 1974).

Protoporphyrin IX, the physiological substrate, has in all cases exhibited the lowest K_m and usually the lowest V_{max}. Hematoporphyrin

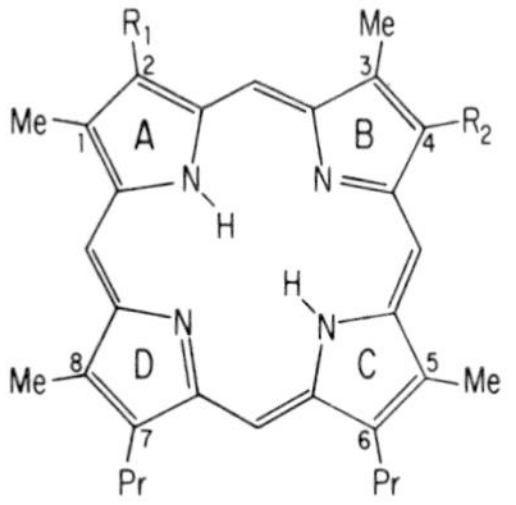

Me = CH$_3$ and Pr = $[CH_2]_2$ CO$_2$H

Porphyrin	R$_1$	R$_2$
Proto-	CH=CH$_2$	CH=CH$_2$
Hemato-	CH(OH)CH$_3$	CH(OH)CH$_3$
2,4-Monohydroxyethyl, monovinyl-*	CH(OH)CH$_3$	CH=CH$_2$
2,4-Monohydroxymethyl, monovinyl-*	CH$_2$OH	CH=CH$_2$
Meso-	CH$_2$CH$_3$	CH$_2$CH$_3$
Deutero-	H	H
2,4-Bis acetal deutero-	CH$_2$CH(OCH$_3$)$_2$	CH$_2$CH(OCH$_3$)$_2$
2,4-Bis glycol deutero-	CH(OH)CH$_2$OH	CH(OH)CH$_2$OH
2,4-Disulfonic deutero-	SO$_3^-$	SO$_3^-$
Copro-III	CH$_2$CH$_2$COOH	CH$_2$CH$_2$COOH

* These are mixtures of isomers.

Figure 3.4 Structures of some IX isomer porphyrins that are commonly used to assay ferrochelatase.

TABLE 3.1 Apparent K_m's for Eukaryotic Ferrochelatases

| Enzyme sources | K_m (μM) | | | | | Reference |
	Iron	Protoporphyrin	Hematoporphyrin	Mesoporphyrin	Deuteroporphyrin	
Human liver	0.5	0.35	—	—	—	Camadro et al., 1984
Mouse liver	—	9.0	9.0	156	247	Dailey et al., 1989
Rat liver	33.1	28.5	—	26.7	—	Taketani and Tokunaga, 1981
Bovine liver	80	11	22	34	47	Dailey and Smith, 1984; Dailey and Fleming, 1983
	46	54	55	46	36	Taketani and Tokunaga, 1982
Sheep liver	—	0.8	—	1.9	4.0	Honeybourne et al., 1979
Chicken erythrocytes	166	37	—	51	80	Hanson and Dailey, 1984
Duck erythrocytes	70	80	—	—	—	Yoneyama et al., 1962

usually has a K_m and V_{max} slightly higher than protoporphyrin, followed by mesoporphyrin, and then deuteroporphyrin. Interestingly, with these substrates one finds increasing K_m and increasing V_{max} when measured in vitro in detergent solutions. While the reason for this remains unclear at present, the increases in V_{max} may reflect the increasing water solubility of this series of porphyrins.

One feature apparent from past studies is that the size of the porphyrin ring side-chain substituents and their positions are critical. Honeybourne et al. (1979) examined the ability of sheep ferrochelatase to use porphyrins with a variety of side-chain substitutions and found that the position of the propionate side chains at positions 6 and 7 on the C and D rings was critical for the porphyrin to serve as a substrate. In comparing protoporphyrin I and mesoporphyrin I, which have propionates at positions 6 and 8, with protoporphyrin IX and mesoporphyrin IX, which have propionates at positions 6 and 7, it was found that the IX but not the I isomers were substrates for the enzyme.

The significance of the 2,4 substituents on the A and B ring has been examined in a variety of species (Yoneyama et al., 1962; Taketani and Tokunaga, 1981, 1982; Dailey, 1982; Dailey and Fleming, 1983; Dailey et al., 1986; Dailey and Smith, 1984; Hanson and Dailey, 1984; Jones and Jones, 1969). The data with sheep ferrochelatase show that the absolute position of these two substituents may be less critical than the 6,7 positions since protoporphyrin XIII (vinyl groups at positions 1,4) works almost as well as protoporphyrin IX (vinyl groups at 2,4) (Honeybourne et al., 1979). However, since only sheep ferrochelatase has been examined with these particular porphyrins, it is not possible to rule out species specificity as the basis for this preference.

Ferrochelatases from four species, chicken, rat, mouse, and bovine, have been examined in some detail with the most extensive studies being done with mouse and bovine liver ferrochelatase. The measured K_m's and apparent K_m's for ferrochelatase show that protoporphyrin IX has the lowest K_m usually in the range of around 10 μM, although highs of over 50 μM and lows of under 1 μM have been reported (see Table 3.1). Hematoporphyrin or 2,4 monovinyl, monohydroxyethyl porphyrin is found to be very similar to protoporphyrin. Mesoporphyrin with ethyl groups at the 2,4 positions has the next highest K_m and also V_{max} with deuteroporphyrin with hydrogens at the 2,4 position usually having the highest V_{max} and K_m. Among the enzymes tested to date, the mouse seems unique in its poor utilization of deuteroporphyrin. In general, it is found that porphyrins with uncharged 2,4 substituents equal in size or smaller than hydroxyethyl will be used in vitro as substrates, while porphyrin with charged or larger substituents at these positions will be found to be competitive inhibitors or very poor substrates.

Table 3.2 shows kinetic data for a variety of porphyrins with mouse and bovine ferrochelatase. By examination it is apparent that significant species-specific differences exist. The fact that a variety of 2,4 substituents can be accommodated by ferrochelatase strongly suggests that these side chains are not involved directly in catalysis, but are most likely involved in spatial orientation of the porphyrin macrocycle. The requirement for both the propionates on rings C and D and the 2,4 substituents on the other two pyrrole rings favors the idea that a four-point orientation of the porphyrin is required to ensure proper alignment of the central nitrogens at the enzyme iron-binding site.

The K_d's for a number of porphyrins and metalloporphyrins with mouse ferrochelatase are shown in Table 3.3. When these values are compared with the K_m's and K_i's for the same enzyme there is little relationship between binding and catalytic efficiency for a given porphyrin. These data would indicate that binding alone is insufficient for catalysis and that orientation of the macrocycle is crucial. In this regard it is apparent that the substituents at the 2,4 positions are critical for this orientation. Minor variations in amino acid residues at the active sites of various species ferrochelatases near the region of the 2,4 side chains could account for the differences seen in substrate specificity. Such changes, while significant and interesting for in vitro studies, would be inconsequential to the in vivo functioning of ferrochelatase since only protoporphyrin IX would ever be seen by the enzyme. Thus, it should

TABLE 3.2   Kinetic Constants for Bovine and Mouse Ferrochelatase*

Porphyrin	Bovine		Mouse	
	K_m (μM)	K_i (μM)	K_m (μM)	K_i (μM)
Protoporphyrin	11	9	—	—
Hematoporphyrin	22	9	—	—
2,4-Monohydroxyethyl, monovinyl porphyrin	23	10	—	—
2,4-Monohydroxymethyl, monovinyl porphyrin	—	62	—	—
Mesoporphyrin	34	156	—	—
Deuteroporphyrin	47	247	—	—
2,4-Bis acetal deuteroporphyrin	—	—	13	36
2,4-Bis glycol deuteroporphyrin	—	—	67	ND[†]
2,4-Disulfonic deuteroporphyrin	—	—	70	ND
N-Methylprotoporphyrin	—	—	0.007	< 0.01
Fe-Protoporphyrin	—	—	—	2.0
Co-Protoporphyrin	—	—	—	3.0
Zn-Protoporphyrin	—	—	—	4.5
Sn-Protoporphyrin	—	—	—	13.0

*Data taken from Dailey and Flemming (1983), Dailey and Smith (1984), and Dailey et al. (1989).
[†]ND—not determined since inhibition was slight and could not be determined accurately.

not be surprising to see relatively wide variations in the acceptability of nonphysiological porphyrins as substrates.

Ferrochelatase will catalyze the insertion of ferrous, but not ferric, iron and divalent cobalt and zinc (Jones and Jones, 1969; Dailey et al., 1986; Mazanowska et al., 1966; Camadro et al., 1984). No other metals have been conclusively shown to be inserted by ferrochelatase, although

TABLE 3.3   Dissociation Constants for Mouse Ferrochelatase*

Porphyrin	K_d (μM)
Protoporphyrin	0.15
Hematoporphyrin	0.15
2,4-Monohydroxymethyl, monovinyl porphyrin	0.25
2,4-Monohydroxymethyl, monovinyl porphyrin	0.20
Mesoporphyrin	0.22
Deuteroporphyrin	0.25
2,4-Bisacetal deuteroporphyrin	0.68
2,4-Bisglycol deuteroporphyrin	0.30
2,4-Disulfonic deuteroporphyrin	0.33
Coproporphyrin III	1.08
N-Methylprotoporphyrin	0.006
Zn-Protoporphyrin	0.65
Sn-Protoporphyrin	0.25

*Taken from Dailey et al. (1989).

a variety of divalent cations are inhibitors of the enzyme. Among these inhibitors are manganese, cadmium, lead, and mercury (Dailey, 1987, and references therein). Among divalent cations that have little or no effect are magnesium, nickel, and copper. Copper is noteworthy since it has been reported to be stimulatory (Wagner and Tephly, 1975), to be inhibitory (Gaertner and Hollebone, 1983), and to have no measurable effect (Dailey, 1987; Dailey et al., 1986; Taketani and Tokunaga, 1981). This range of results may reflect the ability of copper ions to undergo rapid oxidation/reduction reactions which may affect either the sulfhydryl residues of the enzyme or the oxidation state of the iron in the assay mixture.

B. Inhibition of ferrochelatase activity in vitro by heavy metals

Examination of the kinetics of inactivation in a variety of systems has shown that the inhibition by divalent cations is competitive with respect to ferrous iron (Dailey and Fleming, 1983; Dailey, 1987). Mercury is typically the most potent inhibitor of ferrochelatase activity as measured in vitro. Assuming that vicinyl disulfides are involved in binding ferrous iron (see below), then the strong, but sulfhydryl-reversible, inhibition by mercury (as well as arsenite) would easily be explained by its known strong interactions with protein sulfhydryl groups.

Manganese is also a strong inhibitor with K_i reported in the range of 15 μM (Dailey and Fleming, 1983; Dailey, 1987). Similarly, cadmium has strongly inhibitory properties with a K_i of 50 μM (Dailey, 1987). Both of these metals inhibit ferrochelatase in a competitive fashion with respect to ferrous iron. Lead, which is also known to interact with protein sulfhydryls is thought to be an inhibitor of ferrochelatase in vivo. For purified bovine ferrochelatase 10 μM lead inhibits activity in vitro over 60%.

C. N-Methylprotoporphyrin

For a number of years it was recognized that the administration of certain compounds such as 3,5-diethoxycarbonyl-1,4-dihydro-2,4,6-tri-methyl-pyridine (DDC) or griseofulvin to animals resulted in lowered levels of hepatic ferrochelatase activity (Smith and De Matteis, 1980; De Matteis et al., 1987). These same compounds had no effect on enzyme activity when added to cell extracts in vitro and so it was proposed that a metabolite of the added compound, rather than the compound itself, was responsible for enzyme inhibition. This observation was supported by data which showed the cytosolic fraction from DDC-treated mice would inhibit ferrochelatase activity of normal mitochondria in vitro

(Onisawa and Labbe, 1963). Clues to the nature of the inhibitory compound were provided by the observation that in cells where cytochrome P450 was inhibited by SKF 525-A and in newborn animals where cytochrome P450 levels are naturally low, DDC administration did not lead to loss of ferrochelatase activity (De Matteis et al., 1973).

It was noted that in livers in which ferrochelatase activity was reduced by DDC there was an accumulation of a "green pigment." Tephly et al. (1979, 1980, 1981) isolated this green pigment, which was shown to be derived from the heme of cytochrome P450 (Coffman et al., 1982; De Matteis et al., 1982), and demonstrated that it inhibited ferrochelatase activity in vitro. This pigment was identified as N-methylprotoporphyrin, although other compounds may give rise to N-alkylprotoporphyrin with alkyl groups of various sizes. Synthetic N-alkylporphyrins have been produced and the four isomers separated and identified (Ortiz de Montellano, 1980). A number of reviews that outline the discovery, chemical identification, and biological origin of N-alkylporphyrins exist and so this topic will not be covered in much detail here [see Smith and De Matteis (1980), De Matteis et al., (1987), and Cole and Marks (1984)].

The inhibition of ferrochelatase activity by N-alkylporphyrins has been examined in considerable detail in mouse liver by the De Matteis group (De Matteis et al., 1980a, b, 1981, 1982a, b, 1985, 1987; De Matteis and Marks, 1983; Tephly et al., 1979, 1980, 1981) and in chick embryo liver by Marks and co-workers (Marks et al., 1985, 1986, 1987; Cole et al., 1980, 1981a, b, 1982; Cole and Marks, 1980, 1984; Sutherland et al., 1986; McCluskey et al., 1986). In addition, the inhibitory activity of a variety of compounds that may give rise to N-alkylporphyrins have been studied in cell cultures. These cell culture studies by the Marks and Ortiz de Montellano groups (Ortiz de Montellano et al., 1980, 1981, 1986) provide interesting possibilities, but, unfortunately, do not yield unequivocal results since specific compound were not always isolated and demonstrated in vitro to inhibit ferrochelatase.

As documented in a number of papers, the De Matteis group has examined the role of the alkyl group size and position (i.e., which pyrrole ring is alkylated) on the ability of that alkylated porphyrin to inhibit mouse ferrochelatase. What they found was that there are at least three factors involved: (1) the size of the N-alkyl group, (2) the position of the N-alkyl group, and (3) the porphyrin side-chain substituents on the A and B rings at positions 2 and 4 (De Matteis et al., 1985).

With N-methylprotoporphyrin it has been found that ferrochelatase activity in most animal species is about equally inhibited by any of the four possible isomers (De Matteis et al., 1982b). The inhibition of ferrochelatase by N-methylprotoporphyrin has been shown to be via a tight-biding competitive inhibition with a K_i of 7 nM for the bovine enzyme and about 10 nM for the mouse enzyme (Dailey and Fleming,

1983; Dailey et al., 1986a). It should be pointed out that both of these determinations were done with a mixture of the four isomers. However, when the zinc complexes of these isomers are examined one finds substantial differences between those porphyrins with methyl groups on the A or B ring vs. the C or D ring. In this case the C or D ring methylated porphyrins are significantly poorer inhibitors than the A or B ring methylated protoporphyrins (Table 3.4). This finding is quite interesting since formation of the zinc complex is known to result in increased distortion of the porphyrin macrocycle. It has been calculated that the N-methylated pyrrole ring will be canted about 28° from the plane of the macrocycle while insertion of zinc into this same molecule will result in a 38° tilt (Lavallee and Anderson, 1982).

The nature of the 2,4 substituents on the A and B rings also significantly affects the observed inhibitory activity of the four possible N-methylporphyrin isomers with mouse ferrochelatase (De Matteis et al., 1985). While the isomers of N-methylprotoporphyrin are equally potent inhibitors, for N-methylmesoporphyrin, in which the two vinyl groups are replaced by two ethyl groups on the A and B ring, the isomers N-methylated on the A or B ring are about half as inhibitory as those N-methylated on the C or D ring (Table 3.4). The insertion of zinc once again results in a magnification of the difference in inhibitory potency of the C or D vs. A or B alkylated isomers. With deuteroporphyrin, in which the 2,4 vinyl groups have been replaced with hydrogens, there is a significant difference between the N-methylated A or B vs. C or D ring isomers. Thus, the alteration of side chains at the 2,4 positions on the A and B rings, while not affecting the size or orientation of the N-methyl groups, nonetheless has a significant impact on the inhibitory activity of the N-methylated porphyrin.

Increasing the size of the alkyl group in general resulted in decreased inhibitory activity. While the four isomers of N-methylprotoporphyrin are equally inhibitory, increasing the alkyl group size to ethyl decreases

TABLE 3.4   Inhibition of Ferrochelatase by N-Alkylporphyrins*

N-Alkylporphyrin	Inhibitory activity (inhibitory units $\cdot$ nmol^{-1})	
	Isomers A and B	Isomers C and D
N-Methylprotoporphyrin	9.2	10.7
N-Ethylprotoporphyrin	6.7	6.9
N-Propylprotoporphyrin	6.1	0.1
N-Methylmesoporphyrin	8.0	15.0
N-Ethylmesoporphyrin	8.2	0.1
N-Methyldeuteroporphyrin	8.8	0.3
N-Methylprotoporphyrin (zinc complex)	15.7	2.1
N-Methylmesoporphyrin (zinc complex)	6.9	0.5

*Data taken from De Matteis et al. (1985).

the inhibition slightly and N-propylprotoporphyrin has even lower inhibitory activity for the A or B isomers, while the C or D isomers are poor inhibitors. Alteration of the 2,4 positions on the A and B ring for N-ethyl and N-propyl adducts results in the same general changes seen for the N-methylations.

Ortiz de Montellano et al. (1981) reported that for rat ferrochelatase the A or B alkylated isomers of N-ethylprotoporphyrin were stronger inhibitors than the C or D N-alkylated isomers. The difference between this and what was reported for mouse ferrochelatase by De Matteis et al. (1985) may be attributed to either species differences between rat and mouse ferrochelatase or, as suggested by De Matteis, it may reflect differences in the assay procedure since the C or D isomers do inhibit ferrochelatase, but are more readily displaced by substrates than are the A or B isomers. Whatever the explanation, it is obvious that increasing the size of the alkyl groups decreases inhibitory activity and this effect is seen most strongly on the C or D ring alkylations.

A number of studies have been reported for DDC analogues that give rise to N-alkylporphyrins with ethyl and larger alkyl groups in the chick liver embryo system (Marks et al., 1987, and references therein). What is found is that ethyl, propyl, and butyl, but not isopropyl or isobutyl, form N-alkylporphyrins that are inhibitory to ferrochelatase, although the potency of the inhibitor decreases with increasing alkyl size. These data are, then, basically consistent with those found in vitro as described above.

Explanations for the very strong inhibitory nature of N-alkyl-porphyrins and for the isomer-specific inhibition are varied, but usually cite as significant features the size of the alkyl group, the ring over which the alkyl group resides, and the tilt of the ring. However, until the structure of the active site of ferrochelatase is determined it will only be possible to base explanations on proposed active-site models (see below).

D. Ferrochelatase active site

Bovine ferrochelatase has been examined more extensively than any other species although those studies with mouse and chicken ferrochelatase indicate a high degree of similarity. Specifically, four areas have been examined: (1) protein amino acid residues involved in iron binding, (2) protein residues associated with porphyrin binding, (3) fluorescence studies of putative active-site bound fluorophores and endogenous protein fluorescence, and (4) enzyme kinetic studies.

An enzymatic kinetic mechanism for bovine ferrochelatase has been proposed based upon substrate and inhibitor studies (Fig. 3.5) (Dailey and Fleming, 1983). The reaction consists of two substrates, porphyrin and ferrous iron, and two products, protoheme and two protons. The enzyme is proposed to bind initially the divalent iron with the concomi-

tant release of two protons. This is followed by the binding of protoporphyrin. Iron insertion into the porphyrin macrocycle occurs with the
exchange of the two pyrrolic nitrogen protons to the enzyme, thereby,
displacing the ferrous iron chelate. Ferro-protoheme is released, complet-
ing the cycle. Elimination of the second product, the two protons, occurs
only upon initiation of a new catalytic cycle. Therefore, ferrochelatase
has a sequential Bi–Bi mechanism.

Early reports on ferrochelatase documented that it contained a "sulfhydryl" group essential for activity (Labbe and Hubbard, 1960; Porra et
al., 1967). It is a common observation that sulfhydryl reagents such as
iodoacetamide and N-ethylmaleimide rapidly inactivate ferrochelatase.
A better understanding of the basis for this sensitivity was provided
with studies on purified bovine liver ferrochelatase (Dailey, 1984). It was
shown that inactivation was rapid and followed pseudo-first-order kinetics. Interestingly, the bovine enzyme is inhibited most rapidly by N-ethylmaleimide and other less polar sulfhydryl-specific reagents and is
slowly inactivated by iodoacetamide and more polar reagents.

The mechanism of inactivation is consistent with the chemical blocking of sulfhydryl residues involved with the binding of ferrous iron
(Dailey, 1984). Ferrous iron has a protective effect against inactivation
by thiol reagents, while porphyrin substrates yield no protection against
inactivation. The finding that arsenite reversibly inhibits ferrochelatase
was interpreted as support for vicinyl sulfhydryl groups forming a
bidentate complex with ferrous iron. Reversible inhibition by mercuric
chloride is consistent with this suggestion. Pseudo-first-order inactivation by sulfhydryl reagents would then be explained by the fact that
while two sulfhydryls are involved in the chelate, the reaction of a single
sulfhydryl residue is sufficient to inhibit the binding of iron. The stoichiometry of inactivation by N-ethylmaleimide supports this hypothesis.

While chemical modification of sulfhydryl groups affects the binding
of iron, it has no effect on porphyrin binding. Because the number and
position of the porphyrin propionate groups is critical for catalysis, the
possibility of the existence of corresponding charge-pair interactions
between the anionic propionate groups and cationic protein residues was
examined (Dailey and Fleming, 1986). In bovine ferrochelatase it was

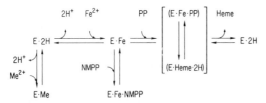

Figure 3.5 Proposed kinetic mechanism for mammalian ferrochelatase [adopted from Dailey and
Fleming (1983)].

found that lysyl group modification had no effect on catalytic parameters, but the reaction of arginyl moieties inactivated the enzyme. This inactivation was rapid and the stoichiometry of inactivation by phenylglyoxal suggests that the reaction of a single guanido group yields maximum inhibition. Interestingly, examination of the kinetic parameters of the modified bovine enzyme shows that arginyl group modification does alter the K_m for porphyrin and not iron, but the apparent K_m is decreased, rather than increased, and the V_{max} is decreased. Such data suggest that while arginyl groups may be significant in porphyrin binding and/or orientation, there must be additional factors involved. Considering the planar, nonpolar nature of protoporphyrin, a reasonable hypothesis would be that hydrophobic interactions between the porphyrin substrate and enzyme active site help to bind this substrate. An arginyl residue in the bovine enzyme (or possibly a lysyl residue in other species), probably in conjunction with another residue, would then be involved, not in binding per se, but in substrate orientation in the active site. Because of the specificity for the 2,4-position substituents, there would also be some type of interaction between the enzyme and the porphyrin A and B rings to aid in the proper alignment.

The fact that maleimides inactivate ferrochelatase by reaction with putative active-site sulfhydryl residues allowed studies with maleimide-bound fluorescent receptors groups. In a series of studies that included fluorescence emission shifts and dynamic quenching, it was concluded that the active site was relatively hydrophobic in nature and poorly accessible to polar external molecules (Dailey, 1985). The polarity of this region appears to be similar to that of the heme binding pocket of globin molecules. The intrinsic protein fluorescence appears to originate mainly from tryptophanyl residues. This fluorescence is characteristic of a residue in an environment that is neither highly polar nor entirely nonpolar. Dynamic quenching indicates that this residue(s) is poorly accessible to the external medium. However, since neither the structure nor the position of tryptophanyl residues is known, it was not possible to conclude that the fluorescence is attributable to active-site residues.

The results of kinetic studies on ferrochelatase are covered above. These, in general, addressed the significance of the position and nature of the porphyrin side-chain substituents on enzyme catalysis (Dailey and Fleming, 1983; Dailey et al., 1986a; Dailey and Smith, 1984). Additionally, the measurement of K_d for porphyrins with mouse ferrochelatase by fluorescence anisotropy demonstrated that significant differences in the ability to bind porphyrins with a variety of side chains did not exist (Table 3.3). These data, along with arginyl modification data, suggest that binding alone is not sufficient to ensure that efficient metalation occurs. Both binding and proper alignment are required for catalysis.

Another line of experimental data also approaches this question, that is, the inhibition of ferrochelatase by N-alkylporphyrins. There are several structural features of N-alkylporphyrins that may be important for inhibition of ferrochelatase. First, and perhaps most significant but frequently overlooked, is the ring distortion that is present in all N-alkylated porphyrins. Model studies have shown that the alkylated ring will be "tilted" about 40° from the plane of the porphyrin ring (Lavallee and Anderson, 1982; Lavallee, 1989). Assuming that ring distortion occurs as part of the normal metalation reaction of ferrochelatase (which is a reasonable hypothesis since distortion of model porphyrin compounds has been shown to increase the rate of chemical metalation 10^3- to 10^5-fold) (Bain-Ackerman and Lavallee, 1979; Lavallee, 1989), then an N-alkylated protoporphyrin molecule would, when the proper ring was alkylated, bind to ferrochelatase as a stable transition-state analogue. This might also explain the high affinity and tight binding that is seen with these porphyrin derivatives. Under these circumstances the enzyme specificity for various N-alkyl isomers would not reflect the steric hindrance attributable to the spatial orientation of the alkyl group, but rather, would reflect a preference for a particular ring distortion. An observation that reinforces this view is the effect of zinc chelation in N-methylprotoporphyrin and mesoporphyrin that is discussed above. It has been pointed out that ring tilt of either the C or D pyrrolic rings will result in spatial displacement of the propionate group on that ring (De Matteis et al., 1982b, 1985). Since porphyrin binding and/or orientation in the active site involves complementary charge pairing with these propionates, this spatial displacement may have a negative impact upon the binding of the C or D isomers. Assuming this to be correct, it may explain in part the decreased efficiency of inhibition by the C or D vs. A or B isomers. However, this particular effect of ring tilt is secondary and can explain only why the C or D isomers do not bind as well as the A or B isomers. The explanation for the tight binding of any of the N-alkylated porphyrins must reside in the actual macrocycle distortion.

One proposal put forward to explain the differential inhibition observed by the Ortiz de Montellano group (1986, 1981) is that the active site of ferrochelatase is relatively open with only the two propionate-containing pyrrolic rings being tightly bound by the enzyme (Fig. 3.6). In such a model, the alkylation of the nitrogens on either the C or D ring would prevent binding of these to ferrochelatase due to steric constraints. Modification of the A or B ring would still allow binding since these rings are outside of the active site. While this model may explain the differential inhibition patterns seen with N-alkylated porphyrins, it does not explain the significant impact that the 2,4 substituents have on the catalytic acceptability of given porphyrins, nor does it address the active-site fluorescence data.

A second model for the active site of ferrochelatase has been suggested that attempts to explain all presently available data (Dailey et al., 1986, and references therein; De Matteis et al., 1985; Lavallee, 1989). In this model the porphyrin binding site resembles the heme binding crevas of globins and cytochromes where the A and B rings are interior and the porphyrin propionates face the exterior, aqueous environment. In this model porphyrin binding would occur mainly from hydrophobic interactions between the macrocycle and nonpolar active-site residues. Protein arginyl groups would interact via charge-pair interactions to orient the porphyrin properly in the active site. Metalation would be mediated via porphyrin ring distortion of the A or B ring. The nature of the 2,4 substituents on the A and B ring would be critical for proper alignment of the A and B rings and may even be involved in ring distortion. Active-site aromatic residues, perhaps tryptophan, present in the back of the pocket may aid in ring bending and/or stabilization of the transition-state puckered porphyrin.

In this model the alkylated porphyrins serve as transition-state analogues. There is sufficient room in the porphyrin binding pocket for short alkyl chains above the porphyrin and, depending upon the geometry of the pocket and the orientation of the alkyl chains with respect to the porphyrin, it may be possible to accommodate larger alkyl groups over the A and B rings than over the C or D rings.

For this model (Fig. 3.7) iron binding occurs via interactions of vicinyl sulfhydryl residues [although Lavallee (1989) has presented arguments for binding utilizing one sulfhydryl and one lysyl residue]. Ferrous iron binding occurs first, followed by porphyrin binding, alignment, and macrocycle bending. Iron exchanges with porphyrin protons and protoheme is released. This model would then be consistent with fluorescence studies of the putative active site, with kinetic studies that emphasize the importance of the substituents at the 2,4 position in determination of K_m but not K_d, as well as the inhibition studies with N-alkylporphyrins.

E. Cellular location and role of lipids

In all eukaryotic cells examined, ferrochelatase is found to be an intrinsic mitochondrial inner membrane protein. Solubilization of enzyme activity

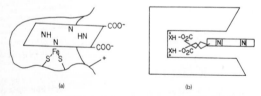

Figure 3.6 Two proposed models for the active site of ferrochelatase. Details are given in the text. (a) Model proposed by Dailey (1985). (b) Model proposed by Ortiz de Montellano (1986).

requires detergents and neigher high nor low salt washes of isolated membrane fractions will solubilize ferrochelatase activity The orientation of ferrochelatase on the membrane has been examined in rat and bovine mitochondria. In the rat enzyme activity in intact mitochondria was found to be "latent" (Jones and Jones, 1969). That is, the measured enzyme activity was low in intact mitochondria, but increased significantly when mitochondria were disrupted. These data were interpreted as demonstrating that the active site of ferrochelatase faces the matrix side of the inner mitochondrial membrane. Later work using more rigorous criteria with bovine ferrochelatase arrived at the same conclusion (Harbin and Dailey, 1985). In the study of the bovine enzyme it was found that a membrane-impermeable sulfhydryl reagent, dimaleimidyl-stilbene disulfonate, which was shown to inactivate solubilized ferrochelatase, did not inactivate ferrochelatase in intact mitochondria, but did inactivate the enzyme in disrupted mitochondria. Since this reagent has been shown to react with a sulfhydryl residue involved in ferrous iron binding, it was concluded that access to the enzyme active site is unavailable to this water-soluble reagent in intact mitochondria or

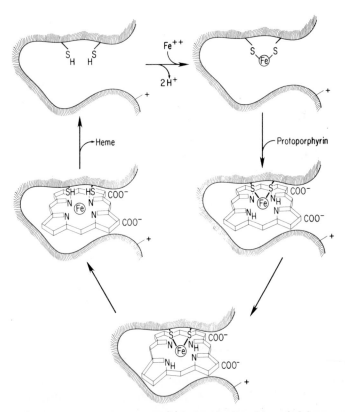

Figure 3.7   Proposal for the catalytic functioning of ferrochelatase.

mitoplasts, thus, supporting the contention that the active site of ferrochelatase is located on the matrix side of the inner mitochondrial membrane. Additional support for this conclusion comes from studies with an enzyme activity-inhibiting antibody. An antibody that inhibited activity of solubilized purified ferrochelatase only inhibited the enzyme in disrupted mitochondria and not in intact mitoplasts.

Additional chemical modification studies with the bovine system also showed that the enzyme spans the inner membrane. Taken together, these data demonstrate that at least a portion of the active site of ferrochelatase is located on the matrix side of the inner mitochondrial membrane although the entire protein spans the membrane.

Recent studies have focused on the in vivo synthesis of ferrochelatase (Karr and Dailey, 1988). The data have shown that the enzyme, as most mitochondrial inner membrane proteins, is nuclear-encoded, synthesized in the cytoplasmic compartment as a precursor form, and then translocated in an energy-requiring step into the inner mitochondrial membrane and proteolytically processed to its final size. Ferrochelatase is synthesized as a precursor with a molecular weight (in mice) of 43,000 and is processed to a final size of 40,000. Somewhat surprising is the inability to sequence the amino terminus of the mature protein suggesting that the amino terminus in the processed enzyme may be blocked.

Since the initial studies on solubilized ferrochelatase there have been a variety of reports on the effects of, or requirements for, lipids for enzyme activity. The results of these studies are far from uniform and range from reports of either no or low stimulation by any lipids to high stimulation by specific fatty acids or phospholipids. Many studies were conducted on relatively crude preparations and because of the possibility of substantial lipid contamination of the preparations, it is difficult to assess the data critically.

Two studies on chicken erythrocyte ferrochelatase have reported stimulation of activity by lipids. Sawada et al. (1969), in a relatively complete examination of a crude enzyme preparation, found strong stimulation by phosphatidyl ethanolamine, phosphatidyl choline, and cardiolipin, with weaker stimulation by phosphatidyl serine and phosphatidyl inositol. In all cases the maximum stimulation was found within a narrow lipid concentration range and the presence of sodium cholate caused a marked decrease in stimulation. Purified chicken erythrocyte ferrochelatase was found to be stimulated by phosphatidyl ethanolamine but not cardiolipin (Hanson and Dailey, 1984). Palmitic and oleic, but not linoleic, acids were also found to stimulate activity. All free fatty acids inhibited enzyme activity at a concentration above 50 μM.

A crude, solubilized pig liver ferrochelatase preparation was reported to be stimulated weakly by various mixtures of phospholipids, although the authors proposed that phosphatidic acid was the stimulatory factor

(Mazanowska et al., 1966). Rat liver ferrochelatase has been shown to be stimulated by lipids. Simpson and Poulson (1977) reported that delipidation by acetone extraction of a crude enzyme preparation resulted in a decrease in ferrochelatase activity, but that a lipid-depleted preparation was stimulated by the addition of linolenic, linoleic, oleic, or stearic acid. The greatest activation was about sixfold over the delipidated enzyme. These authors proposed that the degree of acyl chain desaturation was more crucial than the nature of the polar head group. Taketani and Tokunaga (1981) examined pure, solubilized rat ferrochelatase and also found significant stimulation by lipids. They found that fatty acids stimulated activity more than any phospholipids. In their assays oleic and myristic acids were better stimulators than palmitic and stearic acids. Of the phospholipids, phosphatidylcholine and phosphatidylserine were superior to phosphatidylethanolamine.

Bovine liver ferrochelatase is not stimulated by fatty acids or phospholipids (Dailey and Fleming, 1983; Taketani and Tokunaga, 1982). Mouse liver ferrochelatase has not been extensively studied for the effects of lipids on enzyme activity, but it has been shown that the apparent K_m for deuteroporphyrin is decreased by a factor of 3 when the purified enzyme is reconstituted into soybean phosphatidylcholine (Ferreira and Dailey, 1987).

The proposed roles for lipids in ferrochelatase activity are as diverse as the data. Suggestions that the anionic charge on phosphate groups of phospholipids and carboxyl groups of fatty acids serve to bind iron and bring it closer to the active site (Sawada et al., 1969; Mazanowska et al., 1966), or that the lipid helps to dissolve the porphyrin and present it to the active site (Taketani and Tokunaga, 1981) both seem unlikely since purified systems exist where lipids have no significant effect. It is reasonable that the general detergent action of fatty acids on the usually membrane-bound enzyme is responsible for increases in activity. The role of specific lipids may also be to surround the enzyme with an acceptable hydrophobic milieu, thereby, allowing the protein to assume its proper conformation. Species differences may then be explained as general, nonspecific structural variations that allow different enzymes to have slightly different structural stability in the absence of a lipid membrane. The resolution of this question will require a careful study of the effects of lipid membrane composition on reconstituted purified ferrochelatase.

V. Iron Reduction

Since ferrochelatase has an absolute requirement for ferrous iron, and because biological iron complexes such as transferrin and ferritin chelate ferric iron, a mechanism for ferric iron reduction must exist in the cell. Early work in this area demonstrated that ferric iron, when supplied as ferric chloride or in some microbial siderophores, could be reduced to ferrous iron by mitochondria with NADH or succinate serving as reductants (Barnes and Jones, 1973; Barnes et al., 1972). However, ferritin or transferrin iron was not reduced. The ferrous iron generated in this fashion was used by ferrochelatase for heme biosynthesis when porphyrin was also supplied. The reduction was shown to be coupled to the electron transport chain at the level of NADH and succinate dehydrogenases.

More recently, Taketani et al. (1985, 1986) reexamined this question. They fractionated the bovine heart mitochondrial electron transport chain into complexes I, II, and III and then assayed these complexes to see where ferrochelatase and iron reduction occurred. They found that complex I contained ferrochelatase activity as well as an NADH-dependent ferric-iron-reducing system. The iron reduction was strongly stimulated by FMN.

The ferric iron reduction system is currently poorly characterized. Data do exist, suggesting that this system is sensitive to inhibition at lower concentrations of lead than is ferrochelatase. Assuming that this is true in vivo, then inhibition by lead in animals and the subsequent accumulation of protoporphyrin may be attributed more to the inhibition of iron reduction than the inhibition of ferrochelatase. Additional features of iron metabolism in relation to heme biosynthesis are covered in a later chapter.

VI. Possible Complex of the Terminal Three Enzymes

The location of the terminal three enzymes in the mitochondrion in association with the inner membrane raises interesting questions about the possibility of some type of protein complex. It is attractive to argue for such a complex, whether stable or dynamic in nature, because of the chemical reactivity of the substrates and products of these three steps as well as the close proximity of these enzymes. The isolated enzymes have calculated K_m's in the μM range; a concentration that one would not expect to see normally approached in the cell. In a multiprotein complex the possibility of substrate channeling would eliminate the release of intermediates and obviate the need to justify seemingly high experimentally determined K_m's.

The idea of interactions among the terminal enzymes has been mentioned or suggested by Grandchamp et al. (1978) in their studies on coproporphyrinogen oxidase and by Ferreira et al. (1988) in their work on protoporphyrinogen oxidase and ferrochelatase. While no evidence is available to suggest that a stable ternary complex exists, there are data that are consistent with the presence of at least dynamic interactions.

Coproporphyrinogen oxidase is only loosely associated with the inner mitochondrial membrane and is, therefore, a peripheral membrane protein, while protoporphyrinogen oxidase and ferrochelatase are firmly attached and require detergents for solubilization. In fact, protoporphyrinogen oxidase is solubilized by the same procedures required to solubilize ferrochelatase.

Because of similar membrane-binding properties there is the possibility that a complex may exist among the terminal enzymes of the pathway. Unfortunately, the only data available at present to address this issue are all kinetic data. These data, however, do strongly support a model of protein-protein interaction between at least the terminal two enzymes (Fig. 3.8). Ferreira et al. (1988) demonstrated that substate channeling between these two enzymes does occur in isolated mitochondrial membrane fractions and that this channeling is lost upon solubilization, indicating that any protein complex that may exist in situ must be relatively labile.

VII. Terminal Three Steps in Prokaryotes

The terminal three enzymes of the heme biosynthetic pathway are distinctly different in prokaryotes as opposed to eukaryotes. Unfortunately, there has been considerably less work done on these steps in bacteria than in eukaryotes. The actual steps catalyzed by prokaryotes and eukaryotes are identical, but the manner in which they are carried out varies. A major difference lies in the nature of the electron acceptor for coproporphyrinogen and protoporphyrinogen oxidases. In higher eukaryotic organisms both steps require molecular oxygen as the electron acceptor, whereas in anaerobic prokaryotes numerous cofactors or obligate coupling to the respiratory chain is found. This feature, while adding an interesting dimension to these steps, has created difficulties in

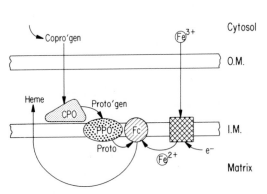

Figure 3.8 Model for the terminal membrane associated steps in the heme biosynthetic pathway. An unidentified iron-reducing component is shown along with ferrochelatase (Fc), protoporphyrinogen oxidase (PPO), and coproporphyrinogen oxidase (CPO) which are associated with the inner mitochondrial membrane. The mode of exit from heme is not shown since present data do not identify a specific transporter nor do they rule out release of heme toward the cytosol by ferrochelatase.

purifying these enzymes due to the problems associated with assaying the individual enzymes.

A. Coproporphyrinogen oxidase

The conversion of coproporphyrinogen III into protoporphyrinogen IX in eukaryotic cells requires the presence of molecular oxygen. In aerobic bacteria this presents no problem, but a large number of anaerobic, microaerophilic, and facultative anaerobes are known to produce copious amounts of protoporphyrin either for heme or bacteriochlorophyll (Le Gall et al., 1979; Gardner et al., 1983; Mori and Sano, 1968; Jacobs, 1974; Odom and Peck, 1981). Unlike bacterial protoporphyrinogen oxidase which couples its substrate oxidation to the cell respiratory chain under anaerobic conditions (below) bacterial coproporphyrinogen oxidase appears to have evolved separate mechanisms to function aerobically vs. anaerobically.

Three prokaryotic organisms have been studied in some detail to determine the requirements for coproporphyrinogen oxidation. These are *Chromatium* (Mori and Sano, 1968), *Rhizobium japonicum* (Keithly and Nadler, 1983), and *Rhodobacter spheroides* (Tait, 1969, 1972; Seehra et al., 1983). These all appear to share similar characteristics with regard to this enzymatic step. All can aerobically oxidize coproporphyrinogen III with molecular oxygen as the electron acceptor and can catalyze the conversion anaerobically with NADP as the acceptor. However, the anaerobic conversion takes place only in the presence of added L-methionine, Mg^{2+}, and ATP (or S-adenosylmethionine). The function of these cofactors is unknown at present. Interestingly, the anaerobic conversion in *R. spheroides* required the presence of both soluble and membrane cell fractions, whereas the aerobic conversion was catalyzed by the soluble fraction alone (Seehra et al., 1983).

In *R. japonicum*, which can exist as a free living bacterium, the additional complication of symbiotic relations between bacteriods and plants exists. Keithly and Nadler (1983) found that these two distinct cell types catalyze coproporphyrinogen III oxidation differently. The free living bacteria produced little protoporphyrin when grown anaerobically, while the formation by bacteriods was unaffected by anaerobiosis. These findings led them to suggest that two distinct mechanisms can exist in this bacterium; one an obligate oxygen-requiring system, and one that utilizes NADP under anaerobic conditions.

Seehra et al. (1983) examined the catalytic mechanism for coproporphyrinogen III oxidation in *R. spheroides*. Previously (see above), it had been proposed that the conversion of the propionate to vinyl side chains proceeded via a β-hydroxypropionate intermediate (Yoshinaga and Sano, 1980; Jackson et al., 1978). Seehra et al. (1983) propose an alternative that does not involve hydroxypropionate intermediates but instead suggests simultaneous hydride ion removal from the β carbon and decarboxylation (Fig. 3.3). One variant of this model invokes the pyrrolic nitrogen electrons as providing the driving force.

To date, coproporphyrinogen oxidase of neither the anaerobic nor aerobic type has been purified to homogeneity from any bacterium so there are no data available about the physical properties of the enzyme.

B. Protoporphyrinogen oxidase

In higher eukaryotes the enzymatic conversion of protoporphyrinogen to protoporphyrin requires molecular oxygen. Among prokaryotes, however, there are a number of anaerobic bacteria which produce large amounts of protoporphyrin for heme and/or bacteriochlorophyll (Gardner et al., 1983; Odom and Peck, 1981). Thus, for these and facultative anaerobes, a system must exist to accept electrons in the absence of oxygen. The manner in which this is done in those prokaryotes examined to date is to couple porphyrinogen oxidation to the organism respiratory chain.

The pioneering work in this field has largely been done by Jacobs and Jacobs in *Escherichia coli* and *R. spheroides* (Jacobs, 1974, and references therein; Jacobs and Jacobs, 1975, 1976, 1977, 1979, 1981, 1984). In bacteria, protoporphyrinogen oxidase, which exhibits the same high specificity for protoporphyrinogen IX as does the eukaryotic enzyme, is membrane-bound and can be solubilized only with the aid of detergents. The enzyme is obligately coupled to the cells respiratory chain and any compound that can serve as a terminal electron acceptor (such as nitrate or fumarate for *E. coli*) will permit porphyrinogen oxidation. Coupling to the respiratory chain has also been demonstrated by the detection of cytochrome reduction in the presence of porphyrinogen and by the effects of classical inhibitors of electron transport chains (Jacobs and Jacobs, 1977).

Because of the obligate coupling to the respiratory chain, purification of protoporphyrinogen oxidase from bacteria presented the difficulty of assaying the solubilized enzyme in the absence of its physiological electron acceptor. Using 2,6-dichlorophenol-indophenol as an electron acceptor, Klemm and Barton (1987) were able to assay the solubilized enzyme and purified protoporphyrinogen oxidase from *Desulfovibrio gigas*. This protein was reported to have a molecular weight of 148,000 and to be composed of three nonidentical subunits. The K_m for protoporphyrinogen is 21 μM and the activation energy above $10°C$ is 1.5 kcal/mol $\cdot$ $°C$. Sulfhydryl reagents inhibit activity and the enzyme displayed a very sharp temperature optimum of $23°C$. To date, this is the only bacterial protoporphyrinogen oxidase that has been purified.

C. Ferrochelatase

Ferrochelatase activity has been reported in a number of bacterial species (Dailey and Lascelles, 1977; Porra and Lascelles, 1965; Porra and Jones, 1963; Jones and Jones, 1970). In general, the level of activity does not appear to be inducible and roughly correlates with the level of heme produced by the cells. However, in *Cyanidium*, ferrochelatase activity increases markedly upon exposure to light (Brown et al., 1984). Under these conditions the cells greatly increase their synthesis of porphyrins and hemes for pigment production. This is unlike *R. spheroides* (Porra and Lascelles, 1965) or *Aquaspirillum itersonii* (Dailey and Lascelles, 1974), where significant changes in hemoprotein content may occur with little or no change in ferrochelatase activity.

Ferrochelatase is all bacteria examined is an intrinsic membrane protein which requires membrane disruption by detergents or chaotropic reagents to solubilize the enzyme. It has been partially purified from *A. itersonii* (Dailey, 1977) and has been purified to homogeneity from *R. spheroides* (Dailey, 1982, 1986). Ferrochelatase of *A. itersonii* has a reported molecular weight of 50,000. Like the eukaryotic enzyme it has a relatively broad substrate specificity using deutero-, meso-, and protoporphyrin and ferrous iron, zinc, and cobalt. The apparent K_m's are listed in Table 3.5. The enzyme is inhibited by sulfhydryl reagents and a variety of divalent cations. Copper was reported to stimulate activity by decreasing the apparent K_m for iron from 20 to 9.5 μM.

Ferrochelatase was purified to homogeneity from the facultative photosynthetic bacterium *R. spheroides* (Dailey, 1982). The enzyme from this organism is unique among those reported to date in that it has a molecular weight of 115,000 which is over double the size of any other ferrochelatase. The reason for this large difference in size is not known and the enzyme has properties very similar to the ferrochelatases of nonphotosynthetic organisms. The possibility that there are distinct regulatory properties is not supported by the present data. This enzyme

TABLE 3.5   Apparent K_m's for Bacterial Ferrochelatase*

	Apparent K_m (μM)	
Substrate	*Rhodobacter spheroides*	*Aquaspirillum itersonii*
Ferrous iron	22	20
Protoporphyrin	18	47
Mesoporphyrin	20	45
Deuteroporphyrin	95	440
2,4-Disulfonic deuteroporphyrin	52	—
2,4-Bisacetal deuteroporphyrin	56	—

*Data taken from Dailey et al. (1986a, b), Dailey and Lascelles (1974); and Dailey (1977).

has been more extensively characterized than any other prokaryotic ferrochelatase (Dailey et al., 1986b; Jones and Jones, 1970; Dailey, 1982, 1986). A variety of porphyrins serve as substrates for this enzyme. Indeed, it appears to have the broadest substrate specificity which regard to the 2,4 positions of any ferrochelatase examined (Table 3.5). A number of porphyrins that are not substrates are competitive inhibitors with respect to the porphyrin substrate. N-Methylprotoporphyrin is also a strong inhibitor of the purified enzyme although a specific K_i has not been reported. It utilizes ferrous iron, cobalt, and zinc, but does not catalyze the chelation of magnesium (Dailey, 1986; Jones and Jones, 1970).

The role of enzyme sulfhydryl residues in catalysis was examined using N-ethylmaleimide and monobromobimane (Dailey et al., 1986b). As with the eukaryotic enzymes, sulfhydryl group modification affected iron binding and the presence of iron had a protective effect. Complete inactivation of ferrochelatase required modification of one or two enzyme sulfhydryl groups. Cationic residues were also examined for their possible role in porphyrin binding. Once again the data are similar to those found with the eukaryotic ferrochelatase. Arginyl group modification had no effect on metal binding, but did increase the K_m for porphyrin suggesting that arginyl residues are involved in porphyrin binding or alignment. Lysyl modification had no effect.

One additional feature that was examined in $R.$ $spheroides$ was the supply of iron for ferrochelatase. Moody and Dailey (1984, 1985) characterized iron uptake and reduction of heme biosynthesis in this organism. Ferric iron in a siderophore complex was taken up in an energy-dependent process, but this is not tightly coupled to heme biosynthesis since inhibition of ferrochelatase with N-methylprotoporphyrin did not affect iron uptake. Iron reduction of ferrisiderophoic complexes appears to be mediated by a specific reductase system and the ferrous iron thus produced is available for insertion into porphyrin by ferrochelatase. Results similar to these have also been reported for a variety of bacteria (Dailey and Lascelles, 1977). In $A.$ $itersonii$ it was demonstrated that ferric iron reduction is coupled to the cells respiratory chain. A feature common to all systems examined, however, is that in vitro iron reduction occurs in excess over the amount required for maximal heme biosynthesis.

REFERENCES

Bain-Ackerman, M. J., and Lavallee, D. K. (1979). Kinetics of metal-ion complexation with N-methyltetraphenylporphyrin: Evidence concerning a general mechanism of porphyrin metalation, $Inorg.$ $Chem.$ **18**:3358–3364.

Barnes, R., Connelly, J. L., and Jones, O. T. G. (1972). The utilization of iron and its complexes by mammalian mitochondria, $Biochem.$ $J.$ **128**:1043–1055.

Barnes, R., and Jones, O. T. G. (1973). The availability of iron from haem synthesis in red blood cells, *Biochim. Biophys. Acta* **304**:304–308.

Batlle, A. M. del C., Benson, A., and Remington, C. (1965). Purification and properties of coproporphyrinogenase, *Biochem. J.* **97**:731–740.

Battersby, A. R., Baldas, J. Collins, J. Grayson, D. H., James, R. J., and McDonald, E. (1972). Mechanism of biosynthesis of the vinyl groups of protoporphyrin IX, *J. Chem. Soc. Chem. Comm.* 1265–1266.

Brown, S. B., Holroyd, J. A., Vernon, D. I., and Jones, O. T. G. (1984). Ferrochelatase activity in the photosynthetic alga *Cyanidium caldarium*. Development of the enzyme during biosynthesis of photosynthetic pigments, *Biochem. J.* **220**:861–863.

Camadro, J. M., Ibraham, N. G., and Levere, R. D. (1984). Kinetic studies of human liver ferrochelatase. Role of endogenous metals, *J. Biol. Chem.* **259**:5678–5682.

Camadro, J. M., Ibraham, N. G., and Levere, R. D. (1985). Kinetic properties of the membrane-bound human liver mitochondrial protoporphyrinogen oxidase, *Arch. Biochem. Biophys.* **242**:206–212.

Chaudhry, I. A., Clezy, P. S., and Diakiw, V. (1977). Chemistry of pyrrolic compounds XXXVI. Some aspects of the chemistry of 2-hydroxypropionate porphyrins: New synthesis of harderoporphyrin trimethyl ester, S-411 porphyrin, tetramethyl ester and related compounds, *Aust. J. Chem.* **30**:879.

Coffman, B. L., Ingall, G., and Tephly, T. R. (1982). The formation of N-alkylprotoporphyrin IX and destruction of cytochrome P-450 in the liver of rats after treatment with 3,5-diethoxycarbonyl-1,4-dihydrocollidine and its 4-ethyl analog, *Arch. Biochem. Biophys.* **218**:220–224.

Cole, S. P., and Marks, G. S. (1980). Structural requirements in dihydropyridines for ferrochelatase inhibition and delta-aminolevulinic acid synthetase induction, *Int. J. Biochem.* **12**:989–992.

Cole, S. P., and Marks, G. S. (1984). Ferrochelatase and N-alkylated porphyrins, *Mol. Cell. Biochem.* **64**:127–137.

Cole, S. P., Marks, G. S., Ortiz de Montellano, P. R., and Kunze, K. L. (1982). Inhibition of ferrochelatase by N-methylprotoporphyrin IX is not accompanied by delta-aminolevulinic acid synthetase induction in chick embryo liver cell culture, *Canad. J. Physiol. Pharmacol.* **60**:212–215.

Cole, S. P., Massey, T. E., Marks, G. S., and Racz, W. J. (1981a). Effects of porphyrin-inducing drugs on ferrochelatase activity in isolated mouse hepatocytes, *Canad. J. Physiol. Pharmacol.* **59**:1155–1158.

Cole, S. P., Whitney, R. A., and Marks, G. S. (1981b). Ferrochelatase-inhibitory and porphyrin-inducing properties 3,5-diethoxycarbonyl-1,4-dihydro-2,4,6-trimethylpyridine and its analogues in chick embryo liver cells, *Mol. Pharmacol.* **20**:395–403.

Cole, S. P., Zelt, D. T., and Marks, G. S. (1980). Comparison of the effects of griseofulvin and 3,5-diethoxycarbonyl-1,4-dihydro-2,4,6-trimethylpyridine on ferrochelatase activity in chick embryo liver, *Mol. Pharmacol.* **19**:477–480.

Dailey, H. A., Jr. (1977). Purification and characterization of the membrane-bound ferrochelatase from *Spirillum itersonii*, *J. Bacteriol.* **132**:302–307.

Dailey, H. A. (1982). Purification and characterization of membrane-bound ferrochelatase from *Rhodopseudomonas sphaeroides*, *J. Biol. Chem.* **257**:14714–14718.

Dailey, H. A. (1984). Effect of sulfhydryl group modification on the activity of bovine ferrochelatase, *J. Biol. Chem.* **259**:2711–2715.

Dailey, H. A. (1985). Spectroscopic examination of the active site of bovine ferrochelatase, *Biochemistry* **24**:1287–1291.

Dailey, H. A. (1986). Purification and characterization of bacterial ferrochelatase, *Methods Enzymol.* **123**:408–415.

Dailey, H. A. (1987). Metal inhibition of ferrochelatase, *Ann. N.Y. Acad. Sci.* **514**:81–86.

Dailey, H. A., and Fleming, J. E. (1983). Bovine ferrochelatase. Kinetic analysis of inhibition by N-methylprotoporphyrin, manganese, and heme, *J. Biol. Chem.* **258**:11453–11459.

Dailey, H. A., and Fleming, J. E. (1986). The role of arginyl residues in porphyrin binding to ferrochelatase, *J. Biol. Chem.* **261**:7902–7905.

Dailey, H. A., Fleming, J. E., and Harbin, B. M. (1986a). Purification and characterization of mammalian and chicken ferrochelatase, *Methods Enzymol.* **123**:401–408.

Dailey, H. A., Fleming, J. E., and Harbin, B. M. (1986b). Ferrochelatase from *Rhodopseudomonas sphaeroides*: Substrate specificity and role of sulfhydryl and arginyl residues, *J. Bacteriol.* **165**:1–5.

Dailey, H. A., Jones, C. S., and Karr, S. W. (1989). Interaction of free porphyrins and metalloporphyrins with mouse ferrochelatase. A model for the active site of ferrochelatase, *Biochem. Biophys. Acta*, in press.

Dailey, H. A., and Karr, S. W. (1987). Purification and characterization of murine protoporphyrinogen oxidase, *Biochemistry* **26**:2697–2701.

Dailey, H. A., Jr., and Lascelles, J. (1974). Ferrochelatase activity in wild-type and mutant strains of *Spirillum itersonii*. Solubilization with chaotropic reagents, *Arch. Biochem. Biophys.* **160**:523–529.

Dailey, H. A., Jr., and Lascelles, J. (1977) Reduction of iron and synthesis of protoheme by *Spirillum itersonii* and other organisms. *J. Bacteriol.* **129**:815–820.

Dailey, H. A., and Smith, A. (1984). Differential interaction of porphyrins used in photoradiation therapy with ferrochelatase, *Biochem. J.* **223**:441–445.

De Matteis, F., Abbritti, G., and Gibbs, A. H. (1973). Decreased liver activity of porphyrin-metal chelatase in hepatic porphyria caused by 3,5-diethyoxycarbonyl-1,4-dihydrocollidine: Studies in rates and mice, *Biochem. J.* **134**:717–727.

De Matteis, F., and Gibbs, A. H. (1980). Drug-induced conversion of liver haem into modified porphyrins. Evidence for two classes of products, *Biochem. J.* **187**:285–288.

De Matteis, F., Gibbs, A. H., Farmer, P. B., and Lamb, J. H. (1981). Liver production of *N*-alkylated porphyrins caused in mice by treatment with substitued dihydropyridines. Evidence that the alkyl group on the pyrrole nitrogen atom originates from the drug, *FEBS Lett.* **129**:328–331.

De Matteis, F., Gibbs, A. H., and Harvey, C. (1985). Studies on the inhibition of ferrochelatase by *N*-alkylated dicarboxylic porphyrins. Steric factors involved and evidence that the inhibition is reversible, *Biochem. J.* **226**:537–544.

De Matteis, F., Gibbs, A. H., and Holley, A. E. (1987). Occurrence and biological properties of *N*-methyl protoporphyrin, *Ann. N.Y. Acad. Sci.* **514**:30–40.

De Matteis, F., Gibbs, A. H., and Smith, A. G. (1980a). Inhibition of protohaem ferro-lyase by *N*-substituted porphyrins, structural requirements for the inhibitory effect, *Biochem. J.* **189**:645–648.

De Matteis, F., Gibbs, A. H., and Tephly, T. R. (1980b). Inhibition of protohaem ferro-lyase in experimental porphyria. Isolation and partial characterization of a modified porphyrin inhibitor. *Biochem. J.* **188**:145–152.

De Matteis, F., Hollands, C., Gibbs, A. H., de Sa, N., Rizzardini, M. (1982a). Inactivation of cytochrome P-450 and production of *N*-alkylated porphyrins caused in isolated hepatocytes by substituted dihydropyridines. Structural requirements for loss of haem and alkylation of the pyrrole nitrogen atom, *FEBS Lett.* **145**:87–92.

De Matteis, F., Jackson, A. H., Gibbs, A. H., Rao, K. R., Atton, J., Weerasinghe, S., and Hollands, C. (1982b). Structural isomerism and chirality of *N*-monosubstituted protoporphyrins, *FEBS Lett.* **142**:44–48.

De Matteis, F., and Marks, G. S. (1983). The effect of N-methylprotoporphyrin and succinyl-acetone on the regulation of heme biosynthesis in chicken hepatocytes in culture, *FEBS Lett.* **159**:127–131.

Deybach, J. C., da Dilva, V., Grandchamp, B., and Nordmann, Y. (1985). The mitochondrial location of protoporphyrinogen oxidase, *Eur. J. Biochem.* **149**:431–435.

Elder, G. H., and Evans, J. O. (1978). Evidence that the coproporphyrinogen oxidase activity of rat liver is situated in the intermembrane space of mitochondria, *Biochem. J.* **172**:345–347.

Elder, G. H., Evans, J. O., Jackson, J. R., and Jackson, A. H. (1978). Factors determining the sequence of oxidative decarboxylation of the 2- and 4-propionate substituents of coproporphyrinogen III by coproporphyrinogen oxidase in rate liver, *Biochem. J.* **169**:215–223.

Fadigan, A., and Dailey, H. A. (1987). Inhibition of ferrochelatase during differentiation of murine erythroleukaemia cells, *Biochem. J.* **243**:419–424.

Ferreira, G. M. A. D. C. (1986). Heme biosynthesis: Characterization of the two terminal membrane-bound enzymes, Ph.D. Dissertation, University of Georgia.

Ferreira, G. C., Andrew, T. L., Karr, S. W., and Dailey, H. A. (1988). Organization of the terminal two enzymes of the heme biosynthetic pathway. Orientation of protoporphyrinogen oxidase and evidence for a membrane complex, *J. Biol. Chem.* **263**:3835–3839.

Ferreira, G. C., and Dailey, H. A. (1987). Reconstitution of the two terminal enzymes of the heme biosynthetic pathway into phospholipid vesicles, *J. Biol. Chem.* **262**:4407–4412.

Ferreira, G. C., and Dailey, H. A. (1988). Mouse protoporphyrinogen oxidase. Kinetic parameters and demonstration of inhibition by bilirubin, *Biochem. J.* **250**:597–603.

Gaertner, R. R., and Hollebone, B. R. (1983). The in vitro inhibition of hepatic ferrochelatase by divalent lead and other soft metal ions, *Canad. J. Biochem. Cell. Biol.* **61**:214–222.

Gardner, R. M., Fuller, M. D., and Caldwell, D. R. (1983). Tetrapyrrole utilization by protoheme-synthesizing anaerobes, *Curr. Microbiol.* **9**:59–62.

Goldberg, A., Ashenbrucker, M., Cartwright, G. E., and Wintrobe, M. M. (1956). Studies on the biosynthesis of heme in vitro by avian erythrocytes, *Blood* **11**:821–833.

Grandchamp, B., Phung, N., and Nordmann, Y. (1978). The mitochondrial localization of coproporphyrinogen III oxidase, *Biochem. J.* **176**:97–102.

Hanson, J. W., and Dailey, H. A. (1984). Purification and characterization of chicken erythrocytes, *Biochem. J.* **222**:695–700.

Harbin, B. M., and Dailey, H. A. (1985). Orientation of ferrochelatase in bovine liver mitochondria, *Biochemistry* **24**:366–370.

Honeybourne, C. L., Jackson, J. T., and Jones, O. T. (1979). The interaction of mitochondrial ferrochelatase with a range of porphyrin substrates, *FEBS Lett.* **98**:207–210.

Jackson, A. H., Elder, G. H., and Smith, S. G. (1978). The metabolism of coproporphyrinogen III into protoporphyrinogen IX, *Int. J. Biochem.* **9**:877–882.

Jackson, A. H., Games, D. E., Couch, P. W., Jackson, J. R., Belcher, R. V., and Smith, S. G. (1974). Conversion of coproporphyrinogen III to protoporphyrin IX, *Enzyme* **17**:81–87.

Jackson, A. H., Jones, D. M., Philip, G., Lash, T. D., Batlle, A. M. del C., and Smith, S. G. (1980). Synthetic and biosynthetic studies of porphyrins. IV. Further studies of the conversion of coproporphyrinogen III to protoporphyrinogen-IX: Mass spectrometric investigations of the incubation of specifically deuteriated coproporphyrinogen-III with chicken red cell haemolysates, *Int. J. Biochem.* **12**:681–688.

Jacobs, N. J. (1974). Biosynthesis of heme, *Microbial Iron Metabolism. A Comprehensive Treatise* (J. B. Neilands, Ed.), Academic, London, pp. 125–148.

Jacobs, N. J., and Jacobs, J. M. (1975). Fumarate as an alternate electron acceptor for the late steps of anaerobic heme synthesis in *Escherichia coli*, *Biochem. Biophys. Res. Comm.* **65**:435–441.

Jacobs, N. J., and Jacobs, J. M. (1976). Nitrate, fumarate and oxygen as electron acceptors for a late step in microbial heme synthesis, *Biochim. Biophys. Acta* **449**:1–9.

Jacobs, N. J., and Jacobs, J. M. (1977). The late steps of anaerobic heme biosynthesis in *E. coli*: Role of quinones in protoporphyrinogen oxidation, *Biochem. Biophys. Res. Comm.* **78**:429–433.

Jacobs, N. J., and Jacobs, J. M. (1979). Microbial oxidation of protoporphyrinogen, an intermediate in heme and chlorophyll biosynthesis, *Arch. Biochem. Biophys.* **197**:396–403.

Jacobs, N. J., and Jacobs, J. M. (1981). Protoporphyrinogen oxidation in *Rhodopseudomonas spheroides*. A step in heme and bacteriochlorophyll synthesis, *Arch. Biochem. Biophys.* **211**:305–311.

Jacobs, N. J., and Jacobs, J. M. (1984). Protoporphyrinogen oxidation, an enzymatic step in heme and chlorophyll synthesis: Partial characterization of the reaction in plant organelles and comparison with mammalian and bacterial systems, *Arch. Biochem. Biophys.* **229**:312–319.

Jones, M. S., and Jones, O. T. G. (1970). Ferrochelatase of *Rhodopseudomonas spheroides*, *Biochem. J.* **119**:453–462.

Jones, M. S., and Jones, O. T. G. (1969). The structural organization of haem synthesis of rata liver mitochondria, *Biochem. J.* **113**:507–514.

Karr, S. R., and Dailey, H. A. (1988). The in vitro and in vivo synthesis of murine ferrochelatase, *Biochem. J.* **254**:799–803.

Kassner, R. J., and Walchak, H. (1973). Heme formation from Fe(II) and porphyrin in the absence of ferrochelatase activity, *Biochim. Biophys. Acta* **304**:294–303.

Keithly, J. H., and Nadler, K. D. (1983). Protoporphyrin formation in *Rhizobium japonicum*, *J. Bacteriol.* **154**:838–845.

Kennedy, G. Y. (1970). Harderoporphyrin—A new porphyrin from the Harderian gland of the rat, *Comp. Biochem. Physiol.* **36**:21–36.

Klemm, D. J., and Barton, L. L. (1987). Purification and properties of protoporphyrinogen oxidase from an anaerobic bacterium, *Desulfovibrio gigas*, *J. Bacteriol.* **169**:5209–5215.

Labbe, R. F., and Hubbard, N. (1960). Preparation and properties of the iron-protoporphyrin chelating enzyme, *Biochim. Biophys. Acta.* **41**:185–191.

Lavallee, D. (1988). *Mechanistic Principles of Enzyme Activity* (J. F. Liedman, and A. Greenberg, Eds.), pp. 279–314. VCH Publishers Inc., New York.

Lavallee, D. K. (1989). Porphyrin metalation reaction in biochemistry, to appear.

Lavallee, D. K., and Anderson, O. P. (1982). Crystal and molecular structure of a free-base N-methylporphyrin : N-methyl-5,10,15,20-tetrakis (p-bromophenyl) porphyrin, *J. Amer. Chem. Soc.* **104**:4707–4708.

Le Gall, J. D., DerVartanian, D. V., and Peck, H. D., Jr. (1979). Flavoproteins, iron proteins and hemoproteins as electron transfer components of the sulfate-reducing bacteria, *Curr. Topics Bioenerg.* **9**:237–265.

Mailer, K., Poulson, R., Dolphin, D., and Hamilton, A. D. (1980). Ferrochelatase: Isolation and purification via affinity chromatography, *Biochem. Biophys. Res. Comm.* **96**:777–784.

Malmstrom, B. G. (1982). Enzymology of oxygen, *Ann. Rev. Biochem.* **51**:21–59.

Marks, G. S., Allen, D. T., Johnston, C. T., Sutherland, E. P., Nakatsu, K., and Whitney, R. A. (1985). Suicidal destruction of cytochrome P-450 and reduction of ferrochelatase activity by 3,5-diethoxycarbonyl-1,4-dihydro-2,4,6-trimethylpyridine and its analogues in chick embryo liver cells, *Mol. Pharmacol.* **27**:459–465.

Marks, G. S., Allen, D. T., Sutherland, E. P., McCluskey, S. A., and Whitney, R. A. (1986). Comparison of the effects of 3-ethoxycarbonyl-1,4-dihydro-2,4-dimethylpyridine and 3,5-diethoxycarbonyl-1,4-dihydro-2,4,6-trimethyl-pyridine on ferrochelatase activity and heme biosynthesis in chick embryo liver cells in culture, *Canad. J. Physiol. Pharmacol.* **64**:483–486.

Marks, G. S., Powles, J., Lyon, M., McCluskey, S., Sutherland, E., and Zelt, D. (1987). Patterns of porphyrin accumulation in response to xenobiotics: Parallels between results in chick embryo and rodents, *Ann. N.Y. Acad. Sci.* **514**:113–127.

Mathews-Roth, M. M., Drouin, G. L., and Duffy, L. (1987). Isolation of human ferrochelatase, *Arch. Dermatol.* **123**:429–430.

Mazanowska, A. M., Neuberger, A., and Tait, G. H. (1966). Effect of lipids and organic solvents on the enzymic formation of zinc protoporphyrin and haem, *Biochem. J.* **98**:117–127.

McCluskey, S. A., Marks, G. S., Sutherland, E. P., Jacobsen, N., and Ortiz de Montellano, P. R. (1986). Ferrochelatase inhibitory activity and N-alkylprotoporphyrin formation with analogues of 3,5-diethoxycarbonyl-1,4-dihydro-2,4,6-trimethylpyridine (DDC) containing extended 4-alkyl groups: Implications for the active site of ferrochelatase, *Mol. Pharmacol.* **30**:252–257.

McColl, K. E. L., Thomspon, G. G., El Omar, E. Moore, M. R., and Goldberg, A. (1987). Porphyrin metabolism and haem biosynthesis in Gilbert's syndrome, *Gut* **28**:125–130.

Moody, M. D., and Dailey, H. A. (1984). Siderophore utilization and iron uptake by *Rhodopseudomonas sphaeroides*, *Arch. Biochem. Biophys.* **234**:178–186.

Moody, M. D., and Dailey, H. A. (1985). Iron transport and its relation to heme biosynthesis in *Rhodopseudomonas sphaeroides*, *J. Bacteriol.* **161**:1074–1079.

Mori, M., and Sano, S. (1968). Protoporphyrin formation from coproporphyrinogen III by *Chromatium* cell extracts, *Biochem. Biophys. Res. Comm.* **32**:610–615.

Odom, J. M., and Peck, H. D., Jr. (1981). Localization of dehydrogenases, reductases and electron transfer components in the sulfate-reducing bacterium *Desulfovibrio gigas*, *J. Bacteriol*, **147**:161–169.

Onisawa, J., and Labbe, R. F. (1963). Effects of diethyl-1,4-dihydro-2,4,6-trimethylpyridine-3,5-dicarboxylate on the metabolism of porphyrins and iron, *J. Biol. Chem.* **228**:724–727.

Ortiz de Montellano, P. R., Costa, A. K., Grab, A., Sutherland, E. P., and Marks, G. S. (1986). Cytochrome P450 destruction and ferrochelatase inhibition, *Porphyrins and Porphyrias* (Y. Nordmann, Ed.), Colloque INSERM, John Libbey Eurotext, London; Vol. 134, pp. 109–117.

Ortiz de Montellano, P. R., Kunze, K. L., Cole, S. P., and Marks, G. S. (1980). Inhibition of hepatic ferrochelatase by the four isomers of N-methylprotoporphyrin IX, *Biochem. Biophys. Res. Comm.* **97**:1436–1442.

Ortiz de Montellano, P. R., Kunze, K. L., Cole, S. P., and Marks, G. S. (1981). Differential inhibition of hepatic ferrochelatase by the isomers of N-ethylprotoporphyrin IX, *Biochem. Biophys. Res. Comm.* **103**:581–586.

Porra, R. J., and Falk, J. E. (1964). The enzymatic conversion of coproporphyrinogen III into protoporphyrin IX, *Biochem. J.* **90**:69–72.

Porra, R. J., and Jones, O. T. G. (1963). Studies on ferrochelatase. 1. Assay and properties of ferrochelatase from a pig liver mitochondrial extract, *Biochem. J.* **87**:181–185.

Porra, R. J., and Lascalles, J. (1965). Haemoproteins and haem synthesis in facultative photosynthetic and denitrifying bacteria, *Biochem. J.* **94**:120–126.

Porra, R. J., Vitols, K. S., Labbe, R. F., and Newton, N. A. (1967). Studies on ferrochelatase. The effects of thiols and other factors on the determination of activity, *Biochem. J.* **104**:321–327.

Poulson, R. (1976). The enzymic conversion of protoporphyrinogen IX to protoporphyrin IX in mammalian mitochondria, *J. Biol. Chem.* **251**:3730–3733.

Poulson, R., and Polglase, W. J. (1975). The enzymic conversion of protoporphyrinogen IX to protoporphyrin IX. Protoporphyrinogen oxidase activity in mitochondrial extracts of *Saccharomyces cerevisiae*, *J. Biol. Chem.* **250**:1269–1274.

Sano, S. (1966). 2,4-bis-(-hydroxypropionic acid) deuteroporphyrinogen IX a possible intermediate between coproporphyrinogen III and protoporphyrin IX, *J. Biol. Chem.* **241**:5276–5283.

Sano, S., and Granick, S. (1961). Mitochondrial coproporphyrinogen oxidase and protoporphyrin formation, *J. Biol. Chem.* **236**:1173–1180.

Sawada, H., Takeshita, M., Sugita, Y., and Yoneyama, Y. (1969). Effect of lipid on protoheme ferro-lyase, *Biochim. Biophys. Acta* **178**:145–155.

Seehra, J. S., Jordan, P. M., and Akhtar, M. (1983). Anaerobic and aerobic coproporphyrinogen III oxidases of *Rhodopseudomonas spheroides*, *Biochem. J.* **209**:709–718.

Siepker, L. J., Ford, M., de Kock, R., and Kramer, S. (1987). Purification of bovine protoporphyrinogen oxidase: Immunological cross-reactivity and structural relationship to ferrochelatase, *Biochim. Biophys. Acta* **913**:349–358.

Simpson, D. M., and Poulson, R. (1977). Effects of lipids on the activity of ferrochelatase, *Biochim. Biophys. Acta* **482**:461–469.

Smith, A. G., and De Matteis, F. (1980). Drugs and the hepatic porphyrias, *Clin. Haematol.* **9**:399–425.

Smith, S. G., and Belcher, R. V. (1974). Distribution of some possible intermediates of the haem biosynthesis, *Enzyme* **17**:1.

Sutherland, E. P., Marks, G. S., Grab, L. A., and Ortiz de Montellano, P. R. (1986). Porphyrinogenic activity and ferrochelatase-inhibitory activity of syndones in chick embryo liver cells, *FEBS Lett.* **197**:17–20.

Tait, G. H. (1969). Coproporphyrinogenase activity in extracts from *Rhodopseudomonas spheroides*, *Biochem. Biophys. Res. Comm.* **37**:166–172.

Tait, G. H. (1972). Coproporphyrinogenase activity in extracts of *Rhodopseudomonas spheroides* and *Chromatium D*, *Biochem. J.* **128**:1159–1169.

Taketani, S., Tanaka-Yoshioka, A., Masaki, R., Tashiro, Y., and Tokunaga, R. (1986). Association of ferrochelatase with complex I in bovine heart mitochondria, *Biochim. Biophys. Acta* **883**:277–283.

Taketani, S., Tanaka, A., and Tokunaga, R. (1985). Reconstitution of heme-synthesizing activity from ferric ion and porphyrins and the effect of lead on the activity, *Arch. Biochem. Biophys.* **242**:291–296.

Taketani, S., and Tokunaga, R. (1981). Rat liver ferrochelatase. Purification, properties, and stimulation by fatty acids, *J. Biol. Chem.* **256**:12748–12753.

Taketani, S., and Tokunaga, R. (1982). Purification and substrate specificity of bovine liver ferrochelatase, *Eur. J. Biochem.* **127**:443–447.

Tephly, T. R., Coffman, B. L., Ingall, G., Abou Zeit-Har, M. S., Goff, H. M., Tabba, H. D., and Smith, K. M. (1981). Identification of *N*-methylprotoporphyrin IX in livers of untreated mice and mice treated with 3,5-diethoxycarbonyl-1,4-dihydrocollidine: Source of the methyl group, *Arch. Biochem. Biophys.* **212**:120–126.

Tephly, T. R., Gibbs, A. H., and De Matteis, F. (1979). Studies on the mechanism of experimental porphyria produced by 3,5-diethoxycarbonyl-1,4-dihydrocollidine: Role of a porphyrin-like inhibitor of protohaem ferro-lyase, *Biochem. J.* **180**:241–244.

Tephly, T. R., Gibbs, A. H., Ingall, G., and De Matteis, F. (1980). Studies on the mechanism of experimental porphyria and ferrochelatase inhibition produced by 3,5-diethoxycarbonyl-1,4-dihydrocollidine, *Int. J. Biochem.* **12**:993–998.

Tokunaga, R., and Sano, S. (1982). Comparative studies on nonenzymatic and enzymic protoheme formation, *Biochim. Biophys. Acta* **264**:263–271.

Wagner, G. S., and Tephly, T. R. (1975). A possible role of copper in the regulation of heme biosynthesis through ferrochelatase, *Adv. Exp. Med. Biol.* **58**:343–354.

Yoneyama, Y., Ohyama, H., Sugeta, Y., and Yoshikawa, H. (1962). Iron-chelating enzyme from duck erythrocytes, *Biochim. Biophys. Acta* **62**:261–268.

Yoneyama, Y., Tamai, A., Yasuda, T., and Yoshikawa, H. (1965). Iron-chelating enzyme from rat liver, *Biochim. Biophys. Acta* **105**:100–105.

Yoshimaga, T., and Sano, S. (1980a). Coproporphyrinogen oxidase. I. Purification, properties, and activation by phospholipids, *J. Biol. Chem.* **255**:4722–4726.

Yoshinaga, T., and Sano, S. (1980b). Coproporphyrinogen oxidase. II. Reaction mechanism and role of tyrosine residues on the activity, *J. Biol. Chem.* **255**:4727–4731.

Zamen, Z., Abboud, M. M., and Akhtar, M. (1972). Mechanism and stereochemistry of vinyl group formation in haem biosynthesis, *J. Chem. Soc. Chem. Comm.* 1263.

Regulation of Heme Biosynthesis in Higher Animals

Tamara L. Andrew

Pascale G. Riley

Harry A. Dailey

I. Introduction

Regulation of heme biosynthesis in higher animals has been extensively studied for over two decades. The data available to date clearly show that there are two distinct regulatory mechanisms, exemplified by erythroid and hepatic (or nonerythroid) cell types. The mode of regulation by nondifferentiating, nonerythroid cell types has been characterized to some degree in hepatocytes. This regulation appears to involve mainly feedback regulation by the product of the pathway, protoheme. In differentiating erythroid cell types, however, the regulatory mechanism is far from being settled experimentally. Diverse groups studying a variety of model systems have proposed a number of possible regulatory schemes that seem only to agree that 5-aminolevulinate synthase (ALAS) is not the sole rate-limiting step of the pathway in these cells.

We will attempt to present a spectrum of the available data concerning the regulation in both erythroid and hepatic cell types. For the hepatic cell type this results in a uniformly accepted regulatory model, whereas for the erythroid cell line the diversity of experimental observations precludes such a consensus model. However, based upon some of the data presented below as well as the newly available molecular approach that is covered in the next chapter, we will attempt to produce a model for discussion.

II. Regulation in Nonerythroid Cells

A. Feedback regulation by heme

The primary regulation of the heme biosynthetic pathway in the liver is a negative feedback effect by the end product of the pathway, heme, on the first and rate-limiting enzyme of the pathway, 5-aminolevulinate synthase (ALAS). The half-life of this enzyme is reported to be much shorter than that of many other mitochondrial enzymes, about 70 min in rat liver (Tschudy et al., 1965), and 3 h in mouse liver (Gayathri et al., 1973) and cultured chick embryo liver cells (Sassa and Granick, 1970). This short enzyme half-life has been postulated to allow the cell to respond rapidly to increases and decreases in the demand for heme. The observed inhibitory effects of aminolevulinic acid on basal and drug-induced ALAS levels in the mouse, rat, and chick embryo in ovo have been attributed to the conversion of aminolevulinic acid to heme in vivo (Granick et al., 1975; Anderson et al., 1981), and the subsequent feedback regulation of ALAS, rather than to a direct effect of aminolevulinic acid itself. While ALAS is normally present at low levels in the cell, all other enzymes and intermediates of the pathway are normally present in non-rate-limiting amounts (Sassa and Kappas, 1981; Kappas et al., 1983; May et al., 1986).

The feedback regulation by heme has been proposed to take place on a number of levels: direct inhibition of ALAS activity, repression of ALAS synthesis at transcriptional and/or translational steps, and inhibition of the translocation and/or processing of cytosolic ALAS into the mito-chondrial form. The oscillations in ALAS activity observed following hemin injection of rats lends support to the idea of a closed negative feedback system mediated by heme (Waxman et al., 1966).

1. Direct feedback inhibition. The possibility that heme might directly feedback-inhibit ALAS has been examined in both cells and with puri-fied enzyme. Hemin treatment of chick liver embryo cells from culture was found not to affect ALAS activity except at nonphysiological con-centrations (Granick, 1966; Sassa and Granick, 1970; Granick and Kappas, 1971). Mitochondrial ALAS purified 95% from drug-induced chick embryo liver was also not inhibited by hemin concentrations as high as 1 mM (Pirola et al., 1984). However, in a partially purified enzyme preparation from rat liver, hemin inhibition of ALAS was observed with a K_i of 2×10^{-5} M (Scholnick et al., 1972). It has been proposed by several investigators that the physical proximity of ALAS and ferrochelatase (Fc) in the mitochondrion might allow for a locally high concentration of heme available for feedback inhibition of ALAS (Sano and Granick, 1961; Jones and Jones, 1970; Whiting and Elliot, 1972), but experiments in intact rat liver mitochondria have established that raising levels of heme generation has no effect on ALAS activity (Wolfson et al., 1979). It is currently thought that feedback inhibition of ALAS activity by heme is not physiologically important (Whiting and Granick, 1976a; Pirola et al., 1984; Bloomer and Straka, 1988).

2. Transcriptional regulation. Observations from a number of groups have suggested that ALAS is regulated at the level of transcription. The possibility that regulation by heme occurs at the transcriptional level is attractive due to the relatively short half-life of ALAS mRNA. The majority of rat liver mRNAs have half-lives of about 40 h (Revel and Hiatt, 1964). In contrast, the half-life of ALAS mRNA in rat liver has been estimated to be about 1 h (Tschudy et al., 1965; Marver et al., 1966a). In chick embryo liver, the half-life of ALAS mRNA is about 5 h (Sassa and Granick, 1970), and in the mouse, 3 h (Gayathri et al., 1973). This short half-life of ALAS mRNA allows for tight feedback repression of ALAS synthesis by heme at the level of transcription.

Hemin administered to rats suppressed drug-mediated induction of ALAS (Hayashi et al., 1968; Hayashi et al., 1972), and also reduced ALAS levels in uninduced rats (Hayashi et al., 1968). In a reticulocyte lysate system, the ability of isolated liver polysomes prepared from induced rats treated with hemin to direct the synthesis of ALAS decreased with a half-life of about 60 min, suggesting that heme inhibits ALAS mRNA synthesis (Yamamoto et al., 1982). In chick embryo liver cell culture, evidence for transcriptional inhibition of ALAS synthesis by nanomolar quantities of heme has been reported (Srivastava et al., 1980a). Hemin was shown to block ALAS synthesis in drug-induced chick embryos in ovo as well (Whiting and Granick, 1976b), and it was suggested that this was probably attributable to depression of ALAS mRNA levels (Whiting, 1976). Thus, the available data from several cell types strongly support transcriptional regulation by heme, but to date the mechanism whereby this heme-mediated inhibition of transcription occurs remains unknown.

3. Translational regulation. While it is well known that heme stimulates general protein synthesis in reticulocyte lysates, there are substantial data available to suggest that heme may serve as a translational inhibitor of ALAS in some cell types. In finely chopped chick embryo liver organ culture, posttranscriptional inhibition of ALAS by heme was found (Tomita et al., 1974). In primary culture of avian hepatocytes, heme was found to exert an effect on drug induction of ALAS similar to that of the protein synthesis inhibitor, cycloheximide, leading to the suggestion that heme was acting at the translational level (Strand et al., 1972). The translational control by heme of ALAS synthesis in chick embryo liver cell culture has also been reported elsewhere (Sassa and Granick, 1970; Tyrrell and Marks, 1972; Sinclair and Granick, 1975). Translational control of heme synthesis has been postulated to take place at the level of ALAS synthesis at the polysomes, or in transport of the newly synthesized ALAS from the polysomes to the mitochondrion (Sinclair and Granick, 1975). Heme may combine with some apoprotein to modulate this translation (Granick et al., 1975). Evidence has been obtained in a cell-free system for a role by heme in the inhibition of ALAS peptide chain elongation (Yamamoto et al., 1983). As with the inhibition of transcription by heme, the molecular details of the translational inhibition of ALAS synthesis by heme remain to be elucidated.

4. Posttranslational regulation.   ALAS, like many mitochondrial proteins, is synthesized in the cytosol in a precursor form and then translocated into the mitochondrion and proteolytically processed into its mature form. In the liver of rats treated with 2-allyl-2-isopropylacetamide (AIA) (Hayashi et al., 1969; Scholnick et al., 1969), and in mice treated with AIA and 3,5-dicarbethoxy-1,4-dihydrocollidine (DDC) (Igarashi et al., 1976), ALAS activity was found to increase in both the mitochondria and the cytosol. Furthermore, it was shown that the cytosolic form is transferred into the mitochondria (Ohashi and Sinohara, 1978); the immunochemical identity of the mitochondrial and cytosolic fractions are identical (Nakakuki et al., 1980), and a catalytically active form of cytosolic ALAS derived from the intact enzyme appears to be the same as the mitochondrial enzyme (Ohashi and Kikuchi, 1979). ALAS in chick embryo liver is also synthesized in the cytosol and then translocated into the mitochondria (Hayashi et al., 1983; Srivastava et al., 1983a). The properties of the two forms are similar (Watanabe et al., 1984), and the processing of the cytosolic form apparently involves cleavage of a 56 N-terminal highly basic amino acid extension (Borthwick et al., 1985a).

  Hemin inhibits the transfer of cytosolic ALAS into the mitochondrion rats (Kurashima et al., 1970; Yamauchi et al., 1980; Hayashi et al., 1980), chick embryo livers (Srivastava et al., 1983b; Hayashi et al., 1983), and cock liver (Ohashi and Kikuchi, 1972). Alternatively, or perhaps additionally, hemin may block the posttranslocational processing of the ALAS precursor form (Ades, 1983). How heme inhibits translocation is presently not known, but it might be imagined that it is simply by the precursor form of ALAS binding free heme, thereby physically inhibiting subsequent translocation due to the secondary and tertiary structure assumed by the pre-ALAS–heme complex. Alternatively, an additional heme binding factor may be involved, or the pre-ALAS–membrane translocator complex may be blocked by heme. One final possibility is that heme in vivo stimulates proteolytic degradation of ALAS. This possibility has yet to be ruled out experimentally, although the accumulation of enzyme in the cytosol argues against this possibility.

B. Free heme pool and the role of glycine

Heme for regulation of the heme biosynthetic pathway has been postulated to arise from a small pool of "free" heme (Yannoni and Robinson, 1975; Grandchamp et al., 1981). This heme is probably "free" only in the sense that it is temporally uncommitted to an identified stable hemoprotein (Israels et al., 1975). This rapidly turning over heme fraction has been suggested to be derived from heme in transit from the mitochondria to hemoproteins (Schmid, 1973) or from heme loosely associated with apoproteins such as apocytochrome P450 and in exchange with other free and loosely bound hemes (Schmid, 1973; Bissell and Hammaker, 1976). The physiological regulatory heme pool has been indirectly estimated to be 10^{-7} to 10^{-9} M (Granick et al., 1975). It has been proposed that the degree of saturation of tryptophan pyrrolase by heme may serve as a gauge of the in vivo regulatory heme pool (Kappas et al., 1985; Yamamoto et al., 1981), but convincing and quantitative data are not currently available.

In the absence of chemical inducers, reducing the intracellular heme concentration by stimulation of heme degradation by heme oxygenase can induce ALAS an isolated chick embryo liver cell suspensions (Srivastava et al., 1980b). Iron chelators, which inhibit heme synthesis by interfering with the insertion of iron into the protoporphyrin IX molecule to form heme, can maintain the drug-initiated induction of ALAS, but do not induce ALAS themselves (Srivastava et al., 1980a; Srivastava et al., 1980b).

The availability of glycine as a substrate for ALAS could also potentially play a role in the regulation of heme biosynthesis. ALAS has a very low affinity for glycine (K_m of 5 to 19 mM for mammalian mitochondrial ALAS) (Tephly et al., 1973; Kappas et al., 1983). The concentration of glycine in the liver is estimated to be lower than this, about 1 mM (Cowtan et al., 1973; Moore and Disler, 1985; May et al., 1986). Substrates for glycine acyltransferase (glycine N-acylase) such as sodium benzoate and para-aminobenzoic acid (PABA) can divert glycine from the heme pathway (K_m of glycine for glycine acyltransferase is 1 M) (Tephly et al., 1973). Treatment of rats with these substrates prevented induction of ALAS by DDC (Tephly et al., 1973) and also reversed this induction (Piper et al., 1973). In the latter case, simultaneous administration of glycine with these compounds prevented the reversal of DDC induction caused by sodium benzoate or PABA (Piper et al., 1973).

C. Effect of steroids

The first group of physiological agents shown to induce porphyrin synthesis in primary culture of chick embryo liver cells were the 5β-H steroid metabolites of neutral C19 and C21 hormones (Granick and Kappas, 1967). These steroids were found to be active in concentrations as low as 10^{-6} to 10^{-8} M. The 5β epimers of these hormones have more inducing activity than do the 5α epimers in chick embryo liver both in ovo (Sassa et al., 1979; Anderson et al., 1982) and in in vitro cell culture (Sassa et al., 1979). Glucuronidation renders these steroids inactive as ALAS inducing agents (Granick and Kappas, 1967; Kappas and Granick, 1968).

Steroids augment the inducing ability of foreign chemicals in vitro only when both are added in suboptimal amounts (Kappas and Granick, 1968), and, as with foreign chemicals, steroid induction of ALAS is inhibited by agents which block protein and nucleic acid synthesis, suggesting that steroids, like foreign chemicals, induce the formation of ALAS rather than enhance its activity (Kappas and Granick, 1968; Kappas et al., 1968). The increase in ALAS induced by steroids has been attributed to an increase in ALAS-specific mRNA (Kappas et al., 1983), and the fact that the 5β-H steroids also induce cytochrome P450 (Anderson et al., 1982) suggests that the induction of ALAS might be attributable to a drop in the "free heme pool" in response to increased apo-P450 synthesis. This hypothesis is supported by the fact that hemin (Sassa et al., 1979; Kappas and Granick, 1968) and other metallopor-phyrins (Kappas and Granick, 1968) inhibit the induction or porphyrin formation by steroids, while CaMgEDTA stimulated the induction by steroids 10-fold, perhaps by inhibiting ferrochelatase and lowering heme concentrations, thereby derepressing ALAS synthesis (Sassa et al., 1979).

In adrenalectomized rats, administration of hydrocortisone was necessary for AIA-mediated induction of ALAS, but hydrocortisone had no effect on the induction in intact rats (Marver et al., 1966b). Cortisol administration to adrenalectomized-ovarectomized rats also facilitated the induction of ALAS by AIA (Padmanaban et al., 1973). Isolated perfused rat liver also required the addition of corticoids to the perfusion medium to allow induction of ALAS by AIA (Bock et al., 1971). The hormones hydrocortisone and triiodothyronine were found to have a "permissive" effect on AIA-induced ALAS levels in rats, but did not induce ALAS by themselves (Matsuoka et al., 1968). In chick embryo liver cells in serum-free media, thyroid hormone and insulin enhanced AIA-induced ALAS synthesis (Morgan et al., 1976); insulin alone, at concentrations of 2 to 3 nM, also augmented AIA induction in these cells (Granick et al., 1975). Dramatic increases in ALAS induction over uninduced controls have been observed in chick embryo liver cells cultured in serum-free media when AIA, hydrocortisone, insulin, and triiodothyronine were used in combination, although these hormones had no effect without AIA (Sassa and Kappas, 1977). The permissive effect of these hormones was also observed in the steroid-mediated induction of ALAS in these cells (Sassa et al., 1979). The exact role that these hormones play in control of heme biosynthesis is unknown, although they have been postulated to act at the transcriptional level through enhancement of mRNA synthesis (Matsuoka et al., 1968; Padmanaban et al., 1973) or at the translational level by stimulation of protein synthesis (Sassa et al., 1979).

D. Glucose effect

The potential role of diet in the induction of heme biosynthesis has been examined in whole animals. The drug-mediated induction of ALAS by AIA is greatly reduced in fed, compared to fasted, rats (Rose et al., 1961; Bock et al, 1971). Administration of glucose (De Matteis, 1964; Marver et al., 1966a; Hickman et al., 1968) or carbohydrates (Tschudy et al., 1964) reduces, but does not eliminate, ALAS induction. This phenomenon has also been observed in uninduced rats (Kim and Kikuchi, 1974) and inbred strains of mice (Gross and Hutton, 1971), and in phenobarbitol-induced rats (Bock et al., 1971). In these animals the inhibition of ALAS induction by drugs was shown to be specific for glucose and closely related sugars; other metabolites such as glycolytic intermediates and TCA cycle intermediates were less effective (Bonkowsky et al., 1973).

The mechanism by which glucose affects ALAS induction is not clear, but one hypothesis is that glucose acts by interfering with the induced synthesis of certain mRNAs (Marver et al., 1966a; Hickman et al., 1968; Bock et al., 1971). In chick embryo liver tissue culture, RNA prepared from the livers of rats treated with AIA and glucose had significantly less effect than RNA from rats treated with AIA alone in increasing porphyrin production in the culture (Hickman et al., 1968). In isolated rat liver cell suspensions (Edwards and Elliot, 1974) and isolated chick embryo liver cells in serum-free media (Srivastava et al., 1979), a dependence of AIA-mediated induction on cAMP was found, leading to an alternate proposal that the in vivo effects of glucose may be related to its effect of lowering hepatic cAMP concentration (Edwards and Elliot,

1974). However, in in vivo studies, cAMP treatment either had no effect (Bonkowsky et al., 1973) or inhibited induction of ALAS by AIA (Kim and Kikuchi, 1972; Kim and Kikuchi, 1974; Bonkowsky et al., 1979).

A third suggestion is that glucose may inhibit porphyrin production in vivo after being metabolized to UDP-glucuronic acid, thereby causing the conversion of inducing steroids to their inactive glucuronide derivatives (Granick and Kappas, 1967; Kappas and Granick, 1968). The glucose effect has also been suggested to be due to an increase in NADPH levels generated by the hexose monophosphate shunt and isocitrate dehydrogenase resulting in the detoxification of the inducing compounds in the liver (Marver, 1969). More recently, a study of porphyrin content in livers of fasting vs. fed pigs led to the proposal that fasting may in some way inhibit the activity of coproporphyrinogen oxidase (Smith and El-Far, 1980), thus lowering heme levels and allowing ALAS induction.

E. Regulation of prenatal and neonatal tissues

The regulation of heme biosynthesis in prenatal and newborn animals has been found to be different from that of their adult counterparts. In prenatal rats, rabbits, and guinea pigs (Woods and Dixon, 1972; Woods, 1974) and neonatal rabbits (Woods and Dixon, 1970), the basal activity of ALAS is elevated to four to eight times normal adult levels. ALAS is also much less sensitive to induction by AIA, DDC, and phenobarbital in prenatal (Song et al., 1971; Woods and Dixon, 1972) and neonatal rats (Song et al., 1971; Maines and Kappas, 1978), and in prenatal and neonatal rabbits (Woods and Dixon, 1970), as well as in maternal rats in later stages of pregnancy (Paul et al., 1974). The refractoriness of ALAS to induction by chemicals was shown not to be due to the presence of inhibitors of ALAS in neonatal livers, or to dietary or endocrine factors (Song et al., 1971). Hemin treatment had little effect on ALAS activity in fetal rat, rabbit, and guinea pig livers (Woods and Dixon, 1972; Woods, 1974; Woods and Murthy, 1975). A semiconstitutive or unrepressed synthesis of ALAS has been postulated for neonatal animals (Woods and Dixon, 1970; Woods and Dixon, 1972). More recently, it was discovered that treatment of neonatal rats with iron chelators allowed induction of ALAS by AIA to adult levels without affecting levels of heme. It was suggested that what appears to be a developmental difference in neonatal ALAS may actually be a chemical repression of its synthesis by endogenous iron released from fetal red blood cells during postparturition hemolysis and subsequent heme oxygenase activity (Maines and Kappas, 1978). However, differences in fetal and adult liver ALAS forms have been reported in the guinea pig (Bishop, 1976).

Following the recent demonstration of two distinct adult forms of ALAS (see Chap. 5), it will be of interest to see which form is predominant in fetal tissue, or if there is either additional fetal ALAS or fetal-specific promoters for the two known ALAS forms.

F. Effects of metals

Several metals have been shown to be effective inhibitors of heme biosynthesis. Foremost among these is cobalt. At low doses (60 mg/kg body weight), $CoCl_2$ reduces ALAS activity in rats (Nakamura et al. 1975; De Matteis and Gibbs, 1977), and it also exerts this effect in chick embryo liver cell culture (Schoenfeld et al., 1984). In addition, $CoCl_2$ can block the induced synthesis of ALAS in vivo and in vitro by AIA (Maines et al., 1976; Maines and Sinclair, 1977; Schoenfeld et al., 1984), DD (De Matteis and Gibbs, 1977; Maines and Sinclair, 1977), and the steroid etiocholanone (Maines and Sinclair, 1977). The effect of cobalt is transitory, with a return to control values of ALAS activity within 24 h (Nakamura et al., 1975; Tephly et al., 1978). Cobalt treatment also appears to induce heme oxygenase (Maines and Kappas, 1975; Maines et al., 1976; De Matteis and Unseld, 1976; Maines and Sinclair, 1977; Yoshinaga et al., 1982) and to suppress cytochrome P450 synthesis (Ravishankar and Padmanaban, 1983; Guzelian and Bissell, 1976). The induction of heme oxygenase by $CoCl_2$ is enhanced in adrenalectomized rats, and hydrocortisone treatment abolishes this effect (Sardana et al., 1980).

The metalloporphyrin Co-protoporphyrin also inhibits drug-mediated induction of ALAS (Igarashi et al., 1978), and following the observation that cobalt treatment causes the accumulation of a nonheme fraction in liver, it was proposed that the observed effects of cobalt were due to its conversion to Co-protoporphyrin (De Matteis and Gibbs, 1977; Igarashi et al., 1978). This proposal was later strengthened both in cell culture (Sinclair et al., 1982b; Schoenfeld et al., 1983; Schoenfeld et al., 1984) and in vivo in rats (Igarashi et al., 1978) by the isolation of Co-protoporphyrin after $CoCl_2$ treatment. Co-Protoporphyrin may thus exert a feedback repression effect analogous to that of the physiological metalloporphyrin, heme (Igarashi et al., 1978; Sinclair et al., 1982b). The alternative possibility, that it is the metal ion itself (either Fe or Co) which affects heme synthesis, has also been raised (Maines and Sinclair, 1977; Maines and Kappas, 1977a, b). In this scheme, the tetrapyrrole molecule acts as a carrier to deliver the metal ion to regulatory sites in the cell.

Co-Protoporphyrin can apparently be incorporated into the apoprotein of cytochrome P450 (Sinclair et al., 1982a; Bonkowsky et al., 1984). The resistance of Co-protoporphyrin (De Matteis and Gibbs, 1977) or the resulting protein (Ravishankar and Padmanaban, 1985) to degradation into bile pigments and their subsequent accumulation in the liver may explain the observed induction by $CoCl_2$ and Co-protoporphyrin of heme oxygenase (De Matteis and Unseld, 1976).

In contrast to the action of Co-protoporphyrin to induce heme degradation in vivo, another metal chelate, Sn-protoporphyrin, inhibits heme oxygenase induction (Kappas et al., 1985), even though the inorganic ions Co^+ and Sn^+ both induce heme oxygenase in vivo, and both Co-protoporphyrin and Sn-protoporphyrin inhibit heme oxygenase activity in vitro (Yoshinaga et al., 1982). Sn-Protoporphyrin inhibits the induction of ALAS by AIA (Galbraith et al., 1985), as does Co-protoporphyrin. Sn-Protoporphyrin, by inhibiting heme oxygenase, lowers the rate of cobalt-induced heme depletion (Kappas et al., 1985). It has been suggested that the metal atom of the porphyrin-metal chelate may determine the in vivo action of the synthetic heme analogues (Kappas and Drummond, 1986).

Iron loading of chick embryo hepatocytes with ferric nitriloacetate (Shedlofsky et al., 1983) and rats with iron dextran (Bonkowsky et al., 1983) or iron citrate (Stein et al., 1970) significantly stimulated ALAS induction by AIA over levels seen with AIA alone. Only in the case of iron dextran was an induction observed without addition of AIA; this induction was attributed to a decrease in ALA dehydratase activity, followed by an increase in ALAS activity (Bonkowsky et al., 1983). Inorganic iron loading of animals (Stein et al., 1970) or cell cultures (Schoenfeld et al., 1984) did not produce any effect on heme synthesis. The synergistic effect of iron citrate on AIA-mediated induction of ALAS is theorized to be due to increased mRNA synthesis (Stein et al., 1969; Bonkowsky et al., 1979).

G. Effects of selected chemicals and drugs

In general, ALAS inducing chemicals are characterized by high lipophilicity and resistance to conversion to compounds of lower lipophilicity (Marks et al., 1975). Inducing chemicals act by increasing enzyme levels, not by enhancing the activity of the enzyme (Whiting and Granick, 1976b). They appear to increase ALAS and cytochrome P450 mRNA, and the increase in ALAS mRNA can be prevented by heme (Borthwick et al., 1985b). All of the known inducing compounds are substrates for cytochrome P450 (Borthwick et al., 1985b). The induction of ALAS may be a direct result of the effect of these lipophilic compounds to induce apocytochrome P450, thereby depleting the regulatory heme pool and allowing derepression of ALAS synthesis (Romeo, 1977; May et al., 1986).

The first evidence that an increase in ALAS activity was responsible for a drug-induced porphyrinogenic response was found for DDC (Granick and Urata, 1963). The induction by DDC can be prevented by simultaneous administration of actinomycin D or hemin in mice (Gayathri et al., 1973). DDC and griseofulvin caused ferrochelatase inhibition and accumulation of protoporphyrin in mouse and rat liver (De Matteis and Gibbs, 1975). Low doses of DDC suppress ferrochelatase activity without inducing ALAS in vivo (Rifkind, 1979) and in chick embryo liver culture (Cole et al., 1981a), suggesting that inhibition of ferrochelatase (Cole et al., 1982) and subsequent heme depletion (Kappas et al., 1983) is not sufficient for ALAS induction.

DDC treatment also decreases cytochrome P450 levels in mice (Wada et al., 1968). In rats and mice induced with DDC, a green porphyrin derivative which is an inhibitor of ferrochelatase was found (Tephly et al., 1979), and this porphyrin could be labeled with ^{14}C-ALA (De Matteis et al., 1980b). Mice treated with griseofulvin also appeared to make a similar porphyrin inhibitor of ferrochelatase (De Matteis and Gibbs, 1980). In contrast, in chick embryo livers in vivo and in vitro, DDC inhibits ferrochelatase activity, but griseofulvin does not (Cole et al., 1981b). The green pigment found in DDC-induced rats has been identified as N-methylprotoporphyrin (Ortiz de Montellano et al., 1981). Rats injected with the ethyl analogue of DDC formed and accumulated N-ethylprotoporphyrin, which also inhibits ferrochelatase (Coffman et al., 1982). DDC is now known to act by transferring its 4-methyl group to the heme moiety of cytochrome P450, causing dissociation of the heme from the apocytochrome, loss of the iron atom, and formation of N-methylprotoporphyrin (Marks et al., 1986). The N-methylprotoporphyrin thus formed inhibits ferrochelatase and, therefore, heme synthesis, thereby causing induction of ALAS (Ortiz de Montellano et al., 1986).

Another potent porphyrinogenic agent is AIA. AIA induces ALAS activity dramatically in chick embryo liver cells in culture (Granick, 1966), perhaps at a transcriptional level (Tomita et al., 1974). In rat liver mitochondria, low concentrations of inhibitors of DNA synthesis such as mitomycin C and actinomycin D inhibited AIA-induced increase of ALAS (Narisawa and Kikuchi, 1966). AIA may stimulate increased ALAS mRNA synthesis (Tyrrell and Marks, 1972; Tomita et al., 1974; Srivastava et al., 1988), increase the stability of ALAS mRNA (Tyrrell and Marks, 1972), or alter the rate of transcription of the ALAS gene (Srivastava et al., 1988). A translational role for AIA-mediated induction of ALAS has also been proposed (Sassa and Granick, 1970). AIA does not affect the rate of ALAS degradation (Sassa and Granick, 1970).

AIA injected into rats increases RNA-dependent ALAS synthesis (Marver et al., 1966a). AIA has been reported to destroy free heme (Sassa and Kappas, 1981) as well as the heme of cytochrome P450 (De Matteis, 1970; Meyer and Marver, 1971; Satyanarayana Rao et al., 1972; Bonkowsky et al., 1984). Pretreatment of rats with phenobarbitone, which stimulates microsomal drug metabolism, doubled cytochrome P450 loss due to AIA. Treatment with SKF525, which inhibits drug-metabolizing enzymes, protected cytochrome P450 against AIA-induced degradation (De Matteis, 1970). Cytochrome P450 destruction by AIA results in the formation of green pigments different from *N*-methylprotoporphyrin which accumulate in the liver (Levin et al., 1972; De Matteis and Unseld, 1976). The heme adduct formed by AIA destruction of cytochrome P450 does not inhibit ferrochelatase (De Matteis et al., 1980b) and cytochrome P450 destroyed by AIA can be partially restored by replacement of the damaged heme moiety with an undamaged one from the regulatory heme pool, thus lowering the heme pool and derepressing ALAS (Correia et al., 1979; Correia et al., 1981; Ortiz de Montellano et al., 1986). In addition, AIA may induce cytochrome P450 apoprotein synthesis (Shedlofsky et al., 1983), thereby creating a further drain on the regulatory heme pool and further derepressing ALAS synthesis. AIA increases P450 mRNA levels, but newly synthesized apoprotein is rapidly degraded unless heme is available to stabilize it (Dwarki et al., 1987). The observed synergistic effects of AIA and DDC on induction of ALAS (Whiting and Granick, 1976a; Brooker et al., 1980) and cytochrome P450 apoprotein (Brooker and O'Connor, 1982) may be due to the combined effects of decreased heme synthesis and depletion of the existing heme pool.

Phenobarbital, and to a lesser extent benzpyrene, are also inducers of ALAS and apocytochrome P450 synthesis (Hasegawa et al., 1970; Baron and Tephly, 1970; Tephly et al., 1971). The drugs are not synergistic, and the mechanism of action of these two drugs appears to be the same for ALAS but not for P450 (Baron and Tephly, 1970). The induction of apocytochrome P450 by phenobarbital is independent of heme synthesis (Correia and Meyer, 1975), and phenobarbital induction of ALAS may partly result from lowered heme levels caused by its action to induce P450 apoprotein (Baron and Tephly, 1970; Rajamanickam et al., 1975; May et al., 1986). Phenobarbital induction of ALAS is reduced by carbohydrate feeding, and is inhibited by actinomycin D, leading to the hypothesis that it acts at a transcriptional level (Marver, 1969).

H. Possibility of multiple genes for ALAS

Because the regulation of hepatic and erythroid heme biosynthesis is so different, it has been postulated that there may be more than one ALAS gene. Immunological evidence for liver and erythroid ALAS isozymes has been found in chicken liver (Watanabe et al., 1983) and rat (Yamamoto et al., 1986). A single copy of the ALAS gene was found in the chicken by Maguire et al. (1986); they did not exclude the possibility of a separate erythroid ALAS gene but did not find any cross hybridization by any other gene with the ALAS gene they isolated. In the mouse (Schoenhaut and Curtis, 1986) and rat (Srivastava et al., 1988), only one ALAS mRNA species has been found. Recently, convincing evidence for the existence of two distinct ALAS forms has been obtained. These data are reviewed in detail in Chap. 5.

I. Hepatic cell type regulation: a model

In Fig. 4.1 a model for the regulation of heme biosynthesis in nondifferentiating nonerythroid cell types is shown. The basis of this model is the regulation of the first enzyme of the pathway, ALAS, by the end product, protoheme. This regulation appears to be expressed most significantly at the level of synthesis of ALAS as well as in the translocation and processing of the precursor form into the mitochondrion. The protoheme responsible is the still hypothetical "free heme pool." Currently, this model suffers from the lack of quantitation and identification of the nature of this heme pool. It would be unreasonable to assume that totally "free" protoheme is present in the cell at appreciable levels, so a major problem that remains is to identify the significant regulatory heme binding agent.

One potential heme binding protein may be the cytoplasmic precursor form of ALAS. It has been shown that heme inhibits the translocation of ALAS into the mitochondrion. It can be envisioned that this occurs either via heme interacting with an ALAS-specific mitochondrial translocator or by heme binding directly to the ALAS precursor, thereby causing it to fold into a conformation that is incompatible with subsequent translocation. Of these possibilities, the first seems least likely since it would require a specific transport system just for ALAS, a

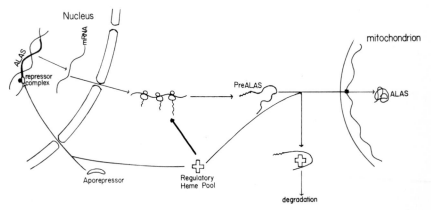

Figure 4.1 Model for control of heme biosynthesis in nonerythroid cells. Details are covered in the text.

protein of relatively low abundance in any circumstances. The second suggestion has several attractive features which include explanations for not only how the hepatic ALAS precursor is prevented from entering the mitochondrion, but also, if only the hepatic ALAS precursor binds heme, for why the effect of heme on erythroid ALAS differs from its effect on hepatic ALAS.

Overall, this model would allow maximum synthesis of ALAS, the rate-limiting enzyme of the pathway, in the absence of a significant regulatory heme pool. In the presence of a regulatory pool, the proto-heme would bind an as yet unidentified aporepressor and turn off the transcription of the ALAS gene. Heme would also bind pre-ALAS that is present in the cytoplasm and thus prevent its translocation into the mitochondrion. The critical regulatory heme pool concentration has been roughly estimated, but it should certainly be no greater than 10^{-6} M since that concentration of heme will inhibit ferrochelatase as well (see Chap. 3).

III. Regulation in Erythroid Cells

A. Role of heme

Because little cell multiplication occurs in the liver, the regulatory mechanism is relatively straightforward, and occurs through negative feedback effects of the final product, heme, on ALAS, the first enzyme of the pathway. In erythroid cells, the regulatory mechanism is not as well defined and different effects of heme have been reported depending on whether one is considering differentiating cells where heme synthesis is undergoing induction, or already hemoglobinized cells such as reticulo-cytes where heme appears to inhibit its own synthesis mainly by direct repression of ALAS (Karibian and London, 1965; Ibrahim et al., 1978), as well as by acting as a translational inhibitor of protein synthesis (Bruns and London, 1965) and by preventing the uptake of transferrin-bound iron into cells (Ponka and Neuwirt, 1969). Results of early investigations on heme biosynthesis in cultured chick blastoderms indicated that these cells have a mechanism similar to that of reticulocytes (Levere and Granick, 1965, 1967). These studies showed that chick blastoderms incubated in vitro start synthesizing heme at about 48 h after incubation has begun and that addition of ALA to the medium causes heme to be synthesized about 12 h earlier (Hoffman et al., 1980; Sassa and Urabe, 1979; Levere et al., 1967; Wainwright and Wainwright, 1966, 1967).

However, more recent studies in mouse erythroleukemia cells and human erythroleukemia cells in culture as well as in normal bone marrow cells have suggested that the mechanism which regulates heme biosynthesis in erythroid cells is more complicated than the one operating in hepatic tissues. This is not surprising as the mechanism regulating heme biosynthesis in erythroid cells needs to adjust to the cells' constantly changing demand for heme. Some evidence for different regulatory mechanisms operating in erythroid and hepatic cells comes from studies of the effects of hemin, Co-protoporphyrin, and dimethylsulfoxide (DMSO) on each of these cells. Hemin suppresses ALAS and heme biosynthetic activity in hepatic cells (Granick and Sassa, 1978) but stimulates heme biosynthesis in erythroid cells such as murine erythroleukemia cells in culture (Ibrahim et al., 1979), and augments the erythroid colony-forming capacity of normal murine bone marrow cells (Porter et al., 1979). Similarly, Co-protoporphyrin, a synthetic metalloporphyrin, stimulates heme biosynthesis in MEL cells (Chang and Sassa, 1982) but inhibits ALAS activity and decreases cytochrome P450 content in rat liver (Drummond and Kappas, 1981). DMSO, a potent inducer of heme oxygenase in liver cells, inhibits heme oxygenase in murine erythroleukemia cells in culture (Sassa, 1983). This finding suggests that in erythroid cells, not only is the biosynthesis of heme under different regulation than in the liver, but that the mechanism for regulating heme oxygenase is also distinct from that operating in liver cells.

B. In vivo studies of heme synthesis

Erythropoiesis and hemoglobin synthesis have been studied in vivo in the spleen of polycythemic mice during erythropoietin-induced erythropoiesis (Nakao et al., 1968), in anemic mutant mice (Sassa et al., 1975b; Sassa and Bernstein, 1977), in the fetal mouse (Rugh, 1968; Freshney and Paul, 1971), and in the avian yolk sac (Levere and Granick, 1965; Wainright and Wainright, 1970; Wilt, 1965). These studies have yielded important information about the induction of heme biosynthetic enzymes and the regulation of heme biosynthesis in whole animals.

Administration of erythropoietin to polycythemic mice results in an increase in RNA synthesis, an increase in the uptake of radiolabeled iron into heme, and an increase in the biosynthesis of heme and in the activity of enzymes of the heme biosynthetic pathway (Nakao et al., 1968). Activity of ALAS increases 8 h after the administration of erythropoietin, followed by an increase in ALA dehydrase activity at 12 h and an increase in ferrochelatase at 28 h (Nakao et al., 1968). Administration of actinomycin D simultaneously with erythropoietin blocks the induction of ALAS but this effect is not observed if actinomycin D is administered at 6 h after treatment with erythropoietin (Nakao et al., 1968). Although these early experiments do not provide much information regarding the regulation of heme biosynthesis in erythroid cells, they do indicate that the enzymes of the heme biosynthetic pathway are induced in a sequential manner in the spleen of polycythemic mice and suggest the importance of ALAS in the heme biosynthetic pathway. They also imply a close relationship between erythropoietin-induced stem cell differentiation and the appearance of ALAS.

Erythropoiesis in the embryonic mouse occurs in the yolk sac from days 1 to 12; from day 12 until a few days before birth erythropoiesis takes place in the liver; and after birth the spleen and bone marrow become the major sites of erythropoiesis (Rugh, 1968; Paul et al., 1969). The most rapid increase in the rate of hemoglobin synthesis occurs during the hepatic phase of erythropoiesis, between days 14 and 15 (Cole and Paul, 1966). During this time an increase in both the synthesis of protein-bound heme and in the levels of adult type hemoglobin are observed (Cole et al., 1968). The activity of the heme-synthesizing enzymes ALAS, ALA dehydrase, and ferrochelatase (heme synthase) may be involved in the control of hepatic erythropoiesis, as the activities of these enzymes have been correlated with the rate of hemoglobin synthesis at various times during gestation. The activity of ALAS, which was about 5 to 6 times higher than that in adult liver for most of the gestational period, reached a peak at 14 days at which point it was 20 times higher than in adult liver and had a specific activity of 3.10 to 6.50 pmol/min/mg protein. ALA dehydrase activity declined between days 12 and 13 of gestation and increased threefold during days 13 to 15. Activity then once again declined to reach normal levels by birth. Ferrochelatase activity declined between days 13 and 14, increased on days 14 and 15, and peaked on day 17. The activity of ferrochelatase had also declined to normal levels at birth. Hemoglobin levels reached a maximum at 15 days (Freshney and Paul, 1971). These results suggest that the activities of ALAS, ALA dehydrase, and ferrochelatase are sequentially induced in the developing mouse embryo and that ferrochelatase is coinduced with hemoglobin synthesis. The considerable delay between maximal induction of ALAS and maximum heme synthesis suggests that ALAS may not be rate-limiting for heme biosynthesis in the mouse embryos as it is in the adult liver.

There is some evidence in the literature that the fetal form of ALAS is similar to the adult erythropoietic form but different form the adult liver form. In contrast to ALAS activity in the adult liver, the activity of ALAS in fetal rodent liver cannot be suppressed by treatment with hemin (Woods and Dixon, 1972; Woods, 1974). However, treatment with aminotriazole suppresses ALAS activity in fetal rodent liver and this suppression can be reversed by concurrent treatment with hemin. This is in contrast to the effect of aminotriazole in adult liver where it causes activity of ALAS to be significantly increased (Woods, 1974). Further evidence that the fetal and the adult form of ALA synthase are different isozymes and regulated by different mechanisms comes from studies involving affinity chromatography on columns composed of AMP

(6-amino) and CoA (sulfhydryl) carboxymethyl cellulose (Bishop et al., 1981).

The temporal separation between maximal ALA dehydrase activity and hemoglobin synthesis indicates that ALA dehydrase would be a more likely candidate for the role of rate-limiting enzyme. The fact that some heme biosynthesis is observed at 15 days whereas maximal induction of ferrochelatase does not occur until 17 days suggests that induction of ferrochelatase may not be the rate-limiting step for heme biosynthesis in the fetal mouse.

C. In vitro studies of erythroid cells

Regulation of heme biosynthesis in erythroid cells has been studied in vitro in cultured chick blastoderm (Levere and Granick, 1965), in chick embryo cells in culture (Sassa and Granick, 1974), in the Philadelphia chromosome positive leukemia cell line, K562 (Hoffman et al., 1980), in Friend virus-transformed murine erythroleukemia cells (Sassa, 1983), human bone marrow cells (Sassa, 1980; Sassa, 1983), and suppressed rat marrow cells induced to undergo differentiation in culture (Beru and Goldwasser, 1985). Investigations with normal erythropoietic cells have been limited by several factors including the inability to establish normal erythroid precursors in long-term culture, the limited availability of genetic variants of significance to differentiation, and the difficulty of establishing a differentiating population synchronized with respect to critical events during differentiation (Marks and Rifkind, 1978). These problems are, for the most part, experimentally overcome by using transformed cells in culture.

The cells of the blood islands of the chick blastoderm are erythroid precursor cells which eventually differentiate into erythrocytes. They provide an excellent system for studying heme and globin synthesis as they can be maintained in culture where they simulate a phase culture of erythroid cells completely devoid of myeloid and lymphoid elements (Levere and Granick, 1965). Under normal circumstances, hemoglobin is first detected in these cells after 14 to 20 h of incubation and is at a maximum between 36 to 48 h; however, treatment of these islands with ALA results in rapid synthesis of large amounts of porphyrins, heme, and globin and causes hemoglobin to appear 12 h earlier (Levere and Granick, 1965, 1967; Levere et al., 1967; Wainwright and Wainwright, 1967).

Treatment of cultured chick blastoderms with steroids such as etiocholanolone or pregnenolone which enhance the de novo synthesis of ALAS also cause an increase in the synthesis of heme and globin and induce the early formation of hemoglobin (Irwing and Mainwaring, 1976; Levere et al., 1967). These results were interpreted to imply that synthesis of heme in erythroid precursor cells is limited by ALAS and that the other enzymes of the pathway are present in nonlimiting amounts (Levere and Granick, 1965, 1967; Levere et al., 1967). Hemoglobin formation can be prevented by addition of inhibitors of protein synthesis, but not by inhibitors of RNA synthesis, whereas heme synthesis is prevented by neither of these (Levere and Granick, 1967). This suggests that heme stimulates the synthesis of globin at the ribosomal level.

The human leukemia cell line K562 is useful for studying erythropoiesis since it represents a system in which erythropoietic stem cells can be maintained for extended periods and induced to undergo erythroid maturation in vitro (Hoffman et al., 1979). When treated simultaneously with sodium butyrate and erythropoietin (Hoffman et al., 1979) or separately with hemin or sodium butyrate (Rutherford et al., 1979a; Hoffman et al., 1980), K562 cells synthesize hemoglobin and undergo the membrane and enzymic changes of normal erythroid cells undergoing differentiation. Treatment with hemin or sodium butyrate not only increases the concentration of hemoglobin in K562 cells but also results in increased activity of ALAS, ALA dehydrase, and ferrochelatase as well as an increase in cellular heme synthesis (Hoffman et al., 1980). Hemin administration also causes a significant decrease in the activity of heme oxygenase, the rate-limiting enzyme in heme catabolism (Hoffman et al., 1980). This is in contrast to what has been reported in vivo in mice with normoblastosis where treatment with hemin causes a marked induction of heme oxygenase (Sassa et al., 1975a), but is in agreement with data reported by Ibrahim et al. (1979) which indicate that heme oxygenase activity is also decreased in erythropoietin-stimulated MEL cells. The significance of these observations is not clear but suggests that a decrease in erythroid heme oxygenase activity is an important feature of the differentiation process and perhaps allows for the conservation of heme to be incorporated into hemoglobin (Hoffman et al., 1980).

Murine erythroleukemia cell lines derived from susceptible mouse spleens infected with the Friend virus complex have been established in continuous cell culture and are useful as an in vitro system for studying the later stages of erythropoiesis. The cells grow in suspension culture as undifferentiated hemocytoblasts which have a low, but measurable, level of spontaneous differentiation depending on the cell strain and the culture media (Singer et al., 1974). When they are treated with dimethylsulfoxide (DMSO) or a variety of other agents including planar polar compounds such as hexamethylene bisacetamide, purines and purine derivatives, hemin, short-chain fatty acids, inhibitors of DNA or RNA synthesis, and uv or x-irradiation (Friend et al., 1971), they undergo differentiation along the erythroid pathway. DMSO-treated leukemia cells show several characteristics of the fully differentiated erythroid cell including erythrocyte membrane antigen (Friend et al., 1971), increased heme (Sassa et al., 1975a) and hemoglobin (Friend et al., 1971), and increased iron uptake (Friend et al., 1971).

During differentiation of some of these cell lines the activities of various enzymes in the heme biosynthetic pathway have been reported to increase in a sequential manner (Sassa et al., 1978). In a Friend cell clone (T3-C1-2) treated with DMSO, increases in ALAS and globin mRNA were seen at 24 h, followed by increases in the activity of ALA dehydrase at 36 h after induction, and PBG deaminase and uroporphyrinogen synthase (URO synthase) at 48 after induction (Ebert and Ikawa, 1974; Sassa et al., 1978; Rutherford et al., 1979b). Levels of ferrochelatase, the enzyme which catalyzes the insertion of iron into heme and is the terminal step in the biosynthesis of heme, rise much more slowly than those of the other enzymes and do not reach a peak until 96 h after induction (Ross et al., 1972; Sassa, 1976; Sassa et al., 1975a; Conder and Dailey, 1989). The increase in ferrochelatase corresponds to the appearance of hemoglobin (Rutherford et al., 1979b).

This sequential induction of the enzymes in the heme biosynthetic pathway has been found to occur in other Friend cell clones and with other inducers of differentiation. In DS19 cells treated with hexamethylene bisacetamide (HMBA), the early and sequential induction of ALA dehydrase, URO synthase, and PBG deaminase occurred more rapidly than in T3-Cl-3 cells treated with DMSO. The activity of ALA dehydrase started increasing at 9 h after induction to reach a maximum at 60 h, and the activities of PBG deaminase and URO synthase started increasing at 18 h after induction and peaked at 72 h (Sassa, 1983). Levels of protoporphyrin IX were significantly increased at 27 h indicating that the activity of protoporphyrinogen oxidase started increasing after that of PBG deaminase (Sassa, 1983). This is in contrast to reports that the increase in PBG deaminase is paralleled by an increase in protoporphyrinogen oxidase (Conder and Dailey, 1989). The percentage of benzidine positive cells increased significantly at 36 h and was 90% by 48 h; this was paralleled by the heme content of the cells (Sassa, 1983). Levels of heme oxygenase, the rate-limiting enzyme in the catabolism of heme, were significantly decreased in DS 19 cells treated with DMSO (Sassa, 1983). This rules out the possibility that induction of heme biosynthesis in cells treated with DMSO is triggered by a deficiency in heme caused by increased degradation of heme by heme oxygenase. Such a mechanism has been described to explain increased heme biosynthesis in the liver (Sassa and Kappas, 1977). The relationship between induction of ALA dehydrase and heme biosynthesis was linear for all MEL clones, as was that between the induction of PBG deaminase and heme biosynthesis. Thus, both ALA dehydrase and PBG deaminase are early inducible and quantitative markers for erythroid differentiation in MEL cells.

In normal human bone marrow cultures induced with erythropoietin, there is also a sequential induction of enzymes in the heme biosynthetic pathway (Gregory and Eaves, 1977; Sassa and Urabe, 1979; Sassa, 1980;

Sassa, 1983). ALAS, ALA dehydrase (Ibrahim et al., 1979), URO synthase, and PBG deaminase are significantly induced by day 4 and hemoglobin first appears on day 7. Levels of PBG deaminase increase linearly with increasing erythropoietin concentration and are proportional to increasing heme concentration (Sassa, 1980). The increase in URO synthase activity was reported to be proportional to the increase in ferrochelatase activity as determined by ^{59}Fe incorporation into heme by intact cells (Sassa and Urabe, 1979). Thus, in human bone marrow cells treated with erythropoietin the induction of ALA dehydrase, PBG deaminase, and URO synthases are early events and a quantitative indication of erythroid differentiation (Sassa and Urabe, 1979).

When suppressed rat marrow cells in culture are induced to undergo erythroid differentiation by treatment with erythropoietin, they respond by increasing their rates of iron uptake and hemoglobin synthesis (Beru and Goldwasser, 1985). The activities of ALAS, ALA dehydrase, and ferrochelatase are not significantly increased by treatment with erythropoietin, whereas the activity of PBG deaminase is greatly increased by the third day of incubation (Beru and Goldwasser, 1985). The increase in PBG deaminase parallels the increase in heme biosynthesis in much the same way as in normal human bone marrow cells (Sassa and Urabe, 1979), suggesting that induction of heme biosynthesis in these cells may be regulated by levels of PBG (Sassa and Urabe, 1979; Beru and Goldwasser, 1985). The data obtained from these studies suggest that regulation of heme biosynthesis in normal erythropoietin-induced erythropoiesis is different from that observed during erythroid differentiation in transformed erythroleukemia cells and is under the control of PBG levels.

D. Effects of inhibitors of heme biosynthesis

An alternate approach to investigate the regulatory role of heme during erythropoiesis has been to block endogenous heme synthesis in differentiating cells. Some studies have involved the use of nonspecific inhibitors such as 3-amino-1,2,3-triazole (Dabney and Beaudet, 1977), isoniazid (Hoffman and Ross, 1980), and penicillamine (Fuchs et al., 1981), but most studies have used more specific inhibitors that inhibit a particular step in heme biosynthesis.

Several divalent cations have been examined for their effect on heme biosynthesis in MEL cells. DMSO-treated cells were supplemented with Mn^{2+}, Cd^{2+}, and Co^{2+} which have been shown to inhibit ferrochelatase activity. All of these cations also strongly inhibited heme biosynthesis even at micromolar concentrations (Fadigan and Dailey, 1987). The fact that similar concentrations of these metals inhibit both ferrochelatase and heme biosynthesis suggests that inhibition of heme synthesis is mediated directly through inhibition of ferrochelatase rather than through effects on the iron uptake mechanism or some other mechanism

(Fadigan and Dailey, 1987) and that levels of ferrochelatase are of some importance in the overall control of heme biosynthesis.

Diethoxycarbonyl-1,4-dihydro-2,4,6-trimethylpyridine (DDC) affects hepatocyte heme biosynthesis by inhibiting ferrochelatase via production of N-methylprotoporphyrin which is a "suicide" inactivator of cytochrome P450 (De Matteis et al., 1980a; Ortiz de Montellano et al., 1986; Cole et al., 1981a; Dailey and Fleming, 1983). Supplementation of DMSO-induced MEL cells with up to 2 μM DDC caused the concentration of heme to increase, whereas heme concentration was decreased at concentrations of DDC from 2 to 6 μM (Fadigan and Dailey, 1987). Cell cultures exposed to 3 μM DDC had a ferrochelatase activity similar to that seen in control cultures, whereas those treated with 6 μM DDC had significantly lower ferrochelatase activity (Fadigan and Dailey, 1987). These data support the theory that ferrochelatase may be a rate-limiting step during the early stages of differentiation in MEL cells. Exogenously supplied N-methylprotoporphyrin had no effect on heme production in MEL cells despite the fact that it drastically inhibited ferrochelatase in enzyme assays. It is possible that MEL cells, like hepatocytes, contain an active DDC-metabolizing form of cytochrome P450 (which will produce in situ the alkylated porphyrin in a suicide reaction) and that this is responsible for elevating the endogenous levels of N-methylprotoporphyrin severalfold above those attained by exogenously supplying N-methylprotoporphyrin (Fadigan and Dailey, 1987).

Succinylacetone (4,6-dioxoheptanoic acid) is a potent inhibitor of ALA dehydrase (Ebert et al., 1979; Ebert et al., 1981). In MEL cells, succinylacetone causes a marked decrease in heme content and prevents the accumulation of hemoglobin (Ebert et al., 1979). These effects can be partially reversed by the addition of exogenous heme in the form of hemin (Ebert et al., 1979; Beaumont et al., 1984) or hematin (Ebert et al., 1981). Succinylacetone is, thus, a useful tool to study the effects of heme depletion on DMSO-mediated induction of the heme biosynthetic enzymes. Succinylacetone potentiates the induction of ALAS by DMSO in MEL cells (clone 745), implying that heme exerts a negative feedback control on ALAS induced by DMSO (Beaumont et al., 1984). This was further substantiated by the fact that addition of hemin reversed this effect. This is the only suggestion in the literature that heme may exert a negative feedback effect on ALAS in erythroid cells, and whether this is similar to negative feedback inhibition of ALAS as seen in the liver is unclear at this point.

The induction of ALA dehydratase in the presence of DMSO and succinylacetone was the same as that seen with DMSO alone as determined by a specific enzyme immunoassay (Beaumont et al., 1984), suggesting that there is no negative feedback inhibition of ALA dehydrase by heme or any intermediate metabolite of the pathway. Succinylacetone completely prevents the DMSO-mediated induction of immunoreactive PBG deaminase, causing the level and activity of this enzyme to remain in the same range as levels in uninduced cells (Beaumont et al., 1984), but does not modify the DMSO-mediated increase in PBG deaminase mRNA (Grandchamp et al., 1985), suggesting that succinylacetone affects the translation of the PBG deaminase message or the stability of the PBG deaminase protein. The effect of succinylacetone on PBG deaminase could not be reversed by hemin and since succinylacetone does not directly inhibit PBG deaminase this effect was difficult to explain. Perhaps PBG plays a necessary role in the induction of PBG deaminase. Such an observation would be in keeping with the "cascade theory" proposed by Sassa (1976) whereby the product of one enzyme activates the gene encoding the next enzyme, but does not explain why the suppression of one step in the heme biosynthetic pathway does not interfere with the enzyme activity in two other steps, namely, uroporphyrinogen decarboxylase (Grandchamp et al., 1985) and ferrochelatase (Beaumont et al., 1984).

Another interesting observation is that succinylacetone does not prevent mouse erythroleukemia cells from losing their proliferative capacity in the presence of DMSO (Grandchamp et al., 1985). This observation is in keeping with recent reports that the commitment of erythroid cells to terminal differentiation, as defined by their loss of proliferative capacity in the presence of DMSO (Gusella et al., 1976), can occur in the absence of hemoglobin synthesis (Gusella et al., 1982; Tsiftgolou et al., 1983). Imidazole, which prevents DMSO-induced differentiation of MEL cells but does not affect their loss of proliferative capacity, effectively dissociates terminal commitment from hemoglobin production by blocking only the latter (Gusella et al., 1982).

E. Role of steroids

The effect of steroids such as hydrocortisone, dexamethasone, aldosterone, deoxycorticosterone, and corticosterone on differentiation in mouse erythroleukemia cells was investigated by Scher et al. (1978), and several were found to be potent inhibitors of DMSO-induced differentiation, although there appeared to be no clear relationship between the inhibitory effect and the biological properties of the compound. The most potent inhibitor was hydrocortisone which was found to inhibit the synthesis of heme and globin and to decrease the hemoglobin content of the cells, as well as inhibiting ALA dehydrase and uroporphyrinogen synthase (Scher et al., 1978). Different effects of hydrocortisone on the synthesis of globin mRNA have been observed depending on the cell line used. For example, Scher et al. (1978) saw an inhibition of globin mRNA, whereas this effect was not observed by others (McLintock and Papaconstantinou, 1974). The mechanism by which heme biosynthesis is inhibited by steroids still remains to be elucidated, although it has been suggested that they act as pretranslational inhibitors of hemoglobin synthesis in much the same way as the halogenated pyrimidine 5-bromo-2'-deoxyuridine (BrdU) (Scher et al., 1972; Preisler et al., 1973; Sassa, 1976; Bick, 1977). BrdU inhibits the synthesis of globin mRNA and hemoglobin (Preisler et al., 1973; Scher et al., 1972) in DMSO-treated Friend leukemia cells. BrdU also prevents increases in ALA dehydrase and uroporphyrinogen synthase if added to the cells within 24 h after induction with DMSO, suggesting that proper transcription is necessary for cell differentiation (Sassa, 1976).

F. Role of iron supply and ferrochelatase

Several researchers have suggested the possibility that heme biosynthesis may be regulated by the iron supply to mitochondrial ferrochelatase, rather than by any of the enzymes in the pathway (Chap. 8; Ponka and Neuwirt, 1974; Ponka and Schulman, 1985). Several steps are involved in the uptake of iron for heme synthesis in erythroid cells and any one of these might be involved in the control mechanism. In reticulocytes iron uptake is coordinated with the utilization of iron for heme synthesis by a negative feedback mechanism in which heme inhibits the uptake of iron from transferrin (Ponka and Neuwirt, 1969; Ponka et al., 1975; Schulman et al., 1974). It appears that this type of control is specific for erythroid cells (Schulman et al., 1981) and seems to suggest that one of the steps in the iron-transferrin cycle may be limiting the overall rate of heme synthesis, possibly at the level of release of iron from transferrin (Morgan, 1981; Schulman et al., 1974; Ponka et al., 1975). In reticulocytes the iron-transferrin cycle can be bypassed by using iron chelators such as Fe-SIH (2-hydroxybenzal isonicotinoyl hydrazone). Increasing the amount of iron taken up by reticulocytes in this way increases the amount of heme synthesized above the maximum seen with saturating amounts of iron-transferrin (Ponka and Schulman, 1985).

Hemin has no effect on iron uptake into noninduced MEL cells but inhibits iron uptake into the cells after treatment with DMSO (Hradilek et al., 1981). Isonicotinic acid hydrazide (INH), which inhibits heme synthesis at the level of ALAS in reticulocytes (Karibian and London, 1965; Neuwirt et al., 1975a), causes an accumulation of iron in the mitochondria of DMSO-induced cells but not noninduced cells (Hradilek et al., 1981). Thus, it appears that there is a specific system for transporting iron into the mitochondria in DMSO-induced cells that is inhibited by hemin (Hradilek et al., 1981). In mutant MEL cells which cannot be induced by DMSO, heme has no effect on iron uptake and addition of INH does not enhance the accumulation of iron in the mitochondria, suggesting that these cells have a defect in their iron transport system.

Such a defect would explain the noninducibility of ferrochelatase in these cells (Hradilek et al., 1981). When Fe-SIH was used as a source of iron in MEL cells derived from clone 745a, it was found that they incorporated iron from Fe-SIH in amounts severalfold higher than from transferrin. In induced cells this results in substantially increased heme production over the maximum possible with transferrin, but in uninduced cells there is only a very slight increase in heme synthesis observed with Fe-SIH (Laskey et al., 1986). Therefore, it appears that iron utilization from transferrin limits the rate of heme production in Friend cells which are actively synthesizing heme but not in uninduced cells. This may be because levels of enzymes of the heme pathway are present in limiting amounts in uninduced cells (Laskey et al., 1986). ALAS may limit the rate of heme synthesis in noninduced MEL cells since addition of ALA to uninduced cells stimulates the rate of heme synthesis. In differentiating Friend cells the rate of heme biosynthesis is under some other control mechanism (Laskey et al., 1986).

Numerous studies have pointed to the importance of ferrochelatase in controlling the rate of heme synthesis in erythroid cells. Sassa (1976) and Rutherford et al. (1979b) observed that in order for Friend cells treated with DMSO to undergo normal differentiation the activity of ferrochelatase first had to be induced. This was true despite the fact that all other enzyme activities in the heme biosynthetic pathway had been induced at a considerably earlier time than ferrochelatase (Granick and Sassa, 1978; Rutherford et al., 1979b; Sassa, 1976). Another factor supporting the regulatory role of ferrochelatase in the regulation of heme biosynthesis in Friend cells is that Friend cells can be induced to differentiate by adding hemin to the media but this response cannot be initiated by adding intermediates such as ALA, porphobilinogen, or protoporphyrin to the media (Dabney and Beaudet, 1977; Granick and Sassa, 1978; Ross and Sautner, 1976).

Since Friend cells are transformed immortal cell lines, it is possible to obtain stable variants which are defective in erythroid differentiation. Analysis of the defects in such variants is useful in helping to identify the control mechanisms involved in erythroid differentiation. DMSO-resistance clones of MEL cells such as 745 Dr-1 do not complete differentiation in the presence of DMSO and do not accumulate heme (Sassa et al., 1978). Dr-1 cells showed greater increases in ALA dehydrase and PBG deaminase activities when treated with DMSO than did wild-type cells. However, there was very little increase in heme content, in the number of benzidine positive cells, or in the rate of globin synthesis (Sassa et al., 1978; Sassa, 1983). Dr-1 cells can be induced to differentiate and synthesize heme by simultaneous treatment with DMSO and hemin (Sassa et al., 1978). Similar results have been observed in other DMSO-resistant MEL clones, $F_4N + 2$ (Eisen et al., 1978), Fw (Rutherford and Harrison, 1979; Rutherford et al., 1979b), and M18 (Mager and

Bernstein, 1979), which also display normal induction of the early enzymes but no increase in heme biosynthesis.

The primary genetic lesion which prevents DMSO-resistant clones of MEL cells from differentiating has not been identified to date. Rutherford and Weatherall (1979) attempted to identify the basis for hemin requirement in Fw cells derived from Charlotte Friend's culture C1A. They attributed the deficiency in heme synthesis to a failure to induce ferrochelatase. ALAS and the intermediate enzymes were present at high levels of activity and were inducible by butyric acid, but ferrochelatase was inducible neither by butyric acid nor by butyric acid and hemin. The growth media was examined for the presence of porphyrin and was found to contain elevated levels of porphyrin, providing further evidence that Fw cells do not accumulate heme due to a block in the pathway at the level of ferrochelatase.

Much of the available evidence pointing toward ferrochelatase as being the rate-limiting enzyme is based on the observation that in differentiating MEL cells levels of ferrochelatase rise much more slowly than those of other enzymes and parallel the increase in heme biosynthesis (Sassa, 1976; Rutherford et al., 1979b), but recent studies have indicated that this may not be so (Beaumont et al., 1984; Fadigan and Dailey, 1987; Conder and Dailey, 1989). Many of the discrepancies between reports from one group of researchers to another have arisen because different laboratories have studied erythropoiesis in different strains of MEL cells and under different culture conditions, or because of the difficulty of measuring very low levels of ferrochelatase such as those seen early on in the induction process. Ferrochelatase was induced at the same rate as the early enzymes when Friend cells (clone 745) were treated with 1.5% DMSO (Beaumont et al., 1984) and levels of ferrochelatase, while low, were significantly induced by 24 h in DS19 cells treated with 2% DMSO (Conder and Dailey, 1989). These observations suggest that the large delay in incorporation of ^{59}Fe into heme after DMSO treatment seen by some researchers may not be related entirely to late induction of ferrochelatase but to some other phenomenon as well, and that ferrochelatase cannot be the rate-limiting enzyme throughout the entire time course of the differentiation process even though it may be rate-limiting for the first 48 h (Fadigan and Dailey, 1987). In spite of the early induction of ferrochelatase, the accumulation of heme did not take place until relatively late in the differentiation process (Beaumont et al., 1984), supporting the theory that another factor becomes rate-limiting during the later stages of differentiation.

Hemin appears to have a fundamental role in promoting maturation and the expression of late markers although the nature of this role is not clear. Although induction of "early erythroid" and "late erythroid" functions can occur independently of one another in MEL cells, both are needed in order for terminal erythroid differentiation to occur.

G. Regulation in differentiating erythroid cells: a model

It has been difficult to reconcile all of the currently available data from in vivo studies and in vitro studies and from studies on transformed cells and nontransformed cells and come up with a reasonable consensus model for the regulation of heme biosynthesis in erythroid cells. It is evident that regulation of heme biosynthesis in differentiating cells is complex and that regulatory mechanisms may be tailored to these cells' individual needs. For example, the mechanism by which heme biosynthesis is regulated in differentiating cells appears to be different from that operating in nondifferentiating cells and regulation in nontransformed cells appears to be different from regulation in transformed cells. Several theories have been put forward which propose that overall heme biosynthesis in erythroid cells is controlled not by ALAS or by ferrochelatase but by one of the intermediate enzymes or by some other mechanism. Laskey et al. (1986) have suggested, on the basis of their experiments, that ALAS may limit the rate of heme synthesis in nondifferentiating MEL cells, whereas iron utilization from transferrin is rate-limiting in differentiating MEL cells. Data from other investigators have pointed toward PBG deaminase as being a possible factor in the regulation of heme biosynthesis in normal erythropoietin-induced erythropoiesis in human bone marrow cells (Sassa and Urabe, 1979) and rat marrow cells (Beru and Goldwasser, 1985) as well as in cultured chick blastoderms (Levere and Granick, 1967) and differentiating MEL cells (Grandchamp et al., 1985). Fadigan and Dailey have proposed a model whereby ferrochelatase activity is rate-limiting for the first 48 h after induction of Friend cells and have suggested that after that time another factor, possibly iron availability, becomes rate-limiting.

Recently it was reported that coproporphyrinogen oxidase activity drops to 50% of its noninduced levels within 24 h after induction of DS-19 cells by DMSO (Conder and Dailey, 1989). This observation, along with the known requirement for PBG to stabilize PBG deaminase (see Chap. 2) and other data discussed above, allow us to construct a model for induction of heme biosynthesis in MEL cells. In this model an initial signal (as yet unknown) induces the early pathway enzymes. Newly synthesized PBG deaminase is unstable and inactive in the absence of sufficient PBG to be incorporated as the enzyme bound dipyrrole and so two mechanisms exist to rapidly raise the intracellular concentration of PBG. One of these is the increase in ALA being produced due to induction of ALA synthase and the second is a decrease in coproporphyrinogen oxidase activity, which will effectively damp the pathway, preventing carbon flow to heme and, indirectly, result in accumulation of PBG via product inhibition. Blockage of the pathway at coproporphyrinogen oxidase will also decrease the demand for iron in heme biosynthesis and allow iron to build up intracellularly to fully induce ALA synthase via an iron responsive promoter element (Chap. 5). Protoporphyrinogen oxidase activity rises rapidly at 24 h so that once protoporphyrinogen IX is being produced at high levels, it will readily be enzymatically converted to protoporphyrin IX. Although ferrochelatase is working at reduced capacity during the initial period postinduction, significant protoporphyrin accumulation does not occur since coproporphyrinogen oxidase activity is low. 48 h post induction all of the early enzymes are induced and ferrochelatase activity is rising. At 72 h ferrochelatase is no longer limiting and is still increasing in specific activity. Thus, control mechanisms may exist at at least four points: (1) ALA synthase, (2) PBG deaminase, (3) coproporphyrinogen oxidase, and (4) ferrochelatase. This represents a form of sequential induction, but of a nature somewhat different than that initially proposed by Sassa (1976).

The recent demonstration that two ALAS enzymes exist, one a proposed "housekeeping" or hepatic-type enzyme and the second an erythroid-specific protein, may help to explain some of the apparently conflicting data previously gathered (see Chap. 5). This discovery will require the critical reexamination of the properties of both ALAS enzymes. An example is the reported difference in the inhibitory activity of heme on ALAS from chick embryo liver cells (Pirola et al., 1984) and its effect on ALAS from adult rat liver (Scholnick et al., 1972).

However, additional key issues remain unresolved. Among these are all of the control elements involved in turning on all of the pathway and delineation of any possible rate-limiting steps. Data discussed in Chaps. 5 and 8 indicate that both heme and iron have potential roles in regulation, but the initial inducer still remains unidentified. It does appear accepted now that the same inducer turns on the entire pathway rather than having a sequential time course for induction. The explanation for temporal variations in actual enzyme activity induction will most likely be found to be a translational, translocational, or protein stability phenomenon rather than transcriptional regulation.

REFERENCES

Ades, I. Z. (1983). Biogenesis of mitochondrial proteins. Regulation of maturation of delta-aminolevulinate synthase by hemin, *Biochem. Biophys. Res. Comm.* **110**:42–47.

Anderson, K. E., Drummond, G. S., Freddara, U., Sardana, M. K., and Sassa, S. (1981). Porphyrogenic effects and induction of heme oxygenase in vivo by δ-aminolevulinic acid, *Biochim. Biophys. Acta* **676**:289–299.

Anderson, K. E., Freddara, U., and Kappas, A. (1982). Induction of hepatic cytochrome P-450 by natural steroids: Relationship to the induction of δ-aminolevulinate synthase and porphyrin accumulation in the avian embryo, *Arch. Biochem. Biophys.* **217**:597–608.

Baron, J., and Tephly, J. R. (1970). Further studies on the relationship of the stimulatory effects of phenobarbital and 3,4-benzpyrene on hepatic heme synthesis to their effects on hepatic microsomal drug oxidations, *Arch. Biochem. Biophys.* **139**:410–420.

Beaumont, C., Deybach, J. C., Grandchamp, B., Da Silva, V., de Verneuil, H., and Nordmann, Y. (1984). Effects of succinylacetone on dimethylsulfoxide-mediated induction of heme pathway enzymes in mouse Friend virus-transformed erythroleukemia cells, *Exp. Cell Res.* **154**:474–484.

Beru, N., and Goldwasser, E. (1985). The regulation of heme biosynthesis during erythropoietin-induced erythroid differentiation, *J. Biol. Chem.* **260**:9251–9257.

Bick, M. D. (1977). Bromodeoxyuridine inhibition of Friend leukemia cell induction, *Biochim. Biophys. Acta* **476**:279–286.

Bishop, D. F. (1976). Differentiation between isozymes of guinea pig δ-aminolevulinate synthase by affinity chromatography, *Fed. Proc.* **35**:1658, Abstract 1542.

Bishop, D. F., Kitchen, H., and Wood, W. A. (1981). Evidence for erythroid and nonerythroid forms of δ-aminolevulinic acid synthetase, *Arch. Biochem. Biophys.* **206**:380–386.

Bissell, D. M., and Hammaker, L. E. (1976). Cytochrome P-450 heme and the regulation of δ-aminolevulinic acid synthetase in the liver, *Arch. Biochem. Biophys.* **176**:103–112.

Bloomer, J. R., and Straka, J. G. (1988). Porphyrin metabolism, *The Liver: Biology and Pathobiology* (I. M. Arias, W. B. Jakoby, H. Popper, D. Schacter, and D. A. Shafritz, Eds.), 2nd ed., Raven, New York, pp. 451–466.

Bock, K. W., Krauss, E., and Fröhling, W. (1971). Regulation of δ-aminolevulinic acid synthetase by drugs and steroids in vivo and in isolated perfused rat liver, *Eur. J. Biochem.* **23**:366–371.

Bonkowsky, H. L., Collins, A., Doherty, J. M., and Tschudy, D. P. (1973). The glucose effect in rat liver: Studies of δ-aminolevulinate synthase and tyrosine aminotransferase, *Biochim. Biophys. Acta* **320**:561–576.

Bonkowsky, H. L., Healey, J. F., Sinclair, P. R., Sinclair, J. R., Shedlofsky, S. I., and Elder, G. H. (1983). Iron and the liver: Acute effects on iron-loading on hepatic heme synthesis of rats. Role of decreased activity of 5-aminolevulinate dehydrase, *J. Clin. Invest.* **71**:1175–1182.

Bonkowsky, H. L., Sinclair, J. F., Healey, J. F., Sinclair, P. R., and Smith, E. L. (1984). Formation of cytochrome P-450 containing heme or cobalt-protoporphyrin in liver homogenates of rats treated with phenobarbital and allylisopropylacetamide, *Biochem. J.* **222**:453–462.

Bonkowsky, H. L., Sinclair, P. R., and Sinclair, J. F. (1979). Hepatic heme metabolism and its control, *Yale J. Biol. Med.* **52**:13–37.

Borthwick, I. A., Srivastava, G., Day, A. R., Pirola, B. A., Snoswell, M. A., May, B. K., and Elliot, W. H. (1985a). Complete nucleotide sequence of hepatic 5-aminolevulinate synthase precursor, *Eur. J. Biochem.* **150**:481–484.

Borthwick, I. A., Srivastava, G., Hobbs, A. A., Pirola, B. A., Mattschoss, L., Steggles, A. W., May, B. K., and Elliot, W. H. (1985b). Control of synthesis of hepatic δ-aminolevulinic acid synthase and cytochrome P-450: Relationship to hepatic porphyrias, *Cellular Regulation and Malignant Growth* (S. Ebashi, Ed.), Japan Sci. Soc. Press, Tokyo/Springer, Berlin, pp. 144–151.

Brooker, J. D., May, B. K., and Elliot, W. H. (1980). Synthesis of δ-aminolaevulinate synthase in vitro using hepatic mRNA from chick embryos with induced porphyria, *Eur. J. Biochem.* **106**:17–24.

Brooker, J. D., and O'Connor, R. (1982). cDNA cloning and analysis of chick-embryo-liver cytochrome P-450 mRNA induced by porphyrinogenic drugs, *Eur. J. Biochem.* **129**:325–333.

Bruns, G. P., and London, I. M. (1965). The effect of hemin on the synthesis of globin, *Biochem. Biophys. Res. Comm.* **18**:236–241.

Chang, C. S., and Sassa, S. (1982). Effects of metalloporphyrins on hemoglobin formation in mouse Friend virus-transformed erythroleukemia cells. Stimulation of heme biosynthesis by cobalt protoporphyrin. *J. Biol. Chem.* **257**:3650–3654.

Coffman, B. L., Ingall, G., and Tephly, T. R. (1982). The formation of N-alkylprotoporphyrin IX and destruction of cytochrome P-450 in the liver of rats after treatment with 3,5-diethoxycarbonyl-1,4-dihydrocollidine and its 4-ethyl analog, *Arch. Biochem. Biophys.* **218**:220–224.

Cole, R. J., Hunter, J., and Paul, J. (1968). Hormonal regulation of pre-natal haemoglobin synthesis by erythropoietin, *Brit. J. Haematol.* **14**:477–488.

Cole, R. J., and Paul, J. (1966). The effects of erythropoietin on haem synthesis in mouse yolk sac and cultured foetal liver cells, *J. Embryol. Exp. Morphol.* **15**:245–260.

Cole, S. P. C., Marks, G. S., Ortiz de Montellano, P. R., and Kunze, K. L. (1982). Inhibition of ferrochelatase by *N*-methylprotoporphyrin IX is not accompanied by δ-aminolevulinic acid synthetase induction in chick embryo liver cell culture, *Canad. J. Physiol. Pharmacol.* **60**:212–225.

Cole, S. P. C., Whitney, R. A., and Marks, G. S. (1981a). Ferrochelatase inhibitory and porphyrin-inducing properties of 3,5-diethoxycarbonyl-1,4-dihydro-2,4,6-trimethylpyridine (DDC) and its analogues in chick embryo liver cells, *Mol. Pharmacol.* **20**:395–403.

Cole, S. P. C., Zelt, D. T., and Marks, G. S. (1981b). Comparison of the effects of griseofulvin and 3,5-diethoxycarbonyl-1,4-dihydro-2,4-6-trimethylpyridine on ferrochelatase activity in chick embryo liver, *Mol. Pharmacol.* **19**:477–480.

Conder, L. H., and Dailey, H. A. (1989). Regulation of heme biosynthesis in murine erythroleukemia cells. Role of the terminal enzymes. Manuscript submitted.

Correia, M. A., Farrell, G. C., Olson, S., Wong, J. S., Schmid, R., Ortiz de Montellano, P. R., Beilan, H. S., Kunze, K. L., and Mica, B. A. (1981). Cytochrome P-450 heme moiety. The specific target in drug-induced heme alkylation, *J. Biol. Chem.* **256**:5466–5470.

Correia, M. A., Farrell, G. C., Schmid, R., Ortiz de Montellano, P. R., Yost, G. C., and Mica, B. A. (1979). Incorporation of exogenous heme into hepatic cytochrome P-450 in vivo, *J. Biol. Chem.* **254**:15–17.

Correia, M. A., and Meyer, U. A. (1975). Apocytochrome P-450: Reconstitution of functional cytochrome with hemin in vitro, *Proc. Nat. Acad. Sci. (U.S.A.)* **72**:400–404.

Cowtan, E. R., Yoda, B., and Israels, L. G. (1973). Cycloheximide enhanced porphyrin synthesis in chick embryo liver: Association with an increase in the hepatic glycine pool, *Arch. Biochem. Biophys.* **155**:194–202.

Dabney, B. J., and Beaudet, A. L. (1977). Increase in globin chains and globin mRNA in erythroleukemia cells in response to hemin, *Arch. Biochem. Biophys.* **179**:106–112.

Dailey, H. A., and Fleming, J. E. (1983). Bovine ferrochelatase. Kinetic analysis of inhibition by *N*-methylprotoporphyrin, manganese and heme, *J. Biol. Chem.* **258**:11453–11459.

De Matteis, F. (1964). Increased synthesis of L-ascorbic acid caused by drugs which induce porphyria, *Biochim. Biophys. Acta* **82**:641–644.

De Matteis, F. (1970). Rapid loss of cytochrome P-450 and haem caused in the liver microsomes by the porphyrogenic agent 2-allyl-2-isopropylacetamide, *FEBS Lett.* **6**:343–345.

De Matteis, F., and Gibbs, A. H. (1975). Stimulation of the pathway of porphyrin synthesis in the liver of rats and mice by griseofulvin, 3,5-diethoxycarbonyl-1,4-dihydrocollidine and related drugs: Evidence for two basically different mechanisms, *Biochem. J.* **146**:285–287.

De Matteis, F., and Gibbs, A. H. (1977). Inhibition of haem synthesis caused by cobalt in rat liver. Evidence for two different sites of action, *Biochem. J.* **162**:213–216.

De Matteis, F., and Gibbs, A. H. (1980). Drug-induced conversion of liver haem into modified porphyrins. Evidence for two classes of products, *Biochem. J.* **187**:285–288.

De Matteis, F., Gibbs, A. H., and Smith, A. G. (1980a). Inhibition of protohaem ferrolyase by *N*-substituted porphyrins, *Biochem. J.* **189**:645–648.

De Matteis, F., Gibbs, A. H., and Tephly, T. R. (1980b). Inhibition of protohaem ferro-lyase in experimental porphyria. Isolation and partial characterization of a modified porphyrin inhibitor, *Biochem. J.* **188**:145–152.

De Matteis, F., and Unseld, A. (1976). Increased liver haem degradation by foreign chemicals a comparison of the effects of 2-allyl-2-isopropylacetamide and cobaltous chloride, *Biochim. Soc. Trans.* **4**:205–209.

Drummond, G. S., and Kappas, A. (1981). Prevention of neonatal hyperbilirubinemia by tin protoporphyrin IX, a potent competitive inhibitor of heme oxygenase, *Proc. Natl. Acad. Sci. (USA).* **78**:6466–6470.

Dwarki, V. J., Francis, V. N. K., Bhat, G. J., and Padmanaban, G. (1987). Regulation of cytochrome P-450 messenger RNA and apoprotein levels by heme, *J. Biol. Chem.* **262**:16958–16962.

Ebert, P. S., Frykholm, B. C., Hess, R. A., and Tschudy, D. P. (1981). Uptake of hematin and growth of malignant murine erythroleukemic cells depleted of endogenous heme by succinylacetone, *Cancer Res.* **41**:937–941.

Ebert, P. S., Hess, R. A., Frykholm, B. C., and Tschudy, D. P. (1979). Succinylacetone, a potent inhibitor of heme biosynthesis: Effect on cell growth, heme content, and δ-aminolevulinic acid dehydratase activity of malignant murine erythroleukemia cells, *Biochem. Biophys. Res. Comm.* **88**:1382–1390.

Ebert, P. S., and Ikawa, Y. (1974). Induction of δ-aminolevulinic acid synthetase during erythroid differentiation of cultured leukemia cells, *Proc. Soc. Exp. Biol. Med.* **146**:601–604.

Edwards, A. M., and Elliott, W. H. (1974). Induction of δ-aminolevulinic acid synthetase in isolated rat liver cell suspensions. Adenosine 3′,5′-monophosphate dependence of induction by drugs, *J. Biol. Chem.* **249**:851–855.

Eisen, H., Keppel-Ballivet, F., Georgopoulos, C. P., Sassa, S., Granick, J., Pragnell, I., and Ostertag, W. (1978). Biochemical and genetic analysis of erythroid differentiation in Friend virus-transformed murine erythroleukemia cells, *Differentiation of Normal and Neoplastic Hemapoietic Cells* (B. Clarkson, P. A. Marks, and J. E. Till, Eds.), Cold Spring Harbor Lab, Cold Spring Harbor Conference on Cell Proliferation, Vol. 5, p. 277.

Fadigan, A. G., and Dailey, H. A. (1987). Inhibition of ferrochelatase during differentiation of murine erythroleukemia cells, *Biochem. J.* **243**:419–424.

Freshney, R. I., and Paul, J. (1971). The activities of three enzymes of haem synthesis during hepatic erythropoiesis in the mouse embryo, *J. Embryol. Exp. Morphol.* **26**:313–322.

Friend, C., Scher, W., Holland, J. G., and Sato, T. (1971). Hemoglobin synthesis in murine virus-induced leukemia cells in vitro. Stimulation of erythroid differentiation of dimethylsulfoxide, *Proc. Nat. Acad. Sci.* (U.S.A.) **68**:378–382.

Fuchs, O., Ponka, P., Borova, J., Neuwirt, J., and Travnicek, M. (1981). Effect of heme on globin messenger RNA synthesis in spleen erythroid cells, *J. Supramol. Struct.* **15**:73–81.

Galbraith, R. A., Drummond, G. S., and Kappas, A. (1985). Sn-Protoporphyrin suppresses chemically induced experimental hepatic porphyria. Potential clinical implications, *J. Clin. Invest.* **76**:2436–2439.

Gayathri, A. K., Satyanarayana Rao, M. R., and Padmanaban, G. (1973). Studies on the induction of δ-aminolevulinic acid synthetase in mouse liver, *Arch. Biochem. Biophys.* **155**:299–306.

Grandchamp, B., Beaumont, C., de Verneuil, H., and Nordmann, Y. (1985). Accumulation of porphobilinogen deaminase, uroporphyrinogen decarboxylase and α- and β-globin mRNAs during differentiation of mouse erythroleukemic cells. Effects of succinylacetone, *J. Biol. Chem.* **260**:9630–9635.

Grandchamp, B., Bissell, D. M., Licko, V., and Schmid, R. (1981). Formation and disposition of newly synthesized heme in adult rat hepatocytes in primary culture, *J. Biol. Chem.* **256**:11677–11683.

Granick, S. (1966). The induction in vitro of the synthesis of δ-aminolevulinic acid synthetase in chemical porphyria: A response to certain drugs, sex hormones, and foreign chemicals, *J. Biol. Chem.* **241**:1359–1375.

Granick, S., and Kappas, A. (1967). Steroid induction of porphyrin synthesis in liver cell culture. I. Structural basis and possible physiological role in the control of heme formation, *J. Biol. Chem.* **242**:4587–4593.

Granick, S., and Kappas, A. (1971). δ-aminolevulinic acid synthetase and the control of heme and chlorophyll synthesis, *Metabolic Pathways. Metabolic Regulation* (H. J. Vogel, Ed.), Academic, New York, Vol. 5, pp. 77–141.

Granick, J. L., and Sassa, S. (1978). Hemin control of heme biosynthesis in mouse Friend virus-transformed erythroleukemia cells in culture, *J. Biol. Chem.* **253**:5402–5406.

Granick, S., Sinclair, P., Sassa, S., and Grieninger, G. (1975). Effects by heme, insulin, and serum albumin on heme and protein synthesis in chick embryo liver cells cultured in a chemically defined medium, and a spectrofluorometric assay for porphyrin composition, *J. Biol. Chem.* **250**:9215–9225.

Granick, S., and Urata, G. (1963). Increase in activity of δ-aminolevulinic acid synthetase in liver mitochondria induced by feeding of 3,5-dicarbethoxy-1,4-dihydrocollidine, *J. Biol. Chem.* **238**:821–827.

Gregory, C. J., and Eaves, A. C. (1977). Human marrow cells capable of erythropoietic differentiation in vitro: Definition of three erythroid colony responses, *Blood* **49**:855–864.

Gross, S. R., and Hutton, J. J. (1971). Induction of hepatic δ-aminolevulinic acid synthetase activity in strains in inbred mice, *J. Biol. Chem.* **246**:606–614.

Gusella, C. J., Geller, R., Clark, B., Weeks, V., and Houseman, D. (1976). Commitment to erythroid differentiation by Friend erythroleukemia cells, *Cell* **9**:221–229.

Gusella, J. F., Tsiftsoglou, A. S., Volloch, V., Weil, S. C., Neumann, J., and Houseman, D. (1982). Dissociation of hemoglobin accumulation and commitment during murine erythroleukemia cell differentiation by treatment with imidazole, *J. Cell. Physiol.* **113**:179–185.

Guzelian, P. S., and Bissell, D. M. (1976). Effect of cobalt on synthesis of heme and cytochrome P-450 in the liver. Studies of adult rat hepatocytes in primary monolayer culture and in vivo, *J. Biol. Chem.* **251**:4421–4427.

Hasegawa, E., Smith, C., and Tephly, T. R. (1970). Induction of hepatic mitochondrial ferrochelatase by phenobarbital, *Biochem. Biophys. Res. Comm.* **40**:517–523.

Hayashi, N., Kurashima, Y., and Kikuchi, G. (1972). Mechanism of allylisopropylacetamide-induced increase of δ-aminolevulinate synthetase in liver mitochondria. V. Mechanism of regulation by hemin of the level of δ-aminolevulinate synthetase in rat liver mitochondria, *Arch. Biochem. Biophys.* **148**:10–21.

Hayashi, N., Terasawa, M., Yamauchi, K., and Kikuchi, G. (1980). Effects of hemin on the synthesis and intracellular translocation of δ-aminolevulinate synthase in the liver of rats treated with 3,5-dicarbethoxy-1,4-dihydrocollidine, *J. Biochem.* **88**:1537–1543.

Hayashi, N., Watanabe, N., and Kikuchi, G. (1983). Inhibition by hemin of in vitro translocation of chicken liver δ-aminolevulinate synthase into mitochondria, *Biochem. Biophys. Res. Comm.* **115**:700–706.

Hayashi, N., Yoda, B., and Kikuchi, G. (1968). Mechanism of allylisopropylacetamide-induced increase of δ-aminolevulinate synthetase in liver mitochondria. II. Effects of hemin and bilirubin on enzyme induction, *J. Biochem.* **63**:446–452.

Hayashi, N., Yoda, B., and Kikuchi, G. (1969). Mechanism of allylisopropylacetamide-induced increase of δ-aminolevulinate synthetase in liver mitochondria. IV. Accumulation of the enzyme in the soluble fraction of rat liver, *Arch. Biochem. Biophys.* **131**:83–91.

Hickman, R., Saunders, S. J., Dowdle, E., and Eales, L. (1968). The effect of carbohydrate on δ-aminolaevulinate synthetase: The role of ribonucleic acid, *Biochem. Biophys. Acta* **161**:197–204.

Hoffman, L. M., and Ross, J. (1980). The role of heme in the maturation of erythroblasts. The effects of inhibition of pyridoxal metabolism. *Blood* **55**:762–771.

Hoffman, R., Ibrahim, N., Murnane, M. J., Diamond, A., Forget, B. G., and Levere, R. D. (1980). Hemin control of heme biosynthesis and catabolism in a human leukemia cell line, *Blood* **56**:567–570.

Hoffman, R., Murnane, M. J., Benz, E. J., Prohaska, R., Floyd, V., Dainiak, N., Forget, B. G., and Furthmay, H. (1979). Induction of erythropoietic colonies in a human chronic myelogenous leukemia cell line, *Blood* **54**:1182–1187.

Hradilek, A., Borova, J., Fuchs, O., and Neuwirt, J. (1981). The effect of heme on intracellular iron pools during differentiation of Friend erythroleukemia cells, *Biochim. Biophys. Acta* **678**:373–380.

Ibrahim, N. G., Gruenspecht, N. R., and Freedman, M. L. (1978). Hemin feedback inhibition of reticulocyte δ-aminolevulinic acid synthetase and δ-aminolevulinic acid dehydratase, *Biochem. Biophys. Res. Comm.* **80**:722–729.

Ibrahim, N. G., Lutton, J. D., and Levere, R. D. (1979). In vitro development of heme enzymes, *Blood* **54** (Suppl.):352.

Igarashi, J., Hayashi, N., and Kikuchi, G. (1976). δ-aminolevulinic acid synthetases in the liver cytosol fraction and mitochondria of mice treated with allylisopropylacetamide and 3,5-dicarbethoxy-1,4-dihydrocollidine, *J. Biochem.* **80**:1091–1099.

Igarashi, J., Hayashi, N., and Kikuchi, G. (1978). Effects of administration of cobalt chloride and cobalt protoporphyrin on δ-aminolevulinate synthase in rat liver, *J. Biochem.* **84**:997–1000.

Irwing, R. A., and Mainwaring, W. I. P. (1976). The regulation of haemoglobin synthesis in cultured chick blastoderm by steroids related to 5β androstane, *Biochem. J.* **45**:344–349.

Israels, L. G., Yoda, B., and Schacter, B. A. (1975). Heme binding and its possible significance in heme movement and availability in the cell, *Ann. N.Y. Acad. Sci.* **244**:651–661.

Jones, M. S., and Jones, O. T. G. (1970). Permeability properties of mitochondrial membranes and the regulation of haem biosynthesis, *Biochem. Biophys. Res. Comm.* **41**:1072–1079.

Kappas, A., and Drummond, G. S. (1986). Control of heme metabolism with synthetic metalloporphyrins, *J. Clin. Invest.* **77**:335–339.

Kappas, A., Drummond, G. S., and Sardana, M. K. (1985). Sn-Protoporphyrin rapidly and markedly enhances the heme saturation of hepatic tryptophan pyrrolase. Evidence that this synthetic metalloporphyrin increases the functional content of heme in the liver, *J. Clin. Invest.* **75**:302–305.

Kappas, A., and Granick, S. (1968). Steroid induction of porphyrin synthesis in liver cell culture. II. The effects of heme, uridine diphosphate glucuronic acid, and inhibitors of nucleic acid and protein synthesis on the induction process, *J. Biol. Chem.* **243**:346–351.

Kappas, A., Sassa, S., and Anderson, K. E. (1983). The porphyrias, *The Metabolic Basis of Inherited Disease*, (J. B. Stanbury, J. B. Wyngaarden, D. S. Frederickson, J. L. Goldstein, and M. S. Brown, Eds.), 5th ed., McGraw-Hill, New York, pp. 1301–1384.

Kappas, A., Song, C. S., Levere, R. D., Sachson, R., and Granick, S. (1968). The induction of δ-aminolevulinic acid synthetase in vivo in chick embryo liver by natural steroids, *Proc. Nat. Acad. Sci. (U.S.A.)* **61**:509–513.

Karibian, D., and London, I. M. (1965). Control of heme biosynthesis by feedback inhibition, *Biochem. Biophys. Res. Comm.* **18**:243–247.

Kim, H. J., and Kikuchi, G. (1972). Possible participation of cyclic AMP in the regulation of δ-aminolevulinic acid synthesis in rat liver, *J. Biochem.* **71**:923–926.

Kim, H. J., and Kikuchi, G. (1974). Mechanism of allylisopropylacetamide-induced increase of δ-aminolevulinate synthetase in liver mitochondria. Effects of administration of glucose, cyclic AMP, and some hormones related to glucose metabolism, *Arch. Biochem. Biophys.* **164**:293–304.

Kurashima, Y., Hayashi, N., and Kikuchi, G. (1970). Mechanism of inhibition by hemin of increase of δ-aminolevulinate-synthetase in liver mitochondria, *J. Biochem.* **67**:863–865.

Laskey, J. D., Ponka, P., and Schulman, H. M. (1986). Control of heme biosynthesis during Friend cell differentiation: Role of iron and transferrin, *J. Cell Physiol.* **129**:185–192.

Levere, R. D., and Granick, S. (1965). Control of hemoglobin synthesis in the cultured chick blastoderm by δ-aminolevulinic acid-synthase: Increase in the rate of hemoglobin formation with δ-aminolevulinic acid, *Proc. Nat. Acad. Sci. (U.S.A.)* **54**:134–137.

Levere, R. D., and Granick, S. (1967). Control of hemoglobin synthesis in the cultured chick blastoderm, *J. Biol. Chem.* **242**:1903–1911.

Levere, R. D., Kappas, A., and Granick, S. (1967). Stimulation of hemoglobin synthesis in chick blastoderms by certain 5β androstane and 5β pregnane steroids, *Proc. Nat. Acad. Sci. (U.S.A.)* **58**:985–990.

Levin, W., Jacobson, M., and Kuntzman, R. (1972). Incorporation of radioactive-δ-aminolevulinic acid into microsomal cytochrome P_{450}: Selective breakdown of the hemoprotein by allylisopropylacetamide and carbon tetrachloride, *Arch. Biochem. Biophys.* **148**:262–269.

Mager, D., and Bernstein, A. (1979). The role of heme in the regulation of the late program of Friend cell erythroid differentiation, *J. Cell Physiol.* **100**:467–480.

Maguire, D. J., Day, A. R., Borthwick, I. A., Srivastava, G., Wigley, P. L., May, B. K., and Elliott, W. H. (1986). Nucleotide sequence of the chicken 5-aminolevulinate synthase gene, *Nucl. Acids Res.* **14**:1379–1391.

Maines, M. D., Janousek, V., Tomio, J. M., and Kappas, A. (1976). Cobalt inhibition of synthesis and induction of δ-aminolevulinate synthase in liver, *Proc. Nat. Acad. Sci. (U.S.A.)* **73**:1499–1503.

Maines, M. D., and Kappas, A. (1975). Cobalt stimulation of heme degradation in the liver. Dissociation of microsomal oxidation of heme from cytochrome P-450, *J. Biol. Chem.* **250**::4171–4177.

Maines, M. D., and Kappas, A. (1977a). Regulation of heme pathway enzymes and cellular glutathione content by metals that do not chelate with tetrapyrroles: Blockade of metal effects by thiols, *Proc. Nat. Acad. Sci. (U.S.A.)* **74**:1875–1878.

Maines, M. D., and Kappas, A. (1977b). Metals as regulators of heme metabolism, *Science* **198**:1215–1221.

Maines, M. D., and Kappas, A. (1978). Prematurely evoked synthesis and of δ-aminolevulinate synthetase in neonatal liver. Evidence for metal ion repression of enzyme formation, *J. Biol. Chem.* **253**:2321–2326.

Maines, M. D., and Sinclair, P. (1977). Cobalt regulation of heme synthesis and degradation in avian embryo liver cell culture, *J. Biol. Chem.* **252**:219–223.

Marks, G. S., Allen, D. T., Sutherland, E. P., McCluskey, S. A., and Whitney, R. A. (1986). Comparison of the effects of 3-ethoxycarbonyl-1,4-dihydro-2,4-dimethylpyrimidine and 3,5-diethoxycarbonyl-1,4-dihydro-2,4,6-tri-methylpyrimidine on ferrochelatase activity and heme biosynthesis in chick embryo liver cells in culture, *Canad. J. Physiol. Pharmacol.* **64**:483–486.

Marks, G. S., Krupa, V., Murphy, F., Taub, H., and Blattel, R. A. (1975). Mechanisms of drug-induced porphyrin biosynthesis, *Ann. N.Y. Acad. Sci.* **244**:472–480.

Marks, P. A., and Rifkind, R. A. (1972). Protein synthesis: Its control in erythropoiesis, *Science* **175**:955–961.

Marks, P. A., and Rifkind, R. A. (1978). Erythroleukemic differentiation, *Ann. Rev. Biochem.* **47**:419–448.

Marver, H. S. (1969). The role of heme in the synthesis and repression of microsomal protein, *Symposium on Microsomes and Drug Oxidations, Bethesda, MD* (Gillette, J. R., A. H. Conney, G. J. Cosmides, R. W. Estabrook, J. R. Fouts, and G. J. Mannering, Eds.), Academic, New York, pp. 495–511.

Marver, H. S., Collins, A., Tschudy, D. P., and Rechcigl, M., Jr. (1966a). δ-Aminolevulinic acid synthetase. II. Induction in rat liver, *J. Biol. Chem.* **241**:4323–4329.

Marver, H. S., Collins, A., and Tschudy, D. P. (1966b). The "permissive" effect of hydrocortisone on the induction of δ-aminolaevulinate synthetase, *Biochem. J.* **99**:31C–33C.

Matsuoka, T., Yoda, B., and Kikuchi, G. (1968). Mechanism of allylisopropylacetamide-induced increase of δ-aminolevulinate synthetase in liver mitochondria. III. Effects of triiodothyronine and hydrocortisone on the induction process, *Arch. Biochem. Biophys.* **126**:530–538.

May, B. K., Borthwick, I. A., Srivastava, G., Pirola, B. A., and Elliot, W. H. (1986). Control of 5-aminolevulinate synthase in animals, *Curr. Topics Cell. Reg.* **28**:233–262.

McLintock, P. R., and Papaconstantinou, J. (1974). Regulation of hemoglobin synthesis in a murine erythroblastic leukemia cell: The requirement for replication to induce hemoglobin synthesis, *Proc. Nat. Acad. Sci. (U.S.A.).* **71**:4551–4554.

Meyer, U. A., and Marver, H. S. (1971). Chemically induced porphyria: Increased microsomal heme turnover after treatment with allylisopropylacetamide, *Science* **171**:64–65.

Moore, M. R., and Disler, P. B. (1985). Chemistry and biochemistry of the porphyrins and porphyrias, *Clinics in Dermatology. Porphyria*, (P. B. Disler and M. R. Moore, Eds.), J. B. Lippincott, Philadelphia, Vol. 3, pp. 7–23.

Morgan, E. H. (1981). Transferrin biochemistry, physiology and clinical significance, *Mol. Aspects Med.* **4**:1–123.

Morgan, R. O., Fischer, P. W. F., Stephens, J. K., and Marks, G. S. (1976). Thyroid hormone enhancement of drug-induced porphyrin biosynthesis in chick embryo liver cells maintained in serum-free Waymouth medium. *Biochem. Pharmacol.* **25**:2609–2612.

Nakakuki, M., Yamauchi, K., Hayashi, N., and Kikuchi, G. (1980). Purification and some properties of δ-aminolevulinate synthase from the rat liver ctyosol fraction and immunochemical identity of the cytosolic enzyme and the mitochondrial enzyme, *J. Biol. Chem.* **255**:1738–1745.

Nakamura, M., Yusukochi, Y., and Minakami, S. (1975). Effect of cobalt on heme biosynthesis in rat liver and spleen, *J. Biochem.* **78**:373–380.

Nakao, K., Sassa, S., Wada, O., and Takaku, F. (1968). Enzymatic studies on erythroid differentiation and proliferation, *Ann. N.Y. Acad. Sci.* **149**:224–228.

Narisawa, K., and Kikuchi, G. (1966). Mechanism of allylisopropylacetamide-induced increase of δ-aminolevulinate synthetase in rat-liver mitochondria, *Biochim. Biophys. Acta* **123**:596–605.

Neuwirt, J., Ponka, P., and Borova, J. (1975a). The role of heme in the regulation of δ-aminolevulinic acid and heme synthesis in rabbit reticulocytes, *Eur. J. Biochem.* **9**:36–41.

Neuwirt, J., Ponka, P., and Borova, J. (1975b). The regulatory role of heme in erythroid cells, *Erythropoiesis, Proc. 4th Int. Conf. on Erythropoiesis* (K. Nakao, J. W. Fisher, and F. Takaku, Eds.), University of Tokyo Press, Tokyo, pp. 413–421.

Ohashi, A., and Kikuchi, G. (1972). Mechanism of allylisopropylacetamide-induced increase of δ-aminolevulinate synthetase in liver mitochondria. VI. Multiple molecular forms of δ-aminolevulinate synthetase in the cytosol and mitochondria of induced cock liver, *Arch. Biochem. Biophys.* 153:34–46.

Ohashi, A., and Kikuchi, G. (1979). Purification and some properties of two forms of δ-aminolevulinate synthase from rat liver cytosol, *J. Biochem.* 85:239–247.

Ohashi, A., and Sinohara, H. (1978). Incorporation of cytosol δ-aminolevulinate synthase of rat liver into the mitochondria in vitro, *Biochem. Biophys. Res. Comm.* 84:76–82.

Ortiz de Montellano, P. R., Berlan, H. S., and Kunze, K. L. (1981). N-Methylproto-porphyrin. IX: Chemical synthesis and identification as the green pigment produced by 3,5-diethoxycarbonyl-1,4-dihydrocollidine treatment, *Proc. Nat. Acad. Sci.* 78:1490–1494.

Ortiz de Montellano, P. R., Costa, A. K., Grab, A., Sutherland, E. P., and Marks, G. S. (1986). Cytochrome P-450 destruction and ferrochelatase inhibition, *Porphyrins and Porphyrias* (Y. Nordmann, Ed.), John Libbey Eurotext, pp. 109–117.

Padmanaban, G., Satyanarayana Rao, M. R., and Malathi, K. (1973). A model for the regulation of δ-aminolaevulinate synthetase induction in rat liver, *Biochem. J.* 134:847–857.

Paul, S., Bickers, D. R., Levere, R. D., and Kappas, A. (1974). Inhibited induction of hepatic δ-aminolevulinate synthetase in pregnancy, *FEBS Lett.* 41:192–194.

Paul, J., Conkie, D., and Freshney, R. I. (1969). Erythropoietic cell population changes during the hepatic phase of erythropoiesis in the foetal mouse, *Cell and Tissue Kinet.* 2:283–294.

Piper, W. N., Condie, L. W., and Tephly, T. R. (1973). The role of substrates for glycine acyltransferase in the reversal of chemically induced porphyria in the rat, *Arch. Biochem. Biophys.* 159:671–677.

Pirola, B. A., Srivastava, G., Borthwick, I. A., Brooker, J. D., May, B. K., and Elliot, W. H. (1984). Effect of heme on the activity of chick embryo liver mitochondrial δ-aminole-vulinate synthase, *FEBS Lett.* 166:298–300.

Ponka, P., and Neuwirt, J. (1969). Regulation of iron entry into reticulocytes. I. Feedback inhibitory effect of heme on iron entry into reticulocytes and on heme synthesis, *Blood* 33:690–707.

Ponka, P., and Neuwirt, J. (1971). Regulation of iron entry into reticulocytes. II. Relationship between hemoglobin synthesis and entry of iron into reticulocytes, *Biochim. Biophys. Acta* 230:381–392.

Ponka, P., Neuwirt, J., and Borova, J. (1975). The role of heme in the release of iron from transferrin in rabbit reticulocytes, *Erythropoiesis, Proc. 4th Int. Conf. on Erythro-poiesis* (K. Nakao, J. W. Fisher and F. Takaku, Eds.), University of Tokyo Press, Tokyo, pp. 403–411.

Ponka, P., Neuwirt, J., Sperl, M., and Brezik, (1970). The ability of exogenous heme to restore globin synthesis in reticulocytes with impaired heme formation, *Biochem. Biophys. Res. Comm.* 38:817–824.

Ponka, P., and Schulman, H. M. (1985). Regulation of heme synthesis in erythroid cells: Hemin inhibits transferrin iron utilization but not protoporphyrin synthesis, *Blood* 65:850–857.

Porter, P. N., Meints, R. H., and Messner, K. (1979). Enhancement of erythroid colony formation in culture by hemin, *Exp. Hematol.* 7:11–16.

Preisler, H. D., Houseman, D., Scher, W., and Friend, C. (1973). Effects of 5-bromo-2'-deoxyuridine on production of globin messenger RNA in dimethylsulfoxide-stimulated Friend leukemia cells, *Proc. Nat. Acad. Sci. (U.S.A.)* 70:2956–2959.

Rajamanickam, C., Satyanarayana Rao, R., and Padmanaban, G. (1975). On the sequence of reactions leading to cytochrome P-450 synthesis—effect of drugs, *J. Biol. Chem.* 250:2305–2310.

Ravishankar, H., and Padmanaban, G. (1983). Effect of cobalt chloride and 3-amino-1,2,4-triazole on the induction of cytochrome P-450 synthesis by phenobarbitone in rat liver, *Arch. Biochem. Biophys.* 225:16–24.

Ravishankar, H., and Padmanaban, G. (1985). Turnover of messenger RNA, apoprotein and haem of cytochrome P-450 b + e induced by phenobarbitone in rat liver, *Biochem. J.* 229:73–79.

Revel, M., and Hiatt, H. H. (1964). The stability of liver messenger RNA, *Proc. Nat. Acad. Sci.* **51**:810–818.

Rifkind, A. B. (1979). Maintenance of microsomal hemoprotein concentrations following inhibition of ferrochelatase activity by 3,5-diethoxy-1,4-dihydrocollidine in chick embryo liver, *J. Biol. Chem.* **254**:4636–4644.

Romeo, G. (1977). Analytical review. Enzymatic defects of hereditary porphyrias: An explanation of dominance at the molecular level, *Hum. Genet.* **39**:261–276.

Rose, G. A., Hellman, E. S., and Tschudy, D. P. (1961). Effect of diet on induction of experimental porphyria, *Metabolism* **10**:514–521.

Ross, J., Ikawa, J., and Leder, P. (1972). Globin messenger-RNA induction during erythroid differentiation of cultured leukemic cells, *Proc. Nat. Acad. Sci. (U.S.A.)* **69**:3620–3623.

Ross, J., and Sautner, D. (1976). Induction of globin mRNA accumulation by hemin in cultured erythroleukemic cells, *Cell* **8**:513–520.

Rugh, R. (1968). In *The Mouse: Its Reproduction and Development*, Burgess, Minneapolis.

Rutherford, T. R., Clegg, J. B., and Weatherall, D. J. (1979a). K562 human leukemic cells synthesize embryonic hemoglobin in response to haemin, *Nature* **208**:164–165.

Rutherford, T. R., and Harrison, P. R. (1979). Globin synthesis and erythroid differentiation in a Friend cell variant deficient in heme synthesis, *Proc. Nat. Acad. Sci.* **76**:5660–5664.

Rutherford, T. R., Thompson, G. C., and Moore, M. R. (1979b). Heme biosynthesis in Friend erythroleukemia cells: Control by ferrochelatase, *Proc. Nat. Acad. Sci. (U.S.A.)* **76**:833–836.

Rutherford, T. R., and Weatherall, D. J. (1979). Deficient heme synthesis as a cause of noninducibility of hemoglobin synthesis in a Friend erythroleukemia cell line, *Cell* **16**:415–423.

Sano, S., and Granick, S. (1961). Mitochondrial coproporphyrinogen oxidase and protoporphyrin formation, *J. Biol. Chem.* **236**:1173–1180.

Sardana, M. K., Sassa, S., and Kappas, A. (1980). Adrenalectomy enhances the induction of heme oxygenase and the degradation of cytochrome P-450 in liver, *J. Biol. Chem.* **255**:11320–11323.

Sassa, S. (1976). Sequential induction of heme pathway enzymes during erythroid differentiation of mouse Friend virus-infected cells, *J. Exp. Med.* **143**:305–315.

Sassa, S. (1980). Control of heme biosynthesis in erythroid cells, *In vivo and in vitro Erythropoiesis: The Friend System* (G. B. Rossi, Ed.), Elsevier/North-Holland Biomedical Press, New York, pp. 219–228.

Sassa, S. (1983). Heme biosynthesis in erythroid cells: Distinctive aspects of the regulatory mechanism, *Regulation of Hemoglobin Synthesis*, Elsevier, New York, pp. 359–383.

Sassa, S., and Bernstein, S. E. (1977). Levels of δ-aminolevulinate dehydratase, uroporphyrinogen-I synthase, and protoporphyrinogen IX in erythrocytes from anemic mutant mice, *Proc. Nat. Acad. Sci. (U.S.A.)* **74**:1181–1184.

Sassa, S., Bradlow, H. L., and Kappas, A. (1979), Steroid induction of δ-aminolevulinic acid synthase and porphyrins in liver. Structure-activity studies and the permissive effects of hormones on the induction process, *J. Biol. Chem.* **254**:10011–10020.

Sassa, S., and Granick, J. L. (1974). Induction of δ-aminolevulinic acid synthetase in chick embryo cells in culture, *Proc. Nat. Acad. Sci. (U.S.A.)* **67**:517–522.

Sassa, S., Granick, J. L., Eisen, H., and Ostertag, W. (1978). Regulation of heme biosynthesis in mouse Friend virus-transformed cells in culture, *In vitro Aspects of Erythropoiesis* (M. J. Murphy, Ed.), Springer, New York, p. 135.

Sassa, S., and Granick, S. (1970). Induction of δ-aminolevulinic acid synthetase in chick embryo liver cells in culture, *Proc. Nat. Acac. Sci.* **67**:517–522.

Sassa, S., Granick, S., Chang, C., and Kappas, A. (1975a). Induction of enzymes of the heme biosynthetic pathway in Friend leukemia cells in culture, *Erythropoiesis, Proc. 4th Int. Conf. on Erythropoiesis* (K. Nakao, J. W. Fisher, and F. Takaku, Eds.), University of Tokyo Press, Tokyo, pp. 383–395.

Sassa, S., and Kappas, A. (1977). Induction of δ-aminolevulinate synthase and porphyrins in cultured liver cells maintained in chemically defined medium. Permissive effects of hormones on induction process, *J. Biol. Chem.* **252**:2428–2436.

Sassa, S., and Kappas, A. (1981). Genetic, metabolic, and biochemical aspects of the porphyrias, *Advances in Human Genetics* (H. Harris and K. Herschhorn, Eds.), Plenum, New York, Vol. 2, pp. 121–231.

Sassa, S., Kappas, A., Bernstein, S. E., and Alvares, A. P. (1975b). Heme biosynthesis and drug metabolism in mice with hereditary hemolytic anemia, *J. Biol. Chem.* **254**:729–735.

Sassa, S., and Urabe, A. (1979). Uroporphyrinogen I synthase induction in normal human bone marrow cultures: An early and quantitative response of erythroid differentiation, *Proc. Nat. Acad. Sci. (U.S.A.)* **76**:5321–5325.

Satyanarayana Rao, M. R., Malathi, K., and Padmanaban, G. (1972). The relationship between δ-aminolaevulinate synthetase induction and the concentrations of cytochrome P-450 and catalase in rat liver, *Biochem. J.* **127**:553–559.

Scher, W., Preisler, H. D., and Friend, C. (1972). Hemoglobin synthesis in murine virus-induced leukemic cells in vitro. III. Effects of 5-bromo-2'-deoxyuridine, dimethylformamide and dimethylsulfoxide, *J. Cell Physiol.* **81**:63–70.

Scher, W., Tsuei, D., Sassa, S., Price, P., Gabelman, N., and Friend, C. (1978). Inhibition of dimethyl sulfoxide-stimulated Friend cell erythrodifferentiation by hydrocortisone and other steroids, *Proc. Nat. Acad. Sci. (U.S.A.)* **75**:3851–3855.

Schmid, R. (1973). Synthesis and degradation of microsomal hemoproteins, *Drug Met. Disp.* **1**:256–258.

Schoenfeld, N., Greenblat, Y., Epstein, O., Tschudy, D. P., and Atsmon, A. (1983). Evidence relating the inhibitory effect of cobalt on the activity of δ-aminolevulinate synthase to the intracellular concentration of porphyrins, *Biochem. Pharmacol.* **32**:2333–2337.

Schoenfeld, N., Wysenbeck, A. J., Greenblat, Y., Epstein, O., Atsmon, A., and Tschudy, D. P. (1984). The effects of metalloporphyrins, porphyrins and metals on the activity of delta-aminolevulinic acid synthase in monolayers of chick embryo liver cells, *Biochem. Pharmacol.* **33**:2783–2788.

Schoenhaut, D. S., and Curtis, P. J. (1986). Nucleotide sequence of mouse 5-aminolevulinic acid synthase cDNA and expression of its gene in hepatic and erythroid tissue, *Gene* **48**:55–63.

Scholnick, P. L., Hammaker, L. E., and Marver, H. S. (1969). Soluble hepatic δ-aminolevulinic acid synthetase: End-product inhibition of the partially purified enzyme, *Proc. Nat. Acad. Sci.* **63**:65–70.

Scholnick, P. L., Hammaker, L. E., and Marver, H. S. (1972). Soluble δ-aminolevulinic acid synthetase of rat liver. II. Studies related to the mechanism of enzyme action and hemin inhibition, *J. Biol. Chem.* **247**:4132–4137.

Schulman, H. M., Martinez-Medellin, J., and Sidloi, R. (1974). The reticulocyte-mediated release of iron and bicarbonate from transferrin. Effect of metabolic inhibitors, *Biochim. Biophys. Acta* **343**:529–535.

Schulman, H. M., Wilczynska, A., and Ponka, P. (1981). Transferrin and iron uptake by human lymphoblastoid and K-562 cells, *Biochem. Biophys. Res. Comm.* **100**:1523–1528.

Shedlofsky, S. I., Bonkowsky, H. L., Sinclair, P. R., Sinclair, J. F., Bement, W. J., and Pomeroy, J. S. (1983). Iron loading of cultured hepatocytes. Effect of iron on 5-aminolaevulinate synthase is independent of lipid peroxidation, *Biochem. J.* **212**:321–330.

Sinclair, J. F., Sinclair, P. R., Healey, J. F., Smith, E. L., and Bonkowsky, H. L. (1982a). Decrease in hepatic cytochrome P-450 by cobalt. Evidence for a role of cobalt protoporphyrin, *Biochem. J.* **204**:103–109.

Sinclair, P. R., and Granick, S. (1975). Heme control on the synthesis in cultured chick embryo liver cells, *Ann. N.Y. Acad. Sci.* **244**:509–520.

Sinclair, P. R., Sinclair, J. F., Bonkowsky, H. L., Gibbs, A. H., and De Matteis, F. (1982b). Formation of cobalt protoporphyrin by chicken hepatocytes in culture. Relationship to decrease of 5-aminolevulinate synthase caused by cobalt, *Biochem. Pharmacol.* **31**:993–999.

Singer, D., Cooper, M., Maniatis, G. M., Marks, P. A., and Rifkind, R. A. (1974). Erythropoietic differentiation in colonies of cells transformed by Friend virus, *Proc. Nat. Acad. Sci. (U.S.A.)* **71**:2668–2670.

Smith, S. G., and El-Far, M. A. (1980). The effect of fasting and protein calorie malnutrition on the liver porphyrins, *Int. J. Biochem.* **12**:979–980.

Song, C. S., Moses, H. L., Rosenthal, A. S., Gelb, N. A., and Kappas, A. (1971). The influence of postnatal development on drug-induced hepatic porphyria and the synthesis of cytochrome P-450. A biochemical and morphological study, *J. Exp. Med.* **134**:1349–1371.

Srivastava, G., Borthwick, I. A., Brooker, J. D., May, B. K., and Elliot, W. H. (1983a). Evidence for a cytosolic precursor of chick embryo liver mitochondrial δ-aminolevulinate synthase, *Biochem. Biophys. Res. Comm.* **110**:23–31.

Srivastava, G., Borthwick, I. A., Brooker, J. D., Wallace, J. C., May, B. K., and Elliot, W. H. (1983b). Hemin inhibits transfer of pre-δ-aminolevulinate synthase into chick embryo liver mitochondria, *Biochem. Biophys. Res. Comm.* **117**:344–349.

Srivastava, G., Borthwick, I. A., Maguire, D. J., Elferink, C. J., Bawden, M. J., Mercer, J. F. B., and May, B. K. (1988). Regulation of 5-aminolevulinate synthase mRNA in different rat tissues, *J. Biol. Chem.* **263**:5202–5209.

Srivastava, G., Brooker, J. D., May, B. K., and Elliot, W. H. (1980a). Haem control in experimental porphyria. The effect of haemin on the induction of δ-aminolaevulinate synthase in isolated chick-embryo liver cells, *Biochem. J.* **188**:781–788.

Srivastava, G., Brooker, J. D., May, B. K., and Elliot, W. H. (1980b). Induction of hepatic δ-aminolelvulinate synthase by heme depletion and its possible significance in the control of drug metabolism, *Biochem. Int.* **1**:64–70.

Srivastava, G., May, B. K., and Elliot, W. H. (1979). cAMP-dependent induction of δ-aminolevulinate synthase in isolated embryonic chick liver cells, *Biochem. Biophys. Res. Comm.* **90**:42–49.

Stein, J., Berk, P., and Tschudy, D. P. (1969). A model for calculating enzyme synthetic rates during induction: Application to the synergistic effect of ferric citrate on the induction of hepatic δ-aminolevulinic acid synthetase, *Life Sci.* **8** (part II):1023–1031.

Stein, J. A., Tschudy, D. P., Corcoran, P. L., and Collins, A. (1970). δ-Aminolevulinic acid synthetase. III. Synergistic effect of chelated iron on induction, *J. Biol. Chem.* **245**:2213–2218.

Strand, L. J., Manning, J., and Marver, H. S. (1972). The induction of δ-aminolevulinic acid synthetase in cultured liver cells. The effects of end product and inhibitors of heme synthesis, *J. Biol. Chem.* **247**:2820–2827.

Tephly, T. R., Gibbs, A. H., and De Matteis, F. (1979). Studies on the mechanism of experimental porphyria produced by 3,5-diethoxycarbonyl-1,4-dihydrocollidine. Role of a porphyrin-like inhibitor of protohaem ferro-lyase, *Biochem. J.* **180**:241–244.

Tephly, J. R., Hasegawa, E., and Baron, J. (1971). Effect of drugs on heme synthesis in the liver, *Metabolism* **20**:200–214.

Tephly, T. R., Wagner, G., Sedman, R., and Piper, W. (1978). Effects of metals on heme biosynthesis and metabolism, *Fed. Proc.* **37**:35–39.

Tephly, T. R., Webb, C., Trussler, P., Kniffen, F., Hasegawa, E., and Piper, W. (1973). The regulation of heme synthesis related to drug metabolism, *Drug Met. Disp.* **1**:259–266.

Tomita, Y., Ohashi, A., and Kikuchi, G. (1974). Induction of δ-aminolevulinate synthetase in organ culture of chick embryo liver by allylisopropylacetamide and 3,5-dicarbothoxy-1,4-dihydrocollidine, *J. Biochem.* **75**:1007–1015.

Tschudy, D. P., Ebert, P. S., Hess, R. A., Frykholm, B. C., and Weinbach, E. (1979). The effect of heme depletion on growth, protein synthesis, and respiration of murine erythroleukemia cells, *Biochem. Pharmacol.* **29**:1825–1831.

Tschudy, D. P., Marver, H. S., and Collins, A. (1965). A model for calculating messenger RNA half-life: Short lived messenger RNA in the induction of mammalian δ-aminolevulinic acid synthetase, *Biochem. Biophys. Res. Comm.* **21**:480–487.

Tschudy, D. P., Welland, F. H., Collins, A., and Hunter, G., Jr. (1964). The effect of carbohydrate feeding on the induction of δ-aminolevulinic acid synthetase, *Metabolism* **13**:396–405.

Tsiftsoglou, A. S., Nunez, M. T., Wong, W., and Robinson, S. H. (1983). Dissociation of iron transport and heme biosynthesis from commitment to terminal maturation of murine erythroleukemia cells, *Proc. Nat. Acad. Sci. (U.S.A.)* **80**:7528–7532.

Tyrrell, D. L. J., and Marks, G. S. (1972). Drug-induced porphyrin biosynthesis. V. Effect of protohemin on the transcriptional and post-transcriptional phases of δ-aminolevulinic acid synthetase induction, *Biochem. Pharmacol.* **21**:2077–2093.

Wada, O., Yanao, Y., Urata, G., and Nakao, K. (1968). Behavior of hepatic microsomal cytochromes after treatment of mice with drugs known to disturb porphyrin metabolism in liver, *Biochem. Pharmacol.* **17**:595–603.

Wainwright, S. D., and Wainwright, L. K. (1966). Regulation of the initiation of hemoglobin synthesis in the blood island cells of chick embryos. II. Qualitative studies on the effects of actinomycin D and δ-aminolevulinic acid, *Canad. J. Biochem.* **45**:1543–1549.

Wainwright, S. D., and Wainwright, L. K. (1967). Regulation of the initiation of hemoglobin synthesis in the blood islands of chick embryos. II. Early onset and stimulation of hemoglobin formation induced by exogenous δ-aminolevulinic acid. *Canad. J. Biochem.* **45**:344–350.

Wainwright, S. D., and Wainwright, L. K. (1970). A kinetic study of the effects of δ-aminolevulinic acid upon the synthesis of embryonic and fetal hemoglobins in the blood island of developing chick blastodisc, *Canad. J. Biochem. Physiol.* **48**:400–406.

Watanabe, N., Hayashi, N., and Kikuchi, G. (1983). δ-Aminolevulinate synthase isozymes in the liver and erythroid cells of chicken, *Biochem. Biophys. Res. Comm.* **113**:377–383.

Watanabe, N., Hayashi, N., and Kikuchi, G. (1984). Relation of the extra-sequence of the precursor form of chicken liver δ-aminolevulinate synthase to its quaternary structure and catalytic properties, *Arch. Biochem. Biophys.* **232**:118–126.

Waxman, A. D., Collins, A., and Tschudy, D. P. (1966). Oscillations of hepatic δ-amino-levulinic acid synthetase produced in vivo by heme, *Biochem. Biophys. Res. Comm.* **24**:675–683.

Whiting, M. J. (1976). Synthesis of δ-aminolaevulinate synthase by isolated liver polyribosomes, *Biochem. J.* **158**:391–400.

Whiting, M. J., and Elliot, W. H. (1972). Purification and properties of solubilized mitochondrial δ-aminolevulinic acid synthetase and comparison with the cytosol enzyme, *J. Biol. Chem.* **247**:6818–6826.

Whiting, M. J., and Granick, S. (1976a). δ-Aminolevulinic acid synthase from chick embryo liver mitochondria. I. Purification and some properties, *J. Biol. Chem.* **251**:1340–1346.

Whiting, M. J., and Granick, S. (1976b). δ-Aminolevulinic acid synthase from chick embryo liver mitochondria. II. Immunochemical correlation between synthesis and activity in induction and repression, *J. Biol. Chem.* **251**:1347–1353.

Wilt, F. H. (1965). Regulation of the initiation of chick embryo hemoglobin synthesis, *J. Mol. Biol.* **12**:331–341.

Wolfson, S. J., Bartczak, A., and Bloomer, J. R. (1979). Effect of endogenous heme generation on δ-aminolevulinic acid synthase activity in rat liver mitochondria, *J. Biol. Chem.* **254**:3543–3546.

Woods, J. S. (1974). Studies on the role of heme in the regulation of δ-aminolevulinic acid synthetase during fetal hepatic development, *Mol. Pharmacol.* **10**:389–397.

Woods, J. S., and Dixon, R. L. (1970). Neonatal differences in the induction of hepatic aminolevulinic acid synthetase, *Biochem. Pharmacol.* **19**:1951–1954.

Woods, J. S., and Dixon, R. L. (1972). Studies of the perinatal differences in the activity of hepatic δ-aminolevulinic acid synthetase, *Biochem. Pharmacol.* **21**:1735–1744.

Woods, J. S., and Murthy, V. V. (1975). δ-Aminolevulinic acid synthetase from fetal rat liver: Studies on the partially purified enzyme, *Mol. Pharmacol.* **11**:70–78.

Yamamoto, M., Fujita, H., Watanabe, N., Hayashi, N., and Kikuchi, G. (1986). An immunochemical study of δ-aminolevulinate synthase and δ-aminolevulinate dehydratase in liver and erythroid cells of rat, *Arch. Biochem. Biophys.* **245**:76–83.

Yamamoto, M., Hayashi, N., and Kikuchi, G. (1981). Regulation of synthesis and intracellular translocation of δ-aminolevulinate synthase by heme and its relation to the heme saturation of tryptophan pyrrolase in rat liver, *Arch. Biochem. Biophys.* **209**:451–459.

Yamamoto, M., Hayashi, N., and Kikuchi, G. (1982). Evidence for the transcriptional inhibition by heme of the synthesis of δ-aminolevulinate synthase in rat liver, *Biochem. Biophys. Res. Comm.* **105**:985–990.

Yamamoto, M., Hayashi, N., and Kikuchi, G. (1983). Translational inhibition by heme of the synthesis of hepatic δ-aminolevulinate synthase in a cell-free system, *Biochem. Biophys. Res. Comm.* **115**:225–231.

Yamauchi, K., Hayashi, N., and Kikuchi, G. (1980). Translocation of δ-aminolevulinate synthase from the cytosol to the mitochondria and its regulation by hemin in the rat liver, *J. Biol. Chem.* **255**:1746–1751.

Yannoni, C. Z., and Robinson, S. H. (1975). Early-labelled haem in erythroid and hepatic cells, *Nature* **258**:330–331.

Yoshinaga, T., Sassa, S., and Kappas, A. (1982). Purification and properties of bovine spleen heme oxygenase. Amino acid composition and sites of action of inhibitors of heme oxidation, *J. Biol. Chem.* **257**:7778–7785.

Molecular Biology of Eukaryotic 5-Aminolevulinate Synthase

Peter Dierks

I. Perspectives and Summary

Iron protoporphyrin IX (heme) functions as the prosthetic group of a complex family of important hemoproteins and is an essential constituent of all animal cells. The "active center" of heme is the central iron atom, which exists in two stable oxidation states: Fe^{2+} and Fe^{3+}. This metal has a high affinity for oxygen (in the ferrous state) and can be reversibly oxidized by the transfer of single electrons to and from its environment. It is well suited, therefore, to function as a single electron carrier in electron transport chains and to serve as a catalyst for ligand binding and redox reactions involving molecular oxygen and certain other oxygen-containing compounds. These capabilities have been applied to a wide variety of biochemical processes associated with the aerobic metabolism of vertebrate organisms, including such prominent functions as the transport and storage of oxygen (hemoglobin and myoglobin), mitochondrial respiration (cytochromes b, c_1, c, a, and a_3), the oxidative metabolism of certain drugs and lipophilic chemicals (xenobiotic-inducible cytochrome P450 monooxygenases), steroid biosynthesis (steroidogenic cytochrome P450 enzymes), the desaturation of fatty acids (microsomal cytochrome b_5), tryptophan catabolism (tryptophan oxygenase), and the enzymatic destruction of peroxides (catalase and peroxidases). In addition, heme has begun to emerge in recent years as in increasingly important and complex regulatory molecule. In reticulocytes, heme controls the activity of a specific protein kinase that phosphorylates the α subunit of eIF2 (Ochoa, 1983; Safer, 1983; London et al., 1987; Edelman et al., 1987); this regulatory circuit plays a central role in coordinating the translation of α- and β-globin chains with the availability of heme during the terminal stages of red blood cell formation. Heme has also been implicated as an important component of the intracellular signaling mechanism (the oxygen sensor) that is used to trigger increased transcription of the erythropoietin gene in response to hypoxia (Goldberg et al., 1988). Moreover, as discussed in this chapter and elsewhere in this volume, heme acts in a number of ways to control the activity of genes involved in its own synthesis and catabolism.

All animal cells synthesize their own heme from simple precursors—glycine, succinyl-CoA, and reduced iron—by the successive action of eight nuclear-encoded enzymes (Fig. 5.1). The rate of heme synthesis is closely regulated in all tissues and coordinated with the expression of numerous apohemoprotein genes. Since the early 1960s, considerable research has been devoted to understanding how this coordination is achieved. Work has focused principally on the regulation of heme synthesis in the liver and in developing red blood cells. In addition to being the major heme-producing organs in vertebrates, these two tissues are the principal sources of excess porphyrin production in a number of inherited and drug-induced disorders of porphyrin synthesis in humans (Ibraham et al., 1983). Consequently, the development of a molecular framework for the regulation of heme and porphyrin synthesis

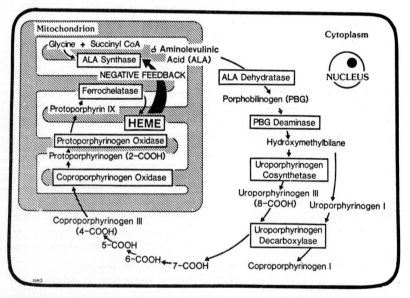

Figure 5.1   Heme biosynthetic pathway in eukaryotic animal cells (*courtesy of M. R. Moore*).

in these tissues is a problem of considerable clinical and fundamental significance.

In the liver, and probably most other fully differentiated tissues, the mechanisms that control the rate of heme synthesis are designed to accommodate transient (i.e., reversible) fluctuations in the rate of apoprotein synthesis. Much of our current understanding of how this is achieved stems from the pioneering work of Granick and colleagues on the regulation of porphyrin synthesis in mammalian and avian liver cells (Granick and Urata, 1963; Granick, 1966). Administration of substances such as barbiturates and dihydropyridines to laboratory animals causes a marked stimulation in the rate of hepatic porphyrin production. These compounds are substrates for a complex group of microsomal enzymes, the cytochrome P450-associated mixed-function oxidases (mono-oxygenases), that direct the oxidative conversion of numerous steroids, drugs, and other lipophilic chemicals (xenobiotics) to water-soluble derivatives [see Whitlock (1986) and Nebert and Gonzalez (1987) for recent reviews]. Collectively, these enzymes consume more than half the heme synthesized in normal liver (Marver and Schmid, 1972). In addition, the expression of each apocytochrome P450 isoenzyme associated with this system is acutely induced by the compounds on which it acts (Whitlock, 1986). An analysis of the effects of one such compound, 3,5-dicarbethoxyl-1,4-dihydrocollidine (DDC), on the activities of the heme pathway enzymes in guinea pig liver showed that it selectively increased the activity of the first enzyme, δ-aminolevulinic acid (ALA) synthase, which catalyzes the formation of ALA from glycine and succinyl-CoA in mitochondria (Granick and Urata, 1963). Since the activities of the remaining enzymes leading to protoporphyrin IX were not significantly altered, it was argued that they were normally present in nonlimiting amounts and that the porphyrinogenic activity of DDC was due to its effect on ALA synthase expression. Shortly thereafter, Granick (1966) reported that the drug-mediated induction of ALA synthase and porphyrin synthesis in cultured chicken embryonic liver cells was sensitive to inhibitors of RNA and protein synthesis and could be blocked by exogenous hemin. [Hemin does not, however, block the drug-mediated induction of cytochrome P450 synthesis (Giger and Meyer, 1981; Hamilton et al., 1988)]. On the strength of these observations, Granick proposed that heme regulates its own rate of synthesis by controlling the production of ALA synthase, the first and rate-limiting enzyme of the pathway. Moreover, since the induction of this enzyme by xenobiotics appeared to occur at the transcriptional level, it seemed reasonable to presume that the inhibition of induction by heme also operated at the level of transcription. Granick (1966), therefore, suggested that heme exerted its effects on ALA synthase expression by functioning as a corepressor of gene transcription.

Over the last 20 or so years extensive biochemical and enzymatic analyses of hepatic heme synthesis have consistently supported three central elements of Granick's model: (1) that ALA synthase is rate-limiting for heme synthesis; (2) that the induction of ALA synthase by xenobiotics is mediated primarily at the transcriptional level; and (3) that heme acts as a negative regulator of ALA synthase expression. However, the mechanisms of feedback regulation by heme appear to be more complex than originally anticipated. There is substantial evidence for at least two levels of control: feedback regulation of ALA synthase transcription, as originally postulated by Granick (1966); and posttranscriptional control of enzyme transport into mitochondria (Yamauchi et al., 1980; Hayashi et al., 1983; Srivastava et al., 1983b). In addition, there has been a moderate amount of debate concerning the exact role of xenobiotics in the induction process. The central issue is whether the induction of ALA synthase by xenobiotics is mediated solely by "derepression," that is, through the reduction of heme levels, or whether these compounds additionally act in a more direct fashion to increase the rate of ALA synthase gene expression. This issue has broad implications concerning the mechanisms that couple heme and apoprotein synthesis and is discussed at length below.

While there is general agreement about the central importance of ALA synthase in controlling the rate of hepatic heme synthesis, the role of this enzyme in erythroid cells has been the subject of considerable controversy. In erythroid cells heme is required primarily for the synthesis of hemoglobin, which accounts for more than 90% of the soluble protein in mature erythrocytes. The production of hemoglobin begins during the terminal stages of erythroid cell differentiation, as erythroid colony-forming (CFU-e) cells undergo differentiation to orthochromatic normablasts, and continues at a significant rate during the postmitotic maturation of these cells to reticulocytes. As with the induction of cytochrome P450 synthesis in the liver, this program is characterized by an acute increase in both the demand for heme and its rate of production. However, unlike the situation in liver, the induction of heme synthesis in this system is accompanied not only by an increase in ALA synthase, but by the activation of most, if not all, of the enzymes in the heme pathway (Sassa, 1976; Rutherford et al., 1979; Beaumont et al., 1984). The generalized activation of this pathway in erythroid cells, together with conflicting data on the exact timing of enzyme induction and the regulatory effects of heme, has led to considerable confusion about the role of ALA synthase and the nature of the kinetic limitation(s) on the rate of heme production. A variety of rate-limiting steps have in fact been proposed, including the formation of ALA (Levere and Granick, 1967; Gardner and Cox, 1988), the formation of heme by ferrochelatase (Sassa, 1976; Rutherford et al., 1979), and the transport of iron (Ponka and Neuwirt, 1970; Ponka and Schulman, 1985; Laskey et al., 1986). Over the last several years, however, the intellectual deadlock that has existed in this field has been largely broken through by an improved understanding of the molecular biology of this pathway. It is now clear that ALA synthase is encoded by at least two distinct genes: a house-keeping gene which is expressed in all tissues and cell types that have been examined, and an erythroid-specific gene which appears to be dedicated to the management of ALA production during the terminal stages of erythroid cell differentiation. Based on our current understanding of the molecular biology of the erythroid ALA synthase gene, the following general outline of events is proposed for the regulation of heme synthesis in developing red blood cells. During the early stages of this process, a developmental signal is generated which activates the expression of all of the genes in the heme biosynthetic pathway, perhaps as a means of recruiting this "housekeeping" pathway into the erythroid program. In the case of ALA synthase this entails the strong transcriptional activation of the erythroid gene; expression of the housekeeping gene is largely unaffected. For porphobilinogen (PBG) deaminase this signal results in the activation of an erythroid-specific promoter embedded within the PBG deaminase "housekeeping" gene (Grandchamp et al., 1987; Chretien et al., 1988). However, as in the liver, control of porphyrin production is proposed to be vested in the first step catalyzed by ALA synthase. Current evidence suggests that the activation of ALA synthase may be attenuated by two separate posttranscriptional feedback controls: one which couples the rate of ALA synthase translation to the availability of iron, and one which allows feedback regulation of enzyme levels by heme. Assuming that none of the downstream enzymes is rate-limiting the former control could be expected to coordinate protoporphyrin IX production with the supply of iron, while the latter may act to coordinate the production of heme with the availability of globin chains. Thus, there are certain strategic similarities between this model and the currently accepted principles for the regulation of heme synthesis in the liver.

II. Molecular and Genetic Characterization: Evidence for a Multigene System

A. Hepatic ALA synthase

1. Molecular characterization of the enzyme. The dramatic induction of hepatic ALA synthase by drugs such as AIA and DDC has greatly facilitated the molecular and genetic characterization of this enzyme. Drug-induced mitochondrial ALA synthase has been purified to apparent homogeneity from embryonic and adult chicken liver (Borthwick et al., 1983; Watanabe et al., 1984) and from adult rat liver (Srivastava et al., 1982). Glutaraldehyde cross-linking studies (Borthwick et al., 1983) and direct electron microscopic analysis of negatively stained enzyme preparations (Pirola et al., 1984) indicate that the solubilized native enzyme from embryonic chicken liver exists as a homodimer. The estimated molecular weights of the subunits as determined by SDS-polyacrylamide gel electrophoresis range from 65,000 (adult chicken liver) to 70,000 (adult rat liver).

Electron microscopic localization of ALA synthase in rat liver using gold-labeled antibodies indicates that the enzyme is attached to the matrix surface of the inner mitochondrial membrane (May et al., 1986). The biogenesis of ALA synthase in the liver is similar to what would be expected from its intramitochondrial location. Most nuclear-encoded mitochondrial proteins are synthesized in the cytoplasm as larger precursors which are then posttranslationally imported in the mitochondria and processed to their mature form [see Hay et al. (1984) for a review]. In general, the precursors contain aminoterminal extensions of 20 to 70 amino acids that target the protein to the mitochondria and participate in intramitochondrial sorting [see Schatz (1987)]. During or after internalization the presequence is generally removed by a metalloprotease. Both the chicken and rat enzymes have been shown to be synthesized in the cytosol on membrane-free polyribosomes as larger precursors which undergo proteolytic maturation during transport into the mitochondrion (Whiting, 1976; Brooker et al., 1980; Ades and Harpe, 1981; Srivastava et al., 1982; Srivastava et al., 1983a; Hayashi et al., 1983; Watanabe et al., 1983). Molecular weight estimates of the chicken precursor range from 70,000 (Whiting, 1976; Brooker et al., 1980) to 75,000 (Ades and Harpe, 1981). The rat precursor has been estimated at 76,000 (Srivastava et al., 1982). The precursor-product relationship of the cytosolic and mitochondrial forms of the enzyme has been established both in vivo by pulse-labelling experiments (Srivastava et al., 1982; Srivastava et al., 1983a) and in vitro by demonstrating the direct posttranslational transfer and concomitant processing of the primary translation product into isolated mitochondria (Hayashi et al., 1983).

An unusual feature of hepatic ALA synthase is the propensity of the precursor to accumulate in the cytosol of drug-treated adult chickens, rats, and mice (Ohashi and Kikuchi, 1972; Yamauchi et al., 1980; Igarashi et al., 1976). In AIA-treated rats the mitochondrial enzyme accumulates rapidly during the first several hours but then levels off. After a slight delay the cytosolic form also increases, but unlike the mature protein it continues to do so throughout the course of the drug treatment (Yamauchi et al., 1980). Although this behavior suggests that the capacity of the mitochondria to transport ALA synthase is limited, much higher levels of mitochondrial ALA synthase can be obtained in embryonic chicken liver without any significant accumulation of the precursor. Consequently, it is uncertain whether this apparent limitation in adult liver mitochondria indicates the existence of a regulatory process aimed specifically at limiting the levels of functional (mitochondrial) enzyme. Nevertheless, both the mechanism and physiological relevance warrant further investigation.

2. cDNA isolation and analysis. In embryonic chicken liver AIA and DDC act synergistically with respect to ALA synthase induction. When administered in combination the activity of the enzyme can be increased as much as 500-fold (Whiting and Granick, 1976a). Under these conditions ALA synthase constitutes 1% or more of the total protein synthesized (Whiting, 1976; Whiting and Granick, 1976b). By analyzing the amount of ALA synthase translated in vitro at the direction of RNA isolated from control and drug-treated livers, Brooker et al. (1980) demonstrated that the increased rate of enzyme synthesis was due at least in part to higher mRNA levels. Based on these observations Borthwick et al. (1984) constructed a cDNA library of drug-induced mRNA isolated from membrane-free polyribosomes and screened the library for putative ALA synthase clones by differential hybridization, using radiolabeled cDNA populations prepared from control and drug-treated liver mRNA as probes. Ninety percent of the clones showing strong hybridization to the probes prepared from drug-treated cells and little or no hybridization to the probe from control cells were found to encode ALA synthase. The amino acid sequence deduced from one full-length clone shows that the precursor contains 635 amino acids and has a calculated molecular weight of 69,852 (Borthwick et al., 1985). Based on the amino acid sequence determined for the N-terminus of the purified mitochondrial enzyme (Borthwick et al., 1985), the mature protein contains 579 amino acids (calculated molecular weight of 63,903) and is preceded by a transit sequence of 56 amino acids.

The cloning of ALA synthase from chicken liver has facilitated the isolation of homologous cDNAs from rat (Srivastava et al., 1988; Yamamoto et al., 1988), human (Bawden et al., 1987; Bishop, personal communication), and mouse liver (Young and Dierks, unpublished). The ALA synthase cDNAs isolated from rat and human liver mRNA encode preproteins of identical length and exhibit a high degree of sequence identity with chicken liver ALA synthase. An alignment of the predicted amino acid sequences of these proteins with that of the chicken enzyme suggests that each preprotein consists of a presequence containing 56 amino acids followed by 586 amino acids of the mature enzyme. The assignment of the cleavage site in the rat preprotein has been confirmed by N-terminal sequence analysis of the purified mitochondrial enzyme

(Srivastava et al., 1988). The amino acid identities of the mature proteins range from 78% (human to chicken) to 83% (human to rat); however, most of the sequence variability resides in the first 110 amino acids of the mature protein. Between amino acid 110 (residue 166 in the precursor) and the C-terminus of the chicken enzyme, 89% of the amino acid residues are identical in the human and chicken proteins, and more that 80% of the nonidentical residues are conservative amino acid substitutions. An additional, and striking, feature of these proteins is the high degree of sequence conservation in the first 38 amino acid residues of the presequence. Within this region there is one amino acid difference between the human and rat sequences (Bawden et al., 1987) and only five differences between human and chicken. The possible biological significance of this conserved region is discussed in a later section. However, the high degree of sequence identity in the enzyme core (C-terminal 75% of the mature protein) and in the N-terminus of the presequence establishes that these cDNAs are derived from homologous genes and provides a basis for classifying the genetic origin of other ALA synthase genes.*

3. Gene structure and expression.   The chick embryonic liver ALA synthase mRNA cloned by Borthwick et al. (1984) is encoded by a single nuclear gene which spans approximately 6.9 kb of chromosomal DNA (Elferink et al., 1987). Sequence analysis of the cloned gene has revealed that the coding regions are distributed over 10 exons which range in size from 156 to 280 bp (Maguire et al., 1986). The results of Northern blot hybridization analyses indicate that the gene encodes a single 2.2 kb mRNA which is present in all tissues that have been examined, including not only normal liver, heart, and brain, but also reticulocytes (Elferink et al., 1987). By all available criteria the structure of the reticulocyte transcript appears to be identical to that found in liver: Primer exten-

---

*The amino acid identities have been calculated based on the sequences reported by Srivastava et al. (1988) and Bawden et al. (1987) for the rat and human precursors, respectively. Between amino acid residues 118 and 134 of the preprotein these two sequences match each other at 13 of 19 positions, but share no sequence identity with the analogous region in the chicken precursor. Recently, Yamamoto et al. (1988) have reported a different amino acid sequence for this region in the rat preprotein due to a shift in reading frame caused by an insertion of a G residue at base position 375 and the absence of a G residue between positions 432 and 433. The sequence deduced by Yamamoto et al. matches the chicken precursor at 13 of 19 positions. Since the sequence of the chicken preprotein in this region has been partially confirmed by peptide sequence analysis (Borthwick et al., 1985), it seems likely that the sequence of Yamamoto et al. is the correct one for this region. A similar shift in reading frame for the human sequence would result in the same degree of amino acid identity between the human and chicken sequences. Hence, the percent identity among these proteins in the aminoterminal regions may be higher than originally anticipated. However, until these conflicts are resolved both sequences must be considered tentative.

sion analyses indicate that it has the same 5′ terminus as the liver RNA, and RNase protection experiments using probes that spanned the entire length of the hepatic ALA synthase mRNA failed to detect any differences in internal sequence organization. In addition, the size of the reticulocyte enzyme, as determined by immunological staining of SDS-polyacrylamide gels with polyclonal antibodies raised against the purified liver enzyme, appears to be identical to that of the liver (Elferink et al., 1987).

Srivastava et al. (1988) have recently reported the results of a similar study in rat, using probes derived from the rat liver cDNA. In agreement with the pattern established in chicken, a single ≈ 2.3 kb mRNA was detected in brain, heart, liver, kidney, testes, and spleen. By RNase protection mapping and primer extension, the structure of these transcripts was identical in each tissue. In addition, these investigators provided quantitative data for each tissue on the relative levels of the transcript in both untreated rats and rats that had been administered various inducers of ALA synthase expression. Basal levels of the RNA in liver and heart were found to be about twice as high as those in brain, kidney, and testes. Treatment of rats with AIA, which selectively induces ALA synthase activity in liver and kidney, resulted in a seven- to eight-fold increase in steady-state transcript levels in both of these tissues, but not in any of the others. Similarly, the amount of ALA synthase mRNA was selectively induced in testes by administration of human chorionic gonadotropin hormone.

These results, together with those described below for mouse liver ALA synthase, demonstrate that a single "hepatic" ALA synthase gene is expressed at a low level in a wide range of different tissues, including those of erythroid origin, and responds in an appropriate manner in liver, kidney, and testes to tissue-specific stimuli that induce ALA synthase expression. Therefore, it seems likely that this gene is active in all animal cells and is responsible for the maintenance of normal housekeeping functions.

B. Erythroid ALA synthase

One of the most controversial areas of investigation in recent years has been the genetic origin of erythroid ALA synthase. As noted above Elferink et al. (1987) have provided compelling evidence that the "hepatic" ALA synthase gene in chickens encodes identical mRNAs and proteins in liver cells and reticulocytes. Similarly, Srivastava et al. (1988) have demonstrated that anemic rat spleen contains an ALA synthase mRNA that is indistinguishable from that found in other tissues. Other investigators, however, have argued that different ALA synthase isozymes are expressed in these two tissues. Bishop et al. (1981) suggested that different forms of ALA synthase are expressed in erythroid and hepatic cells of guinea pig based on the differential binding of partially purified enzyme from these two sources of AMP-agarose. In direct contrast to the results of Elferink et al. (1987), Watanabe et al. (1983) reported that the ALA synthases in chicken liver and reticulocytes differ in size both as mature proteins and as precursors. In these studies polyclonal antibodies raised against purified hepatic ALA synthase were used to examine the apparent molecular weights of both the mature and precursor forms of the enzymes in hepatic and erythroid cells. In extracts of liver mitochondria the enzyme had an apparent molecular weight of 65,000, which is in good agreement with the molecular weight estimates (63,000 to 68,000) of the purified hepatic enzyme and the calculated molecular weight (63,903) of the mature protein. In contrast, the only cross-reacting protein in extracts of erythroid mitochondria had an apparent molecular weight of 53,000. Estimates of the sizes of the preproteins were obtained by analyzing the immunoreactive in vitro translation products synthesized by polyribosomes isolated from each cell type. Liver polysomes directed the synthesis of a precursor (molecular weight 73,000), which is close to the calculated molecular weight of 70,209, while erythroid polysomes produced a protein with an apparent molecular weight of 55,000.

While there was no question as to the accuracy of the estimated molecular weights of the mature and precursor forms of the hepatic enzyme in these experiments, the size estimates of the erythroid forms were the subject of considerable debate. Since hepatic ALA synthase in chickens and rats is known to be highly susceptible to proteolysis and easily converted to smaller polypeptides (molecular weight 49,000 for chicken and 51,000 for rat) that retain enzymatic activity [see May et al. (1986) for discussion], Elferink et al. (1987) suggested that the smaller erythroid forms detected by Watanabe et al. (1983) were likely due to proteolysis of the mature and precursor forms of the same protein that is expressed in liver. However, analyses conducted at the nucleic acid level suggested that this was not the case. Yamamoto et al. (1985) used the polyclonal antiserum described by Watanabe et al. (1983) to identify several putative ALA synthase cDNA clones in a reticulocyte cDNA expression library. One of the cDNAs identified in this approach was shown to hybridize selectively to a reticulocyte mRNA encoding the expected preprotein (molecular weight 55,000). This cDNA hybridized to a unique ≈ 2 kb mRNA that was expressed in reticulocytes but not in liver. In addition, under low stringency hybridization conditions this clone detected a larger noncognate transcript in liver. However, since two smaller liver transcripts, neither of which was large enough to encode ALA synthase, were also detected in these analyses, it is uncertain whether the larger liver transcript is the 2.2 kb ALA synthase mRNA described by Elferink et al. (1987). Moreover, while it seemed safe to conclude that the erythroid primary translation product (molecular weight 55,000) detected by Watanabe et al. (1983) was not encoded by the hepatic ALA synthase gene, but rather by a distinct gene which is differentially expressed in erythroid cells, no formal evidence was presented that the mature protein (molecular weight 53,000) encoded by this gene was in fact an erythroid-specific form of ALA synthase. This issue has recently been resolved, however, by the isolation and analysis of a nearly full length cDNA copy of the erythroid ALA synthase mRNA (Riddle et al., 1989). Sequence analysis of this clone showed that it encodes a preprotein (molecular weight 54,800, 518 amino acids) that shares substantial amino acid sequence identity with the hepatic protein (56% identity over the C-terminal 75% of the molecule). Genomic DNA blotting experiments and RNase protection assays further showed that this cDNA is encoded by a distinct ALA synthase gene which is expressed only in erythroid cells. In agreement with Elferink et al. (1987), these investigators also showed that the hepatic ALA synthase gene is coexpressed in erythroid cells, but at a level that is only 1 to 2% of the erythroid gene.

Similar confusion was initially encountered concerning the number of mouse genes encoding ALA synthase. In 1986 Schoenhaut and Curtis reported the successful use of a novel genetic complementation approach to isolate cDNAs encoding ALA synthase in BALB/c mouse. In this approach an amplified cDNA library was constructed from AIA-treated mouse liver RNA and transferred into an *E. coli hemA* mutant, which lacks endogenous ALA synthase activity and requires exogenous ALA for growth. Bacteria harboring recombinant plasmids that expressed sufficient ALA synthase activity to overcome the *hemA* mutation were then selected by growth on medium lacking exogenous ALA. To exclude the possibility that ALA-independent growth was due to a host mutation, plasmid DNA was isolated from several of the surviving colonies and reintroduced into the *hemA* strain, with the result that 80 to 100% of the transformants exhibited ALA-independent growth. In addition, a comparison of the ALA synthase activity of the parental *hemA* strain and each of the secondary (or tertiary) transformants confirmed that the plasmids directed the synthesis of enzymatically active ALA synthase. One of the resulting cDNAs was then characterized by partial DNA sequence analysis and used to isolate homologous sequences from an anemic spleen cDNA library. A comparison of the DNA sequences of several of the anemic spleen cDNAs with that of the AIA-treated liver cDNA showed that all were identical over ≈ 1 kb of DNA that was surveyed. In RNA blot hybridization experiments using the anemic spleen cDNA as the hybridization probe, a single band corresponding to a ≈ 2.3 kb mRNA was detected in samples obtained from liver, anemic spleen, and MEL cells. Additionally, the level of this mRNA was elevated in AIA-treated livers and in DMSO-induced MEL cells.

Although Schoenhaut and Curtis (1986) were careful not to exclude the possibility that there might be two closely related genes, or alternative promotes and/or splicing patterns within a single gene, the simplest interpretation of their data was that ALA synthase is encoded by a single gene in BALB/c mouse. The only discordant feature of their results, however, was that the nucleotide sequence and coding capacity of the BALB/c mouse ALA synthase cDNA were significantly different from those of the human, rat, and chicken clones. While the human and rat preproteins contain 642 amino acids, the mouse cDNA encodes a preprotein of only 572 amino acids. Although amino acid sequence data are not available for the murine erythroid isozyme, Schoenhaut and Curtis (1986) have suggested from the sequence of the corresponding cDNA that the mature protein may have a molecular weight of 56,400. An alignment of the predicted amino acid sequence of the BALB/c precursor with the human precursor using the LFASTA algorithm of Pearson and Lipman (1988) indicates that the two sequences are homologous over a region of 443 amino acids in the C-terminal 80% of the protein. However, the level of amino acid identity in this region is only 70%, as compared to a value of 90% when the same regions of the chicken and human sequences are compared. There is also a statistically significant similarity between residues 4 to 41 in the chicken precursor and residues 7 to 46 of the predicted mouse precursor, but the degree of sequence identity is only 23%, as compared to values ranging from 82 to 100% when the same regions of the human, rat, and chicken are compared.

More recently, Young and Dierks (unpublished data) used a different approach to isolate ALA synthase cDNAs from DBA/2 mouse and have found that the enzyme is encoded by two distinct genes which are differentially regulated in erythroid and nonerythroid cells. In this approach an ALA synthase cDNA clone was isolated from AIA/DDC-treated embryonic chicken liver and used as a hybridization probe to identify related RNA sequences in DBA/2 mouse tissues and in line 707 murine erythroleukemia (MEL) cells, which are also of DBA/2 origin. Partial DNA sequence analysis of the embryonic chicken liver ALA synthase cDNA showed that it was derived from the same drug-inducible mRNA that had been described previously by Borthwick et al. (1984, 1985). When this probe was used to examine Northern blots of poly(A)-containing RNA isolated from control and differentiated MEL cells and from control and DDC-treated DBA/2 mouse liver, two species of cross-hybridizing RNA was detected: a ≈ 2.1 kb RNA which was expressed at high levels in the differentiated MEL cells, and a ≈ 2.2 kb RNA which was expressed at high levels in DDC-treated liver. Partial cDNA clones (1.7 kb for the 2.1 kb mRNA and 1.4 kb for the 2.2 kb mRNA) of each of the mRNAs have been isolated and characterized by DNA sequence analysis. Comparison of these sequences with those reported for other ALA synthase cDNAs revealed that the ≈ 2.1 kb mRNA expressed in MEL cells is almost identical in sequence to the BALB/c ALA synthase cDNA reported by Schoenhaut and Curtis (1986), while the ≈ 2.2 kb mRNA expressed in DDC-treated liver is highly homologous to the chicken, human, and rat hepatic ALA synthase cDNAs: The degree of nucleotide sequence identity ranges from 79% (mouse to chicken) to 92% (mouse to rat). Although the complete sequences of these mRNAs have not yet been deduced from full-length cDNAs, genomic mapping studies conducted under stringent hybridization conditions and a comparison of the sequences of the partial cDNAs have indicated that the two mRNAs are encoded by distinct genes.

The results of nuclease S1 protection experiments, using DNA probes that were specific for each of these mRNAs, demonstrated that the "hepatic" DBA/2 ALA synthase mRNA is present at a low level in all tissues and cell types that have been tested, including bone marrow, anemic spleen, and both undifferentiated and differentiated MEL cells (Young and Dierks, unpublished data). Furthermore, it is clear from these analyses that the expression of this mRNA is selectively induced in DDC-treated liver and chronically elevated in the harderian glands of both male and female DBA/2 mice. Although the tissue distribution of this mRNA has not been exhaustively pursued, these results are consistent in all respects with the expression profiles of the rat and chicken hepatic ALA synthase genes (Srivastava et al., 1988; Elferink et al., 1987). The erythroid ALA synthase mRNA is coexpressed with the hepatic mRNA in uninduced MEL cells; however, during the course of MEL cell differentiation the level of this mRNA increases dramatically (50- to 75-fold), while that of the "hepatic" transcript remains relatively unchanged on a mass basis. High-level expression of this mRNA was also evident in bone marrow and anemic spleen. The distribution of the erythroid-inducible mRNA in other tissues is uncertain at the present time. Transcripts were detected in all tissues that were assayed, but none of these tissues were perfused prior to removal from the animals, raising the possibility that the transcripts detected were derived from circulating reticulocytes. This view is supported by the observation that there is no detectable expression of the erythroid-inducible ALA synthase mRNA in Hepa 1c1c7 mouse hepatoma cells (Young and Dierks, unpublished data). Nevertheless, it is clear that further studies are required to resolve this issue formally.

Based on these data, it seems likely that the genetic complementation approach used by Schoenhaut and Curtis (1986) introduced a strong bias for the recovery of clones encoding the erythroid-inducible form of the enzyme, thereby creating the false impression that the drug-inducible hepatic ALA synthase mRNA was the same as the mRNA expressed at high levels in differentiating erythroid cells. This view has been largely substantiated by nuclease S1 protection experiments, which have demonstrated the existence of the hepatic ALA synthase mRNA in BALB/c liver, spleen, brain, and harderian gland (Young and Gierks, unpublished data). These analyses have also shown that the level of the hepatic ALA synthase mRNA is markedly elevated in the livers of DDC-treated BALB/c mice. Therefore, there appears to be no significant discrepancy between these two inbred mouse strains with regard to the genetics and expression of ALA synthase.

C. Sequence comparisons: definition of the enzyme core

In addition to the cDNAs encoding the human (Bawden et al., 1987), rat (Srivastava et al., 1988; Yamamoto et al., 1988), and chicken (Borthwick et al., 1985) housekeeping enzymes and the murine (Schoenhaut and Curtis, 1986), and chicken (Riddle et al., 1989) erythroid isozymes, the complete nucleotide sequences of ALA synthase genes in *Saccharomyces cerevisiae* (*HEM*1 gene, Urban-Grimal et al., 1986) and *Bradyrhizobium japonicum* (*HemA* gene, McClung et al., 1987) have been determined. An alignment of the predicted amino acid sequences of these proteins using the LFASTA algorithm (Pearson and Lipman, 1988) indicates that the mammalian enzymes are composed of at least two domains. The C-terminal 70% of the mammalian precursors consists largely of a domain that likely represents the ancestral core of the enzyme. The N-terminus of this domain appears to be located near residue 192 in the chicken precursor. This position corresponds to the N-terminus (excluding leading methionines) of the enzymes found in *B. japonicum* and *Rhizobium meliloti* (partial sequence, Leong et al., 1985). In addition, the degree of sequence identity among the three eukaryotic enzymes falls off rapidly above this position. Between residues 192 and 573 in the chicken precursor, 30% of the positions are invariant among the seven genes and another 18% are identical in six of the seven sequences. Aside from a few small deletions the only significant disruption in these alignments is a 22 amino acid insertion in the yeast enzyme at residue 426. It is interesting to note that the molecular weight of the C-terminal domain in the chicken enzyme ($\approx 49,000$) is the same as that of the catalytically active degraded form obtained in a limit digest of the intact enzyme with papain (Borthwick et al., 1983). May et al. (1986) have reported that attempts to sequence the N-terminus of the degraded enzyme were unsuccessful, ostensibly due to heterogeneity of the ends, and proposed that proteolysis resulted in the loss of the N-terminal portion of the mature protein. Inspection of the hydropathy plots of these enzymes shows that the N-terminus of the conserved region (amino acids 203 to 208) is the most hydrophillic region in the protein and is likely to be a suitable target for protease digestion. It would seem reasonable, therefore, to expect that the C-terminal domain is both necessary and sufficient for catalytic activity.

In addition to the core region each of the eukaryotic precursors contains an aminoterminal domain, which varies in length from 72 residues (yeast) to 200 residues (human housekeeping). In contrast to the C-terminal domain, there is essentially no significant sequence homology in this region between yeast and any of the mammalian precursors. Consequently, aside from the role of the presequences in directing the enzyme to the mitochondrial matrix, the function, if any, of this region is unknown.

III. Regulatory Mechanisms in Hepatic Cells

A. Induction of gene transcription

Granick and co-workers demonstrated that a variety of drugs, endogenous steroids, and other chemicals which stimulate the rate of porphyrin synthesis in avian and mammalian liver cells also cause an increase in the activity of ALA synthase (Granick, 1966; Granick and Urata, 1963). There is now substantial evidence that the drug-mediated induction of ALA synthase activity is due to de novo synthesis of the enzyme. Moreover, this can be attributed almost exclusively to increased transcription of the hepatic ALA synthase gene. The potential importance of transcriptional controls was originally noted by Granick (1966) who showed that the AIA-mediated induction of ALA synthase in cultured enıbryonic chicken hepatocytes was sensitive to inhibitors of RNA and protein synthesis. Subsequently, Whiting and Granick (1976b) used antibodies directed against the chick mitochondrial enzyme to compare the amount of immunologically reactive protein with the activity of the enzyme in control and AIA/DDC-treated livers. Under all conditions tested, the concentration of enzyme antigen was directly proportional to enzyme activity. In addition, the relative rate of enzyme synthesis in vivo, as determined by immunoprecipitation of pulse-labeled proteins, was closely correlated with enzyme activity, suggesting that the induction of ALA synthase was due largely, if not exclusively, to de novo synthesis of the enzyme and not to activation of preformed mitochondrial ALA synthase, as had been suggested by others (Patton and Beattie, 1973). This conclusion was further supported by in vitro analyses of the relative capacity of polyribosomes isolated from drug-induced and control liver to direct the synthesis of the ALA synthase precursor.

Whereas polyribosomes isolated from drug-induced chick embryos (Whiting, 1976) and rats (Yamamoto et al., 1983) directed the translation of large amounts of the precursor, little or no precursor could be detected using polyribosomes isolated from control liver. The possibility that these results might simply reflect a difference in the number of ribosomes on each mRNA was eliminated by showing that the outcome was the same when purified poly(A)-containing mRNA from control and drug-treated livers was translated in vitro (Brooker et al., 1980; Ades and Harpe, 1981). Consequently, these early studies provided substantial, though indirect, evidence that inducers of ALA synthase caused an increase in the level of ALA synthase mRNA. This was recently confirmed by Srivastava et al. (1988), who used a cloned rat liver ALA synthase cDNA to quantitate directly the effects of AIA on hepatic mRNA levels and the relative rate of ALA synthase transcription. Administration of AIA for 12 h resulted in a 7-fold increase in the level of hybridizable mRNA and a 10-fold increase in the relative rate of ALA synthase transcription, as measured by RNA polymerase run-on assays in isolated nuclei. Both responses were reported to be closely correlated with the induction of enzyme activity. Moreover, the induction of ALA synthase expression by AIA was specific, since there was no change in either the mRNA levels or rates of transcription of the rat serum albumin or β-actin genes. Hence, these analyses have provided unequivocal evidence that the induction of hepatic ALA synthase by porphyrinogenic compounds is mediated largely, if not exclusively, by an increase in the rate of gene transcription.

B. Mechanisms of repression

In some cases the extent of ALA synthase induction can be quite dramatic. Treatment of chick embryos with a combination of AIA and DDC has been reported to stimulate ALA synthase levels 500-fold or more (Whiting and Granick, 1976a). Regardless of the magnitude, however, the induction of ALA synthase can be completely prevented if heme is added at the same time as the inducer (Granick, 1966; Srivastava et al., 1980; Hamilton et al., 1988). The mechanisms underlying the feedback repression of ALA synthase have been the subject of considerable investigation. Two mechanisms are well documented: repression of ALA synthase gene transcription, and feedback regulation of enzyme translocation into mitochondria. In addition, Yamamoto et al. (1983) suggested that heme may also act at the translational level. In these experiments high concentrations of hemin (greater than $20\mu M$) were found to inhibit selectively the synthesis of ALA synthase when rat liver polysomes were elongated in a rabbit reticulocyte lysate in vitro. However, other investigators have failed to detect any significant inhibition of ALA synthase translation from polysomes, even with concentrations of hemin as high as 100 μM (Whiting, 1976; May et al., 1986). Hence, there is presently little support for feedback regulation at the elongation step of translation. The possible involvement of heme at the initiation of ALA synthase translation has not been investigated.

1. Repression of transcription. Granick (1966) originally postulated that heme might function as a corepressor of ALA synthase transcription. This hypothesis was not founded on any particular experimental evidence, but rather on the belief that heme would most likely function to counteract the process of enzyme induction, which was sensitive to inhibitors of RNA and protein synthesis. This proposal was supported, however, by subsequent work which showed that heme largely suppressed the drug-mediated induction of enzyme synthesis (Whiting and Granick, 1976b) and the accumulation of translatable ALA synthase mRNA in chicken (Whiting, 1976) and rat liver polysomes (Yamamoto et al., 1982). The suggestion that the reduced synthesis of ALA synthase in these early studies was due to lower mRNA levels has been directly confirmed (at least in rat) by quantitative hybridization studies. Yamamoto et al. (1988) reported that hepatic ALA synthase mRNA levels began to decrease within 10 to 20 min following the intravenous administration of hemin to AIA-treated rats. Moreover, the kinetics of mRNA turnover following the administration of hemin alone, α-amanitin alone, or α-amanitin plus hemin were essentially identical, indicating that heme was as effective in inhibiting ALA synthase gene transcription as α-amanitin (Yamamoto et al., 1988). Similarly, Srivastava et al., (1988) showed that simultaneous administration of AIA and hemin or AIA and ALA completely blocked the AIA-mediated induction of ALA synthase gene transcription and mRNA accumulation in rat liver. In this case it was demonstrated that the effects of hemin and ALA on both the steady-state level of ALA synthase mRNA and the rate of gene transcription were not specific to the induction process per se since these agents also reduced the basal level of gene expression in nondrug-treated (i.e., control) rats to about half its normally low value.

The effectiveness of repression as a means of controlling the expression of the ALA synthase gene is dependent not only on how well the gene can be shut off, but also on the concentration of heme required to achieve repression and the half-life of the mRNA. Since all of the rat studies have been conducted in vivo the concentration of heme required to achieve effective repression of the gene is unknown. However, the studies of Yamamoto et al. (1988) showed that, following complete repression of transcription with hemin, actinomycin D, or α-amanitin, the half-time of disappearance of the mRNA in liver is about 20 min. The reason why this mRNA is so unstable is not known, but the lack of stability provides additional support for the proposal that transcriptional processes play an important role in controlling ALA synthase expression.

In contrast to the situation in the rat, there has been considerable uncertainty concerning the effectiveness of repression as a means of controlling ALA synthase expression in drug-treated embryonic chicken liver cells. Hamilton et al. (1988) have reported evidence that heme is only partially effective in blocking the drug-mediated induction of ALA synthase mRNA accumulation in cultured hepatocytes. In these experiments the dose-dependent effect of heme on the induction of ALA synthase and cytochrome P450 was measured in cells that had been treated with the xenobiotic 2-propyl-2-isopropylacetamide (PIA) in the presence of desferrioxamine (Des, an iron chelator). In the absence of exogenous heme, PIA/Des treatment resulted in about an eight-fold increase in ALA synthase and apocytochrome P450 mRNA levels, and about a six-fold increase in the activity of ALA synthase. No increase in the level of spectrally detected cytochrome P450 was seen in the absence of exogenous heme, indicating that the desferrioxamine had effectively inhibited de novo heme synthesis. As expected, addition of heme (at the same time as PIA/Des) had no effect on the PIA-mediated induction of apocytochrome P450 mRNA, but did lead to an increase in spectrally detected cytochrome P450, indicating that heme was available for binding to apocytochrome P450. The induction of cytochrome P450 holoenzyme formation reached a maximum at about 0.75 μM heme. At the same concentration of heme the induction of ALA synthase activity was completely abolished; however, ALA synthase mRNA levels were only reduced by 50%. Increasing the heme concentration to 2.0 μM neither increased the amount of cytochrome P450 formed nor decreased the amount of ALA synthase mRNA. It is clear from these experiments, therefore, that under conditions in which there was sufficient heme available to block completely the drug-mediated induction of ALA synthase activity and allow for maximum levels of cytochrome P450 synthesis, there was only a partial reduction in ALA synthase mRNA levels. A similar phenomenon was reported by Drew and Ades (1986) who showed that addition of 2.0 μM hemin caused only a 50% reduction in the AIA- or testosterone-mediated induction of ALA synthase mRNA in chicken embryonic liver cells. Since complete inhibition of enzyme induction occurred without a corresponding reduction in mRNA levels, it seems likely that in this system heme is controlling ALA synthase expression predominantly at the level of enzyme translocation into mitochondria (described below), rather than at the level of transcription. Clearly, however, additional work will be needed to understand why the apparent effectiveness of repression in these two systems appears to be different.

2. Inhibition of enzyme translocation into mitochondria. When rats are treated with large doses of AIA there is an initial rise in mitochondrial ALA synthase activity, which is followed after a brief lag by the accumulation of catalytically active enzyme in the cytosol (Yamauchi et al., 1980). Hayashi et al. (1972) demonstrated that intravenous administration of hemin of AIA-treated rats did not immediately alter the total level of ALA synthase activity in the liver, but did change the distribution of enzyme activity between the cytosolic and mitochondrial compartments: Mitochondrial ALA synthase activity decrease to one-half its original level in about 30 min, while the activity in the cytosol tripled. Based on these observations, it was suggested that the cytosolic protein was a precursor to the mitochondrial enzyme and that translocation of the precursor into mitochondria could be blocked by heme. This view was further supported by examining the effects of heme on the apparent half-lives of the cytosolic and mitochondrial enzymes and on the distribution of newly synthesized enzyme. Estimates of the half-lives of the cytosolic and mitochondrial enzymes with cycloheximide indicated that the cytosolic form decayed with a half-life of about 20 min, while the half-life of the mitochondrial enzyme was estimated to be 60 to 70 min (Hayashi et al., 1980). If the decay of the cytosolic form were due to transport of a precursor into mitochondria, one would predict that an inhibition of transport might lead to some stabilization of the cytosolic enzyme and a faster apparent rate of enzyme turnover in mitochondria. This pattern of behavior was in fact observed when AIA-treated rats were administered cycloheximide in the presence of hemin: The cytosolic enzyme showed little evidence of decay, while the half-life of the enzyme in mitochondria decreased to about 35 min (Hayashi et al., 1980). Similarly, Yamauchi et al. (1980) examined the effect of hemin on the distribution of newly synthesized enzyme by pulse-labeling rats with [^{3}H]leucine during the first 10 to 30 min following the administration of hemin. Hemin had no significant effect on the net rate of enzyme synthesis during this time, but largely suppressed the accumulation of newly synthesized enzyme in mitochondria.

Studies conducted with chicken embryonic liver cells, either in ovo or in culture, have provided more direct evidence that heme acts in a specific manner to block both the translocation and processing of the ALA synthase precursor. Although the preprotein does not normally accumulate in the cytosol of drug-treated embryos or cultured hepatocytes, it is the only form of newly synthesized enzyme that can be detected following the administration of hemin to drug-treated hepatocytes (Ades, 1983) or intact embryos (Srivastava et al., 1983b); that is, no newly synthesized enzyme is found in mitochondria and no processed precursor is found in the cytosol (Srivastava et al., 1983b). Moreover, the effects of heme on precursor translocation and processing appear to be specific to ALA synthase. Srivastava et al. (1983b) showed that while hemin completely blocked the formation of mature ALA synthase in chick embryonic liver in ovo it had no significant effect on the transport and processing of another mitochondrial matrix enzyme, pyruvate decarboxylase.

The mechanisms underlying the inhibition of precursor transport and processing by heme are presently unknown. Hayashi et al. (1983) analyzed the posttranslational transport of ALA synthase into liver mitochondria in vitro and showed that it could be inhibited by hemin. While these studies established the feasibility of using in vitro systems to examine this problem, no follow-up experiments have been reported. Nevertheless, recent developments in the transport field as well as our understanding of the structure of the housekeeping ALA synthase mRNA suggest a possible mechanism for this type of control. In recent years there has been mounting evidence that proteins must be partially unfolded in order to pass through a variety of biological membranes, including the inner membrane of mitochondria [reviewed by Eilers and Schatz (1988)]. Eilers and Schatz (1986) showed that several folate analogues blocked mitochondrial import of an artificial precursor composed of a mitochondrial presequence fused to mouse dihydrofolate reducatase (DHFR). These compounds bind tightly to DHFR and inhibit unfolding. In contrast, the import of DHFR into mitochondria was accelerated following treatment with urea (Eilers et al., 1988). By way of analogy to these experiments, one could speculate that the binding of heme to the ALA synthase precursor might stabilize the protein in a configuration that is resistant to ATP-dependent "unfoldases" (Eilers and Schatz, 1988) and thereby block translocation. Although direct binding of heme to the precursor has never been reported, it would seem reasonable to anticipate that it might involve regions of the protein lying outside the catalytic domain that are highly conserved among the various housekeeping preproteins. As mentioned earlier, the amino-terminal sequences of the mammalian housekeeping genes have diverged significantly except for two regions: residues 1 to 38 in the transit peptide and residues 100 to 107. Residues 100 to 105 (KCPFLA) are almost identical to residues 7 to 12 ($CPFL_S^A$) and may be related to the proposed heme binding sites ($_R^K CP_V^r DH$) of the heme-activated yeast transcription factor $HAP1$ that controls expression of the $CYC1$ and $CYC7$ genes (Pfeifer et al., 1989). These sequences are not present in the yeast ALA synthase precursor, which does not appear to be subject to this type of feedback control (Urban-Grimal et al., 1986). While this mechanism is purely speculative, it would provide an intuitively satisfying explanation for the selectivity of heme in blocking mitochondrial import of ALA synthase and may also explain why these regions have been so well conserved.

C. Mechanisms of induction by xenobiotics. The mechanisms by which chemical inducers cause an increase in the rate of ALA synthase gene expression has attracted considerable attention, particularly since many of these compounds are known to precipitate attacks of acute porphyria in genetically susceptible humans. Two basic models have been proposed to account for the action of these compounds. In Granick's original studies on embryonic chicken liver cells the extent of inhibition of porphyrin synthesis by heme was dependent upon the concentrations of both the inducing agent (AIA) and heme. On the assumption that this signified competition between these compounds, as well as some evidence of structural similarity between barbiturate and collidine inducers and the pyrrole subunits of heme, Granick (1966) suggested that inducers might function as heme analogues which compete with heme for a gene-controlling aporepressor. This model and related variants indicate that the inducer plays an active role in the induction process and should be able to stimulate gene transcription even when heme is present. The alternative model, which has been discussed at length by May et al. (1986), is that transcription of the ALA synthase gene is regulated solely by intracellular heme levels. According to this view, xenobiotics exert their effect on ALA synthase gene expression indirectly by decreasing intracellular heme levels. This can be achieved in several ways. All compounds that act as inducers of hepatic ALA synthase are known to be substrates for, and inducers of, one or more apocytochrome P450 genes (Whitlock, 1986). In addition, inducers such as AIA and DDC belong to a broad group of compounds that cause the mechanism-based destruction of cytochrome P450 heme and/or produce metabolites that interfere with the operation of the heme biosynthetic pathway. During the oxidative metabolism of AIA and DDC, the heme moiety of cytochrome P450 is destroyed at a high frequency by the transfer of an alkyl group from the substrate to one of the pyrrole nitrogens, to yield an N-alkylated derivative of protoporphyrin IX which is subsequently released from the enzyme (Ortiz de Montellano and Correia, 1983). Since the resulting apoprotein can be reconstituted with heme (Correia et al., 1979), this suicide reaction has the potential to amplify the effective level of apocytochrome P450 beyond that which is due to de novo synthesis alone. In addition, the N-methylprotoporphyrin formed during the metabolism of DDC is a strong competitive inhibitor of the terminal enzyme in the pathway, ferrochelatase (Dailey and Fleming, 1983).

A clear requirement of the "indirect" model of xenobiotic function is that a reduction in heme levels, brought about by any circumstances, should not only relieve the system from feedback repression, but should in and of itself cause derepression (induction) of ALA synthase expression. Srivastava et al. (1980) presented evidence that the derepressed state, once it has been established by treating embryonic chicken hepatocytes with the xenobiotic AIA, can at least be propagated in the absence of AIA, provided that upon removal of the inducer further heme synthesis is blocked. In this system, ALA synthase activity was elevated within 1 hr after adding AIA and continued to increase for the next 7 h. When the drug was removed after only 3 h of induction by washing the cells with fresh medium the activity of the enzyme continued to increase for about 1 h, then leveled off and began to decline by 8 h. However, when the AIA was replaced after 3 h of induction by the iron chelator desferrioxamine, which blocks heme synthesis at the last step of the pathway, ALA synthase activity continued to increase at an unaltered rate. Since desferrioxamine by itself did not induce ALA synthase expression, these results suggested that once heme levels had been reduced by AIA treatment high-level expression of the gene could be maintained in the absence of the drug only if subsequent heme synthesis was blocked by desferrioxamine. An implicit assumption in this experiment, however, is that the reduction in enzyme activity following the removal of AIA reflects a reduction in mRNA levels due to reduced rates of transcription. Since heme can also act posttranscriptionally to reduce ALA synthase activity, it is unclear whether this assumption is valid. Subsequently, however, Schoenfeld et al. (1982) showed that the activity of ALA synthase could be increased in embryonic chicken hepatocytes by prolonged exposure to succinylacetone, which inhibits heme synthesis by inactivating ALA dehydratase. Although this study was also conducted at the enzyme level, the basic conclusion that inhibition of heme synthesis with succinylacetone can derepress ALA synthase transcription is supported by recent studies of the effects of this drug on mRNA levels in mouse hepatoma cells (Young and Dierks, unpublished observation). Assuming that succinylacetone does not function as a xenobiotic (i.e., induce apocytochrome P450 synthesis), it appears that a reduction of cellular heme levels is by itself sufficient to cause derepression of ALA synthase gene transcription.

While the experiments described above indicate that it may be feasible for xenobiotics to exert their effects on ALA synthase indirectly, this does not preclude the possibility that they could play a direct role in the induction process, as originally postulated by Granick (1966). Recently, Hamilton et al. (1988) have provided persuasive evidence for the direct involvement of PIA in the induction of ALA synthase in embryonic chicken liver cells. If the induction of ALA synthase by PIA were driven indirectly by the increased synthesis of apocytochrome P450 synthesis, one might expect that induction of apocytochrome P450 synthesis should both precede and be necessary for an increase in ALA synthase expression. However, a kinetic analysis of mRNA accumulation showed that both mRNAs increased rapidly and simultaneously following PIA treatment. Moreover, in agreement with the conclusions of earlier indirect analyses (Sassa and Granick, 1970; Tyrrell and Marks, 1972), the PIA-mediated induction of ALA synthase mRNA accumulation was enhanced, rather than inhibited, by pretreatment of the cells with cycloheximide. Although cycloheximide treatment is known to increase the stability of labile mRNAs (Shaw and Kamen, 1986), it had no effect on ALA synthase mRNA levels in the absence of PIA. Both of these results indicate that the activation of apocytochrome P450 synthesis is not essential for PIA-mediated induction of ALA synthase mRNA accumulation. More importantly, however, when enough exogenous hemin was added to achieve maximal levels of cytochrome P450 holoenzyme formation and to suppress completely any increase in ALA synthase enzyme activity, the induction of ALA synthase mRNA accumulation by PIA was inhibited by only 50%. This result is clearly inconsistent with the "indirect" mode of induction and strongly suggests that PIA plays a direct role in the activation of ALA synthase transcription. Whether this behavior is unique to this class of xenobiotics or is characteristic of the mechanisms that are used to coordinate ALA synthase expression with any of the apocytochrome P450 genes is an important point that remains to be determined.

IV. Regulatory Mechanisms in Erythroid Cells

The production of hemoglobin begins during the terminal stages of red blood cell development, as erythroid colony-forming (CFU-e) cells undergo differentiation into reticulocytes. Reticulocytes are easily isolated from the circulating blood of anemic animals and have been used extensively to characterize heme synthesis during the postmitotic phase of the program. By the reticulocyte stage of development, however, the nucleus has either been lost (mammalian reticulocytes) or is largely heterochromatic and quiescent (avian reticulocytes). To understand the mechanisms that coordinate the synthesis of heme with the developmental activation of globin genes, it is necessary to focus on the earlier mitotic phase of the program. CFU-e cells, however, typically constitute about 0.1% of the nucleated cells in adult bone marrow, and until recently they have been difficult to purify in large numbers (Nijhof and Wierenga, 1983). As a result, investigations of the early phases of this program have relied heavily on the use of cultured erythroid cell lines, such as murine erythroleukemia (MEL) cells, which can be manipulated to reproduce the differentiation of CFU-e cells to at least the orthochromatic stage of development in vitro (Marks and Rifkind, 1978; Volloch and Housman, 1982; Harrison, 1984).

A. Induction and repression of ALA synthase in MEL cells

Erythroid differentiation in MEL cells is triggered by exposing the cells to chemical agents such as dimethylsulfoxide (DMSO) or hexamethylenebisacetamide (HMBA). In DMSO-treated cells the onset of hemoglobin accumulation occurs midway through the developmental program, and results in a 50-fold increase in cellular heme levels (Sassa, 1976). As noted earlier, this process is accompanied by an increase in the activities of most, if not all, of the enzymes in the heme biosynthetic pathway (Sassa, 1976; Rutherford et al., 1979; Beaumont et al., 1984). For many of the enzymes, including ALA synthase, the magnitude of this increase is relatively modest. Under normal induction conditions the activity of ALA synthase begins to increase between 24 and 48 h after DMSO addition and reaches a maximum that is about 3 to 5 times higher than the preinduced level by 72 to 96 h. However, Beaumont et al. (1984) showed that the extent of ALA synthase induction could be significantly altered by manipulating the availability of heme in differentiating cells. Addition of 10 μM hemin at the beginning of the induction procedure almost completely blocked the differentiation-dependent increase in ALA synthase activity. To assess how the enzyme would respond to a reduction in heme levels, the cells were treated with DMSO in the presence of succinylacetone (4,6-dioxoheptanoic acid), which is a potent inhibitor of ALA dehydratase that allows induction of globin mRNA expression and commitment of cells to terminal cell division (Grandchamp et al., 1965) but blocks the accumulation of hemoglobin (Ebert et al., 1979). Under these conditions the activity of ALA synthase increased at a slightly higher rate than normal during the first 48 h and then rose sharply, reaching a maximum by 96 h that was about six times higher than the level achieved with DMSO alone. Hemin added at 72 h aborted the "superinduction" of ALA synthase and reduced its activity over the next 24 h to about the same level achieved with DMSO alone. These results indicate that the activity of ALA synthase in differentiating MEL cells is sensitive to the intracellular heme balance. Strategically, therefore, this type of feedback regulation resembles the control of ALA synthase in liver and suggests that this enzyme also plays a central role in governing the rate of heme and/or porphyrin synthesis in erythroid cells.

B. Mechanism of induction

As noted earlier, the housekeeping and erythroid ALA synthase genes are coexpressed in undifferentiated MEL cells. While the level of housekeeping gene transcripts remains relatively unchanged during the program of differentiation, the number of erythroid ALA synthase mRNAs per cell increases dramatically, reaching levels that are about 50 to 75 times above baseline by 96 h of induction (Fraser and Curtis, 1987; Young and Dierks, unpublished observations). Fraser and Curtis (1987) have demonstrated that most, if not all, of this increase can be attributed to higher rates of ALA synthase gene transcription. The kinetics of transcript accumulation and transcriptional activation of this gene roughly parallel those of the mouse β-globin gene.

The existence of heme-sensitive feedback controls for regulating ALA synthase activity in MEL cells suggests two possible models for the induction of erythroid gene transcription. The first is a simple derepression model in which expression of the erythroid ALA synthase gene is regulated solely by heme. This model, like its counterpart for the housekeeping ALA synthase gene, predicts that the activation of the erythroid gene in differentiating MEL cells is caused by a reduction in cellular heme levels brought about by a rapid rise in the production of globin chains. Alternatively, one could propose that the induction of ALA synthase is caused by a developmental signal generated early during the program of differentiation, and that feedback mechanism(s) act to coordinate the magnitude of this response with other aspects of the program. These two models have been tested by manipulating the availability of heme in both undifferentiated and differentiated cells and assaying how these alterations affect the expression of the erythroid gene (Young and Dierks, unpublished observations). If the derepression model were correct one might expect that expression of the erythroid gene could be activated in the absence of differentiation by depleting the cells of heme. This has been tested by culturing undifferentiated cells in the presence of succinylacetone in medium made with heme-depleted serum (Dierks, unpublished procedure). Under these conditions the cells undergo an average of three to four cell divisions and then enter a state of growth arrest. This arrest is dependent upon succinylacetone and can be prevented by supplementing the culture with exogenous hemin (10 μM). Moreover, addition of hemin to arrested cultures restores growth ability. These cells appear, therefore, to be functionally depleted of heme. Despite this treatment, however, the level of erythroid ALA synthase transcripts was essentially identical to that observed in cells which had been grown either in the absence of succinylacetone or in the presence of succinylacetone and 10 μM hemin (in both normal and heme-depleted serum). Hence, the expression of the erythroid gene cannot be activated in undifferentiated cells by depleting the cells of heme. A similar series of experiments was performed with cells that had been induced to differentiate with DMSO. In agreement with the results of Beaumont et al. (1984), it was found that succinylacetone caused a hemin-reversible inhibition of hemoglobin formation, and resulted in superinduction of ALA synthase activity to levels that were approximately 50 times higher than untreated (undifferentiated) controls and about 10 times higher than in cells treated with DMSO alone. However, S1 mapping analyses showed that the kinetics of erythroid ALA synthase transcript accumulation were essentially unaffected by succinylacetone, hemin, or the type of serum used, either individually or in any combination. It was concluded, therefore, that the induction of erythroid ALA synthase gene transcription in this system is a developmentally regulated response, which is largely unaffected by the intracellular heme balance. Moreover, these analyses also demonstrated that the extent of ALA synthase mRNA induction (50- to 75-fold increase) is much greater than the normal 5-fold increase in enzyme activity. Hence, it would appear that this transcriptional response is attenuated posttranscriptionally by mechanisms that are sensitive to the presence of succinylacetone or hemin.

C. Mechanisms of posttranscriptional control

The simplest interpretation of the opposing effects of succinylacetone and hemin on the level of ALA synthase activity in MEL cells is that the rate of translation and/or transport of ALA synthase is under negative control by heme. Thus, depletion of the heme pool by succinylacetone would be expected to increase the rate of enzyme production, while addition of hemin would be expected to have the opposite effect. However, inspection of the structure of the erythroid ALA synthase mRNA suggests that more than one level of posttranscriptional control may be involved. Residues 6 to 40 in 5' untranslated region (UTR) of this mRNA exhibit striking structural and sequence similarity to the cis-acting iron responsive elements (IRE) that are used to coordinate production of the heavy and light subunits of ferritin (Aziz and Munro, 1987; Hentze et al., 1987) and synthesis of the transferrin receptor (Casey et al., 1988) with the availability of iron. Based on a comparison of putative IREs in a number of ferritin and transferrin receptor mRNAs Casey et al. (1988) have suggested that these elements are characterized by (1) a 6-nucleotide loop containing the sequence CAGUGX, (2) an upper stem of five paired bases, (3) an unpaired 5' C residue separated by five bases from the loop, and (4) a lower stem of variable length. All of these elements are present in the putative IRE in the 5'-UTR of the mouse erythroid ALA synthase mRNA (Fig. 5.2). (The sequence data currently available on the chicken erythroid ALA synthase mRNA cover only a small portion of 5'-UTR; it is, therefore, not clear whether a similar element exists in that gene. However, no such element is present in any of the housekeeping ALA synthase genes that have examined to date.)

The synthesis of the iron-storage protein ferritin is regulated at the translational level by the availability of iron. The mRNAs for both subunits are stored as inactive ribonucleoprotein particles, which can be recruited for translation when iron enters the cell (Rogers and Munro, 1987; Zähringer et al., 1976; Aziz and Munro, 1986). The redistribution of these mRNAs into polysomes in the presence of iron is believed to be mediated by cis-acting sequences (the IRE) found in the 5'-UTR of both the heavy and light subunit mRNAs. Fusion of the 5'-UTR derived from either of these genes to a chloramphenicol acetyltransferase (CAT) reporter gene has been shown to confer iron-dependent control of CAT gene expression (Aziz and Munro, 1987; Hentze et al., 1987). Recently, Liebold and Munro (1988) have reported the detection of a cytoplasmic protein in rat tissues and hepatoma cells that exhibits iron-sensitive binding in vitro to the 5'-UTR of both mRNAs. Based on these results, it has been proposed that when iron levels are low, a cytoplasmic protein selectively binds to the 5'-IRE in the ferritin mRNAs and blocks translation. When iron enters the cell these complexes are disrupted, allowing access of the 5'-UTR to ribosomes, and translation of the mRNA ensues. In the case of the transferrin receptor, it is believed that as many as five IREs may be located in the 3'-UTR (Casey et al., 1988). In contrast to ferritin, the synthesis of transferrin receptors is stimulated when intracellular iron levels are low, presumably as a means of increasing the rate of iron acquisition. This response is mediated at least in part by post-transcriptional stabilization of the transferrin receptor mRNA (Rao et al., 1986), and requires sequences located in the 3'-UTR (Casey et al., 1988). It is believed that the same types of protein interactions which control the rate of translation in ferritin mRNAs may occur with the IREs in the 3'-UTR of the transferrin receptor mRNA, thereby protecting the message from degradation and leading to increased mRNA levels and increased rates of transferrin receptor synthesis. The functional equivalence of these 3'-IREs to those located in the 5'-UTR of

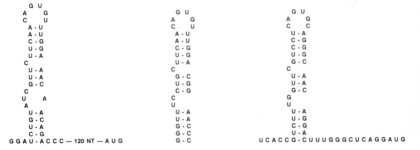

Figure 5.2 Iron-responsive elements of ferritin subunit mRNAs (Liebold and Munro, 1987; Costanzo et al., 1987) and the proposed iron-responsive element for mouse erythroid ALA synthase mRNA (Schoenhaut and Curtis, 1986; P. Curtis, personal communication). Structures are depicted according to the convention of Casey et al. (1988).

ferritin mRNAs has been demonstrated by showing that placement of one of such element in the 5′-UTR region of the human growth hormone gene conferred ferritin-like iron regulation of human growth hormone production (Casey et al., 1988).

In light of those observations, it seems probable that translation of the erythroid ALA synthase mRNA is coupled to the availability of iron. Although formal proof of this hypothesis is currently lacking, there is at least circumstantial evidence that DMSO-induced MEL cells may have an iron-poor environment, which would be expected to attenuate the translational efficiency of the erythroid mRNA. In addition to causing increased globin and heme biosynthesis, treatment of MEL cells with DMSO results in about a six-fold increase in the number of transferrin receptors expressed on the cell surface (Wilczynska et al., 1984). Moreover, the induction of transferrin receptor expression in MEL cells has been reported to be blocked by heme (Wilczynska et al., 1984). Heme has been used routinely as a source of iron for many of the transferrin receptor studies conducted in nonerythroid systems (Casey et al., 1988). Assuming that the same mechanisms are used to regulate transferrin receptor synthesis in MEL cells, this behavior would be consistent with the idea that intracellular iron levels are reduced during differentiation. Further support for this notion has been obtained by examining the effects of increasing the rate of iron transport during differentiation. The transferrin receptor-dependent iron transport system can be circumvented by using the synthetic iron chelator salicylaldehyde isonicotinoyl hydrazone (SIH), which is a more effective iron delivery system than transferrin for both uninduced and induced MEL cells (Laskey et al., 1986). When Fe-SIH, rather than Fe-transferrin, was used as the iron source, the rate of incorporation of [2-^{14}C]glycine into heme in DMSO-treated cells was increased about 3.6-fold (Laskey et al., 1986). Similarly, addition of ALA to DMSO-treated cells had no effect on the rate of ^{59}Fe incorporation into heme when ^{59}Fe-transferrin was used as the iron donor, but did increase the rate of iron incorporation when ^{59}Fe-SIH was the donor. These experiments indicate that it is the rate of iron transport, rather than the synthesis of ALA, that limits the production of heme in differentiating MEL cells. Accordingly, one can image that the strong transcriptional response of the erythroid ALA synthase is attenuated at the level of translation by the availability of iron as a means of coordinating the rate of protoporphyrin IX synthesis with the rate of iron transport. If this view is correct, then the superinduction of ALA synthase by succinylacetone may reflect not a reduction in heme levels per se, but rather increased levels of iron due to the inhibition of protoporphyrin IX production.

While an iron-sensitive feedback loop at the level of translation can account for the effects of succinylacetone, it cannot explain the inhibition of ALA synthase expression by heme. At the present time there are no data to indicate what the function of this feedback control is or how it may operate. The only clear fact is that it must act past the level of transciption. The most likely speculation would be that this feedback circuit acts to coordinate the rate of heme synthesis with the availability of globin chains. Moreover, given the well-documented role of heme in controlling the import of the housekeeping isozyme into mitochondria, it may be that such a control mechanism may operate on the erythroid isozyme as well. Clearly, however, much work remains to be done before this point can be resolved.

REFERENCES

Ades, I. Z. (1983). Biogenesis of mitochondrial proteins: Regulation of maturation of delta-aminolevulinate synthase by hemin, *Biochem. Biophys. Res. Comm.* **110**:42–47.

Ades, I. Z., and Harpe, K. G. (1981). Biogenesis of mitochondrial proteins: Identification of the mature and precursor forms of the subunit of δ-aminolevulinate synthase from embryonic chick liver, *J. Biol. Chem.* **256**:9329–9333.

Aziz, N., and Munro, H. N. (1986). Both subunits of rat liver ferritin are regulated at a translational level by iron induction, *Nucl. Acids Res.* **14**:915–927.

Aziz, N., and Munro, H. N. (1987). Iron regulates ferritin mRNA translation through a segment of its 5' untranslated region, *Proc. Nat. Acad. Sci.* **84**:8478–8482.

Bawden, M. J., Borthwick, I. A., Healy, H. M., Morris, C. P., May, B. K., and Elliott, W. H. (1987). Sequence of human 5-aminolevulinate synthase cDNA, *Nucl. Acids Res.* **15**:8563.

Beaumont, C., Deybach, J.-C., Grandchamp, B., Da Silva, V., de Verneuil, H., and Nordmann, Y. (1984). Effects of succinylacetone on dimethylsulfoxide-mediated induction of heme pathway enzymes in mouse Friend virus-transformed erythroleukemia cells, *Exp. Cell Res.* **154**:474–484.

Bishop, D. F., Kitchen, H., and Wood, W. A. (1981). Evidence for erythroid and nonerythroid forms of δ-aminolevulinate synthase, *Arch. Biochem. Biophys.* **206**:380–391.

Borthwick, I. A., Srivastava, G., Brooker, J. D., May, B. K., and Elliott, W. H. (1983). Purification of 5-aminolevulinate synthase from liver mitochondria of chick embryo, *Eur. J. Biochem.* **129**:615–620.

Borthwick, I. A., Srivastava, G., Day, A. R., Pirola, B. A., Snoswell, M. A., May, B. K., and Elliott, W. H. (1985). Complete nucleotide sequence of hepatic 5-aminolevulinate synthase precursor, *Eur. J. Biochem.* **150**:481–484.

Borthwick, I., Srivastava, G., Hobbs, A. A., Pirola, B. A., Brooker, J. D., May, B. K., and Elliott, W. H. (1984). Molecular cloning of hepatic 5-aminolevulinate synthase, *Eur. J. Biochem.* **144**:95–99.

Brooker, J. D., May, B. K., and Elliott, W. H. (1980). Synthesis of δ-aminolevulinate synthase in vitro using hepatic mRNA from chick embryos with induced porphyria, *Eur. J. Biochem.* **106**:17–24.

Casey, J. L., Hentze, M. W., Koeller, D. M., Caughman, S. W., Rouault, T. A., Klausner, R. D., and Harford, J. B. (1988). Iron-responsive elements: Regulatory RNA sequences that control mRNA levels and translation, *Science* **240**:924–928.

Chretien, S., Dubart, A., Beaupain, D., Raich, N., Grandchamp, B., Rosa, J., Gossens, M., and Romeo, P.-H. (1988). Alternative transcription and splicing of the human porphobilinogen deaminase gene result either in tissue-specific or in housekeeping expression, *Proc. Nat. Acad. Sci.* **85**:6–10.

Correia, M. A., Farrell, G. C., Schmid, R., Ortiz de Montellano, P. R., Yost, G. S., and Mico, B. A. (1979). Incorporation of exogenous heme into hepatic cytochrome P450, in vivo, *J. Biol. Chem.* **254**:15–17.

Costanzo, F., Columbo, M., Staempfli, S., Santoro, C., Marone, M., Frank, R., Delius, H., and Cortese, R. (1986). Structure of gene and pseudogenes of human apoferritin H, *Nucl. Acids Res.* **14**:721–735.

Dailey, H. A., and Fleming, J. E. (1983). Bovine ferrochelatase, *J. Biol. Chem.* **258**:11453–11459.

Drew, P. D., and Ades, I. Z. (1986). Regulation of production of embryonic chick liver delta-aminolevulinate synthase: Effects of testosterone and of hemin on the mRNA of the enzyme, *Biochem. Biophys. Res. Comm.* **140**:81–87.

Ebert, P. S., Hess, R. A., Frykholm, B. C., and Tschudy, D. P. (1979). Succinylacetone, a potent inhibitor of heme biosynthesis: Effect on cell growth, heme content and δ-aminolevulinic acid dehydratase activity of malignant murine erythroleukemia cells, *Biochem. Biophys. Res. Comm.* **88**:1382–1390.

Edelman, A. M., Blumenthal, D. K., and Krebs, E. G. (1987). Protein serine/threonine kinases, *Ann. Rev. Biochem.* **56**:567–613.

Eilers, M., Hwang, S., and Schatz, G. (1988). Unfolding and refolding of a purified precursor protein during import into isolated mitochondria, *EMBO J.* **7**:1139–1145.

Eilers, M., and Schatz, G. (1986). Binding of a specific ligand inhibits import of a purified precursor protein into mitochondria, *Nature* **322**:228–232.

Eilers, M., and Schatz, G. (1988). Protein unfolding and the energetics of protein translocation across biological membranes, *Cell* **52**:481–483.

Elferink, C. J., Srivastava, G., Maguire, D. J., Borthwick, I. A., May, B. K., and Elliott, W. H. (1987). A unique gene for 5-aminolevulinate synthase in chickens: Evidence for expression of an identical messenger RNA in hepatic and erythroid tissues, *J. Biol. Chem.* **262**:3988–3992.

Fraser, P. J., and Curtis, P. J. (1987). Specific pattern of gene expression during induction of mouse erythroleukemia cells, *Genes and Dev.* **1**:855–861.

Gardner, L. C., and Cox, T. M. (1988). Biosynthesis of heme in immature erythroid cells, *J. Biol. Chem.* **264**:6678–6682.

Giger, M., and Meyer, M. A. (1981). Induction of δ-aminolevulinate synthase and cytochrome P-450 hemoproteins in hepatocyte culture, *J. Biol. Chem.* **256**:11182–11190.

Goldberg, M. A., Dunning, S. P., and Bunn, H. F. (1988). Regulation of the erythropoietin gene: Evidence that the oxygen sensor is a heme protein, *Science* **244**:1412–1415.

Grandchamp, B., Beaumont, C., de Verneuil, H., and Nordmann, Y. (1985). Accumulation of porphobilinogen deaminase, uroporphyrinogen decarboxylase, and α- and β-globin mRNAs during differentiation of mouse erythroleukemic cells: Effects of succinylacetone, *J. Biol. Chem.* **260**:9630–9635.

Grandchamp, B., de Verneuil, H., Beaumont, C., Chretien, S., Walter, O., and Nordmann, Y. (1987). Tissue-specific expression of porphobilinogen deaminase, *Eur. J. Biochem.* **162**:105–110.

Granick, S. (1966). The induction in vitro of the synthesis of δ-aminolevulinic acid synthase in chemical porphyria: A response to certain drugs, sex hormones, and foreign chemicals, *J. Biol. Chem.* **241**:1359–1375.

Granick, S., and Urata, G. (1963). Increase in activity of δ-aminolevulinic acid synthase in liver mitochondria induced by feeding of 3,5-dicarbethoxy-1,4-dihydrocollidine, *J. Biol. Chem.* **238**:821–827.

Hamilton, J. W., Bement, W. J., Sinclair, P. R., Sinclair, J. F., and Wetterhahn, K. E. (1988). Expression of 5-aminolaevulinate synthase and cytochrome P-450 mRNAs in chicken embryo hepatocytes in vivo and in culture, *Biochem. J.* **255**:267–275.

Harrison, P. R. (1984). Molecular analysis of erythropoiesis. A current appraisal, *Exp. Cell. Res.* **155**:321–344.

Hay, R., Böhni, P., and Gasser, S. (1984). How mitochondria import proteins, *Biochim. Biophys. Acta* **779**:65–87.

Hayashi, N., Kurashima, Y., and Kikuchi, G. (1972). Mechanism of allylisopropylacetamide-induced increase of δ-aminolevulinate synthetase in liver mitochondria. V. Mechanism of regulation by hemin of the level of δ-aminolevulinate synthetase in rat liver mitochondria, *Arch. Biochem. Biophys.* **148**:10–21.

Hayashi, N., Terasawa, M., and Kikuchi, G. (1980). Immunochemical studies of the turnover of δ-aminolevulinate synthase in rat liver mitochondria and the effect of hemin on it, *J. Biochem.* **88**:921–926.

Hayashi, N., Watanabe, N., and Kikuchi, G. (1983). Inhibition by hemin of in vitro translocation of chicken liver δ-aminolevulinate synthase into mitochondria, *Biochem. Biophys. Res. Comm.* **115**:700–706.

Hentze, M. W., Rouault, T. A., Caughman, S. W., Dancis, A., Harford, J. B., and Klausner, R. D. (1987). A cis-acting element is necessary and sufficient for translational regulation of human ferritin expression in response to iron, *Proc. Nat. Acad. Sci.* **84**:6730–6734.

Ibraham, N. G., Friedland, M. L., and Levere, R. D. (1983). Heme metabolism in erythroid and hepatic cells, *Prog. Hematol.* **13**:75–130.

Igarashi, J., Hayashi, N., Kikuchi, G. (1976). δ-Aminolevulinate synthetases in the liver cytosol fraction and mitochondria of mice treated with allylisopropylacetamide and 3,5-discarbethoxy-1,4-dihydrocollidine, *J. Biochem.* **80**:1091–1099.

Laskey, J. D., Ponka, P., and Schulman, H. M. (1986). Control of heme synthesis during Friend cell differentiation: Role of iron and transferrin, *J. Cell Physiol.* **129**:185–192.

Leong, S. A., Williams, P. H., and Ditta, G. S. (1985). Analysis of the 5′ regulatory region of the gene for δ-aminolevulinic acid synthetase of *Rhizobium meliloti*, *Nucl. Acids Res.* **13**:5965–5976.

Levere, R. D., and Granick, S. (1967). Control of hemoglobin synthesis in the cultured chick blastoderm, *J. Biol. Chem.* **242**:1903–1911.

Liebold, E. A., and Munro, H. N. (1987). Characterization and evolution of the expressed rat ferritin light subunit gene and its pseudogene family, *J. Biol. Chem.* **262**:7335–7341.

Liebold, E. A., and Munro, H. N. (1988). Cytoplasmic protein binds in vitro to a highly conserved sequence in the 5′ untranslated region of ferritin heavy- and light-subunit mRNAs, *Proc. Nat. Acad. Sci.* **85**:2171–2175.

London, I. M., Levin, D. H., Matts, R. L., Thomas, N. S. B., Petryshyn, R., and Chen, J.-J. (1987). Regulation of protein synthesis, *The Enzymes* **18**:359–380.

Maguire, D. J., Day, A. R., Borthwick, I. A., Srivastava, G., Wigley, P. L., May, B. K., and Elliott, W. H. (1986). Nucleotide sequence of the chicken 5-aminolevulinate synthase gene, *Nucl. Acids Res.* **14**:1379–1391.

Marks, P., and Rifkind, R. (1978). Erythroleukemic differentiation, *Ann. Rev. Biochem.* **47**:419–448.

Marver, H. S., and Schmid, R. (1972). The porphyrias, *The Metabolic Basis of Inherited Disease* (J. B. Stanbury, J. B. Wyngaarden, and D. S. Frederickson, Eds.), 3rd ed., McGraw-Hill, New York, pp. 1087–1140.

May, B. K., Borthwick, I. A., Srivastava, G., Pirola, B. A., and Elliott, W. H. (1986). Control of 5-aminolevulinate synthase in animals, *Curr. Topics Cell. Reg.* **28**:233–262.

McClung, C. R., Somerville, J. E., Guerinot, M. L., and Chelm, B. K. (1987). Structure of *Bradyrhizobium japonicum* gene *hemA* encoding 5-aminolevulinic acid synthase, *Gene* **54**:133–139.

Nebert, D. W., and Gonzalez, F. J. (1987). P450 genes: Structure, evolution, and regulation, *Ann. Rev. Biochem.* **56**:945–993.

Nijhof, W., and Wierenga, P. K. (1983). Isolation and characterization of the erythroid progenitor cells: CFU-E, *J. Cell. Biol.* **96**:386–392.

Ochoa, S. (1983). Regulation of protein synthesis initiation in eucaryotes, *Arch. Biochem. Biophys.* **223**:325–349.

Ohashi, A. and Kikuchi, G. (1972). Mechanism of allylisopropylacetamide-induced increase of δ-aminolevulinate synthetase in liver mitochondria. VI. Multiple molecular forms of δ-aminolevulinate synthetase in the cytosol and mitochondria of induced cock liver, *Arch. Biochem. Biophys.* **153**:34–46.

Ortiz de Montellano, P. R., and Correia, M. A. (1983). Suicidal destruction of cytochrome P-450 during oxidative drug metabolism, *Ann. Rev. Pharmacol. Toxicol.* **23**:481–503.

Patton, G. M., and Beattie, D. S. (1973). Studies on hepatic δ-aminolevulinic acid synthetase, *J. Biol. Chem.* **248**:4467–4474.

Pearson, W. R., and Lipman, D. J. (1988). Improved tools for biological sequence comparison, *Proc. Nat. Acad. Sci.* **85**:2444–2448.

Pfeifer, K., Kim, K.-S., Kogan, S., and Guarante, L. (1989). Functional dissection and sequence of yeast HAP1 activator, *Cell* **56**:291–301.

Pirola, B. A., Mayer, F., Borthwick, I. A., Srivastava, G., May, B. K., and Elliott, W. H. (1984). Electron microscopic studies on 5-aminolevulinate synthase, *Eur. J. Biochem.* **144**:577–579.

Ponka, P., and Neuwirt, J. (1970). The use of reticulocytes with non-haem iron pool for studies of regulation of haem synthesis, *Brit. J. Haematol.* **19**:593–604.

Ponka, P., and Schulman, H. M. (1985). Acquisition of iron from transferrin regulates reticulocyte heme synthesis, *J. Biol. Chem.* **260**:14717–14721.

Rao, K., Harford, J. B., Rouault, T., McClelland, A., Ruddle, F. H., and Klausner, R. D. (1986). Transcriptional regulation by iron of the gene for the transferrin receptor, *Mol. Cell. Biol.* **6**:236–240.

Riddle, R. D., Yamamoto, M., and Engel, J. D. (1989). Expression of δ-aminolevulinate synthase in avian cells: Separate genes encode erythroid-specific and basal isozymes, *Proc. Nat. Acad. Sci.*, **86**:792–796.

Rogers, J., and Munro, H. (1987). Translation of ferritin light and heavy subunit mRNAs is regulated by intracellular chelatable iron levels in rat hepatoma cells, *Proc. Nat. Acad. Sci.* **84**:2277–2281.

Rutherford, T., Thompson, G. G., and Moore, M. R. (1979). Heme biosynthesis in Friend erythroleukemia cells: Control by ferrochelatase, *Proc. Nat. Acad. Sci.* **76**:833–836.

Safer, B. (1983). 2B or not 2B: Regulation of the catalytic utilization of eIF-2, *Cell* **33**:7–8.

Sassa, S. (1976). Sequential induction of heme pathway enzymes during erythroid differentiation of mouse Friend leukemia virus-infected cells, *J. Exp. Med.* **143**:305–315

Sassa, S., and Granick, S. (1970). Induction of δ-aminolevulinic acid synthetase in chick embryo liver cells in culture, *Proc. Nat. Acad. Sci.* **67**:517–522.

Schatz, G. (1987). Signals guiding proteins to their correct locations in mitochondria, *Eur. J. Biochem.* **165**:1–6.

Schoenfeld, N., Greenblat, Y., Epstein, O., and Atsman, A. (1982). The effects of succinylacetone (4,6-dioxoheptanoic acid) on δ-aminolevulinate synthase activity and the content of heme in monolayers of chick embryo liver cells, *Biochim. Biophys. Acta* **721**:408–417.

Schoenhaut, D. S., and Curtis, P. J. (1986). Nucleotide sequence of mouse 5-aminolevulinic acid synthase cDNA and expression of its gene in hepatic and erythroid tissues, *Gene* **48**:55–63.

Shaw, G., and Kamen, R. (1986). A conserved AU sequence from the 3′ untranslated region of GM-CSF mRNA mediates selective mRNA degradation, *Cell* **46**:659–667.

Srivastava, G., Borthwick, I. A., Brooker, J. D., May, B. K., and Elliott, W. H. (1982). Purification of rat liver mitochondrial δ-aminolevulinate synthase, *Biochem. Biophys. Res. Comm.* **109**:305–312.

Srivastava, G., Borthwick, I. A., Brooker, J. D., May, B. K., and Elliott, W. H. (1983a). Evidence for a cytosolic precursor of chick embryo liver δ-aminolevulinate synthase, *Biochem. Biophys. Res. Comm.* **110**:23–31.

Srivastava, G., Borthwick, I. A., Brooker, J. D., Wallace, J. C., May, B. K., and Elliott, W. H. (1983b). Hemin inhibits transfer of pre-δ-aminolevulinate synthase into chick embryo liver mitochondria, *Biochem. Biophys. Res. Comm.* **117**:344–349.

Srivastava, G., Borthwick, I. A., Maguire, D. J., Elferink, C. J., Bawden, M. J., Mercer, J. F. B., and May, B. K. (1988). Regulation of 5-aminolevulinate synthase mRNA in different rat tissues, *J. Biol. Chem.* **263**:5202–5209.

Srivastava, G., Brooker, J. D., May, B. K., and Elliott, W. H. (1980). Haem control in experimental porphyria. The effect of hemin on the induction of δ-aminolevulinate synthase in isolated chick-embryo liver cells, *Biochem. J.* **188**:781–788.

Tyrrell, D. L. J., and Marks, G. S. (1972). Drug-induced porphyrin biosynthesis. V. Effect of protohemin on the transcriptional and post-transcriptional phases of δ-aminolevulinic acid synthetase induction, *Biochem. Pharmacol.* **21**:2077–2093.

Urban-Grimal, D., Volland, C., Garnier, T., Dehoux, P., and Labbe-Bois, R. (1986). The nucleotide sequence of the *HEM*1 gene and evidence for a precursor form of the mitochondrial 5-aminolevulinate synthase in *Saccharomyces cerevisiae*, *Eur. J. Biochem.* **156**:511–519.

Volloch, V., and Housman, D. (1982). Terminal differentiation of murine erythroleukemia cells: Physical stabilization of end-stage cells, *J. Cell. Biol.* **93**:390–394.

Watanabe, N., Hayashi, N., and Kikuchi, G. (1983). δ-Aminolevulinate synthase isozymes in the liver and erythroid cells of chicken, *Biochem. Biophys. Res. Comm.* **113**:377–383.

Watanabe, N., Hayashi, N., and Kikuchi, G. (1984). Relation of the extra-sequence of the precursor form of chicken liver δ-aminolevulinate synthase to its quarternary structure and catalytic properties, *Arch. Biochem. Biophys.* **232**:118–126.

Whiting, M. J. (1976). Synthesis of δ-aminolevulinate synthase by isolated liver polyribosomes, *Biochem. J.* **158**:391–400.

Whiting, M. J., and Granick, S. (1976a). δ-Aminolevulinic acid synthase from chick embryo liver mitochondria. I. Purification and some properties, *J. Biol. Chem.* **251**:1340–1346.

Whiting, M. J., and Granick, S. (1976b). δ-Aminolevulinic acid synthase from chick embryo liver mitochondria. II. Immunochemical correlation between synthesis and activity in induction and repression, *J. Biol. Chem.* **251**:1347–1353.

Whitlock, J. P., Jr. (1986). The regulation of cytochrome P-450 gene expression, *Ann. Rev. Pharmacol. Toxicol.* **26**:333–369.

Wilczynska, A., Ponka, P., and Schulman, H. M. (1984). Transferrin receptors and iron utilization in DMSO-inducible and -uninducible Friend erythroleukemia cells, *Exp. Cell Res.* **154**:561–566.

Yamamoto, M., Hayashi, N., and Kikuchi, G. (1982). Evidence for the transcriptional inhibition by heme of the synthesis of δ-aminolevulinate synthase in rat liver, *Biochem. Biophys. Res. Comm.* **105**:985–990.

Yamamoto, M., Hayashi, N., and Kikuchi, G. (1983). Translational inhibition by heme of the synthesis of hepatic δ-aminolevulinate synthase in a cell-free system, *Biochem. Biophys. Res. Comm.* **115**:225–231.

Yamamoto, M., Kure, S., Engel, J. D., and Hiraga, K. (1988). Structure, turnover, and heme-mediated suppression of the level of mRNA encoding rat liver δ-aminolevulinate synthase, *J. Biol. Chem.* **263**:15973–15979.

Yamamoto, M., Yew, N. S., Federspiel, M., Dodgson, J. B., Hayashi, N., and Engel, J. D. (1985). Isolation of recombinant cDNAs encoding chicken erythroid δ-aminolevulinate synthase, *Proc. Nat. Acad. Sci.* **82**:3702–3706.

Yamauchi, K., Hayashi, N., and Kikuchi, G. (1980). Translocation of δ-aminolevulinate synthase from the cytosol to the mitochondria and its regulation by hemin in rat liver, *J. Biol. Chem.* **255**:1746–1751.

Zähringer, J., Baliga, B. S., and Munro, H. N. (1976). Novel mechanisms for translational control in regulation of ferritin synthesis by iron, *Proc. Nat. Acad. Sci.* **73**:857–861.

6

Tetrapyrrole and Heme Biosynthesis in the Yeast *Saccharomyces Cerevisiae*

Rosine Labbe-Bois

Pierre Labbe

I. Introduction

The history of the heme pathway in yeast is strictly related to that of sugar catabolism. That story started in the middle of the nineteenth century when Pasteur (1876) showed that yeast cells are able to grow under anaerobic conditions but that for the same amount of sugar the cell mass produced is much greater for aerobically grown cells. The explanation given by Pasteur was proved long after to be exact: The energy available from alcoholic fermentation being low, much more sugar is needed for synthesizing the same amount of cell mass. It was later demonstrated that when oxygen is added to an anaerobic suspension of highly fermenting resting cells, the rate of glucose consumption decreases dramatically to a small percentage of its anaerobic rate; this correlated with the cessation of fermentation product accumulation. That phenomenon, which was named the "Pasteur effect," is a general property of all facultative aerobic cells, including those of higher animals. These findings were in many aspects the starting point for a tremendous increase in important discoveries concerning essentially anaerobic sugar catabolism. At that time, and after the important discovery by the Buchner's in 1897 (Florkin and Stotz, 1975) that cell-free extracts are still able to perform alcoholic fermentation, baker's and brewer's yeasts became the favorite of the pioneers in biochemistry. However, the role of oxygen in aerobic sugar metabolism (and in the "Pasteur effect") remained unanswered until the 1920s when the role of cytochromes as oxidation-reduction intermediates in yeast respiration was unequivocally proved by the classical experiments of Keilin in 1925 and Warburg in 1928 (Florkin and Stotz, 1975). Therefore, it became clear that yeast—at least aerobically grown cells—do contain all the enzymatic machinery to synthesize the heme moieties of the cy- tochromes (protoheme, heme c, heme a). However, the presence of the so-called cytochromes "a_1" and "b_1" in anaerobically grown cells which was described by Ephrussi and Slonimski (1950) raised the problem of their physiological roles. These authors suggested that those hemopro- teins might represent the "precursors" of the cytochromes of the respira- tory chain during the phenomenon of "respiratory adaptation." In "respiratory adaptation" experiments, *resting cells* of anaerobically grown yeast incubated with glucose and oxygen synthesize in a few hours active mitochondria in terms of whole cell cyanide-sensitive oxygen uptake and enzymatic activities of the respiratory chain. However, the most spectacular manifestation of "respiratory adaptation" lies in the progressive appearance of the absorption bands of a + a_3, b, c_1, and c cytochromes.

This simple experimental system became very attractive mostly be- cause the results were supposed to be not complicated by cell growth. Thus, for many years, *intact* yeast cells were used to detect and to quantify the intracellular cytochromes and tetrapyrroles or to catalyze the synthesis of cytochromes from simple radioactive precursors. At that time, all of the experiments were concerned with the synthesis of the protein moiety of the cytochromes and little attention was paid to heme, and by extension to yeast as a simple eukaryotic model to study heme biosynthesis. In fact, the heme pathway was elicited mainly by Shemin, Neuberger, and Granick during the period 1945–1960 by using essen- tially animal cells (Florkin and Stotz, 1979). Concerning intact yeast cells, the experiments of Ycas and Drabkin (1957) using [^{14}C]glycine and especially those of Barrett (1969) using [^{14}C]glycine and [^{14}C]ALA led to the decisive conclusion that during "respiratory adaptation" the whole molecule of cytochromes (hemes + proteins) is synthesized de novo; in other words, cytochromes "b_1" and "a_1" could no longer be considered as precursors of the respiratory chain-linked cytochromes. Nonetheless, the synthesis of the heme moieties of cytochromes "a_1" and "b_1" by anaero- bically grown cells, which moreover excrete coproporphyrin(ogen) (Slonimski, 1953), raised the problem of the constitutivity of a heme pathway in a facultative aerobe. Later, the nature of the physiological electron acceptor used for protoporphyrin formation from porphyrinogen by anaerobically grown cells, and therefore the capability of these cells to make heme, became a much debated question.

After these experiments with intact cells, cell-free extracts were used to detect global and/or individual activities involved in heme synthesis. It took approximately 12 years to show that heme synthesis in yeast was similar to that described in higher eukaryotes, starting from succinyl-CoA and glycine. In 1963 Chaix and Labbe (1965) showed that cell-free extracts of anaerobically and aerobically grown yeast were able to synthesize protoporphyrin when incubated in the presence of oxygen but in the absence of any heme precursor. This indicated that these extracts contain not only the enzymes of the heme pathway but also some precursor(s); it was shown later (Labbe, 1971) that ALA was that precursor. It was also shown that yeast ferrochelatase was a membrane-bound enzyme able to incorporate either Fe^{2+} or Zn^{2+} into protoporphyrin. In 1967 De Barreiro (1967) was able to measure the activity of PBG synthase in cell-free extracts and to detect ALA synthase by using [^{14}C]glycine. In 1968 Miyake and Sugimura (1968) measured a coproporphyrinogen oxidase activity in soluble cellular extracts which was much higher in extracts from anaerobically grown cells and from a respiratory-deficient mutant; this led these authors to suggest a possible repression by heme of the synthesis of that enzyme. In 1971 Labbe (1971) measured the activities of some of the enzymes of the heme pathway in cellular extracts of yeast cells grown aerobically (under different conditions of repression of their respiratory system) as well as anaerobically; this definitely proved that the heme pathway is constitutive in *Saccharomyces cerevisiae*. At last, Poulson and Polglase (1975) were the first to measure a protoporphyrinogen oxidase activity in yeast mitochondria.

The fact that *S. cerevisiae* is a facultative aerobe made that unicellular eukaryotic organism a powerful tool for isolating respiratory-deficient mutants defective in heme synthesis. By using different methods of selection and/or enrichment in heme mutants, Gollub et al. (1977) and Urban-Grimal and Labbe-Bois (1981) succeeded in isolating mutants each blocked in one of each seven steps of heme biosynthesis; no mutant affecting uroporphyrinogen III synthase has yet been described. These mutants have provided valuable information concerning the regulation of the heme pathway. They have also been used very successfully to study the regulation by heme of the synthesis of cytochromes and heme-proteins and the mechanism of their assembly. In 1983 the gene coding for ALA synthase was isolated (Arrese et al., 1983), one year later ALA synthase was purified (Volland and Felix, 1984), and today four genes and five enzymes of the yeast biosynthetic pathway have been isolated.

The present review begins with a description of the tetrapyrrolic pigments and heme-proteins present in *S. cerevisiae*, with a brief description of the roles of heme and oxygen in the synthesis of the apoheme-proteins. We next present an overview of the heme pathway and its modulation depending upon the physiological status of the cells. A section dealing with heme-deficient mutants follows. Then, each individual enzyme is considered in detail. Finally, tentative conclusions and prospects for future research are presented.

We shall confine ourselves to the heme biosynthetic pathway of the yeast *S. cerevisiae*. Current knowledge concerning this pathway in other organisms is detailed in other parts of this volume. Information concerning the life cycle, genetics, and metabolism, in particular other anabolic pathways of *S. cerevisiae*, can be found in Strathern et al. (1981, 1982).

II. Tetrapyrroles and Heme-Proteins of *S. Cerevisiae*

Because of the early spectral studies of yeast in the 1930s [for reference see Slonimski (1953)], it is known that the nature and the amount of the tetrapyrrolic pigments and the heme-containing proteins made by the cells are highly dependent upon the cultivation conditions.

A. A catalog

Let us first list the porphyric and heme compounds found in *S. cerevisiae*. In addition to the "classical" cytochromes a + a_3, b, c, and c_1 associated with the respiratory chain bound to the inner membrane, yeast mitochondria contain two other hemoproteins: the cytochrome c peroxidase and the cytochrome b_2 (L-lactate dehydrogenase), located in the intermembrane space (Daum et al., 1982). Two catalases, A and T, are present in the cytosol, catalase A being associated with the peroxisomes (Skoneczny et al., 1988). Two cytochromes, b_5 and P450, are present in the microsomal fraction. Cytochrome b_5 corresponds to the cytochrome originally called b_1 (Yoshida et al., 1974) and is involved in the oxidative desaturation of fatty acids (Tamura et al., 1976). Cytochrome P450 (designated cytochrome $P450_{14DM}$) catalyzes the oxidative removal of the 14α-methyl group of lanosterol, the initial step of ergosterol biosynthesis from lanosterol (Aoyama et al., 1987); there are indications, however, that more than one form of cytochrome P450 might exist (Kappeli, 1986; King and Wiseman, 1987). The presence of a siroheme-containing sulfite reductase (Yoshimoto and Sato, 1970), catalyzing an early step in methionine biosynthesis, can be inferred from the absence of that activity in the mutants blocked in the heme pathway prior to urogen III (the precursor of siroheme), which leads to methionine auxotrophy (Gollub et al., 1977). The same reasoning leads us to think that *S. cerevisiae* does not synthesize vitamin B12: The cells do not require vitamin B12 or a precursor as a nutritional supplement for growth, and the hemeless mutants do not develop a vitamin B12 auxotrophy.

Spectral analysis of whole cells (and subcellular fractions) grown under various conditions revealed the presence of additional pigments which have been attributed to different heme precursors or heme-proteins by the different authors who described them. Soluble pigment(s) P420, able to bind carbon monoxide when reduced to give an absorption band near 420 nm, has been attributed to a "reduced protohemin compound" (Lindenmayer and Smith, 1964), "unidentified hemoprotein" (Ishidate et al., 1969), "hemoglobin" (Mok et al., 1969), or "unassigned or sequestered free protoheme" (Labbe-Bois et al., 1983). An absorption band near 585 nm has been assigned to cytochrome a_1 (Ephrussi and Slonimski, 1950) or to hemoglobin (Keilin, 1953; Ycas, 1956); but Chaix and Labbe (1965) showed that it was more likely to be due to Zn-protoporphyrin. In fact, from our experience, the presence of absorption bands around 575 nm and 585–590 nm, which depends on the strains, genetic backgrounds, and physiological state of the cells, is merely due to porphyrins and Zn-porphyrins. Finally, whole cells contain a pigment, P503, with a single absorption maximum at 503 to 505 nm, first described by Lindenmayer and Smith (1964). On the basis of its chemical reactivity, Labbe et al. (1967) suggested that P503 was a tetrahydroprotoporphyrin (or protoporphomethene), an intermediate in the oxidation of protoporphyrinogen to protoporphyrin. A similar conclusion was reached by Poulson and Polglase (1973). However, this assumption is no longer tenable for the following reasons (Labbe and Chambon, unpublished results): (1) in growing cells the addition of methionine and aminopterine in the medium prevented the presence of P503, while the addition of glycine increased it; (2) in resting cells the addition of glucose caused a rapid increase of P503 in 5 to 10 min up to about 300 nmol/g D.W. [using the extinction coefficient given by Poulson and Polglase (1973)], whether the cells contained it or not initially; here also, methionine prevented it and glycine increased it; (3) it has never been possible to extract P503 as protoporphyrin; (4) to explain the rapid glucose-induced increase of P503 in resting cells, it was necessary to postulate the existence of a pool of porphyrinogens; however, all the attempts to extract them have been unsuccessful; (5) all the *hem* mutants isolated in our laboratory and which are blocked in different enzymic steps of the heme pathway contained P503 which could be further increased by glucose as in wild-type strains. All these data are inconsistent with the proposal that P503 is protoporphomethene. Since they show some relationship between the presence of P503 and the metabolism of tetrahydrofolate, one could propose now that this absorption at 503 nm is due to the quinonoid intermediates formed by many enzymes with pyridoxal phosphate, tetrahydrofolate, and substrates, as has been well documented in the case of the enzyme serine-hydroxymethyltransferase (Schirch and Jenkins, 1964).

In addition to tetrapyrrole pigments, yeast cells were shown to contain high concentrations of ALA (0.3 to 1.5 mM in the cell sap) whatever the growth conditions (Labbe, 1971; Labbe-Bois and Volland, 1977a).

B. Glucose repression and oxygen induction (respiratory adaptation)

It has long been known that glucose and oxygen are the major regulatory factors which control the amount of the different heme-proteins made by S. cerevisiae. That amount is the highest in *derepressed* cells, that is, cells grown with vigourous aeration and a nonfermentable carbon source (such as ethanol, glycerol, or lactate), or a slowly fermentable sugar (such as galactose), or a low amount of glucose. High concentrations of glucose *repress* mitochondrial cytochrome synthesis and mitochondria development (Ephrussi et al., 1956; Yotsuyanagi, 1962; Jayaraman et al., 1966). Cytochrome b$_2$ (Guiard, 1985) and catalases A and T (Hortner et al., 1982) are also repressed by glucose. On the contrary, the production of cytochrome P450 and the P420 CO-binding pigments is increased in the glucose-repressed cells as compared to the derepressed cells where they are barely detectable (Kappeli, 1986; King and Wiseman, 1987; Dehoux, 1978).

When the cells are grown under *anaerobiosis*, the only spectrally detectable heme-proteins are the cytochromes b$_5$ (formerly b$_1$) and P450 and the P420 pigments (Slonimski, 1953, and references therein for earlier work; Lindenmayer and Estabrook, 1958; Heyman-Blanchet and Chaix, 1959; Lindenmayer and Smith, 1964; Ishidate et al., 1969; Criddle and Schatz, 1969). However, these cytochromes do not function in vivo because of oxygen limitation; that explains why ergosterol and oleic acid (delivered as Tween 80, i.e., polyoxyethylene sorbitane monooleate) are nutritional requirements for anaerobic growth (Andreasen and Stier, 1953, 1954). Anaerobic cells accumulate Zn-protoporphyrin and, in the stationary phase, neutral protoporphyrin (Chaix and Labbe, 1965), while they excrete in the medium coproporphyrin(ogen) (Slonimski, 1953; Pretlow and Sherman, 1967; Porra et al., 1972; Charalampous, 1974; Labbe-Bois and Volland, 1977a). The presence of heme compounds and protoporphyrin was observed in spite of the care taken by the different authors to avoid any contamination with oxygen during the growth and the harvesting of the cells [see also Somlo and Fukuhara (1965); Pretlow and Sherman (1967), Ohaniance and Chaix (1966), Labbe-Bois and Volland (1977a), and Lukaszkiewicz and Bilinski (1979)]. In fact, we calculated that as little as 50 μL of air is sufficient to account for the amount of heme made by the cells grown in a 1-L culture for 24 h; such a low amount of air can be due to its diffusion through the tubings and the glass walls.

Anaerobically grown cells, which lack the respiratory chain-linked cytochromes, are able to synthesize them upon exposure to oxygen and glucose under nongrowing (resting) conditions (Ephrussi and Slonimski, 1950). The speed of the respiratory adaptation, that is, the increase in the respiratory activity and the appearance of the cytochromes a + a_3, b, c, and c_1, depends on both the carbon source used for anaerobic growth and the growth phase at which the cells were harvested. The adaptive process takes hours when the cells are harvested in the exponential phase of growth on glucose; it is much more rapid and does not require exogenous glucose with cells harvested in the early stationary phase of glucose growth, or with cells grown with galactose whatever the growth phase (Lindenmayer and Estabrook, 1958; Heyman-Blanchet and Chaix, 1959; Somlo and Fukuhara, 1965). A relationship between the rate of respiratory adaptation and the glycogen content of the cells has been reported, but its physiological significance is unclear (Labbe-Bois et al., 1973). Also unclear is the inhibitory effect of zinc on the oxygen-induced biosynthesis of respiratory cytochromes (Ohaniance and Chaix, 1966, 1970).

The purification of almost all the heme-proteins of *S. cerevisiae* and the obtention of specific antibodies, the isolation and sequencing of most of their structural genes together with the isolation of regulatory mutations, have permitted tremendous progress to be made in the understanding of the molecular mechanisms governing the synthesis of these heme-proteins. The use of heme-deficient mutants has further shown that the synthesis of many of them was also controlled by heme. The main results concerning the regulation by oxygen and heme will be summarized in the next section. The repression by glucose is a very complex system (Entian, 1986) and affects different metabolisms besides the synthesis of the apoheme-proteins. Although exogenous heme, or heme analogues (such as deuteroheme and Co-protoporphyrin) can alleviate glucose repression (Guarente et al., 1984; Gopalan and Rajamanickam, 1986), there does not yet exist strong evidence that glucose repression of respiratory cytochromes and other heme-proteins is due to heme deficiency (Hortner et al., 1982).

C. Regulation of heme-protein synthesis by oxygen and heme

Is it a matter of chance or the result of a rational design that the synthesis of the different heme-proteins is regulated differently by oxygen and heme?

It was Schatz who initiated that study by analyzing with new immunological methods the presence of the protein moieties of different cytochromes and heme-proteins in anaerobically grown cells and in a mutant deficient in heme formation due to the absence of ALA synthase activity. The apoproteins whose synthesis is apparently unaffected by heme deficiency, anaerobiosis, or both include the following: (1) the cytoplasmically made cytochrome c peroxidase (Djavadi-Ohaniance et al., 1978; Saltzgaber-Muller and Schatz, 1978) and cytochrome c_1 (Ross and Schatz, 1976; Saltzgaber-Muller and Schatz, 1978; Lin et al., 1982); the latter, however, has been shown to depend on heme for its proteolytic maturation during its import into mitochondria (Ohashi et al., 1982); (2) the mitochondrially synthesized cytochrome b (Saltzgaber-Muller and Schatz, 1978; Clejan et al., 1980; Lin et al., 1982). Why apoproteins and not holoenzymes are made under anaerobiosis is still an unresolved question. The rather low efficiency of anaerobic heme production might be an explanation, although it is large enough to make holocytochromes b_5 and P450, the P420 pigments, and holocatalases in some mutants (Bilinski et al., 1980). Why is that heme found associated mainly with the microsomal and soluble fraction, when it is produced in the mitochondria?

The case of the cytochrome c oxidase is much more complex. It comprises nine subunits. The three largest ones (subunits I, II, and III) are made on mitochondrial ribosomes, whereas the others are made in the cytoplasm. Early, rather complicated and tricky, experiments led the authors to conclude that coproporphyrin III is the inhibitor of the synthesis of cytochrome oxidase in anaerobic yeast protoplasts and that oxygen regulates its de novo synthesis by abolishing the inhibition by coproporphyrin (Charalampous and Chen, 1974; Charalampous, 1974). These results have never been confirmed. More recently, Schatz and co-workers have shown that both heme and oxygen are required for the assembly of the cytochrome oxidase subunits into the membrane, and that the accumulation of each subunit is affected to different extents by the absence of heme or oxygen (Saltzgaber-Muller and Schatz, 1978; Woodrow and Schatz, 1979).

The apoproteins and enzymes whose synthesis is regulated at the transcriptional level by heme and oxygen are listed in Table 6.1. The reader will find in the legend the last or main references of the different contributions to the field, in which references to earlier work can be found. Therefore, we shall present here only a brief survey emphasizing the important features of these regulations. Evidence for a regulation, either positive or negative, came first by analyzing the amount of immunodetectable protein and corresponding mRNA (by in vitro translation and Northern blot analysis). The fusion of the promoter sequences of these regulated genes with the β-galactosidase coding sequence and

TABLE 6.1 *S. Cerevisiae* Genes Transcriptionally Regulated by Oxygen and Heme

Gene designation	Gene product	Regulation by* Heme	Regulation by* Oxygen	Cis-acting regulatory sequences	Trans-acting regulatory mutations	References†
CYC1	Iso-1-cytochrome c	+	+	Yes	CYP1(= HAP1), ROX1 Factors RC2, RAF	1–7
CYP3 (= CYC7)	Iso-2-cytochrome c	0/+	+	Yes	CYP1	3, 5, 7, 8
CYB2	Cytochrome b2	+	+	Yes	CYP1	References in 5, 9
CTT1	Catalase T	+	+	Yes	CAS1, CGR4	1, 10, 11, 12
CTA1	Catalase A	+	+			1, 13
COX5	Subunit V of cytochrome oxidase	+				14, 15
—	Subunit VII of cytochrome oxidase	+				14
SOD	Mn superoxide dismutase	+	+		ROX1, CYP1	4, 8, 16
COR1	44,000-dalton subunit of complex III	+				15
ANB1	Unknown	−	−		ROX1	4, 17
HEM13	Coproporphyrinogen oxidase	−	−		CYP1	This review

* +, positive control; −, negative control, 0, no control. In all columns, a blank means not determined.

† 1: Hortner et al., 1982; 2: Guarente et al., 1984; 3: Laz et al., 1984; 4: Lowry and Zitomer, 1984; 5: Verdiere et al., 1985; 6: Verdiere et al., 1986; 7: Guarente, 1987; 8: Zitomer et al., 1987; 9: Guiard, manuscript in preparation; 10: Bilinski et al., 1980; 11: Sledziewski et al., 1981; 12: Spevak et al., 1986; 13: Cohen et al., 1985; 14: Gollub and Dayan, 1985; 15: Myers et al., 1987; 16: Marres et al., 1985; 17: Lowry and Lieber, 1986.

the introduction of the resultant chimeric gene into yeast cells facilitated these studies: The activity of the promoter could be analyzed simply by measuring the level of β-galactosidase activity. Deletion analysis of the promoter regions led to the identification of cis-acting sequences, the so-called UASs (upstream activation sites), which are responsible for these regulations. UASs of the $CYC1$ gene are functional when inverted, thus sharing some similarity with eukaryotic enhancers. A combination of genetic and biochemical approaches led to the discovery of trans-acting factors which mediate these regulations; some have been shown to bind in vitro to short sequences within the UASs. The gene of one of these regulatory factors, $CYP1$ ($= HAP1$), has been cloned (Verdiere et al., 1985) and its sequence recently determined (Creusot, Verdiere, Gaisne, and Slonimski, unpublished results). It codes for a large protein with two interesting features: a DNA-binding "Zn finger" at its NH_2 terminus, and several tandemly repeated sequences which might play a role in "sensing" directly or indirectly the presence of heme or oxygen and then controlling the regulatory activity of the protein.

Impressive though these results are, they have not answered some crucial questions. Since it is highly unlikely that oxygen itself is the effector molecule, how is its presence sensed and transduced by the cells? Do oxygen and heme act independently or via a common metabolite or mechanism? Does oxygen act solely as a substrate for the synthesis of heme which then would be the genuine effector? Were this correct, why are not the apoproteins transcribed in anaerobic cells which may contain as much heme as aerobic cells?

As regards cytochrome P450, its production depends on both high glucose and oxygen limitation for reasons which remain unclear (King and Wiseman, 1987). There is also some indication that the apoprotein is not made in the absence of heme (Meussdoerffer and Fiechter, 1986). The recent isolation of its gene should help to clarify these questions (Kalb et al., 1987).

Finally, one may ask whether the transcriptional regulation by heme is limited to (heme)-proteins involved in oxygen metabolism and whether heme does not interfere also at other stages of protein synthesis. The answer to the former question seems to be yes (Schmalix et al., 1986), although as noted by the authors "the search is complicated by the fact that heme, via the assembly of a functional respiratory chain, also leads to a general activation of the cellular metabolism." As to the latter question, only specific controls by heme occurring at the level of translation have been reported in the cases of catalases A and T (Hamilton et al., 1982) and a chimeric heterologous gene (Jensen et al., 1986). The molecular mechanism mediating these heme-dependent translational effects in yeast is unknown. It is unlikely that the phosphorylation state of the initiation factor eIF-2α is involved, as documented in higher eukary-

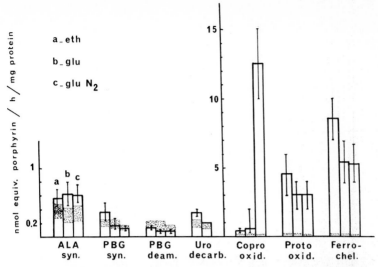

Figure 6.2 Steady-state levels of enzymic activities measured in acellular extracts from *S. cerevisiae* cells growing aerobically with (a) ethanol or (b) glucose and (c) anaerobically with glucose. ALA syn., ALA synthase; PBG syn., PBG synthase; PBG deam., PBG deaminase; uro decarb., uroporphyrinogen decarboxylase; copro oxid., coproporphyrinogen III oxidase; proto oxid., protoporphyrinogen IX oxidase; ferrochel., ferrochelatase. The deviations represent the range of values measured with different wild-type strains in our laboratory or taken and recalculated when possible from the literature. The dotted parts of the bars represent the activities estimated in vivo (see the text).

nose-derepressed cells have a higher ALA synthase activity as compared to ethanol- or glucose-grown cells). (4) The two membrane-bound enzymes, protogen oxidase and ferrochelatase, function in vivo at only a small percentage of their maximal velocity measured in vitro, while the other enzymes work in vivo roughly near their maximal velocity.

Much less is known about the enzymic steps catalyzing the formation of heme c and heme a. Mutations at two different loci, *CYC2* and *CYC3*, have been uncovered which cause partial or complete deficiency, respectively, in only both isocytochromes c without affecting cytochrome c_1. Since the mutants contain apoisocytochrome c, it was proposed, to explain their different phenotypes, that "the *CYC3* locus codes for a heme attachment activity, while the *CYC2* gene product may be a protein which facilitates apocytochrome c transport across the outer mitochondrial membrane or enhances the heme attachment activity" (Matner and Sherman, 1982). Recently, the *CYC3* gene has been isolated and sequenced and demonstrated to encode cytochrome c heme lyase, the enzyme catalyzing the covalent attachment of heme to apocytochrome c (Dumont et al., 1987).

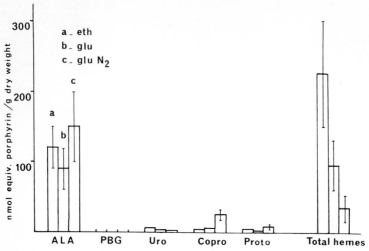

Figure 6.3   Amounts of heme(s) and heme precursors present in *S. cerevisiae* cells growing aerobically with (a) ethanol or (b) glucose and (c) anaerobically with glucose. ALA, intracellular 5-aminolevulinic acid; PBG, intracellular porphobilinogen (not detectable); uro, intracellular uroporphyrin and its decarboxylation products 7-, 6-, 5-COOH porphyrin; copro, coproporphyrin(ogen) present in the cells and excreted in the medium; proto, protoporphyrin and Zn-protoporphyrin in cells and medium; total hemes, protoheme + heme c + heme a determined spectrophotometrically from cytochromic or pyridine hemochrome spectra. All measurements were carried out with midlogarithmic phase cultures.

As for the synthesis of heme a, it needs the metabolization of the methyl group at position 8 to a formyl group and the addition of a hydroxyfarnesyl group to the vinyl group at position 2 of the protoporphyrin ring. Mevalonic acid, a precursor of farnesyl pyrophosphate, has been shown to be incorporated into the heme a moiety of cytochrome oxidase in *S. cerevisiae* (Keyhani and Keyhani, 1978). Cryptoheme a, an ill-defined analogue of heme a, has been found in yeast adapting to oxygen (Barrett, 1969), but it is not clear whether it is a precursor or a degradation product of heme a. It is not clear also whether protoporphyrin or protoheme is the true precursor for heme a formation. That protoporphyrin is first metabolized to porphyrin a which is then converted to heme a has been suggested by Keyhani and Keyhani (1980a, b) who described the presence of porphyrin a in yeast cells deficient in cytochrome oxidase because of either copper deficiency or mitochondrial mutations. But there exists some experimental evidence favoring protoheme as the precursor: Liver ferrochelatase cannot incorporate iron in vitro into porphyrin a (Porra and Jones, 1963b); heme a is found radiolabeled in heme-deficient bacterial mutants fed with exogenous radiolabeled protoheme (Sinclair et al., 1967); respiratory activity and spectrally detectable cytochrome oxidase are restored in hemeless mutants by supplementing the growth medium with heme (Gollub et al., 1977; Labbe-Bois, unpublished results). It may be relevant to recall here that in the course of chlorophyll biosynthesis, magnesium is inserted into protoporphyrin before the reactions modifying the side chains take place.

Virtually nothing is known about yeast concerning the fate of heme once made in the inner mitochondrial membrane and about its eventual catabolism, in contrast to the situation in mammalian cells. Is newly synthesized heme immediately transferred to a small cytosolic pool of "regulatory free heme" in equilibrium with the different heme-proteins? Do there exist specific heme-binding proteins for carrying heme to its final destinations in the different compartments? There is some indication that extra-heme bound to unspecified ligands is made under certain circumstances (Labbe-Bois et al., 1983), but its physiological significance is highly questionable. Regarding heme catabolism, neither the heme oxygenase system nor the presence of its reaction products have been described in yeast. But an obvious question for which there is as yet no answer may be raised at this point. Is there any physiological evidence that yeast must possess a heme-degrading system? It is generally accepted that the turnover rate of components of a microorganism is kept at its minimum in rapidly growing cells. During derepressed aerobic growth, synthesis of heme and heme-proteins are apparently poised and heme production stops when cells are in the stationary phase; however, as mentioned above, a surplus amount of heme is made under conditions hindering normal apoprotein synthesis (anaerobiosis, glucose repression, rho$^-$ state). On the other hand, gradual elimination of "excess" respiratory cytochromes has been reported by Luzikov [see Luzikov (1986) for references]. Selective loss of certain cytochromes occurs during the cell-division cycle and accompanies the derepressed-glucose repressed or anaerobic-aerobic transitions (Lloyd, 1974). These data, taken among others, illustrate how little is known about heme intracellular traffic in yeast, a process essential in fulfilling its structural and regulatory functions.

B. Genetic approach

Since the heme-proteins present in *S. cerevisiae* have functions in various cellular metabolisms, the absence of heme is expected to be highly pleiotropic and, in fact, serendipity accounted for the isolation of most mutants which have been shown afterward to be affected in heme synthesis.

Heme-deficient mutants are respiratory incompetent due to a lack of mitochondrial cytochromes and, therefore, grow only on fermentable sugars and form *petite* colonies on agar plates. They require unsaturated fatty acids and ergosterol for growth owing to the absence of cytochromes b_5 and P450; and because of the ergosterol deficiency they show nystatin resistance. They also lack catalase activity. In addition, the mutants affected in the early steps of the heme pathway have an extra methionine auxotrophy, while those affected at the late steps are fluorescent under uv light due to the accumulation of porphyrin intermediates. Supplementation with heme alleviates respiratory deficiency and auxotrophies. All these phenotypic characteristics have been employed as selection methods to isolate the mutant cells after mutagenesis (except methionine auxotrophy). This explains the variety of names given to the mutants or used for gene designation (Table 6.2). Since the frequency of obtention of the mutants previously described in the literature was rather low, Grimal and Labbe-Bois (1980) developed an enrichment procedure based specifically on the properties of the heme pathway: A selective photooxidative killing of the wild-type cells, sensitized by Zn-protoporphyrin, synthesized and accumulated in wild-type cells under defined conditions (Sec. IV-G). It is worth noting that, taken all together, (1) many more mutants have been obtained which are blocked in the early steps of the heme pathway than blocked in the last ones; (2) many mutants do not have all the features of the phenotype described above, suggesting that the mutations are leaky to some extent, although they are respiratory deficient.

Partial mutants have also been isolated which could respire and grow on nonfermentable carbon sources (ethanol) while accumulating large amounts of porphyrins making them fluorescent under uv light. They were expected to be partially defective in the last steps of the heme

TABLE 6.2 *S. Cerevisiae* **Genes Coding for Heme Biosynthetic Enzymes**

Gene	Other designations	Gene product	References*
HEM1	*ole3, CYD1, HEMA*[†]	ALA synthase	1–6
HEM2	*ole4, olerg4, HEM10*	PBG synthase	2, 4, 6, 7
HEM3	*ole2, olerg2, HEM11, HEMC*	PBG deaminase	2, 4–7
HEM12	*HEM6, POP3, POP1?*[‡]	Urogen decarboxylase	4, 6, 8–12
HEM13	*HEMG, HEM4?, cyt?*	Coprogen oxidase	4, 6, 13, 14
HEM15	*HEM5? POP2?*	Ferrochelatase	4, 6, 8, 11

*1: Sanders et al., 1973; 2: Bard et al., 1974; 3: Woods et al., 1975; 4: Gollub et al., 1977; 5: Labbe-Bois et al., 1977; 6: Urban-Grimal and Labbe-Bois, 1981; 7: Karst and Lacroute, 1973; 8: Pretlow and Sherman, 1967; 9: Arrese et al., 1982; 10: Rytka et al., 1984; 11: Kurlandzka and Rytka, 1985; 12: Kurlandzka et al., 1988; 13: Miyake and Sugimura, 1968; 14: Bilinski et al., 1981.

[†]*HEMA* previously reported as being not allelic to *ole3* (ref. 5) has been shown later to be allelic with *HEM1* (Rytka, unpublished results).

[‡]A question mark means that allelism with other mutations of the same group has not been reported. However, biochemical characteristics suggest that they belong to that group.

pathway or changed in its regulation (Rytka et al., 1984; Kurlandzka and Rytka, 1985).

Genetic and biochemical analysis of these heme-deficient mutants revealed that most of them carry mutations in nuclear gene coding for one of the enzymes of the heme pathway. Six such loci, listed in Table 6.2, have been uncovered at the present time. They are not linked (Gollub et al., 1977; Urban-Grimal, unpublished results) except for *HEM*12 and *HEM*13 separated by a map interval of 10 c*M* and localized on chromosome IV (Kurlandzka et al., 1988). *HEM*2 has been mapped on chromosome VII (Urban-Grimal and Labbe-Bois, 1981). All the mutations described so far at these loci are recessive. A nuclear mutant lacking protogen oxidase activity has been described (Camadro et al., 1982); but, since it has been shown later to be impaired in iron metabolism (Sec. IV-F), the nature of the primary genetic lesion is not ascertained. On the other hand, there is no genetic evidence that protogen oxidase is made in the mitochondria, contrary to an early proposal by Poulson and Polglase (1974b). The rho⁻ mutation, which leads to the loss of mitochondrial funtions, does not bring any gross changes in the heme synthesis enzymes (Labbe-Bois and Volland, 1977b), including protogen oxidase (Camadro et al., 1982). No mutant with a phenotype suggestive of urogen III synthase deficiency has been reported yet.

A few other mutations have been described, which are not alleles of the *HEM* structural genes but interfere specifically with the functioning of some *HEM* gene products. These mutations will be considered in detail in the next section, inasmuch as they enlighten the in vivo operation of some enzymes. Although suggested by preliminary analysis of some catalase-deficient mutants (Labbe-Bois et al., 1977), there is no evidence at present for a coordinated regulation of the whole pathway.

The systematic analysis of the enzymic activities of the heme pathway in an isogenic collection of hemeless mutants (Urban-Grimal and Labbe-Bois, 1981; Camadro et al., 1982) and also in partial mutants (Labbe-Bois et al., 1980; Rytka et al., 1984) suggested possible modes of regulation of heme synthesis at the level of some individual enzymes. When compared to the activities measured in their respective parental strains: (1) ALA synthase activity was unchanged in all completely blocked mutants, suggesting no heme feedback repression. However, a two- to threefold increase was measured in mutants partially affected in the last steps of heme synthesis and this was accompanied by a considerable rise in ALA intracellular content. (2) PBG deaminase activity was nil in ALA and PBG synthase mutants, suggesting a possible induction of that enzyme by its substrate PBG. (3) Coprogen and protogen oxidase activities were increased in all mutants, 5- to 50-fold for coprogen oxidase, depending upon the parental strain, twofold for protogen oxidase. This suggested a possible repression by heme of these two enzymes.

The availability of *hem* mutants permitted the straightforward cloning of the *HEM* genes by screening yeast genomic libraries, using transformation procedures developed for yeast cells, for recombinant plasmids that complemented the respiratory defect or the auxotrophies. The mutant cells transformed by a plasmid bearing the *HEM* gene recovered the ability to grow on glycerol or glucose media in the absence of exogenous heme or unsaturated fatty acid and ergosterol supplements. In return, the isolation of the *HEM* genes provided new tools to study the regulation of the enzymes they were coding for. At present, four *HEM* genes have been isolated which code for ALA synthase (Sec. IV-A), PBG synthase (Sec. IV-B), coprogen oxidase (Sec. IV-E), and PBG deaminase (Sec. IV-C), the first three of which have been sequenced. We can anticipate that the isolation of other *HEM* genes should follow soon.

IV. Individual Enzymes: Enzymology, Genetics, and Regulations

In this section we shall consider in detail each enzyme, with particular emphasis on its implication in the control of heme production. References to other systems, humans, animals, or bacteria, will be kept at a minimum, since these are treated in other parts of this volume.

A. 5-Aminolevulinic acid (ALA) synthase

As the first committed enzyme of the heme pathway and, as such thought to play an important role in controlling heme synthesis, ALA synthase is the enzyme of the pathway which has received the most attention.

De Barreiro (1967) first reported an incorporation of radiolabeled glycine in ALA catalyzed by yeast cellular extracts. Thereafter, Labbe (1971), Tuppy and Wiche (1971), Jayaraman et al. (1971), and Porra et al. (1972) described the presence of an ALA synthase activity in extracts prepared from cells grown in different conditions and from rho⁻ mutants. Moreover, Labbe (1971) showed that succinyl-CoA, substrate of the enzyme, could be formed from either succinate or α-ketoglutarate and that pyridoxal-phosphate was required for the activity. In this connection it is interesting to note that pyridoxine deficiency in *Saccharomyces carlsbergensis* leads to the absence of cytochromes and to decreased levels of unsaturated fatty acids and ergosterol (Nakamura et al., 1974). ALA synthase activity was found predominantly in the cytosolic fraction by Tuppy and Wiche (1971), whereas Porra et al. (1972) and Poulson (1976b) found it mainly associated with the mitochondria of aerobic cells, and the cytosol of anaerobic cells. No attempt to isolate the enzyme was reported until 1984, when Volland and Felix

(1984) succeeded in purifying it to homogeneity about 7000-fold with an overall yield of 40%. They also demonstrated that the enzyme is located entirely in the mitochondria, whatever the growth conditions.

Purified yeast ALA synthase had a specific activity of 39,000 nmol of ALA per hour and per milligram of protein at 30°C, with an optimal pH around 7.5 (Table 6.3). The enzyme activity was sensitive to thiol-blocking reagents, but the inhibition was prevented by pyridoxal-phosphate. It was 50% inhibited by 6 μM oxidized heme but not by reduced heme, which is more likely to be the physiological state of heme found in mitochondria. Pyridoxal-phosphate was an essential cofactor and a K_d value of 5 μM was estimated. The affinity for its substrates was measured and K_m values obtained are 2 μM for succinyl-CoA and 3 mM for glycine. Such a low affinity of ALA synthase for glycine might explain why a mutant impaired in glycine metabolism was deficient in cytochrome c and catalase which could be restored to normal by protoporphyrin or glycine supplementation (Ycas and Starr, 1953). A severe shortage of succinyl-CoA supply due to a defect in α-ketoglutarate dehydrogenase can also lead to the absence of cytochromes (reversed by exogenous ALA) in a *hem*16 nuclear mutant which has a normal mitochondrially located ALA synthase (Labbe-Bois et al., 1983). The exact nature of the defect, which might also be nutritional, has not yet been elucidated in the *cyc*4 mutant which has normal level of ALA synthase activity but low ALA and cytochrome cellular contents (Sanders et al., 1973; Woods et al., 1975; Mattoon et al., 1978; Malamud et al., 1983).

The pure enzyme was composed of two identical subunits of a relative molecular mass of 53,000 daltons, identical to that found for the native protein (Volland and Felix, 1984; Urban-Grimal et al., 1986). That the enzyme is a homodimer agrees with the previous finding of a phenomenon of functional interallelic complementation between some of the *hem*1 mutants: The products of the two different mutated *hem*1 alleles can form a hybrid enzyme which regained part of the activity, the defects in each subunit correcting each other (Urban-Grimal and Labbe-Bois, 1981; Labbe-Bois et al., 1983).

The *HEM*1 gene coding for ALA synthase has been isolated (Arrese et al., 1983; Bard and Ingolia, 1984; Urban-Grimal et al., 1984). Interestingly enough, the transformed cells carrying the *HEM*1 gene borne on a multicopy plasmid did not present higher-than-normal content of cytochromes, heme, or porphyrins although they showed a large increase in ALA synthase activity and ALA intracellular content. The complete sequence of the *HEM*1 gene and its flanking regions were determined (Urban-Grimal et al., 1986; Keng et al., 1986; Keng and Guarente, 1987). It codes for a protein of 548 amino acids with a calculated molecular weight of 59,275, and the deduced amino acid sequence shows clear homologies with the sequence of the ALA synthase from chick embryo

TABLE 6.3 Molecular and Catalytic Properties of *S. Cerevisiae* Heme Biosynthetic Enzymes

	ALA synthase	PBG synthase	Urogen decarboxylase	Coprogen oxidase	Protogen oxidase	Ferro-chelatase
Specific Activity*	39,000	4,700§	2,000¶	3,600	12,000	35,000 (Fe) 27,000 (Zn)
Turnover number†	60			4.2	11.2	23
Molecular weight, Molecular weight precursor form	Homodimer 2 × 53,000 56,500		38,000	Homodimer 2 × 35,000	56,000 59,000	40,000 44,000
K_m (μM)	glycine: 3,000 succinyl-CoA: 2	ALA: 1,500–2,600 (pH 9.6, 45–55°C)	Urogen I or Urogen III: ~ 0.01	coprogen: 0.05 oxygen: ?	protogen: 0.5 Oxygen: ?	proto: 0.09 Fe^{2+}: 0.16 Zn^{2+}: 0.25
Cofactor	Pyridoxal-P	Zn^{2+}		Fe?	?	
Inhibitors	—SH reagents oxidized heme	—SH reagents o-phenanthroline levulinic acid	—SH reagents	—SH reagents		—SH reagents
Activators				Phospholipids		Fatty acids
Amino acid sequence	Deduced from sequencing *HEM1*	Deduced from sequencing *HEM2*		Deduced from sequencing *HEM13*		N terminus of purified protein
References‡	1, 2	3, 4, 5, 6	7	8, 9	10	11

*Nanomoles of product per hour per milligram of protein, at 30°C and pH ~ 7.5.
†Mole of product per mole enzyme per minute, at 30°C.
‡1: Volland and Felix, 1984; 2: Urban-Grimal et al., 1986; 3: De Barreiro, 1967; 4: Labbe, 1971; 5: Borralho et al., 1983; 6: Myers et al., 1987; 7: Felix and Brouillet, manuscript in preparation; 8: Camadro et al., 1986; 9: Zagorec et al., 1988; 10: Camadro, Chambon, Jomary, and Labbe, manuscript in preparation; 11: Camadro and Labbe, 1988.
§Measured with an enzyme preparation probably only partially purified and under undefined conditions of pH and temperature (ref. 3).
¶Estimated as nmoles coproporphyrin I formed from urogen I per hour per milligram of protein, at 37°C.

liver cells. The amino-terminal region of the protein presents all the features of the cleavable presequences which direct the proteins imported into mitochondria; and it was shown that it is indeed the case. ALA synthase was synthesized both in vitro and in vivo as a precursor of larger molecular size (about 3500 daltons higher) which is processed to the mature form during its import in the mitochondria; import was not inhibited by exogenous heme (Urban-Grimal et al., 1986). By fusing β-galactosidase gene to various lengths of $HEM1$ gene corresponding to amino-terminal fragments of ALA synthase, and analyzing the final location of each of these fusion proteins in the cell, Keng et al. (1986) showed that the nine amino-terminal residues of ALA synthase are sufficient to direct the foreign protein to the mitochondrial matrix. But Volland and Urban-Grimal (1988) found that an ALA synthase deleted of its first 75 amino acids, thus deprived of its presequence and with a new atypical NH_2 terminus, could be directed in vivo to the mitochondria, although it was unable to reach the mitochondrial matrix and was locked in the membranes. Their results suggest that topogenic sequence(s) exists in the mature part of the protein which can replace the presequence but with lower efficiency and accuracy.

The studies on the regulation of ALA synthase have not always proceeded in a systematic fashion and this has resulted in a mass of rather confusing and even conflicting data. The experimental approaches were different, as were the methodologies for measuring ALA synthase and the strains used. From all the data available in the literature, there does not seem to exist in wild-type strains a clear and simple relationship between the state of derepression of the cells or the amount of heme made and the level of ALA synthase activity measured in acellular extracts from growing cells. But relative changes have been observed in cells undergoing transitions between different states. During the growth cycle on glucose, ALA synthase activity increases (twofold maximum) at the end of the exponential phase of growth before falling to very low values when the cells are fully derepressed (Jayaraman et al., 1971; Labbe-Bois and Volland, 1977a); this is accompanied by a rise and fall of intracellular ALA content (Labbe-Bois and Volland, 1977a; Mattoon et al., 1978). A transient increase in ALA synthase activity has also been observed when cells previously grown under glucose-repressing conditions are transferred into derepression medium containing nitrogen sources and low glucose; it was prevented by cycloheximide and high glucose (Mahler and Lin, 1974; Jayaraman et al., 1971), the latter effect being reversed by exogenous cyclic AMP* (Mahler and Lin, 1978a). But

---

*It must be stressed here that it is advisable to be very cautious when interpreting these effects of cyclic AMP since it is generally accepted now that, first, normal wild-type cells are not permeable to cyclic AMP, and second, cyclic AMP does not reverse glucose-catabolite repression in yeast.

Poulson (1976b) found an increased ALA synthase activity, prevented by cyclic AMP, in anaerobic protoplasts adapting to oxygen in the presence of high glucose. On the other hand, Labbe et al. (1972) reported a rapid loss of ALA synthase activity when glucose-grown cells are incubated with glucose but without any nitrogen source; this loss (degradation?, inactivation?) did not occur in the absence of glucose, whereas it did occur in the presence or absence of glucose with galactose-grown cells. At last, an effect of both glucose and respiratory competency on the expression of ALA synthase has been proposed to explain the phenotypic behavior of a leaky mutation *cyd*1, allelic to *hem*1 and giving a labile enzyme (Sanders et al., 1973; Woods et al., 1975; Lancashire and Mattoon, 1979).

There is no strong evidence at present for a control of ALA synthase by heme via some feedback mechanism. A normal level of ALA synthase activity was observed in some mutants totally deficient in heme synthesis (Urban-Grimal and Labbe-Bois, 1981), but in some others the activity was either increased or decreased (Gollub et al., 1977; Bilinski et al., 1981). A two- to threefold increase in activity has been described in mutants with a partial block in the last steps of heme synthesis (Rytka et al., 1984), together with an increase in accumulation of intracellular ALA (Malamud et al., 1983; Rytka et al., 1984). Finally, an almost twofold decrease of ALA synthase activity has been reported when wild-type cells are grown in the presence of exogenous heme (Poulson, 1976b).

It must be pointed out that all these studies were concerned only in measuring steady-state levels of ALA synthase activity. Therefore, it is not known whether these activity changes reflect changes in the synthesis of the protein, at a transcriptional or translational level, or changes in the turnover of the protein, or even both. Recently, Keng and Guarente (1987) analyzed the expression of the *HEM*1 gene (fused to β-galactosidase) in cells grown under a variety of conditions. They found that it was no more than about twofold higher in derepressed cells as compared to glucose-repressed or heme-deficient cells. But paradoxically, the expression of *HEM*1 was activated by the products of the *HAP2-HAP3* genes, a global regulatory system controlling the expression of some apocytochromes and whose absence leads to respiratory incompetence. Dissection of the *HEM*1 promoter revealed that the apparent constitutive expression was, indeed, the result of the presence of two oppositely regulated sites: a positive one, close to or even identical to the *HAP2-HAP3* target sequence, which "keeps *HEM*1 turned on" in the absence of heme; and a negative one "that counteracts derepression" in a lactate medium. These results suggest that *HEM*1 expression is subject to a complex set of regulations whose physiological signals and the protein factors which mediate them are still unknown. It would be amazing if these regulations were merely coincidental. One can speculate that they respond to the need for the cells to keep a tight but composite control on ALA formation in order to supply it, when required, in concentrations saturating or not for the next cytosolic enzyme, PBG synthase, which is considered to be a rate-limiting step for heme synthesis.

All these data concerning ALA synthesis provide strong evidence that ALA is produced solely via ALA synthase and that the glutamate pathway described in plants or the dioxovalerate-transamination pathway reported in mammals do not exist in *S. cerevisiae*. This is further substantiated by the fact that the disruption or deletion of the chromosomal copy of the *HEM1* gene leads to the absence of any functionally detectable heme and even, in some strains, to the incapability of the cells to grow in the absence of minute amount of exogenous ALA [see Keng and Guarente (1987) and Guiard and Urban-Grimal, personal communications].

B. PBG synthase

PBG synthase activity, also named ALA dehydratase, was first measured in yeast by De Barreiro (1967) who also presented the only report to date on the purification of the enzyme. The 900-fold purified enzyme appeared fairly free of contaminating material after gel electrophoresis and its specific activity was 4700 nmol PBG formed per hour and per milligram of protein (pH and temperature not specified by the author). But no molecular properties of the enzyme were given and the catalytic characteristics were determined with a crude preparation. The activity was heat stable up to 55°C and had a sharp optimal pH at 9.6. When measured under these optimal conditions, a K_m value of 1.5 mM was obtained for ALA. Similar values were reported later, when measured (45°C, pH 9.6) with permeabilized cells or cell free extracts (Borralho et al., 1983). The activity was inhibited by thiol-directed reagents, but only partially by EDTA. An inhibition by excess cysteine was shown later (De Barreiro, 1969) to be probably due to a reaction between ALA and SH-cysteine. Then, zinc was shown to be required for the activity (Labbe, 1971) and o-phenanthroline was described as a better inhibitor than EDTA (Labbe, 1971; Brouillet et al., 1975).

Levulinic acid, a relatively weak competitive inhibitor of PBG synthase from other sources, has been shown to interfere also with heme synthesis in yeast. Provided the medium was kept at low pH to permit its entrance in the cells, high concentrations (50 to 100 mM) of levulinic acid inhibited growth on ethanol. Mutants resistant to 50 mM levulinic acid in a glycerol medium were isolated, but the nature of the mutation has not been further characterized (Mattoon et al., 1978). With cells growing on glucose, increasing amounts of levulinic acid caused an accumulation of ALA and a concomitant decrease of cytochromes, suggesting that its site of action is PBG synthase (Malamud et al., 1979). Indeed, the addition of levulinic acid to growing cells has been used to analyze the effects of heme depletion in a wild-type background (Ohashi et al., 1982). Succinylacetone (4,6-dioxoheptanoic acid), a very potent inhibitor of mammalian PBG synthase, has not been tested on whole cells, but preliminary experiments with cellular extracts (Labbe-Bois, unpublished data) suggest that if succinylacetone itself is a poor inhibitor, succinylacetone pyrrole formed by condensation of succinylacetone with ALA might be a potent inhibitor of yeast enzyme, as described to be the case with *Clostridium tetanomorphum* PBG synthase (Brumm and Friedmann, 1981).

The *HEM*2 gene coding for PBG synthase was isolated recently and shown to code for a protein of 342 amino acids with a calculated molecular weight of 37,837. The yeast enzyme and human PBG synthase share 52% overall homology with highly conserved regions, especially the domain proposed to constitute the zinc-binding site (Myers et al., 1987). Disruption of the chromosomal copy of *HEM*2 led to viable cells which are respiratory incompetent and require oleic acid, ergosterol, and methionine for growth. The overproduction of PBG synthase in cells carrying multiple copies of *HEM*2 should facilitate the purification of the protein and permit a detailed investigation of its molecular and catalytic properties.

All reports agreed in finding a two- to fourfold lower steady-state level of PBG synthase activity in extracts from glucose-repressed cells than from derepressed cells. Moreover, a two- to fourfold increase in PBG synthase activity was observed when repressed cells were shifted to a derepression medium or when cells, anaerobically grown on either glucose or galactose, where adapted to oxygen under nonproliferating conditions (presence of glucose but absence of nitrogen sources) (Labbe, 1971; Jayaraman et al., 1971; Labbe et al., 1972; Poulson, 1976b; Labbe-Bois and Volland, 1977a; Mahler and Lin, 1978a, b; Borralho et al., 1983). The increase of PBG synthase activity in derepression experiments or during respiratory adaptation was shown to require both RNA (Mahler and Lin, 1978b) and protein (Labbe et al., 1972; Mahler and Lin, 1978b) synthesis, while independent of mitochondrial function(s) (Mahler and Lin, 1978b; Labbe-Bois and Volland, 1977a). That increase was prevented by glucose, this effect being overcome by exogenous cyclic AMP (Poulson, 1976b; Mahler and Lin, 1978a). These results were taken as evidence that PBG synthase was subject to glucose (catabolite) repression. Further support for this came from the analysis of PBG synthase activity in a mutant carrying the *hex*2 mutation which leads to glucose-repression resistance of many sugar-utilizing enzymes: The mutant exhibited derepressed levels of enzyme activity throughout the growth on glucose, in contrast to wild-type strains which had a lower activity as long as glucose was present in the medium (Borralho et al., 1983). However, the regulatory events underlying these changes in PBG synthase activity are still unknown: Is it the synthesis or the activity of the protein which is regulated?

The low level of PBG synthase activity as compared to the level of ALA synthase, and its sluggish affinity for its substrate can explain the accumulation of ALA in the cells; its concentration, which is 0.2 to 0.4 mM (assuming no subcellular compartmentation) in growing wild-type cells, reaches 1.5 mM in partial mutants (Rytka et al., 1984). This suggests strongly that PBG synthase is a rate-limiting step for porphyrin production, whose activity in vivo depends on intracellular ALA concentration which itself depends on the functioning of ALA synthase. In this context, it is not impossible that the exit of ALA out of the mitochondria and its local concentration in the cytosol might also interfere. Such a role for PBG synthase has also been reported in *Neurospora crassa* (Chandrika and Padmanaban, 1980). But it is the opposite of the situation in liver cells for instance, where PBG synthase is in excess, ALA never accumulates and ALA synthase is considered to be the rate-limiting step of the pathway.

C. PBG deaminase and uroporphyrinogen III synthase

These are the least documented enzymes of the heme biosynthetic pathways in yeast. They have not been purified and nothing is known at present about their kinetic and catalytic properties. PBG deaminase activity, estimated as the amount of porphyrins made in cellular extracts incubated in the presence of ALA or PBG, was generally a little higher in derepressed cells than in repressed or anaerobic cells (Labbe, 1971; Labbe-Bois and Volland, 1977a). The activity disappeared rapidly upon incubation of glucose-grown cells with glucose but without nitrogen source; it was stable in galactose-grown cells (Labbe et al., 1972). The absence of PBG deaminase activity has been reported in some, but not all, mutants deficient in ALA and PBG synthases (Gollub et al., 1977; Labbe-Bois et al., 1980; Urban-Grimal and Labbe-Bois, 1981). The recovery of the activity in a *hem*1 mutant upon supplementation by ALA required protein synthesis (Labbe-Bois et al., 1980). Although these results might suggest an induction of PBG deaminase by its substrate PBG, they can as well be explained by an increased instability of the enzyme in the absence of its substrate, leading to an accelerated turnover, as shown to be the case in mammalian cells (Beaumont et al., 1986).

A plasmid has been isolated which carries a yeast DNA fragment capable of complementing the respiratory deficiency and auxotrophies of a *hem*3 mutant lacking PBG deaminase activity (Gellerfors et al., 1986). The activity was 10-fold increased in the transformed cells as compared to the wild-type strains, and the in vitro translation of mRNA selected by hybridization with the plasmid gave a protein with a molecular weight of 43,000, close to the molecular weight of the mammalian enzyme. Therefore, it is highly likely, although not positively demonstrated, that the *HEM*3 gene encoding yeast PBG deaminase was isolated.

PBG deaminase is now known to catalyze the formation of preurogen, a linear hydroxymethylbilane, which either cyclizes very rapidly and nonenzymically to yield urogen I, or is converted into urogen III in the presence of urogen III synthase. The only report of the presence of urogen III synthase in yeast came from Jordan and Berry (1980) who measured in cell-free extract a specific activity of 2.3 nmol of urogen III formed (per hour per milligram of protein, 37°C) with preurogen as the substrate. This activity appears, thus, to be in excess over PBG deaminase which catalyzes at most the formation of 0.2 nmol of total porphyrins (per hour per milligram of protein, 30°C) from PBG. Although this latter activity is rather low, there is no indication to date that it might play a role in limiting the formation of porphyrins (see Figs. 6.2 and 6.3).

D. Uroporphyrinogen decarboxylase

Genetic and biochemical data obtained with yeast mutants indicate that a single enzyme specified by the locus *HEM*12 catalyzes the four decarboxylation steps leading from urogen III to coprogen III, as has been shown with the enzyme purified from mammalian sources.

Uro(gen) and its intermediary decarboxylation products, the hepta-, hexa-, and pentacarboxyporphyrin(ogen)s, do not accumulate significantly in wild-type cells whatever their physiological status (Fig. 6.3). But their presence was reported in cell free extracts incubated with ALA or PBG (Labbe, 1971; Brouillet et al., 1975), and in whole cells of mutant strains (Pretlow and Sherman, 1967; Urban-Grimal and Labbe-Bois, 1981; Arrese et al., 1982; Rytka et al., 1984; Kurlandzka and Rytka, 1985; Labbe-Bois et al., 1986; Kurlandzka et al., 1988). Genetic analysis of these mutants revealed that most of them were allelic at the locus *HEM*12, within which the mutation sites have been mapped (Kurlandzka et al., 1988), while a few others carried different mutations although they had the same phenotype as the *hem*12 mutants.

The *hem*12 mutants are characterized by the presence of two strong bands near 540 and 575 nm in the whole-cell absorption spectra, indicative of an accumulation of Zn-porphyrins. That Zn-porphyrins rather than porphyrinogens accumulated most probably results from the nonenzymic oxidation of porphyrinogens and the nonenzymic insertion of Zn into the porphyrins. When the mutants are grown under anaerobic conditions, the Zn-porphyrins are no more detectable although the amount and the nature of the porphyrin(ogen)s extracted from the cells are identical to those made in aerobiosis (Labbe-Bois, unpublished observations). Only uroporphyrin III was present in mutants totally heme-deficient, in agreement with the lack of detectable urogen decarboxylase activity in the cellular extracts (Urban-Grimal and Labbe-Bois, 1981; Kurlandzka et al., 1988).

Regarding the partially affected *hem*12 mutants which could grow on ethanol (Rytka et al., 1984; Labbe-Bois et al., 1986; Kurlandzka et al., 1988), they accumulated mainly uroporphyrin, hepta-, and hexacarboxyporphyrins mostly of the isomer-III type, whereas they excreted mainly pentacarboxyporphyrin or dehydroisocoproporphyrin. The presence of dehydroisocoproporphyrin has been suggested to arise, in mammalian cells, from the oxidative decarboxylation of the 2-propionate side chain of pentacarboxyporphyrinogen III catalyzed by coprogen oxidase. This is also the case in yeast, since double mutants carrying the partial defect in urogen decarboxylase plus a total block in coprogen oxidase were no longer able to synthesize dehydroisocoproporphyrin (Kurlandzka, Zoladek, Chelstowska, Rytka, and Labbe-Bois, 1988). Heme synthesis was very low in the mutant cells when grown on glucose, and they also accumulated less porphyrins than did cells grown on ethanol. Also, the less heme made by the different mutants growing on ethanol, the more porphyrins were accumulated. But for each mutant, the sum of heme(s) plus porphyrins was roughly the same in both the parent and the mutant cells grown on either glucose or ethanol, which indicates a similar production of tetrapyrroles by both the parent and mutant strains. This suggests that the diminished production of heme in the parent strains and of porphyrins in the mutants when the cells are grown on glucose is caused by some glucose-dependent regulatory event(s) occurring in the early steps of the pathway. The decrease of heme synthesis in the different mutants correlated fairly well with the decrease of urogen decarboxylase activity measured in cell-free extracts, ranging from 50 to 90%. Moreover, the relative rates of the four decarboxylation steps were shown to be modified differently with the various mutant enzymes, although the pattern of porphyrins accumulated in vivo did not differ significantly among the different mutants. A more-detailed kinetic study of the decarboxylations catalyzed by these mutationally defective enzymes should allow a better understanding of the functioning of urogen decarboxylase and, in particular, deciding whether the decarboxylations take place at one or more catalytic sites. That could also be learnt from the analysis of the (in)ability of the inactive enzyme present in some totally blocked *hem*12 mutants [detected by immune replica with an antiserum raised against purified yeast urogen decarboxylase (Felix and Brouillet, unpublished observations)] to decarboxylate all possible intermediates between urogen I or III and coprogen I or III.

A number of mutations have been described, which lead to the accumulation of uroporphyrin and its partial decarboxylation products, although they are not at the *HEM*12 locus. This is the case of the recessive nuclear *pop*4 mutation which is also characterized by the absence of cytochrome oxidase although the other respiratory chain cytochromes were made (Arrese et al., 1982). This double phenotype led the investigators to suggest that the mutation interfered specifically with heme a synthesis, possibly at the level of "a urogen decarboxylase isoenzyme specifically involved in heme a production." However, this was not substantiated by further biochemical analysis and the nature of the *pop*4 mutation remains obscure. Kurlandzka and Rytka (1985) reported the isolation of three mutants which complemented each other and also complemented all *hem* mutants tested. Genetic analysis revealed a complex pattern of porphyrin-accumulation segregation, indicating that more than two genes controlled the mutant phenotype (Rytka, unpublished data). Similar observations were made by Pretlow and Sherman (1967) who found that the porphyrin accumulation due to the *pop*1 mutation (whose allelism to *hem*12 is unknown) was "partially suppressed by at least one dominant gene and perhaps by one or more additionally genes." Finally, a mutation, *ipa*1, was uncovered which specifically increased porphyrin accumulation in one of the partial *hem*12 mutants (Kurlandzka et al., 1988). All these results indicate that factors other than, or adding further to, a reduction in urogen decarboxylase activity can lead to "uroporphyric" yeast cells. This is reminiscent of the situation encountered in human porphyria cutanea tarda where different etiologic agents have been implicated in the expression of an acquired or inherited deficiency in urogen decarboxylase (this volume). Also noteworthy is the finding that chick embryo fibroblasts accumulate uroporphyrin in place of protoporphyrin after long-term treatment with compounds which impair mitochondrial functions (De Muys and Morais, 1984).

Yeast urogen decarboxylase was recently purified in our laboratory about 8- to 10,000-fold with a 55% yield (Felix and Brouillet, unpublished observations). The enzyme, a protein with a molecular mass of 38,000 daltons and a pI at 6.2, had a specific activity of 2000 nmol copro(gen) I per hour per milligram of protein from urogen I at 37°C. The activity was sensitive to SH reagents but no cofactor (pyridoxal-P, thiamine) was found. The affinity for both urogen I and III was very high ($K_m \simeq 0.01 \ \mu M$).

There is no indication at present that urogen decarboxylase might be a rate-limiting step in the pathway. Its activity, although low, appears to cope with the flow of metabolites, probably within a multienzyme complex comprising the cytosolic enzymes of the pathway. One can even imagine that this complex would be located close to the mitochondria to ensure a minimum of loss in the supply of protogen to the membrane-bound late enzymes. But direct experimental evidence for such a complex is still lacking. Its presence is only suggested from indirect observations. For instance, it is difficult to understand otherwise the dysfunction of PBG deaminase after breakage of the cells of mutants having defective urogen decarboxylase or coprogen oxidase enzymes (Urban-Grimal and Labbe-Bois, 1981; Bilinski et al., 1981; Rytka et al., 1984).

E. Coproporphyrinogen III oxidase

The first report of the presence of coprogen oxidase in yeast was from Miyake and Sugimura (1968) in their attempt to understand the phenotypic expression of a nuclear mutation, *cyt*, they had previously isolated: This thermosensitive mutant was wild-type when grown at 20°C, but at 35°C it was respiratory deficient, lacked all cytochromes, and accumulated large amounts of coproporphyrin. They found, unexpectedly, that coprogen oxidase was 10 times higher in the mutant grown at 35°C than in wild-type strains or in the mutant grown at 20°C. Moreover, the enzymes from the mutant and the wild-type strains were indistinguishable for all of their properties tested: K_m for coprogen, optimal pH, heat stability, sensitivity to thiol reagents, localization mainly in the soluble fraction. Since the activity was also 10-fold increased in wild-type cells grown under anaerobiosis, the authors concluded that the "phenotype of the *cyt* mutant cannot be an enzymatic lesion at the site of coproporphyrinogenase" and they further suggested that heme might repress the synthesis of the enzyme. The nature of the *cyt* mutation is still obscure today, and it is not even known if it is an allele of the *HEM*13 gene, the structural gene of coprogen oxidase.

Then, Poulson and Polglase (1974a) reported that the specific activity of coprogen oxidase was slightly higher in mitochondria than in the cytoplasmic fraction and concluded that the enzyme was located in the mitochondria from which they purified it 150-fold. The molecular mass of the active enzyme was estimated at 75,000 daltons by gel filtration. Almost the same level of activity was found in extracts from aerobically and anaerobically grown cells. Furthermore, coprogen oxidase in these two extracts and in the purified preparation was found to function equally well with, as electron acceptor, either oxygen ("aerobic" activity) or, under anaerobiosis, $NADP^+$ provided that ATP, methionine, and a divalent metal anion were present ("anaerobic" activity). Such an "anaerobic" coprogen oxidase activity had been previously described by

Tait (1969) in semi-anaerobically grown *Rhodobacter spheroides*, but it could not be measured in aerobically grown cells. A physiological argument for methionine playing a role in (an)aerobic coprogen oxidase activity was provided by Demain and White (1971) who showed that ethionine supplementation during aerobic growth of *Paracoccus denitrificans* inhibited vitamin B12 overproduction and led to excretion of large amounts of coproporphyrin III, which suggested "interference by ethionine with the activity of methionine in coproporphyrinogenase action"; unfortunately, no attempt to measure that activity in cellular extracts was made. But Mori and Sano (1972) could not measure the "anaerobic" activity in cellular extracts of anaerobically grown *Chromatium* whatever the electron acceptor used, although an "aerobic" activity was present; similar results were reported by Jacobs et al. (1970) for cellular extracts of anaerobically grown *P. denitrificans*.

The uncertainties concerning both the participation of oxygen in the enzymic reaction and the intracellular localization of the enzyme led Camadro et al. (1986) to reexamine yeast coprogen oxidase. The enzyme, definitively proved to be located in the cytosol, was purified to homogeneity and shown to be a homodimer with a subunit molecular weight of 35,000. This last result was ascertained by the unique N-terminal amino acid sequence and was consistent with the finding of interallelic complementation between some *hem*13 mutants. Two iron atoms per molecule of native protein were detected but their involvement in the catalytic activity could not be demonstrated. The K_m value for coprogen was found to be very low (0.05 μM), compared to the much higher values reported previously by Miyake and Sugimura (1968) and by Poulson and Polglase (1974a) (15 and 30 μM, respectively). This is most probably due to the much more sensitive test used in the latter studies. Since thiol-directed reagents partially inhibited the enzyme, SH group(s) are probably required for the activity. The yeast enzyme was activated two- to threefold by phospholipids or neutral detergents, as described for the bovine liver enzyme (Yoshinaga and Sano, 1980). Despite considerable technical efforts, the "anaerobic" activity previously reported by Poulson and Polglase (1974a) could not be measured either with the pure enzyme or with cellular extracts of anaerobically or aerobically grown cells. The nonreproducible, erratic, protein-independent, and very low formation of protogen could be attributed to contamination by traces of atmospheric air when pipetting, which allowed coprogen oxidase to use oxygen with a very high affinity. Although the K_m for oxygen could not be measured owing to technical difficulties, it was estimated to be very low (≤ 0.1 μM). Thus, these results do not favor the hypothesis that $NADP^+$ (+methionine + ATP) is the electron acceptor for coprogen oxidase when molecular oxygen is not available. The experimental conditions of the assay used at that time by Poulson and Polglase (1974a) were not rigorous enough to avoid any traces of oxygen, a problem far from being trivial when working with oxidases having such an high affinity for oxygen.

The cytosolic localization of coprogen oxidase in yeast, in contrast to its location in the mitochondrial intermembrane space in liver cells (Grandchamp and Nordmann, 1978; Elder and Evans, 1978), raises the problem of the supply of protogen to the next two enzymes of the pathway which are firmly associated with the inner mitochondrial membrane (Jomary and Labbe, unpublished results). The lipophilic, highly autooxidizable protogen must then cross an extra membrane (the outer membrane of mitochondria) to reach its site of enzymic oxidation. Since there is no experimental evidence to support the possible accumulation of protogen in vivo and in vitro, it is probable that the obligatory crossing of the outer membrane by protogen is realized by some transitory interaction of coprogen oxidase with the mitochondrial surface, possibly at contact sites between the two membranes. Such an interaction has been described in other enzymic systems (Ostlund et al., 1983). The activation of pure yeast coprogen oxidase by phospholipids and neutral detergents supports this thesis. The advantage for the cells to have coprogen oxidase in the cytosol is not evident. Is it pertinent to the fact that *S. cerevisiae* is a facultative anaerobe? Is it a vestige of the old times when the organisms were slowly adapting to oxygen?

The *HEM*13 gene was isolated recently and its nucleotide sequence determined (Zagorec et al., 1988). It encodes a protein of 328 amino acids. Its calculated molecular mass (37,673 daltons), amino acid composition, and *N*-terminal sequence predicted from the DNA sequence were in agreement with those determined for the purified enzyme. But the amino acid sequence itself was not very informative in the absence of any other sequence information. The 5' ends of the *HEM*13 transcripts were identified; the same initiation sites of transcription were used upon induction.

As suggested 20 years ago by Miyake and Sugimura (1968), recent studies confirmed that the synthesis of coprogen oxidase is regulated negatively by heme and oxygen. The activity was increased in all mutants deficient in heme synthesis, whatever the enzymic block (Labbe-Bois et al., 1980; Urban-Grimal and Labbe-Bois, 1981; Rytka et al., 1984), and this effect could be partially reversed by the addition of heme to the growth medium (Zagorec and Labbe-Bois, 1986). The same high level of activity was reached in all mutants, but the increase relative to their parental strains varies between 5- and 50-fold. Similar increases were found in wild-type cells grown anaerobically, but they could not be reversed by exogenous heme. No further increase in activity occurred when the mutants were grown anaerobically indicating that the effects of heme and oxygen deficiency are not additive. These activity changes were paralleled by similar changes in (1) the steady-state amounts of protein detected by an antiserum raised against yeast coprogen oxidase and (2) the steady-state concentrations of coprogen oxidase mRNA estimated by in vitro translation/immunoprecipitation or by hybridization with the HEM13 gene (Northern blots) (Zagorec and Labbe-Bois, 1986; Zagorec et al., 1988). This demonstrated that the negative regulation by heme and oxygen operates at the level of transcription. Moreover, analysis of the effects of deletions in the promoter region of HEM13 on coprogen oxidase expression in cells grown aerobically and anaerobically revealed that DNA sequence located upstream 409 nucleotides from the initiating ATG was needed for induction under anaerobiosis.

What is the physiological significance of this negative regulation of coprogen oxidase expression by heme and oxygen? The loss of induction of coprogen oxidase activity under oxygen deficiency, as a result of deletions in the HEM13 promoter, was shown to cause a considerable decrease in the heme content of anaerobic cells, which became barely detectable (Zagorec et al., 1988). This means that in cells growing anaerobically coprogen oxidase was a rate-limiting step for heme synthesis, probably as a consequence of the very low amount of oxygen present in these cells since oxygen is required for the enzyme activity. The cells respond to oxygen limitation by increasing the amount of enzyme. But the meaning of the regulation by heme in aerobiosis is less clear, since there is no evidence for a rate-limiting function of coprogen oxidase for heme production in aerobic cells. The activation of HEM13 expression by heme or oxygen deficiency was found to require the product of the CYP1 gene, a regulatory protein mediating the activation by heme or oxygen of the synthesis of many apocytochromes and proteins (See Sec. II-C) (Zagorec, 1986; Verdière and Labbe-Bois, unpublished results). One could then imagine the CYP1 protein as a "sensor" of the heme status of the cells, acting as a link coordinating heme and protein synthesis in an opposite fashion: It would activate heme synthesis via coprogen oxidase in the case of heme limitation, while triggering apoprotein synthesis only in the case of heme sufficiency. Or, the CYP1 protein could "sense" a certain redox state of the cells which would be similar under both heme or oxygen deprivation. Obviously, more experimental support is needed before understanding the mechanism of these regulations at the molecular level.

F. Protoporphyrinogen IX oxidase

The first experimental data giving some support for an enzymatic oxidation of protogen was provided by Sano and Granick (1961) during their pioneering work on mammalian coprogen oxidase when they discovered that the rate of protogen oxidation in vitro at neutral pH was increased by addition of freeze-thawed liver cells mitochondria. That oxidative activity was later found in ox liver mitochondrial extracts by Porra and Falk (1961) who gave to that enzymatic activity its current name and showed that oxygen was the unique hydrogen acceptor during conversion of coprogen to protoporphyrin (Porra and Falk, 1964). However, 10 years elapsed before the definitive identification of that enzyme by Poulson and Polglase in yeast (1975) and mammalian mitochondria (Poulson, 1976a). The yeast enzyme, tightly bound to mitochondrial membranes, was solubilized by a neutral detergent (Tween 80). The molecular mass of the 70-fold purified enzyme, estimated by gel filtration, was $180,000 \pm 18,000$ daltons. The enzymatic activity was destroyed by heating above 40°C, proteolytic digestion or irreversible denaturation outside the pH range 4.0 to 9.5; pH optimum was 7.5 and K_m for protogen was 4.8 μM. Yeast protogen oxidase did not catalyze oxidation of coprogen I and III and urogen I and III. The presence of thiol groups in the enzyme system was suggested, but no metal ion or other cofactor requirement was demonstrated. Enzyme activity was partially inhibited by Cu^{2+}, Co^{2+}, and heme (within the range 20 to 100 μM).

Recently, purification of yeast protogen oxidase was achieved in our laboratory and some properties of the enzyme were determined (Camadro, Chambon, Jomary, and Labbe, manuscript in preparation). Protogen oxidase was purified 800-fold with a 15% yield from baker's yeast mitochondrial membranes according to a procedure adapted from that used for purification of yeast ferrochelatase (Camadro and Labbe, 1988). The presence of dithiothreitol during the whole purification procedure was essential for recovering active enzyme. The pure enzyme was found to be a 56,000-dalton polypeptide with a specific activity of 12,000 nmol of protoporphyrin formed per hour per milligram of protein at 30°C; the pI of the enzyme was 8.5 and its optimum pH was 7.2. The same molecular mass was found for the enzyme detected in total protein extracts by an immune-replica method using antibodies raised against the purified protein, or after immunoprecipitation of the enzyme radiolabeled *in vivo*. This demonstrated that the purified enzyme was not a degraded form of the native protein. However, when total RNAs were translated in vitro the immunoprecipitated newly synthesized protogen oxidase exhibited a higher molecular mass (59,000 daltons), suggesting that it is synthesized as a precursor with an extension which is cleaved during its import into the mitochondria.

The Michaelis constant of the purified enzyme for protogen was rather low ($K_m = 0.5 \mu M$), a further argument for a channeling of protogen from coprogen oxidase to protogen oxidase through the mitochondrial outer membrane and intermembrane space. Although the topology of the yeast enzyme in the inner membrane was not investigated, as done in detail for the liver enzyme (Deybach et al., 1985), it is likely to be an intrinsic component of the membrane. Molecular oxygen was required as the electron acceptor for the functioning of both the membrane-bound and the purified protogen oxidase. Neither fumarate nor nitrate, which were shown to play that role for the *E. coli* enzyme (Jacobs and Jacobs, 1976), could replace oxygen. Unless alternate electron acceptors, which would work with low efficiency, are uncovered in the future for both coprogen and protogen oxidases, the formation of protoporphyrin and heme in anaerobic cells can reasonably be explained now by the presence of contaminating traces of oxygen ($\leq 0.1 \ \mu M$) in "anaerobic" cultures, which are practically inevitable under the conditions used routinely in laboratories. In our opinion, the apparently absolute requirement for oxygen of coprogen and protogen oxidase activities determined in vitro over short periods of time (30 min) cannot be used as an argument, often read in the literature, for the absence of heme in cells growing anaerobically (or microaerobically?) for hours.

A *hem*14 mutant has been isolated which lacks cytochromes, accumulates protoporphyrin, is devoid of protogen oxidase activity (Urban-Grimal and Labbe-Bois, 1981; Camadro et al., 1982), and makes normal amounts of immunodetectable protein and protogen oxidase mRNA estimated by in vitro translation/immunoprecipitation (Camadro, Chambon, Jomary, and Labbe, manuscript in preparation). But further analysis of this mutant revealed that it was also impaired in iron metabolism as compared to wild-type strains and other hemeless mutants. The *hem*14 mutant cells differed essentially at the level of mitochondria which contained about 35 times less "free" iron, which, in addition, was found mainly in the oxidized state ("free" iron is unassigned iron, i.e., iron not associated with heme or iron-sulfur clusters) (Jomary, Ohnishi, Labbe, and Labbe-Bois, unpublished experiments). Whether the primary mutational event is in protogen oxidase or in some step of iron metabolism is unknown at present. But the latter hypothesis seems more probable, since it is easier to imagine the loss of protogen oxidase activity as a consequence of iron-metabolism perturbation than the reverse, which then implies that iron is involved in the functioning of the enzyme.

Protogen oxidase has been proposed to be the site of repression by glucose of heme biosynthesis (Poulson and Polglase, 1974b; Poulson, 1976b). This was based on (1) the accumulation of pigment P503 thought at that time to be an intermediate between protogen and protoporphyrin (see Sec. II-A); (2) the absence of detectable protogen oxidase activity in glucose-repressed and anaerobic cells; (3) its increase during respiratory adaptation of protoplasts in presence of low glucose, the inhibitory effect of high glucose being prevented by exogenous cyclic AMP. However, this proposal is no longer tenable since the first assumption proved to be incorrect and the second argument was most probably due to the fact that the assay used to measure the activity was not as reliable as the one described later by Brenner and Bloomer (1980). By using a sensitive two-step enzymatic assay developed to overcome some technical problems of the previous ones, Camadro et al. (1982) showed that protogen oxidase was indeed present in glucose-repressed and anaerobic cells, but with a specific activity twice lower than in derepressed cells and in heme-deficient mutants. The causes of these activity changes are unknown and any speculation would be imprudent at the present time since they might also reflect changes in the synthesis of the enzyme as modulation of its activity via changes in its membranous environment brought about by the metabolic state of the cells. In any case, the physiological meaning of an eventual regulation of protogen oxidase synthesis is not obvious, since it is far from functioning at its maximal velocity in vivo (Fig. 6.2). Incidentally, that might be the reason why protogen oxidase is not induced under oxygen limitation, in contrast to coprogen oxidase.

G. Ferrochelatase

The history of yeast ferrochelatase looks like a long search, punctuated with technical improvements of the enzymic assays, for understanding the functioning of the enzyme in vivo and its possible participation in the regulation of heme synthesis. In particular, the capability of the cells to synthesize Zn-protoporphyrin focused attention on the relationships between iron and zinc and the "metal-chelatase" activities of ferrochelatase. In this section we shall consider separately the properties of the membrane-bound enzyme and those of the purified protein. Current knowledge concerning iron metabolism in S. cerevisiae will be presented at the end.

1. Properties of membrane-found ferrochelatase. The presence of ferrochelatase activity in cellular extracts of anaerobically and aerobically grown yeast was first described by Chaix and Labbe (1965) who showed that the enzyme was membrane-bound, could be solubilized by a neutral detergent (Tween 80), and was able to incorporate either ferrous iron or zinc into protoporphyrin to form heme or Zn-protoporphyrin, respectively. This last property permitted one to attribute the absorption band detected near 583 nm in anaerobic cells to the presence of Zn-protoporphyrin. The intracellular concentration of Zn-protoporphyrin can be tremendously increased when (an)aerobically grown cells are incubated without glucose at pH 7 to 8 in aerated buffer. This Zn-protoporphyrin was found to accumulate in the mitochondrial membranes, leading to a total inhibition of the respiratory activity of isolated mitochondria and to photolethality of whole cells (Gilardi et al., 1971). Such a photolethality had been reported earlier by Elkind and Sutton (1957a, b) who presented the absorption spectrum of the sensitizer but did not identify it at that time.

Later, Labbe et al., (1968), using the popular but rather insensitive pyridine-hemochromogen assay (Porra and Jones, 1963a), described some properties of ferrochelatase bound to mitochondrial membranes. Zinc and ferrous iron were incorporated into protoporphyrin at nearly the same rate and both activities required mitochondrial lipids. Although it was clear that the formation of heme and Zn-protoporphyrin was enzymatic, it could not be decided at that time if iron- and zinc-chelatase activities were carried by the same protein. More recently, Camadro and Labbe (1982), reinvestigating that problem with a more-sensitive spectrophotometric assay (Jones and Jones, 1969), provided strong evidence that a single enzyme catalyzed both reactions. First, a heme-deficient mutant carrying a single nuclear mutation at the locus *HEM*15 lacked both iron- and zinc-chelatase activities in vitro and in vivo. Second, iron and zinc were found to act as competitive substrates of ferrochelatase. Ferrous iron was a much more potent inhibitor of zinc-chelatase activity than was zinc for iron-chelatase activity (Table 6.4). Ferric iron, not the substrate itself, was a poor inhibitor ($K_i \simeq 0.1$ mM) of both reactions. Moreover, yeast mitochondrial membranes were shown to contain measurable amounts of unassigned iron and zinc which acted as reciprocal competitors in ferrochelatase reactions. These pools of "free" iron and zinc in the membranes (0.5 to 2 nmol/mg protein) could be utilized for the chelatase reactions. Interestingly, 30 to 50% of the iron pool consisted of ferrous iron, as in mammalian mitochondria (Tangeras et al., 1980). Such amounts of "free" metals within the membranes are, in fact, far from being negligible when expressed in moles/volume of membranes (0.1 to 1 mM).

The kinetic parameters of membrane-bound ferrochelatase and the high content of endogenous metal ions suggest important regulatory mechanisms of heme synthesis implicating the amount and the redox state of iron or compartmentation of both iron and zinc within the membranes. For instance, the above-mentioned synthesis of Zn-protoporphyrin in aerated resting cells could be explained by a depletion of the ferrous iron pool at the site of ferrochelatase which would relieve zinc-chelatase inhibition, allowing Zn-protoporphyrin to be made. This depletion might be caused by an oxidation of ferrous iron or by the nonfunctioning of an "iron-reductase" activity due to the loss of its substrates upon starvation. Such an "iron-reductase" activity has been measured in yeast mitochondrial membranes and found to depend partially on the functioning of the NADH or succinate dehydrogenase of the respiratory chain: Its specific activity (0.5 to 1 nmol ferric iron

TABLE 6.4 Kinetic Parameters of *S. cerevisiae* Ferrochelatase

Material	Method	K_m (μM) for			References
		Protoporphyrin	Fe^{2+}	Zn^{2+}	
Mitochondrial membranes	Spectrophotometric measurement of pyridine hemochromogen or Zn-protoporphyrin formation	66	30	1000	Labbe et al., 1968
Mitochondrial membranes	Spectrophotometric determination of protoporphyrin disappearance or Zn-protoporphyrin formation	5.9 (Fe) 3.6 (Zn)	1.6 $K_i^{Zn^{2+}}$: 1.5	0.16 $K_i^{Fe^{2+}}$: 0.07	Camadro and Labbe, 1982
Mitochondrial membranes	Fluorometric determination of protoporphyrin disappearance (proto. endogenously generated)	0.07 (Fe) 0.25 (Zn)			Camadro and Labbe, unpublished
Purified enzyme	Fluorometric determination of protoporphyrin disappearance or Zn-protoporphyrin formation	0.09 (Fe, Zn)	9 0.25 (— DTT *)		Camadro and Labbe, 1988

*DTT, dithiothreitol.

reduced/per hour per milligram of protein) was much weaker than ferrochelatase activity ($\sim$ 20 nmol heme/per hour per milligram of protein) but of the same order of magnitude as the rate of production of heme estimated in vivo ($\sim$ 0.2 nmol heme/per hour per milligram of protein) (Fig. 6.2). But similar reasoning cannot explain why protoporphyrin and Zn-protoporphyrin accumulate in anaerobically growing cells, while only a limited amount of heme is made. Probably, other factors, besides the supply of its substrates, can interfere with the functioning of ferrochelatase, such as the release of heme and its subsequent transport which might depend on the availability of the different apoproteins. This problem is even more complex if ferrochelatase and "iron-reductase" are located on the matrix side of the inner membrane, as proposed for the liver enzymes (Jones and Jones, 1969; McKay et al., 1969; Barnes et al., 1972).

The affinity of membrane-bound ferrochelatase for protoporphyrin was rather low when measured in these assays, with exogenous protoporphyrin added as a "solution" in a neutral detergent (Table 6.4). This probably reflects the difficulty to determine the concentration in the membrane of monomeric protoporphyrin, thought to be the true substrate of the enzyme. In fact, the balance of protoporphyrin monomers between detergent micelles, membrane, and possibly hydrosoluble dimers depends on the concentration of protoporphyrin and other factors (Rotenberg and Margalit, 1987 and references therein). By using a two-step fluorometric assay (Labbe et al., 1985), very low amounts of protoporphyrin can be enzymatically generated inside the membrane through the consecutive action of the soluble coprogen oxidase and the membrane-bound protogen oxidase. In situ generated protoporphyrin is very probably located in the lipid bilayer of the membrane since its absorption spectrum is characteristic of monomeric protoporphyrin in apolar solvents (hexane, diethyl ether). This technique allowed Camadro and Labbe (unpublished experiments) to measure an extremely low K_m for protoporphyrin for either iron- or zinc-chelatase activities (Table 6.4). These values obtained under physiological conditions are highly likely to be representative of the situation prevailing in vivo and, in fact, they are almost identical to the values measured with the pure enzyme.

The level of ferrochelatase activity is usually two- to fourfold higher in mitochondrial membranes from derepressed cells than from glucose-repressed or anaerobic cells (Labbe, 1971; Labbe et al., 1972; Poulson, 1976b). This led Poulson (1976b) to propose that ferrochelatase is subject to glucose repression. However, these activity changes are less likely to be due to changes in the amount of enzyme made than to changes in the lipid environment of the enzyme in the membrane. This interpretation is supported by the following observations. First, ferrochelatase activity, together with protogen oxidase, is in large excess compared to the activities of the other enzymes of the pathway (Fig. 6.2). Second, the activity of ferrochelatase is highly dependent on the presence of lipids. Third, ferrochelatase activity of membranes from repressed cells is increased upon adding to the assay a crude extract of lipids from derepressed mitochondria.

2. Properties of isolated ferrochelatase. Almost a quarter of a century separated the only two reports on yeast ferrochelatase purification. Riethmuller and Tuppy (1964) first described a 75-fold purification of the enzyme after its extraction from mitochondrial membranes by Triton X100. Then, on the basis of the technique introduced by Taketani and Tokunaga (1981) for the rat liver enzyme, yeast ferrochelatase was purified to homogeneity (1800-fold) from mitochondrial membranes with an overall yield of 43% (Camadro and Labbe, 1988). The enzyme, a polypeptide of 40,000 daltons with a pI at 6.3, had a specific activity of 35,000 nmol heme/per hour per milligram of protein and 27,000 nmol Zn-protoporphyrin/per hour per milligram of protein. This proved definitively that the same protein catalyzes the incorporation of both iron and zinc into protoporphyrin at nearly the same rate. As described previously for the rat liver enzyme, purified yeast ferrochelatase had an absolute requirement for fatty acids to be active in vitro. The Michaelis constants could be measured for protoporphyrin, ferrous iron, and zinc, in the presence of dithiothreitol to keep iron reduced and after removal of contaminating zinc from all chemicals used (Table 6.4). The affinity of the enzyme for zinc was lower in the presence of dithiothreitol than in its absence. That might be relevant to ferrochelatase activity control, all the more so since sulfhydryl groups were shown to be involved in the activity.

The molecular mass of ferrochelatase (40,000 daltons) was identical for the pure enzyme and the enzyme detected in total protein extracts by immune-replica. But a precursor form of ferrochelatase with a higher molecular weight (44,000 daltons) was detected after in vitro translation of total RNAs. This precursor form, which is very rapidly matured to the 40,000 molecular weight form, was also observed in vivo in pulse-labeled cells. That ferrochelatase is synthesized with an extension which is cleaved off during its import into the mitochondria is consistent with the fact that the N-terminal amino acid sequence of the purified protein was found to be frayed. Interestingly, when ferrochelatase was first immunoprecipitated from cells metabolically labeled, many contaminating proteins were coprecipitated with it, suggesting that it precipitates as part of a complex representing the surroundings of the enzyme in situ. This is in agreement with the finding of Taketani et al. (1986) that bovine liver ferrochelatase is associated with complex I of the respiratory chain, which might be of physiological significance in the problem of iron reduction.

All these results concerning the catalytic properties of membrane-bound and purified ferrochelatase indicate that the last enzyme of the pathway is expected to play an important role in governing the production of heme.

3. Iron metabolism of *S. cerevisiae*.

As the supplier of the last substrate of the heme pathway, iron metabolism is directly linked to heme production by the calls. The major question, not yet resolved in detail whatever the system studied, is how does iron travel throughout the cell from the extracellular medium where it is found in the oxidized state to the site of ferrochelatase where it must be in the reduced state. The presence of a pool of "free" reduced iron in the mitochondrial membranes also raises a number of questions. How is that pool kept reduced? How is it replenished, for example, what is the chemical nature of the cytosolic donor? How can it coexist inside the inner membrane with the hydrophobic oxygen molecule needed for the oxidases and the hydrosoluble reduced iron: differential sequestration, chelation of ferrous iron?

Curiously, nothing was known before 1987 about the metabolization of iron by the yeast *S. cerevisiae*. The excretion of specific iron-chelator compounds (siderophores) in response to iron limitation, as it occurs in most microorganisms including fungi and some species of yeast, could not be detected in *S. cerevisiae*. However, by analogy with what had been described in bacteria and fungi [see Winkelman et al. (1987) for a review], one could surmise that there exist in *S. cerevisiae* chelator(s), membrane-bound receptor(s), membrane-bound or cytosolic reductase(s), and carrier and storage proteins to account for iron assimilation by this yeast.

The first well-documented report on iron metabolism in *S. cerevisiae* was provided by Lesuisse et al. (1987) who studied iron uptake by these cells. They showed that iron was taken up essentially in its soluble reduced form and that the cells were able to reduce various extracellular ferric chelates, including bacterial ferrisiderophores, by a cytoplasmic membrane-bound redox system which was increased more than 30-fold in cells grown in iron-deficient medium. It was thus proposed that iron must be reduced outside the cell by a ferri-reductase activity bound to the cytoplasmic membrane before entering the cells via a transporter which might be common to other divalent cations. Once in the cells, iron was located preferentially in the vacuoles and although a ferritin-like protein was isolated from iron-loaded cells, its iron content was very low and not representative of the cellular iron content: This suggested that the vacuoles, rather than ferritin, are involved in the storage of iron (Raguzzi et al., 1988).

More recent experiments with heme-deficient mutants shed new light on iron-uptake mechanisms (Lesuisse and Labbe, 1989). Hemeless cells were found to exhibit a very low, residual ferri-reductase activity, which moreover was no more inducible by iron limitation. However, iron uptake from the bacterial siderophore ferrioxamine, but not from iron-citrate, was not impaired, indicating that other mechanisms besides iron reduction could exist to take up iron. And, indeed, a receptor-mediated transport of ferrioxamine was found also in wild-type cells which was inducible under iron-deficiency conditions. Therefore, it appears that in *S. cerevisiae* two systems coexist for iron uptake, a reductive mechanism of low affinity and specificity, and a specific high-affinity transport system for ferrioxamine-like siderophores. Such an opportunist siderophore-mediated transport system in a cell which itself does not excrete any siderophore has been described in some plants [see Winkelman et al. (1987)].

The effects of iron-limited growth on the mitochondrial respiratory chain and the energy conservation mechanism have been reported in the case of the obligate aerobic yeast *Candida utilis* (Light, 1972; Clegg and Skyrme, 1973). But the metabolic alterations brought about by iron limitation or iron overload are largely unknown in *S. cerevisiae* (Lesuisse, 1987), especially at the level of the heme biosynthetic pathway.

V. Conclusions

From both biochemical and genetic data, a picture of the functioning and the regulation of the heme biosynthetic pathway in yeast is beginning to emerge. The five enzymes that have been purified have molecular and catalytic properties very similar to those described for the higher eukaryote enzymes. They are present in rather low amounts under normal conditions, each representing about 0.005 to 0.01% of total proteins, and appear to be in roughly equimolar ratio. Apparently, this low expression is not a necessity for the cells since they are capable of a very high level of expression when the *HEM* genes are borne on multicopy plasmids, at least for the four genes which have been isolated to date. The regulation of the expression of two genes, *HEM*1 and *HEM*13 coding for ALA synthase and coprogen oxidase, has been shown to be mediated by regulatory proteins controlling also the synthesis of some (apo)proteins: It is tempting to speculate that this provides for linkage of metabolic flow through the heme pathway to oxidative energy metabolism. The other enzymes have two- to fourfold increased specific activities when the cells are grown in a respiratory mode, but the causes of these changes are unclear. Although these "repression-derepression" responses to metabolic conditions are modest, as found also for many enzymes of other anabolic pathways (Strathern, 1982; Hinnebusch, 1986), it would be interesting to reinvestigate them now that new tools (antibodies, genes) are available. Further studies of the molecular mechanisms and physiological effectors governing the negative regulation by heme and oxygen of coprogen oxidase synthesis should help in understanding these important and general regulations, which also occur in other organisms.

Sequencing of the many missense mutated alleles of the *HEM* genes described in the literature should provide a basis for examining the effects of site-specific modifications on structure-functional relationships in the heme biosynthetic enzymes. Yeast could also be used as the host for high-level production and large-scale purification of heme biosynthetic enzymes, either homologous or heterologous, thus facilitating structural studies on these enzymes.

Other interesting problems related to the heme pathway could be approached in yeast as, for instance, the fate of newly synthesized heme and the control of its distribution into the different heme-proteins in response to changing requirements of the cell. The study of assimilation and metabolization of iron by *S. cerevisiae*, combining the biochemical and genetic approaches, could provide valuable information on iron metabolism in relationship to heme biosynthesis in an eukaryotic system which does not excrete siderophores and does not use extracellular iron-protein. Finally, it might be interesting to analyze the heme pathway enzymes and the heme-protein synthesis and degradation in relation to the cell cycle, especially in mutants affected in its control.

Nomenclature

ALA	5-aminolevulinic acid
PBG	porphobilinogen
Urogen	uroporphyrinogen
Coprogen	coproporphyrinogen III
Protogen	protoporphyrinogen IX
Heme	protoheme, or heme b: protoporphyrin IX–iron chelate, with iron in the ferrous state. If the iron is in the ferric state, it is called hemin. However, we have used the term "heme" loosely to refer to protoheme whatever the oxidation state of the iron, and also to refer to total hemes (heme a, b, c) in order to avoid repetitions
Rho	respiratory-deficient mutant due to very large deletions in the mitochondrial genome

ACKNOWLEDGMENTS

We thank our co-workers, past and present. We are grateful to Joanna Rytka, Jacqueline Verdière, and Bernard Guiard who have made available their results prior to publication.

The work reported from this laboratory was supported by grants from CNRS, Université Paris VII, Ministère de la Recherche, and Fondation pour la Recherche Médicale.

REFERENCES

Andreasen, A., and Stier, T. (1953). Anaerobic nutrition of *Saccharomyces cerevisiae*. I. Ergosterol requirement for growth in a defined medium, *J. Cell. Comp. Physiol.* **41**:23–36.

Andreasen, A., and Stier, T. (1954). Anaerobic nutrition of *Saccharomyces cerevisiae*. II. Unsaturated fatty acid requirement for growth in defined medium, *J. Cell. Comp. Physiol.* **43**:271–281.

Aoyama, Y., Yoshida, Y., Sonoda, Y., and Sato Y. (1987). Metabolism of 32-hydroxy-24,25,dihydrolanosterol by purified cytochrome $P450_{14DM}$ from yeast. Evidence for contribution of the cytochrome to whole process of lanosterol 14α-demethylation, *J. Biol. Chem.* **262**:1239–1243.

Arrese, M., Carvajal, E., Robison, S., Sambunaris, A., Panek, A., and Mattoon, J. (1983). Cloning of the δ-aminolevulinic acid synthase structural gene in yeast, *Curr. Genet.* **7**:175–183.

Arrese, M. R., Vojensky, D., and Mattoon, J. R. (1982). Characterization of a cytochrome oxidase-deficient yeast mutant which accumulates porphyrins, *Biochem. Biophys. Res. Comm.* **107**:848–855.

Bard, M., and Ingolia, T. D. (1984). Plasmid-mediated complementation of a Δ-aminolevulinic-acid-requiring *Saccharomyces cerevisiae* mutant, *Gene* **28**:195–199.

Bard, M., Woods, R. A., and Haslam, J. M. (1974). Porphyrin mutants of *Saccharomyces cerevisiae*: Correlated lesions in sterol and fatty acid biosynthesis, *Biochem. Biophys. Res. Comm.* **56**:324–330.

Barnes, R., Connelly, J. L., and Jones, O. T. G. (1972). The utilization of iron and its complexes by mammalian mitochondria, *Biochem. J.* **128**:1043–1055.

Barrett, J. (1969). The incorporation of [2-^{14}C]-glycine and 5-amino [4-^{14}C]-laevulinic acid into the prosthetic groups of cytochrome oxidase and other cytochromes in yeast adapting to oxygen, *Biochim. Biophys. Acta* **177**:443–455.

Beaumont, C., Grandchamp, B., Bogard, M., de Verneuil, H., and Nordmann, Y. (1986). Porphobilinogen deaminase is unstable in the absence of its substrate, *Biochim. Biophys. Acta* **882**:384–388.

Bilinski, T., Litwinksa, J., Lukaszkiewicz, J., Rytka, J., Simon, M., and Labbe-Bois, R. (1981). Characterization of two mutant strains of *Saccharomyces cerevisiae* deficient in coproporphyrinogen III oxidase activity, *J. Gen. Microbiol.* **122**:79–87.

Bilinski, T., Litwinska, J., Sledziewski, A., and Rytka, J. (1980). Hemoprotein formation in yeast. VII. Genetic analysis of pleiotropic mutants affected in the response to glucose repression and anoxia, *Acta Microbiol. Polon.* **29**:199–212.

Borralho, L. M., Panek, A. D., Malamud, D. R., Sanders, H. K., and Mattoon, J. R. (1983). In situ assay for 5-aminolevulinate dehydratase and application to the study of a catabolite repression-resistant *Saccharomyces cerevisiae* mutant, *J. Bacteriol.* **156**:141–147.

Brenner, D. A., and Bloomer, J. R. (1980). A fluorometric assay for measurement of protoporphyrinogen oxidase activity in mammalian tissue, *Clin. Chim. Acta* **100**:259–266.

Brouillet, N., Arselin-Dechateaubodeau, G., and Volland, C. (1975). Studies on protoporphyrin biosynthetic pathway in *Saccharomyces cerevisiae*: Characterization of the tetrapyrrole intermediates, *Biochimie* **57**:647–655.

Brumm, P. J., and Friedmann, H. C. (1981). Succinylacetone pyrrole, a powerful inhibitor of vitamin B12 biosynthesis: Effect of δ-aminolevulinic acid dehydratase, *Biochem. Biophys. Res. Comm.* **102**:854–859.

Camadro, J. M., Chambon, H., Jolles, J., and Labbe, P. (1986). Purification and properties of coproporphyrinogen oxidase from the yeast *Saccharomyces cerevisiae*, *Eur. J. Biochem.* **156**:579–587.

Camadro, J. M., and Labbe, P. (1982). Kinetic studies of ferrochelatase in yeast. Zinc and iron as competing substrates, *Biochim. Biophys. Acta* **707**:280–288.

Camadro, J. M., and Labbe, P. (1988). Purification and properties of ferrochelatase from the yeast *Saccharomyces cerevisiae*. Evidence for a precursor form of the protein. *J. Biol. Chem.* **263**:11675–11682.

Camadro, J. M., Urban-Grimal, D., and Labbe, P. (1982). A new assay for protoporphyrinogen oxidase. Evidence for a total deficiency in that activity in a heme-less mutant of *Saccharomyces cerevisiae, Biochem. Biophys. Res. Comm.* **106**:724–730.

Chaix, P., and Labbe, P. (1965). A propos de l'interprétation du spectre d'absorption de cellules de levures récoltées à la fin ou après la phase exponentielle de leur croissance anaérobie, *Colloque International sur les Mécanismes de Régulation des Activités Cellulaires chez les Microorganismes, Marseille 1963* (C.N.R.S., Ed.), Paris, pp. 481–489.

Chandrika, S. R., and Padmanaban, G. (1980). Purification, properties and synthesis of δ-aminolaevulinate dehydratase from *Neurospora crassa, Biochem. J.* **191**:29–36.

Charalampous, F. C. (1974). Coproporphyrin III, inhibitor of the synthesis of cytochrome oxidase in anaerobic yeast protoplasts, *J. Biol. Chem.* **249**:1014–1021.

Charalampous, F. C., and Chen, W. L. (1974). Anaerobic synthesis of apocytochrome oxidase and assembly of the holoenzyme in yeast protoplasts, *J. Biol. Chem.* **249**:1007–1013.

Clegg, R. A., and Skyrme, J. E. (1973). The effects of iron-limited growth on the reduced nicotinamide-adenine dinucleotide dehydrogenase activity and the membrane proteins of *Candida utilis* mitochondria, *Biochem. J.*, **136**:1029–1037.

Clejan, L., Beattie, D. S., Gollub, E. G., Liu, K. P., and Sprinson, D. B. (1980). Synthesis of the apoprotein of cytochrome b in heme-deficient yeast cells, *J. Biol. Chem.* **255**:1312–1316.

Cohen, G., Fessl, F., Traczyk, A., Rytka, J., and Ruis, H. (1985). Isolation of the catalase A gene of *Saccharomyces cerevisiae* by complementation of the *cta*1 mutation, *Mol. Gen. Genet.* **200**:74–79.

Criddle, R. S., and Schatz, G. (1969). Promitochondria of anaerobically grown yeast. I. Isolation and biochemical properties, *Biochemistry* **8**:322–334.

Daum, G., Bohni, P. C., and Schatz, G. (1982). Import of proteins into mitochondria. Cytochrome b2 and cytochrome c peroxidase are located in the intermembrane space of yeast mitochondria, *J. Biol. Chem.* **257**:13028–13033.

De Barreiro, O. L. C. (1967). 5-Aminolaevulinate hydro-lyase from yeast. Isolation and purification, *Biochim. Biophys. Acta* **139**:479–486.

De Barreiro, O. L. C. (1969). Effect of sulfhydryl groups on 5-aminolaevulinate dehydratase activity, *Biochim. Biophys. Acta* **178**:412–415.

Dehoux, P. (1978). Ph.D. Thesis, University of Paris VII, Paris.

Demain, A. L., and White, R. F. (1971). Porphyrin overproduction by *Pseudomonas denitrificans*: Essentiality of betaine and stimulation by ethionine, *J. Bacteriol.* **107**:456–460.

De Muys, J. M., and Morais, R. (1984). Uroporphyria development in cultured chick embryo fibroblasts long-term treated with chloramphenicol and ethidium bromide, *FEBS Lett.* **173**:142–146.

Deybach, J. C., Da Silva, V., Grandchamp, B., and Nordmann, Y. (1985). The mitochondrial location of protoporphyrinogen oxidase, *Eur. J. Biochem.* **149**:431–435.

Djavadi-Ohaniance, L., Rudin, Y., and Schatz, G. (1978). Identification of enzymically inactive apocytochrome c peroxidase in anaerobically grown *Saccharomyces cerevisiae*, *J. Biol. Chem.* **253**:4402–4407.

Dumont, M. E., Ernst, J. F., Hampsey, D. M., and Sherman, F. (1987). Identification and sequence of the gene encoding cytochrome c heme lyase in the yeast *Saccharomyces cerevisiae, EMBO J.* **6**:235–241.

Elder, G. H., and Evans, J. O. (1978). Evidence that the coproporphyrinogen oxidase activity of rat liver is situated in the intermembrane space of mitochondria, *Biochem. J.* **172**:345–347.

Elkind, M. M., and Sutton, H. (1957a). Lethal effect of visible light on a mutant strain of haploid yeast. I. General dependencies, *Arch. Biochem. Biophys.* **72**:84–95.

Elkind, M. M., and Sutton, H. (1957b). Lethal effect of visible light on a mutant strain of haploid yeast. II. Absorption and action spectra, *Arch. Biochem. Biophys.* **72**:96–111.

Entian, K. D. (1986). Glucose repression: A complex regulatory system in yeast, *Microbiol. Sci.* **3**:366–371.

Ephrussi, B., and Slonimski, P. P. (1950). La synthèse adaptative des cytochromes chez la levure de boulangerie, *Biochim. Biophys. Acta* **6**:256–267.

Ephrussi, B., Slonimski, P. P., Yotsuyanagi, Y., and Tavlitzki, J. (1956). Variations physiologiques et cytologiques de la levure au cours du cycle de la croissance aérobie, *C. R. Lab. Carlsberg Ser. Physiol.* **26**:87–102.

Florkin, M., and Stotz, E. H. (1975). *Comprehensive Biochemistry*, Elsevier, Amsterdam, Vol. 31.

Florkin, M., and Stotz, E. H. (1979). *Comprehensive Biochemistry*, Elsevier, Amsterdam, Vol. 33A, pp. 193–238.

Gellerfors, P. L., and Saltzgaber-Muller, J., and Douglas, M. G. (1986). Selection by genetic complementation and characterization of the gene coding for the yeast porphobilinogen deaminase, *Biochem. J.* **240**:673–677.

Gilardi, A., Djavadi-Ohaniance, L., Labbe, P., and Chaix, P. (1971). Effet de l'accumulation de Zn-protoporphyrine par la cellule de levure sur la synthèse et le fonctionnement de son système respiratoire, *Biochim. Biophys. Acta* **234**:446–457.

Gollub, E. G., and Dayan, J. (1985). Regulation by heme of the synthesis of cytochrome c oxidase subunits V and VII in yeast, *Biochem. Biophys. Res. Comm.* **128**:1447–1454.

Gollub, E. G., Liu, K. P., Dayan, J., Adlersberg, M., and Sprinson, D. B. (1977). Yeast mutants deficient in heme biosynthesis and a heme mutant additionally blocked in cyclisation of 2,3-oxidosqualene, *J. Biol. Chem.* **252**:2846–2854.

Gopalan, G., and Rajamanickam, C. (1986). Role of exogenous hemin in the synthesis of hemoproteins and non heme proteins during glucose repression in *Saccharomyces cerevisiae*, *Arch. Biochem. Biophys.* **248**:210–214.

Grandchamp, B., and Nordmann, Y. (1978). The mitochondrial localization of coproporphyrinogen III oxidase, *Biochem. J.* **176**:97–102.

Grimal, D., and Labbe-Bois, R. (1980). An enrichment method for heme-less mutants of *Saccharomyces cerevisiae* based on photodynamic properties of Zn-protoporphyrin, *Mol. Gen. Genet.* **178**:713–716.

Guarente, L. (1987). Regulatory proteins in yeast, *Ann. Rev. Genet.* **21**:425–452.

Guarente, L., Lalonde, B., Gifford, P., and Alani, E. (1984). Distinctly regulated tandem upstream activation sites mediate catabolite repression of the *CYC1* gene of *S. cerevisiae*, *Cell* **36**:503–511.

Guiard, B. (1985). Structure, expression and regulation of a nuclear gene encoding a mitochondrial protein: The yeast $L(+)$-lactate cytochrome c oxidoreductase (cytochrome b_2), *EMBO J.* **4**:3265–3272.

Hamilton, B., Hofbauer, R., and Ruis, H. (1982). Translational control of catalase synthesis by hemin in the yeast *Saccharomyces cerevisiae*, *Proc. Nat. Acad. Sci. (U.S.A)* **79**:7609–7613.

Heyman-Blanchet, T., and Chaix, P. (1959). Variations du spectre cytochromique de la levure cultivée en anaérobiose en fonction de ses phases de croissance, *Biochim. Biophys. Acta* **35**:85–93.

Hinnebusch, A. G. (1986). The general control of amino acid biosynthetic genes in the yeast *Saccharomyces cerevisiae*, *CRC Critical Rev. Biochem.* **21**:277–317.

Hortner, H., Ammerer, G., Hartter, E., Hamilton, B., Rytka, J., Bilinski, T., and Ruis, H. (1982). Regulation of synthesis of catalase and iso-1 cytochrome c in *Saccharomyces cerevisiae* by glucose, oxygen and heme, *Eur. J. Biochem.* **128**:179–184.

Ishidate, K., Kawaguchi, K., Tagawa, K., and Hagihara, B. (1969). Hemoproteins in anaerobically grown yeast cells, *J. Biochem.* **65**:375–383.

Jacobs, N. J., and Jacobs, J. M. (1976). Nitrate, fumarate and oxygen as electron acceptors for a late step in microbiol heme synthesis, *Biochim. Biophys. Acta* **449**:1–9.

Jacobs, N. J., Jacobs, J. M., and Brent, P. (1970). Formation of protoporphyrin from coproporphyrinogen in extracts of various bacteria, *J. Bacteriol.* **102**:398–403.

Jayaraman, J., Cotman, C., Mahler, H. R., and Sharp, C. W. (1966). Biochemical correlates of respiratory deficiency. VII. Glucose repression, *Arch. Biochem. Biophys.* **116**:224–251.

Jayaraman, J., Padmanaban, G., Malathi, K., and Sarma, P. S. (1971). Haem synthesis during mitochondriogenesis in yeast, *Biochem. J.* **121**:531–535.

Jenson, E. O., Marcker, K. A., and Villadsen, I. S. (1986). Heme regulates the expression in *Saccharomyces cerevisiae* of chimaeric genes containing 5′-flanking soybean leghemoglobin sequences, *EMBO J.* **5**:843–847.

Jones, M. S., and Jones, O. T. G. (1969). The structural organization of haem synthesis in rat liver mitochondria, *Biochem. J.* **113**:507–514.

Jordan, P. M., and Berry, A. (1980). Preuroporphyrinogen, a universal intermediate in the biosynthesis of uroporphyrinogen III, *FEBS Lett.* **112**:86–88.

Kalb, V. F., Woods, C. W., Turi, T. G., Dey, C. R., Sutter, T. R., and Loper, J. C. (1987). Primary structure of the P450 lanosterol demethylase gene from *Saccharomyces cerevisiae*, *DNA* **6**:529–537.

Kappeli, O. (1986). Cytochromes P-450 of yeasts, *Microbiol. Rev.* **50**:244–258.

Karst, F., and Lacroute, F. (1973). Isolation of pleiotropic yeast mutants requiring ergosterol for growth, *Biochem. Biophys. Res. Comm.* **52**:741–747.

Keilin, D. (1953). Occurrence of hemoglobin in yeast and the supposed stabilization of the oxygenated cytochrome oxidase, *Nature* **172**:390–393.

Keng, T., Alani, E., and Guarente, L. (1986). The nine amino-terminal residues of δ-aminolevulinate synthase direct β-galactosidase into the mitochondrial matrix, *Mol. Cell. Biol.* **6**:355–364.

Keng, T., and Guarente, L. (1987). Constitutive expression of the yeast *HEM1* gene is actually a composite of activation and repression, *Proc. Nat. Acad. Sci. (U.S.A.)* **84**:9113–9117.

Keyhani, E., and Keyhani, J. (1980a). Identification of porphyrin present in apo-cytochrome c oxidase of copper-deficient yeast cells, *Biochim. Biophys. Acta.* **663**:221–227.

Keyhani, E., and Keyhani, J. (1980b). Defect in heme a biosynthesis of *OXI* mutants of the yeast *Saccharomyces cerevisiae*, *The Organization and Expression of the Mitochondrial Genome* (A. M. Kroon and G. Saccone, Eds.), Elsevier, Amsterdam, pp. 369–374.

Keyhani, J., and Keyhani, E. (1978). Mevalonic acid as a precursor for the alkyl side chain of heme a of cytochrome c oxidase in yeast *Saccharomyces cerevisiae*, *FEBS Lett.* **93**:271–274.

King, D. J., and Wiseman, A. (1987). Yeast cytochrome P448 enzymes and the activation of mutagens, including carcinogens, *Enzyme Induction, Mutagen Activation and Carcinogen Testing in Yeast* (A. Wiseman, Ed.), Ellis Horwood, Chichester, UK, pp. 115–167.

Kurlandzka, A., and Rytka, J. (1985). Mutants of *Saccharomyces cerevisiae* partially defective in the last steps of the haem biosynthetic pathway: Isolation and genetical characterization, *J. Gen. Microbiol.* **131**:2909–2918.

Kurlandzka, A., Zoladek, T., Rytka, J., Labbe-Bois, R., and Urban-Grimal, D. (1988). The in vivo effects of mutationally modified uroporphyrinogen decarboxylase in different *hem12* mutants of *Saccharomyces cerevisiae*, *Biochem. J.* **253**:109–116.

Labbe, P. (1971). Synthèse du protohème par la levure *Saccharomyces cerevisiae*. I. Mise en évidence de différentes étapes de la synthèse du protohème chez la levure cultivée en aérobiose et en anaérobiose. Influence des conditions de culture sur cette synthèse, *Biochimie* **53**:1001–1014.

Labbe, P., Camadro, J. M., and Chambon, H. (1985). Fluorometric assays for coproporphyrinogen oxidase and protoporphyrinogen oxidase, *Anal. Biochem.* **149**:248–260.

Labbe, P., Dechateaubodeau, G., and Labbe-Bois, R. (1972). Synthèse du protohème par la levure *Saccharomyces cerevisiae*. II. Influence exercée par le glucose sur l'adaptation respiratoire, *Biochimie* **54**:513–528.

Labbe, P., Volland, C., and Chaix, P. (1967). A propos de la nature et du role d'un pigment absorbant à 503 nm chez certaines levures, *Biochim. Biophys. Acta* **143**:70–78.

Labbe, P., Volland, C., and Chaix, P. (1968). Etude de l'activité ferrochélatase des mitochondries de levure, *Biochim. Biophys. Acta* **159**:527–539.

Labbe-Bois, R., Brouillet, N., Camadro, J. M., Chambon, H., Felix, F., Labbe, P., Rytka, J., Simon-Casteras, C., Urban-Grimal, D., Volland, C., and Zagorec, M. (1986). Molecular approaches to heme biosynthesis in the yeast *Saccharomyces cerevisiae*, *Porphyrins and Porphyrias* (Y. Nordmann, Ed.), John Libbey, London, pp. 15–23.

Labbe-Bois, R., Rytka, J., Litwinska, J., and Bilinski, T. (1977). Analysis of heme biosynthesis in catalase and cytochrome deficient yeast mutants, *Mol. Gen. Genet.* **156**:177–183.

Labbe-Bois, R., Simon, M., Rytka, J., Litwinska, J., and Bilinski, T. (1980). Effect of 5-aminolevulinic acid synthesis deficiency on expression of other enzymes of heme pathway in yeast, *Biochem. Biophys. Res. Comm.* **95**:1357–1363.

Labbe-Bois, R., Urban-Grimal, D., Volland, C., Camadro, J. M., and Dehoux, P. (1983). About the regulation of protoheme synthesis in *Saccharomyces cervisiae*, *Mitochondria 1983* (R. J. Schweyen, K. Wolf, and F. Kaudewitz, Eds.), Walter de Gruyter, Berlin, pp. 523–534.

Labbe-Bois, R., and Volland, C. (1977a). Changes in the activities of the protoheme-synthesizing system during the growth of yeast under different conditions, *Arch. Biochem. Biophys.* **179**:565–577.

Labbe-Bois, R., and Volland, C. (1977b). Protoheme synthesis system in the cytoplasmic "petite" mutant of *Saccharomyces cerevisiae*, *Biochimie* **59**:539–541.

Labbe-Bois, R., Volland, C., Forestier, J. P., and Labbe, P. (1973). Protohaem synthesis by the yeast *Saccharomyces cerevisiae* during respiratory adaptation. Relationship with glycogen metabolism, *Enzyme* **16**:9–20.

Lancashire, W. E., and Mattoon, J. R. (1979). Genetic manipulation of a latent defect in yeast cytochrome biosynthesis utilizing cytoduction, *Biochem. Biophys. Res. Comm.* **90**:801–809.

Laz, T. M., Pietras, D. F., and Sherman, F. (1984). Differential regulation of the duplicated isocytochrome c genes in yeast, *Proc. Nat. Acad. Sci. (U.S.A.)* **81**:4475–4479.

Lesuisse, E. (1987). Ph.D. Thesis, Louvain-La-Neuve, Belgium.

Lesuisse, E., and Labbe, P. (1989). Reductive and nonreductive mechanisms of iron assimilation by the yeast *Saccharomyces cerevisiae*, *J. Gen. Microbiol.* **135**:257–263.

Lesuisse, E., Raguzzi, F., and Crichton, R. R. (1987). Iron uptake by the yeast *Saccharomyces cerevisiae*: Involvement of a reduction step, *J. Gen. Microbiol.* **133**:3229–3336.

Light, P. A. (1972). Influence of environment on mitochondrial function in yeast, *J. Appl. Chem. Biotechnol.* **22**:509–526.

Lin, C. P., Gollub, E. G., and Beattie, D. S. (1982). Synthesis of the proteins of complex III of the mitochondrial respiratory chain in heme-deficient cells, *Eur. J. Biochem.* **128**:309–313.

Lindenmayer, A., and Estabrook, R. W. (1958). Low temperature spectral studies on the biosynthesis of cytochromes in baker's yeast, *Arch. Biochem. Biophys.* **78**:66–82.

Lindenmayer, A., and Smith, L. (1964). Cytochromes and other pigments of baker's yeast grown aerobically and anaerobically, *Biochim. Biophys. Acta* **93**:445–461.

Lloyd, D. (1974). *The Mitochondria of Microorganisms*, Academic Press, London.

Lowry, C. V., and Lieber, R. H. (1986). Negative regulation of the *Saccharomyces cerevisiae ANB*1 gene by heme, as mediated by the *ROX*1 gene product, *Mol. Cell. Biol.* **6**:4145–4148.

Lowry, C. V., and Zitomer, R. S. (1984). Oxygen regulation of anaerobic and aerobic genes mediated by a common factor in yeast, *Proc. Nat. Acad. Sci. (U.S.A.)* **81**:6129–6133.

Lukaszkiewicz, J., and Bilinski, T. (1979). Effect of anaerobiosis and glucose on the content of haem and its precursors in intact yeast cells, *Acta Biochim. Polon.* **26**:161–168.

Luzikov, V. N. (1986). Proteolytic control over topogenesis of membrane proteins, *FEBS Lett.* **200**:259–264.

Mahler, H. R., and Lin, C. C. (1974). The derepression of Δ-aminolevulinate synthetase in yeast, *Biochem. Biophys. Res. Comm.* **61**:963–970.

Mahler, H. R., and Lin, C. C. (1978a). Exogenous adenosine $3':5'$-monophosphate can release yeast from catabolite repression, *Biochem. Biophys. Res. Comm.* **83**:1039–1047.

Mahler, H. R., and Lin, C. C. (1978b). Molecular events during the release of δ-aminolevulinate dehydratase from catabolite repression, *J. Bacteriol.* **135**:54–61.

Malamud, D. R., Borralho, L. M., Panek, A. D., and Mattoon, J. R. (1979). Modulation of cytochrome biosynthesis in yeast by antimetabolic action of levulinic acid, *J. Bacteriol.* **138**:799–804.

Malamud, D. R., Padrao, G. R. B., Borralho, L. M., Arrese, M., Panek, A. D., and Mattoon, J. R. (1983). Regulation of porphyrin biosynthesis in yeast. Level of δ-aminolevulinic acid in porphyrin mutants of *Saccharomyces cerevisiae*, *Brazilian J. Med. Biol. Res.* **16**:203–213.

Marres, C. A. M., Van Loon, A. P. G. M., Oudshoorn, P., Van Steeg, H., Grivell, L. A., and Slater, E. C. (1985). Nucleotide sequence analysis of the nuclear gene coding for manganese superoxide dismutase of yeast mitochondria, a gene previously assumed to code for the Rieske iron-sulphur protein, *Eur. J. Biochem.* **147**:153–161.

Matner, R. R., and Sherman, F. (1982). Differential accumulation of two apo-isocytochromes c in processing mutants of yeast, *J. Biol. Chem.* **257**:9811–9821.

Mattoon, J. R., Malamud, D. R., Brunner, A., Braz, G., Carjaval, E., Lancashire, W. E., and Panek, A. D. (1978). Regulation of heme formation and cytochrome biosynthesis in normal and mutant yeast, *Biochemistry and Genetics of Yeast, Pure and Applied Aspects* (M. Bacila, B. L. Horecker, and A. O. M. Stoppani, Eds.), Academic Press, New York, pp. 317–337.

McKay, R., Druyan, R., Getz, G. S., and Rabinowitz, M. (1969). Intramitochondrial localization of 5-aminolevulinate synthetase and ferrochelatase in rat liver, *Biochem. J.* **114**:455–461.

Meussdoerffer, F., and Fiechter, A. (1986). Effect of mitochondrial cytochromes and haem content on cytochrome P450 in *Saccharomyces cerevisiae*, *J. Gen. Microbiol.* **132**:2187–2193.

Miyake, S., and Sugimura, T. (1968). Coproporphyrinogenase in a respiration-deficient mutant of yeast lacking all cytochromes and accumulating coproporphyrin, *J. Bacteriol.* **96**:1997–2003.

Mok, T. C. K., Richard, P. A. D., and Moss, F. J. (1969). The carbon monoxide-reactive haemoproteins of yeast, *Biochim. Biophys. Acta* **172**:438–449.

Mori, M., and Sano, S. (1972). Studies on the formation of protoporphyrin IX by anaerobic bacteria, *Biochim. Biophys. Acta* **264**:252–262.

Myers, A. M., Crivellone, M. D., Koerner, T. J., and Tzagoloff, A. (1987). Characterization of the yeast *HEM* 2 gene and transcriptional regulation of *COX*5 and *COR*1 by heme, *J. Biol. Chem.* **262**:16822–16829.

Nakamura, I., Nishikawa, Y., Kamihara, T., and Fukui, S. (1974). Respiratory deficiency in *Saccharomyces carlsbergensis* 4228 caused by thiamin and its prevention by pyridoxine, *Biochem. Biophys. Res. Comm.* **59**:771–776.

Ohaniance, L., and Chaix, P. (1966). Effet inhibiteur de Zn^{2+} sur la biosynthèse induite par l'oxygène des enzymes respiratoires de la levure, *Biochim. Biophys. Acta* **128**:228–238.

Ohaniance, L., and Chaix, P. (1970). Cinétique de la formation des iso-cytochromes c au cours de la synthèse induite par l'oxygène des enzymes respiratoires de levure provenant de cultures additionnees ou non de Zn^{++}, *Bull. Soc. Chim. Biol.* **52**:1105–1110.

Ohashi, A., Gibson, J., Gregor, I., and Schatz, G. (1982). Import of proteins into mitochondria. The precursor of cytochrome c_1 is processed in two steps, one of them heme-dependent, *J. Biol. Chem.* **257**:13042–13047.

Ostlund, A. K., Gohring, U., Krause, J., and Brdiczka, D. (1983). The binding of glycerol kinase to the outer membrane of rat liver mitochondria: Its importance in metabolic regulation, *Biochem. Med.* **30**:231–245.

Pasteur, L. (1876). Etudes sur la bière, Oeuvres réunies, Vol. V, 1928, Masson, Paris.

Porra, R. J., Barnes, R., and Jones, O. T. G. (1972). The level and sub-cellular distribution of δ-aminolaevulinate synthase activity in semi-anaerobic and aerobic yeast, *Hoppe-Seyler's Z. Physiol. Chem.* **353** (Supplement):1365–1368.

Porra, R. J., and Falk, J. E. (1961). Protein-bound porphyrins associated with protoporphyrin biosynthesis, *Biochem. Biophys. Res. Comm.* **5**:179–184.

Porra, R. J., and Falk, J. E. (1964). The enzymatic conversion of coproporphyrinogen III to protoporphyrin IX, *Biochem. J.* **90**:69–75.

Porra, R. J., and Jones, O. T. G. (1963a). Studies on ferrochelatase. I. Assay and properties of ferrochelatase from a pig-liver mitochondrial extract, *Biochem. J.* **87**:181–185.

Porra, R. J., and Jones, O. T. G. (1963b). Studies on ferrochelatase. 2. An investigation of the role of ferrochelatase in the biosynthesis of various haem prosthetic groups, *Biochem. J.* **87**:186–192.

Poulson, R. (1976a). The enzymic conversion of protoporphyrinogen IX to protoporphyrin IX in mammalian mitochondria, *J. Biol. Chem.* **251**:3730–3733.

Poulson, R. (1976b). The regulation of heme synthesis, *Ann. Clin. Res.* **8**:56–63.

Poulson, R., and Polglase, W. J. (1973). Evidence for the identification of P503 with prototetrahydroporphyrin IX, *Biochim. Biophys. Acta* **329**:256–263.

Poulson, R., and Polglase, W. J. (1974a). Aerobic and anaerobic coproporphyrinogenase activities in extracts from *Saccharomyces cerevisiae*, *J. Biol. Chem.* **249**:6367–6371.

Poulson, R., and Polglase, W. J. (1974b). Site of glucose repression of heme biosynthesis, *FEBS Lett.* **40**:258–260.

Poulson, R., and Polglase, W. J. (1975). The enzymatic conversion of protoporphyrinogen IX to protoporphyrin IX. Protoporphyrinogen oxidase activity in mitochondrial extracts of *Saccharomyces cerevisiae*, *J. Biol. Chem.* **250**:1269–1274.

Pretlow, T. P., and Sherman, F. (1967). Porphyrins and zinc-porphyrins in normal and mutant strains of yeast, *Biochim. Biophys. Acta* **148**:629–644.

Raguzzi, F., Lesuisse, E., and Crichton, R. R. (1988). Iron storage in *Saccharomyces cerevisiae*, *FEBS Lett.* **231**:253–258.

Riethmuller, G., and Tuppy, H. (1964). Haem synthetase (ferrochelatase) in *Saccharomyces cerevisiae* nach aerobem und anaerobem Wachstum, *Biochem. Z.* **340**:413–420.

Romero, D. R., and Dahlberg, A. E. (1986). The alpha subunit of initiation factor 2 is phosphorylated in vivo in the yeast *Saccharomyces cerevisiae*, *Mol. Cell. Biol.* **6**:1044–1049.

Ross, E., and Schatz, G. (1976). Cytochrome c_1 of baker's yeast. II. Synthesis of cytoplasmic ribosomes and influences of oxygen and heme on accumulation of the apoprotein, *J. Biol. Chem.* **251**:1997–2004.

Rotenberg, M., and Margalit, R. (1987). Porphyrin-membrane interactions: Binding or partition?, *Biochim. Biophys. Acta* **905**:173–180.

Rytka, J., Bilinski, T., and Labbe-Bois, R. (1984). Modified uroporphyrinogen decarboxylase activity in a yeast mutant which mimics porphyria cutanea tarda, *Biochem. J.* **218**:405–413.

Saltzgaber-Muller, J., and Schatz, G. (1978). Heme is necessary for the accumulation and assembly of cytochrome c oxidase subunits in *Saccharomyces cerevisiae*, *J. Biol. Chem.* **253**:305–310.

Sanders, H. K., Mied, P. A., Briquet, M., Hernandez-Rodriguez, J., Gottal, R. F., and Mattoon, J. R. (1973). Regulation of mitochondrial biogenesis: Yeast mutants deficient in synthesis of δ-aminolevulinic acid, *J. Mol. Biol.* **80**:17–39.

Sano, S., and Granick, S. (1961). Mitochondrial coproporphyrinogen oxidase and protoporphyrin formation, *J. Biol. Chem.* **236**:1173–1180.

Schirch, L., and Jenkins, W. T. (1964). Serine transhydroxymethylase. Properties of the enzyme-substrate complexes of D-alanine and glycine, *J. Biol. Chem.* **239**:3801–3807.

Schmalix, W., Oechsner, U., Magdolen, V., and Bandlow, W. (1986). Kinetics of the intracellular availability of heme after supplementing of heme-deficient yeast mutant with 5-aminolevulinate, *Biol. Chem. Hoppe-Seyler* **367**:379–385.

Sinclair, P., White, D. C., and Barrett, J. (1967). The conversion of protoheme to heme a in *Staphylococcus*, *Biochim. Biophys. Acta* **143**:427–428.

Skoneczny, N., Cheltowska, A., and Rytka, J. (1988). Studies of the coinduction by fatty acids of catalase A and acylCoA oxidase in standard and mutant *Saccharomyces cerevisiae* strains, *Eur. J. Biochem.* **174**:297–302.

Sledziewski, A., Rytka, J., Bilinski, T., Hortner, H., and Ruis, H. (1981). Postranscriptional heme control of catalase synthesis in the yeast *Saccharomyces cerevisiae*, *Curr. Genet.* **4**:19–23.

Slonimski, P. (1953). *La Formation des Enzymes Respiratoires chez la Levure*, Desoer, Liege.

Somlo, M., and Fukuhara, H. (1965). On the necessity of molecular oxygen for the synthesis of respiratory enzymes in yeast, *Biochem. Biophys. Res. Comm.* **19**:587–591.

Spevak, W., Hartig, A., Meindl, P., and Ruis, H. (1986). Heme control region of the catalase T gene of the yeast *Saccharomyces cerevisiae*, *Mol. Gen. Genet.* **203**:73–78.

Strathern, J. N., Jones, E. W., and Broach, J. R. (Eds.). (1981) *The Molecular Biology of the Yeast Saccharomyces. Life Cycle and Inheritance*, Cold Spring Harbor Laboratory, Cold Spring Harbor, N.Y.

Strathern, J. N., Jones, E. W., and Broach, J. R. (Eds.) (1982). *The Molecular Biology of the Yeast Saccharomyces. Metabolism and Gene Expression*, Cold Spring Harbor Laboratory, Cold Spring Harbor, N.Y.

Taketani, S., Tanaka-Yoshioka, A., Masaki, R., Tashiro, Y., and Tokunaga, R. (1986). Association of ferrochelatase with complex I in bovine heart mitochondria, *Biochim. Biophys. Acta* **883**:277–283.

Taketani, S., and Tokunaga, R. (1981). Rat liver ferrochelatase. Purification, properties and stimulation by fatty acids, *J. Biol. Chem.* **256**:12748–12753.

Tait, G. H. (1969). Coproporphyrinogenase activity in extracts from *Rhodopseudomonas spheroides, Biochem. Biophys. Res. Comm.* **37**:116–122.

Tamura, Y., Yoshida, Y., Sato, R., and Kumaoka, H. (1976). Fatty acid desaturase system of yeast microsomes. Involvement of cytochrome b_5-containing electron-transport chain, *Arch. Biochem. Biophys.* **175**:284–294.

Tangeras, A., Flatmark, T., Bachstrom, D., and Ehrenberg, A. (1980). Mitochondrial iron not bound in heme and iron-sulfur centers. Estimation, compartmentation and redox state, *Biochim. Biophys. Acta* **589**:162–175.

Tuppy, H., and Wiche, G. (1971). δ-Aminolävulinsäure-synthetase in backerhefe. Vergleichende Untersuchung des enzyms in wildstamm und petite-mutante, *Monats. fur Chemie* **102**:1305–1310.

Urban-Grimal, D., and Labbe-Bois, R. (1981). Genetic and biochemical characterization of mutants of *Saccharomyces cerevisiae* blocked in six different steps of heme biosynthesis, *Mol. Gen. Genet.* **183**:85–92.

Urban-Grimal, D., Ribes, V., and Labbe-Bois, R. (1984). Cloning by genetic complementation and restriction mapping of the yeast *HEM1* gene coding for 5-aminolevulinate synthase, *Curr. Genet.* **8**:327–331.

Urban-Grimal, D., Volland, C., Garnier, T., Dehoux, P., and Labbe-Bois, R. (1986). The nucleotide sequence of the *HEM1* gene and evidence for a precursor form of the mitochondrial 5-aminolevulinate synthase in *Saccharomyces cerevisiae, Eur. J. Biochem.* **156**:511–519.

Verdière, J., Creusot, F., Guarente, L., and Slonimski, P. P. (1986). The overproducing *CYP1* and the underproducing *hap1* mutations are alleles of the same gene which regulates in *trans* the expression of the structural genes encoding iso-cytochromes c, *Curr. Genet.* **10**:339–342.

Verdière, J., Creusot, F., and Guérineau, M. (1985). Regulation of the expression of iso-2-cytochrome c gene in *S. cerevisiae*: Cloning of the positive regulatory gene *CYP1* and identification of the region of its target sequence on the structural gene *CYP3, Mol. Gen. Genet.* **199**:524–533.

Volland, C., and Felix, F. (1984). Isolation and properties of 5-aminolevulinate synthase from the yeast *Saccharomyces cerevisiae, Eur. J. Biochem.* **142**:551–557.

Volland, C., Labbe-Bois, R., and Labbe, P. (1975). Assay in situ of yeast enzymes involved in protohaem synthesis, *Biochimie* **57**:117–120.

Volland, C., and Urban-Grimal, D. (1988). The presequence of yeast 5-aminolevulinate synthase is not required for targeting to mitochondria, *J. Biol. Chem.* **263**:8294–8299.

Winkelman, G., Van der Helm, D., and Neilands, J. B. (Eds.) (1987). *Iron Transport in Microbes, Plants, and Animals*, VCH Verlagsgesellschaft mBH, D6940, Weinheim, FGA.

Woodrow, G., and Schatz, G. (1979). The role of oxygen in the biosynthesis of cytochrome c oxidase of yeast mitochondria, *J. Biol. Chem.* **254**:6088–6093.

Woods, R. A., Sanders, H. K., Briquet, M., Foury, F., Drysdale, B. E., and Mattoon, J. R. (1975). Regulation of mitochondrial biogenesis: Enzymatic changes in cytochrome-deficient yeast mutants requiring δ-aminolevulinic acid, *J. Biol. Chem.* **250**:9090–9098.

Ycas, M. (1956). Formation of hemoglobin and the cytochromes by yeast in the presence of antimycin A, *Exp. Cell. Res.* **11**:1–6.

Ycas, M., and Drabkin, D. L. (1957). The biosynthesis of cytochrome c in yeast adapting to oxygen, *J. Biol. Chem.* **244**:921–933.

Ycas, M., and Starr, T. J. (1953). The effect of glycine and protoporphyrin on a cytochrome deficient yeast, *J. Bacteriol.* **65**:83–88.

Yoshida, Y., Kumaoka, H., and Sato, R. (1974). Studies on the microsomal electron-transport system of anaerobically grown yeast. II. Purification and characterization of cytochrome b₅, *J. Biochem.* **75**:1211–1219.

Yoshimoto, A., and Sato, R. (1970). Studies on yeast sulfite reductase. III. Further characterization, *Biochim. Biophys. Acta* **220**:190–205.

Yoshinaga, T., and Sano, S. (1980). Coproporphyrinogen oxidase. I. Purification, properties, and activation by phospholipids, *J. Biol. Chem.* **255**:4722–4726.

Yotsuyanagi, Y. (1962). Étude sur le chondriome de la levure. I. Variations de l'ultrastructure du chondriome au cours du cycle de la croissance aérobie, *J. Ultrastructure Res.* **7**:121–140.

Zagorec, M. (1986). Ph.D. Thesis, University of Paris VI, Paris.

Zagorec, M., Buhler, J. M., Treich, I., Keng, T., Guarente, L., and Labbe-Bois, R. (1988). Isolation, sequence and regulation by oxygen of the yeast *HEM*13 gene coding for coproporphyrinogen oxidase, *J. Biol. Chem.* **263**:9718–9724.

Zagorec, M., and Labbe-Bois, R. (1986). Negative control of yeast coproporphyrinogen oxidase synthesis by heme and oxygen, *J. Biol. Chem.* **261**:2506–2509.

Zitomer, R. S., Sellers, J. W., McCarter, D. W., Hastings, G. A., Wick, P., and Lowry, C. V. (1987). Elements involved in oxygen regulation of the *Saccharomyces cerevisiae CYC7* gene, *Mol. Cell. Biol.* **7**:2212–2220.

Tetrapyrrole Metabolism in Photosynthetic Organisms

Samuel I. Beale

Jon D. Weinstein

I. Variety and Functions of Tetrapyrroles in Photosynthetic Organisms

The greatest diversity of naturally occurring tetrapyrroles is found among species capable of carrying out photosynthesis. These species share with other organisms the need for heme-containing cytochromes and oxidases and, in addition, employ tetrapyrroles as pigments for the photosynthetic processes of trapping light energy and converting it to chemical energy.

The tetrapyrrole pigments that are characteristic of photosynthetic species fall into two structural groups: Mg-containing closed-macrocycle chlorophylls and their structural relatives, and open-macrocycle bilins. In this chapter the biosynthesis of tetrapyrroles in photosynthetic organisms will be discussed with emphasis on those processes and end products that are unique to photosynthetic organisms or whose metabolism has been most thoroughly characterized in these species.

A. Introduction to the branched tetrapyrrole biosynthetic pathway

Figure 7.1 illustrates the biosynthetic relationships among the major groups of tetrapyrrole pigments characteristic of photosynthetic organisms. The earliest well-characterized precursor that is committed to the tetrapyrrole pathway is ALA (5-aminoleuulinate synthase). A major branch point occurs at protoporphyrin IX, the last common intermediate leading to both the chlorophylls and the other major products. Another important branch point occurs at protoheme, which is the last common intermediate leading to both other hemes and the phycobilins (including the phytochrome chromophore). A third branch point occurs at uroporphyrinogen III, the last common intermediate that leads to siroheme and the corrinoids.

B. Chlorophylls and bacteriochlorophylls

Tetrapyrrole pigments that are grouped under the general classification of chlorophylls all contain Mg as the centrally chelated metal (Fig. 7.2). All chlorophylls also contain a fifth, so-called isocyclic, ring. The macrocycle oxidation state may be that of a porphyrin (as in the chlorophylls c), dihydroporphyrin (chlorophylls a and b, and bacteriochlorophylls c, d, and e), or tetrahydroporphyrin (bacteriochlorophylls a, b, and g). In all cases the macrocycle is aromatic and contains a complete conjugated double-bond system.

C. Hemes

Plant and algal cells contain all three common heme types found in nonphotosynthetic organisms: protoheme (heme b) is a constituent of

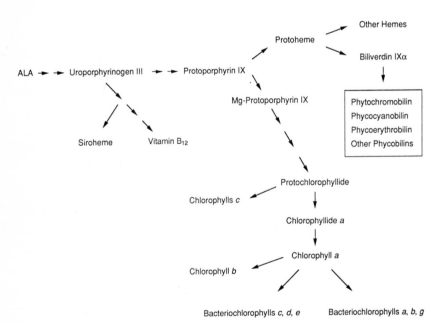

Figure 7.1 Outline of the tetrapyrrole biosynthetic pathway, illustrating the end products characteristic of photosynthetic organisms, and their biosynthetic relationships.

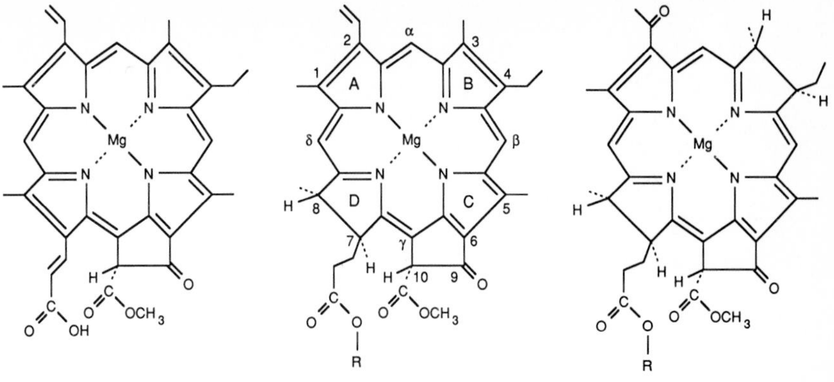

Chlorophyll c_1

Chlorophyll a

Bacteriochlorophyll a

Figure 7.2 Three "chlorophyll" pigments having different degrees of reduction of the macrocyclic ring: chlorophyll c_1 (a porphyrin), chlorophyll a (a dihydroporphyrin), bacteriochlorophyll a (a tetrahydroporphyrin). R is usually phytyl in chlorophyll a, and can be either phytyl or geranylgeranyl in bacteriochlorophyll a. Chlorophyll a is illustrated with the conventional designations for the pyrrole rings by capital letters, pyrrole substituent positions by numbers, and meso positions by lowercase Greek letters.

respiratory cytochromes, photosynthetic electron transport chain components, peroxidases, plant microsomal cytochrome P450 (Werck-Reichhart et al., 1988), and other oxidative enzymes; heme a is found in plants as the prosthetic group of mitochondrial cytochrome c oxidase (Schneegurt and Beale, 1986); heme c is found in cytochromes that function in the electron transport chains of both mitochondria (cytochrome c) and plastids (cytochrome f).

D. Phycobilins and phytochrome chromophore

In plants and algae, unlike the situation in most other organisms, bilins are functional tetrapyrrole end products. Cyanobacteria, red algae, and cryptophytes employ bilins as primary light-harvesting photosynthetic pigments, and higher plants and some green algae contain another bilin as the chromophore of the important photomorphogenetic pigment phytochrome. Thus, in many photosynthetic species, the bilins must be included in discussions of tetrapyrrole biosynthesis.

Phycobilins are open-chain tetrapyrroles that function as photosynthetic light-harvesting pigments when covalently linked to specific proteins (Fig. 7.3). Two major classes of phycobiliproteins are phycocyanins and phycoerythrins, which are, respectively, colored blue and red. These pigments are largely responsible for the characteristic colors of the organisms which contain them. The different colors arise from slightly

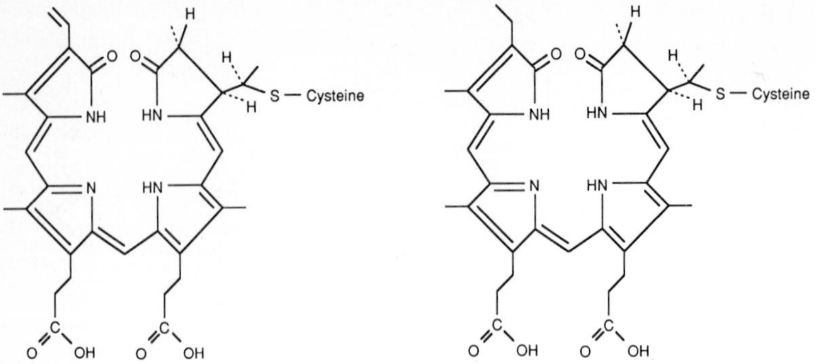

Phytochrome Chromophore

Phycocyanin Chromophore

Figure 7.3 Chromophores of phytochrome and phycocyanin illustrated with covalent thioether bond linkage to the apoproteins.

different phycobilin chromophores. In blue-green and red algae, phycobiliproteins form functional aggregates, called phycobilisomes, which decorate the external surface of thylakoid membranes and mediate efficient light absorption and excitation transfer to the photosynthetic reaction centers. The cryptomonad algae also contain phycobiliproteins and utilize them for light harvesting, but in these organisms the phycobiliproteins occur within the inner loculi of the thylakoid membranes. Phycocyanobilin may occur alone as the only phycobilin in some algal species, or it may occur together with other phycobilins, but in all cases, it is the centrally important chromophore necessary for utilization of light energy absorbed by other phycobilin pigments.

The photomorphogenetic pigment phytochrome is a biliprotein whose chromophore structure closely resembles the phycobilins, and whose biosynthesis may share features with the latter. Phytochrome is ubiquitous in higher plants and also occurs in some algae.

E. Other tetrapyrroles found in photosynthetic organisms

Plant cells contain siroheme as the prosthetic group of nitrite and sulfite reductases (Zumft, 1972; Murphy et al., 1974; Hucklesby et al., 1976). Many prokaryotic photosynthetic species are also capable of synthesizing corrinoids. The biosynthesis of these uroporphyrinogen-derived molecules will not be specifically addressed in this chapter.

There are still other tetrapyrroles found in photosynthetic species, which are more restricted in their distribution. Among these are the dinoflagellate luciferin, which is a bilin that has been proposed to be derived from chlorophyll (Dunlap et al., 1981).

II. Biosynthetic Route

The tetrapyrrole biosynthetic pathway in photosynthetic organisms can be considered to begin from two roots, each giving rise to the precursor ALA by a different mechanism, followed by a common trunk leading from ALA to protoporphyrin IX, then splitting into three branches which give rise to hemes, bilins, and chlorophylls (Fig. 7.1). There is also a minor branch from the trunk leading to siroheme and the corrinoids.

A. ALA formation

The earliest well-characterized committed tetrapyrrole precursor is ALA. Two distinct mechanisms exist in photosynthetic species for the diversion of general metabolic intermediates into the tetrapyrrole biosynthetic pathway by transformation to ALA. In plants, algae (including the prokaryotic cyanobacteria), and some photosynthetic bacteria, ALA is formed from the intact carbon skeleton of glutamic acid, in a process requiring three enzymatic reactions and tRNA^{glu} (Fig. 7.4). In other photosynthetic bacteria ALA is formed by condensation of glycine and succinyl-CoA in a reaction analogous to that occurring in yeast and animal mitochondria (Fig. 7.5).

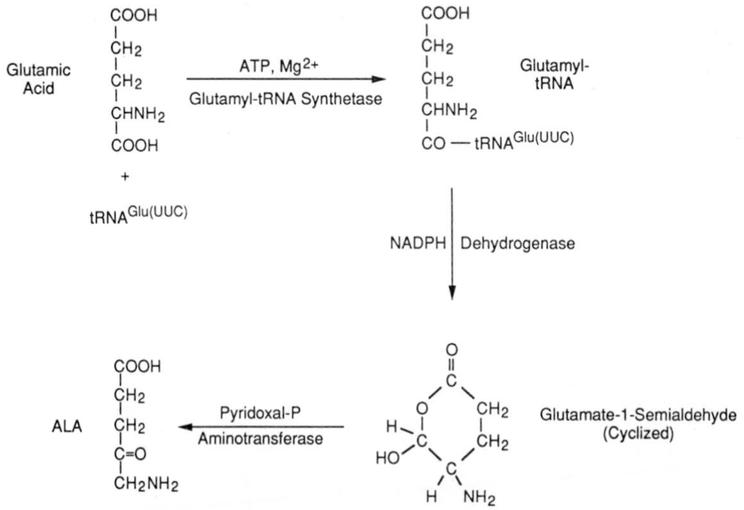

Figure 7.4   ALA biosynthesis from glutamate. The cyclic compound illustrated is one of several structures proposed for the product of the dehydrogenase reaction.

1. ALA biosynthesis from glutamate

a. In vivo evidence for ALA and tetrapyrrole formation from glutamate. When ALA dehydratase inhibitors are administered to greening etiolated plant tissues, ALA accumulates. Radioactivity from ^{14}C-labeled exogenous compounds is incorporated into the accumulated ALA. In greening etiolated plant tissues, glycine and succinate were relatively inefficient contributors of label to ALA, whereas the five-carbon compounds glutamate, α-ketoglutarate, and glutamine were much better contributors (Beale and Castelfranco, 1974b; Meller et al., 1975; Ramaswamy and Nair, 1976). Based on the uniform degree of incorporation of all of the carbons of glutamate, and the carbon-to-carbon correspondence of label position in precursor and product molecules, a number of hypothetical routes were proposed for the transformation of the intact carbon skeleton of glutamate or α-ketoglutarate into ALA (Beale et al., 1975; Meller et al., 1975). Preferential and specific transfer of label from glutamate or α-ketoglutarate to ALA formed in vivo, in the presence of levulinic acid, has been found in a variety of cell types, including blue-green (Avissar, 1980; Kipe-Nolt and Stevens, 1980; Meller and Harel, 1978), red (Jurgenson et al., 1976), and green (Meller and Harel, 1978) algae, and many higher plant tissues (Beale and Castelfranco, 1974b; Beale et al., 1975; Meller et al., 1975).

Evidence supporting the physiological role of a five-carbon pathway in providing ALA for photosynthetic pigments was first provided by Castelfranco and Jones (1975). They demonstrated that both protoheme and chlorophyll were labeled most efficiently by five-carbon precursors in greening barley. Similarly, ^{14}C-labeled α-ketoglutarate was superior to glycine or succinate in contributing label to phycocyanobilin in growing cultures of *Anacystis nidulans* (Laycock and Wright, 1981). Based on the relative abilities of C_1- or C_2-labeled acetate to contribute label to chlorophyll and glutamate in *Synechococcus* 630I, McKie et al. (1981) concluded that the five-carbon pathway operates exclusively in tetrapyr-

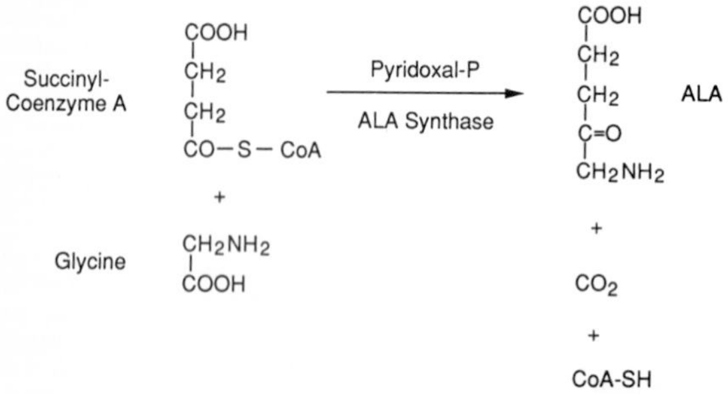

Figure 7.5   ALA biosynthesis from glycine and succinyl-CoA.

role precursor formation. Finally, Oh-hama et al. (1982) performed ^{13}C nmr analysis on chlorophyll formed from ^{13}C-labeled glycine or glutamate in *Scenedesmus obliquus*. Glycine was shown to contribute label only to the methoxyl group adjacent to the isocyclic ring, while glutamate contributed label in a manner that was consistent with the exclusive operation of the five-carbon pathway in ALA formation. This result was confirmed in maize (Porra et al., 1983), and similar results were obtained with the photosynthetic bacteria *Chromatium* (Oh-hama et al., 1986a) and *Prosthecochloris* (Oh-hama et al., 1986b; Smith and Huster, 1987).

It is now generally accepted that a five-carbon pathway is the route of synthesis for ALA destined for all cellular tetrapyrroles in plants and most algae. By measuring the relative ability of ^{14}C-labeled glycine and glutamate to contribute radioactivity to heme a, the prosthetic group of mitochondrial cytochrome oxidase, it was determined that glutamate is the source of the carbon for this heme in etiolated maize epicotyl sections (Schneegurt and Beale, 1986) and in the unicellular red alga *Cyanidium caldarium* (Weinstein and Beale, 1984). Other cellular hemes also appear to be made from glutamate in plants. Peroxidase is excreted into the medium by peanut cell suspension cultures. In these cultures the heme moiety was more efficiently labeled with five-carbon ALA precursors than with ALA synthase precursors (Chibbar and van Huystee, 1983). Likewise plant microsomal cytochrome P450 heme appears to be made from glutamate, as deduced from the inhibition of its biosynthesis by gabaculine (3-amino-2,3-dihydrobenzoic acid), a potent, specific inhibitor of the aminotransferase step in the conversion of glutamate to ALA (see below) (Werck-Reichhart et al., 1988).

b. Mechanism of ALA formation from glutamate. Much of the earlier work on ALA formation from five-carbon precursors by intact chloroplasts and unpurified cell extracts has been summarized previously (Beale, 1984). Particulate-free cell extracts capable of converting glutamate to ALA have been obtained from barley (Gough and Kannangara, 1977), *Euglena* (Mayer et al., 1987), the green algae *Chlamydomonas* (Wang et al., 1984) and *Chlorella* (Weinstein and Beale, 1985a), the red alga *Cyanidium* (Weinstein et al., 1986a), the cyanobacteria *Synechocystis* and *Synechococcus* (Rieble and Beale, 1988), the prochlorophyte *Prochlorothrix* (Rieble and Beale, 1988), and the photosynthetic bacterium *Chlorobium* (Rieble et al., 1988). Similar or identical reaction mechanisms appear to operate in all cases, and reaction components from some heterologous sources can be mixed to reconstitute activity in fractionated systems.

A minimum of three enzyme reactions is required for transformation of glutamate to ALA. In the first, glutamate is ligated to tRNA in a reaction identical or very similar to the charging reaction in protein biosynthesis. Like aminoacyl-tRNA formation in general, this reaction requires ATP and Mg^{2+}. Next, the tRNA-bound glutamate is converted to a reduced form in a reaction that requires a reduced pyridine nucleotide. The product of this reduction has been characterized as glutamate-1-semialdehyde (Houen et al., 1983) or its hydrated hemiacetal form (Hoober et al., 1988). However, some of the reported properties of the product are inconsistent with the presence of an α-aminoaldehyde group, and other structures have been proposed (P.M. Jordan, personal communication). Finally, the positions of the nitrogen and oxo atoms of the reduced five-carbon intermediate are interchanged to form ALA.

Consistent with the above scheme, the ALA-forming systems extracted from barley (Bruyant and Kannangara, 1987) and *Chlorella* (Weinstein et al., 1987) have each been separated into four macromolecular components, all of which must be present to catalyze in vitro ALA formation from glutamate. Three of these are enzymes and the fourth is a low-molecular-weight RNA.

i. tRNA^{glu}. In vitro ALA-forming activity in extracts from barley plastids (Kannangara et al., 1984) and whole cells of *Chlamydomonas reinhardtii* (Huang et al., 1984) and *Chlorella vulgaris* (Weinstein and Beale, 1985b) was blocked by preincubation of the extracts with RNase A. Addition of RNase inhibitor plus low-molecular-weight RNA from the same species restored activity. More recently, RNA was also found to be required for ALA formation from glutamate in extracts of cyanobacteria and a prochlorophyte (Rieble and Beale, 1988), and the green photosynthetic bacterium *Chlorobium* (Rieble et al., 1988). In the barley chloroplast system, the required RNA was purified, sequenced, and characterized as tRNA^{glu}, bearing the UUC glutamate anticodon (Schön et al., 1986). Two of the anticodon bases bear modifications: The first U is 5-methylaminomethyl-2-thiouridine, and the second is pseudouridine. Although the extent of the modifications in the anticodon region is greater than previously reported for any tRNA^{glu}, this species is the only tRNA^{glu} found in barley chloroplasts (Schön et al., 1988), and, thus, it must take part in both protein synthesis and ALA formation. Two other glutamate-accepting tRNAs in barley chloroplasts were found to carry glutamine anticodons (Schön et al., 1988), and it was concluded that in barley chloroplasts, as in *Bacillus subtilis* (Lapointe et al., 1986), glutaminyl-tRNA is formed by ligation of tRNA^{gln} with glutamate, and subsequent amidation of the γ carbon of glutamate to form the glutaminyl moiety while the molecule is bound to the tRNA.

In several plant and algal species examined, the tRNA required for ALA formation was found to contain the UUC glutamate anticodon. This was determined by affinity purification using an affinity ligand directed against the UUC glutamate anticodon (Schneegurt and Beale, 1988). In the prokaryotic cyanobacterium *Synechocystis*, the tRNA required for ALA formation was first purified by affinity chromatography directed against the UUC anticodon. The purified UUC anticodon-bearing tRNA was then further fractionated into two components by mixed-mode (anion exchange and hydrophobic interaction) HPLC (Beale et al., 1988). Each homogeneous tRNA was tested for the ability to be charged with glutamate and to participate in ALA formation and protein synthesis in extracts derived from *Synechocystis*. The results indicated that the same species of tRNA can participate in both processes. In vitro, the two tRNAs differ functionally only in their relative abilities to be charged with glutamate by *Synechocystis* extracts. Once charged, they both participate equally well in both ALA formation and protein synthesis. The two tRNA^{glu}s were reported to have the same nucleotide sequence, and to differ by some unspecified base modification (O'Neill et al., 1988).

ii. Glutamyl-tRNA.   Activity of barley tRNA^{glu} in ALA formation required the presence of the 3'-terminal CCA, suggesting that the tRNA functions as a glutamate acceptor in the ALA-forming system (Schön et al., 1986). Glutamyl-tRNA served as a substrate for ALA formation in *Chlamydomonas* extracts (Huang and Wang, 1986a). However, the efficiency of incorporation of label from ^{14}C-glutamyl-tRNA into ALA was low, and the extracts to which the ^{14}C-glutamyl-tRNA was added still had the ability to form ALA from glutamate. More direct proof for the intermediacy of glutamyl-tRNA was obtained with fractionated *Chlorella* extract. Glutamyl-tRNA, but not free glutamate, could serve as precursor to ALA in a partially reconstituted system lacking one fraction. The missing enzyme fraction had glutamyl-tRNA synthetase activity (Avissar and Beale, 1988).

iii. Glutamyl-tRNA synthetase.   A single glutamyl-tRNA synthetase was detected in barley chloroplasts (Bruyant and Kannangara, 1987). The synthetase was purified by immunoaffinity chromatography. The purified 54,000 molecular weight enzyme was capable of linking glutamate to the tRNA^{glu} and both tRNA^{gln} species present in chloroplasts. The aminoacylation reaction required ATP. The presence of this enzyme was required for ALA synthesis from glutamate in the presence of other enzyme fractions. The glutamyl-tRNA synthetase in *Chlorella* extracts that participates in ALA formation was separated from the other enzyme components by serial affinity chromatography on Blue-Sepharose and ADP-agarose (Weinstein et al., 1987). In the absence of this enzyme fraction, ALA was formed from glutamyl-tRNA, but not from free glutamate (Avissar and Beale, 1988). The *Chlorella* enzyme that is required for the reaction to proceed starting from free glutamate has a molecular weight of 73,000.

iv. Glutamate-1-semialdehyde.   Glutamate-1-semialdehyde was reported to be chemically synthesized and used as a substrate for the in vitro enzyme system (Kannangara and Gough, 1978, 1979). The conversion required only the enzyme system plus glutamate-1-semial-dehyde, and was inhibited by the aminotransferase inhibitors, aminooxy-acetate and cycloserine. These results were questioned by Meisch and Maus (1983), who synthesized glutamate-1-semialdehyde and found it to be extremely unstable in solution. They also concluded on theoretical grounds that the method published by Kannangara and Gough (1978) could not have yielded glutamate-1-semialdehyde. In response to the above criticisms, a more-stable derivative of glutamate-1-semialdehyde, the diethyl acetal, was synthesized and its structure confirmed by mass spectrometry and by carbon and proton magnetic resonance (Houen et al., 1983). The diethyl acetal of glutamate-1-semialdehyde could be hydrolyzed in dilute acid to a compound that was converted to ALA by the soluble barley chloroplast enzyme system. The hydrolyzed product was chromatographically indistinguishable from glutamate-1-semial-dehyde prepared by the previous method (Kannangara and Gough, 1978). Other investigators have reported the conversion of glutamate-1-semialdehyde to ALA in in vitro preparations (Harel and Ne'eman, 1983; Wang et al., 1984). In these cases the glutamate-1-semialdehyde was supplied by Kannangara and co-workers. Material identical to chemi-cally synthesized glutamate-1-semialdehyde was reported to accumulate in greening barley leaves when treated with gabaculine, a mechanism-based inhibitor of ω-aminotransferases that blocks chlorophyll synthesis (Kannangara and Schouboe, 1985).

Recently, Jordan and co-workers have reported that the compound synthesized by the procedure of Kannangara and Gough is not gluta-mate-1-semialdehyde, but the cyclic ester between the γ-carboxyl group and the hydrated aldehyde group (P.M. Jordan, personal communica-tion). The cyclic structure does not contain free aldehyde or carboxylic acid functions, and is more compatible with the previously reported properties of the chemically synthesized product (stability in aqueous solution, heat stability) than the free α-aminoaldehyde. The cyclic compound, and not glutamate-1-semialdehyde, was reported to be the product of the dehydrogenase enzyme and the substrate of the barley aminotransferase.

v. Dehydrogenase.   In unfractionated or reconstituted ALA-forming systems from algae or barley chloroplasts, a reduced pyridine nucleotide is required for activity. In *Chlorella* extracts NADH is about half as effective as NADPH (Weinstein and Beale, 1985a), in *Euglena gracilis* extracts the two reduced pyridine nucleotides are about equally effective (Mayer et al., 1987), and in *Synechocystis* extracts NADPH is more effective at low concentrations but becomes inhibitory above 1 mM, and NADH is more effective at 5 mM (Rieble and Beale, 1988).

For technical reasons, the dehydrogenase activity is usually measured in coupled enzyme assays where the substrate is generated in vitro from glutamate plus tRNA, and/or the product is converted in situ to ALA.

The isolated dehydrogenase reaction, conversion of glutamyl-tRNA to a product identical to chemically synthesized glutamate-1-semialdehyde, was reported in *Chlamydomonas* extracts when the conversion of the dehydrogenase product to ALA was blocked by separation of aminotransferase enzyme from the other two enzymes by affinity chromatography prior to incubation (Huang and Wang, 1986a). In this preparation, glutamyl-tRNA synthetase activity was not physically separated from the dehydrogenase.

The enzyme component that utilizes the pyridine nucleotide cofactor was physically separated from the other enzyme components by affinity chromatography (Weinstein et al., 1987), and this enzyme was shown to be active in ALA formation from glutamyl-tRNA in the absence of glutamyl-tRNA synthetase (Avissar and Beale, 1988). Barley dehydrogenase was also separated from glutamyl-tRNA synthetase by immunoaffinity chromatography and chromatography on salicylate-Sepharose, and found to retain activity when recombined with the glutamyl-tRNA synthetase fraction (Bruyant and Kannangara, 1987). Earlier, aminotransferase activity was physically separated from the other enzymes in barley extracts by Blue-Sepharose affinity chromatography. The product formed by incubation of the other enzymes with glutamate, ATP, Mg^{2+}, and NADPH copurified with chemically synthesized glutamate-1-semialdehyde (Wang et al., 1981).

vi. Aminotransferase. An enzyme capable of converting chemically synthesized glutamate-1-semialdehyde to ALA was purified from extracts of barley chloroplasts (Kannangara and Gough, 1978; Wang et al., 1981) and *Chlamydomonas* cells (Wang et al., 1984) by affinity chromatography. The transamination reaction requires no added substrate or cofactor other than glutamate-1-semialdehyde. Barley aminotransferase has a molecular weight of 80,000 (Kannangara et al., 1981, 1988) and is inhibited by very low concentrations of gabaculine (Hoober et al., 1988). Gabaculine-resistant mutants of *Chlamydomonas* contain elevated levels of aminotransferase activity (Kahn and Kannangara, 1987).

The question of whether the migration of the amino group in the conversion of glutamate to ALA involves an intramolecular or intermolecular transfer was examined in *Chlamydomonas* extracts by the use of ^{13}C- and ^{15}N-labeled glutamate. When the heavy isotope labels were present on separate substrate molecules, a significant proportion of the ALA product molecules contained two heavy atoms, suggesting that the conversion occurs by intermolecular nitrogen transfer (Mau and Wang, 1988). However, the isotopic stability of ALA in the incubations was not measured, leaving open the possibility that the observed redistribution of heavy isotopes among product molecules occurred after the initial formation of ALA.

In most reports on in vitro transformation of glutamate to ALA, pyridoxal phosphate was included in all media used for cell homogenization, enzyme fractionation, and incubation, even though dependence upon added pyridoxal phosphate for activity could not be demonstrated (Kannangara and Gough, 1978; Wang et al., 1981; Wang et al., 1984). The evidence for the involvement of pyridoxal phosphate as a cofactor for the aminotransferase step consisted of the observation that in vitro ALA formation was inhibited by compounds such as aminooxyacetate and gabaculine, which are considered to be pyridoxal antagonists (Kannangara and Schouboe, 1985; Weinstein and Beale, 1985a). However, when cell disruption and enzyme fractionation were carried out in the absence of added pyridoxal phosphate, and the relative proportion of the enzymes in the reconstituted ALA-forming assay was adjusted so that the aminotransferase was rate-limiting, strong pyridoxal phosphate dependence of ALA formation could be directly demonstrated (Avissar and Beale, 1989).

2. ALA biosynthesis from glycine and succinyl-CoA. In vitro ALA formation was first reported in extracts of anaerobically grown cells of the facultatively aerobic photosynthetic bacterium *Rhodobacter spheroides*, which synthesize large quantities of bacteriochlorophyll as well as lesser amounts of heme and corrinoids (Kikuchi et al., 1958; Sawyer and Smith, 1958). ALA is formed in these cells by the condensation of succinyl-CoA and glycine, mediated by the pyridoxal phosphate-requiring enzyme, ALA synthase [succinyl-CoA : Glycine C-succinyltransferase (decarboxylating) EC 2.3.1.37]. In the reaction the carboxyl carbon of glycine is lost as CO_2 and the remainder is incorporated into the ALA.

ALA synthase was purified over 1600-fold from *R. spheroides* (Nandi and Shemin, 1977). The native enzyme has a molecular weight of 80,000 and consists of two subunits of 41,000 to 45,000 molecular weight. A native molecular weight of 61,000 to 65,000 was derived for ALA synthase from *Rhodopseudomonas palustris* (Viale et al., 1987).

The ALA synthase reaction mechanism was studied with the *R. spheroides* enzyme. During the reaction, the glycine 2-H atom having the pro-*R* configuration is specifically removed and the pro-2*S* H atom occupies the *S* position at C-5 of ALA (Zaman et al., 1973; Abboud et al., 1974). In the absence of succinyl-CoA, the enzyme catalyzes the exchange of one of the C-2 hydrogen atoms of glycine with the medium (Laghai and Jordan, 1976), and in the absence of either substrate, the enzyme catalyzes the exchange of one of the C-5 hydrogen atoms of ALA with the medium (Laghai and Jordan, 1977). The powerful allosteric inhibitor heme has little effect on these exchange reactions.

The presence of ALA synthase in plants and algae has remained doubtful. One early brief report of activity in spinach leaf extracts (Miller and Teng, 1967) was never confirmed. Certain atypical plant cells, such as nongreening soybean callus cultures (Barreiro, 1975; Batlle et al., 1975; Wider de Xifra et al., 1971, 1978) and greening peels of cold-stored potatoes (Ramaswamy and Nair, 1973, 1974, 1976), have been reported to contain ALA synthase. Indirect evidence supporting the existence of ALA synthase was reported in dark-grown barley (Meller and Gassman, 1982), some algae (Klein and Senger, 1978a, b; Meller and Harel, 1978; Porra and Grimme, 1974), and one moss (Harel, 1978a). Operation of ALA synthase was inferred from the relative rates of in vivo label incorporation into ALA from specifically ^{14}C-labeled exogenous presumptive substrates. ALA synthase activity was reported to be present in extracts of certain pigment mutants of the unicellular green alga S. obliquus, but the reports were too brief to allow evaluation of the nature of the reaction and product (Humbeck and Senger, 1981; Kah et al., 1981). On the other hand, it has been determined that the unicellular red alga C. caldarium (Weinstein and Beale, 1984) and etiolated maize epicotyl sections (Schneegurt and Beale, 1986) synthesize all cellular hemes, including the heme a prosthetic group of mitochondrial cytochrome oxidase, from ALA that is generated exclusively from glutamate.

ALA synthase activity was found in extracts of the green photosynthetic phytoflagellate Euglena (Beale et al., 1981). An examination of the physical and kinetic properties of the enzyme (Dzelzkalns et al., 1982) and the regulation of its activity (Beale and Foley, 1982; Foley et al., 1982) led to the conclusion that in Euglena, ALA synthase functions exclusively to provide precursors for nonplastid tetrapyrroles. This conclusion was subsequently proven directly by measuring incorporation of labeled precursors into isolated tetrapyrroles specific to plastids and mitochondria (Weinstein and Beale, 1983). Under all growth conditions examined, heme a of mitochondrial cytochrome c oxidase was formed from glycine, even while in cells growing under conditions permitting chlorophyll formation, the plastid pigments were formed exclusively from glutamate. Thus, unlike higher plants and other algae examined, Euglena has both ALA-forming pathways, each separately compartmented and responsible for synthesizing distinct pools of precursors for different classes of tetrapyrrole end products.

3. Distribution of the two ALA-forming pathways among photosynthetic species. The in vivo and in vitro results discussed earlier indicate that in higher plants, green algae, red algae, and cyanobacteria, all cellular tetrapyrroles are formed from glutamate. Some photosynthetic bacteria have the glutamate pathway, while others have the glycine pathway. Euglena is uniquely able to form plastid tetrapyrroles from glutamate while simultaneously forming mitochondrial hemes from glycine and succinate.

Recently, all of the photosynthetic bacterial groups were surveyed for the mode of ALA formation by in vitro measurement of label transfer to ALA from [1-^{14}C]glutamate and [2-^{14}C]glycine, and by measurement of the effect of RNase on the label transfer (Avissar et al., 1988). The results indicated that the pathway from glutamate is widely distributed among the bacterial groups and is probably the more primitive and evolutionarily earlier pathway. Genera containing the glutamate pathway include green sulfur bacteria (*Chlorobium*), green nonsulfur bacteria (*Chloroflexus*), gram-positive green bacteria (*Heliospirillum*), purple sulfur bacteria (*Chromatium*), and *Desulfovibrio* (which is not photosynthetic but may be closely related to photosynthetic groups). The glycine pathway was found only in the purple nonsulfur bacteria (*R. spheroides, Rhodospirillum rubrum*). The mode of ALA formation has not been determined in any of the several strains of bacteria that have been reported to form bacteriochlorophyll a under aerobic growth conditions (Pierson and Castenholz, 1971; Sato, 1978; Harashima et al., 1978; Fleischmann et al., 1988). It should also be noted that the five-carbon ALA biosynthetic pathway is not restricted to photosynthetic organisms. The operation of this pathway has been demonstrated in vivo and in extracts of *Clostridium thermoaceticum* (Oh-hama et al., 1988) and *Methanobacterium thermoautotrophicum* (Friedmann and Thauer, 1986; Friedmann et al., 1987).

B. Pathway from ALA to protoporphyrin IX

The steps leading from ALA to protoporphyrin, and the enzymes catalyzing the reactions, in photosynthetic organisms are generally identical or very similar to those in nonphotosynthetic species. An important consideration in higher plants and eukaryotic algae is the intracellular distribution of the enzymes. Isolated chloroplasts are capable of synthesizing protochlorophyllide from exogenous glutamate (Fuesler et al., 1984a; Huang and Castelfranco, 1986). Thus, they must contain all of the enzymes catalyzing the reactions leading from glutamate to porphyrins. It is not yet clear how many of the biosynthetic steps leading to hemes may also occur in other cellular regions, and, for those that do, whether the properties of the nonplastid enzymes differ from those of the plastids. Knowledge gained in this area will shed light on the degree of cellular dependence on the plastids for tetrapyrrole biosynthesis and have implications for the functions of the plastid metabolism and its regulation, especially in nonphotosynthetic tissues.

1. ALA dehydratase. Plant ALA dehydratase has been studied extensively. Spinach leaf ALA dehydratase is a hexamer of about 300,000 molecular weight (Liedgens et al., 1980). The enzyme from *R. spheroides* is also a hexamer (van Heyningen and Shemin, 1971). These results are in contrast to the octameric structure of the animal enzyme. Another apparent difference among the enzymes from different sources is the metal requirement. Whereas the animal enzyme requires Zn^{2+} for activity, the plant and bacterial enzymes require Mg^{2+} (Nandi and Waygood, 1967; Shetty and Miller, 1969; Shibata and Ochiai, 1977; Tamai et al., 1979; Liedgens et al., 1980). The similarity of plant and bacterial ALA dehydratases suggests that the plant enzyme is of the prokaryotic type and located within the plastids. Most of the ALA dehydratase activity in greening radish cotyledons is associated with the plastid stroma, but a portion is bound to the thylakoid membranes (Nasri et al., 1988). The significance of this intraplastid distribution is unknown. Whether green plant cells also contain an additional, animal-like ALA dehydratase in a nonplastic region is not known. One report localizes ALA dehydratase in the plastids of pea leaves and *Arum* spadices (Smith, 1988). The latter tissue is nongreening. However, it is interesting that ALA dehydratase from nongreening soybean callus cells was reported to share with the animal cytoplasmic enzyme a requirement for Zn^{2+}, rather than Mg^{2+} (Tigier et al., 1970).

In single-turnover experiments, Jordan and Seehra (1980) established that in the reaction catalyzed by ALA dehydratase from *R. spheroides*, the first bound ALA molecule is the one that contributes the propionic acid side chain of the product. In the formation of PBG, the removal of hydrogen to form the aromatic pyrrole ring must occur on the enzyme, as is indicated by the stereospecific retention of one of the two hydrogens derived from the C-5 hydrogens of ALA (Abboud and Akhtar, 1976).

2. PBG deaminase. PBG deaminase condenses four PGB molecules to form the first tetrapyrrole, uroporphyrinogen. The initial product of the enzymic catalysis is the linear tetrapyrrole, hydroxymethylbilane, which, in the absence of uroporphyrinogen III cosynthase, spontaneously cyclizes to form uroporphyrinogen I. Biosynthesis of the biologically relevant isomer, uroporphyrinogen III, requires the presence of uroporphyrinogen III cosynthase during, or immediately after, release of the initial tetrapyrrole product of PBG deaminase.

PBG deaminase was purified 200-fold from *Euglena* (Williams et al., 1981). The native enzyme, a monomer of 41,000 molecular weight, does not contain a chromophoric prosthetic group or require metal ions for activity. This appears to conflict with a report of the isolation of a pteridine compound from *Euglena* cells which stimulates *Euglena* PBG deaminase activity in vitro (Juknat et al., 1988a, b). PGB deaminase from wheat germ and spinach leaves also has a molecular weight of about 40,000 (Higuchi and Bogorad, 1975). The molecular weight of the enzyme from *Chlorella regularis* was 35,000 (Shioi et al., 1980) and that of *R. spheroides* 36,000 (Jordan and Shemin, 1973), while the molecular weight of PBG deaminase from *R. palustris* was reported to be 74,000 (Kotler et al., 1987).

PBG deaminases from *R. spheroides* and *Euglena* were used to establish that the order of assembly of the four PBG units is ABCD, as they appear in uroporphyrinogen (Jordan and Seehra, 1979; Battersby et al., 1979b). Covalently enzyme-bound mono- through tetrapyrrole intermediates are formed (Jordan and Berry, 1981; Battersby et al., 1983) and then hydroxymethylbilane is released (Battersby et al., 1979a; Scott et al., 1980).

The nascent mono- through tetrapyrrole enzyme complexes have been shown to be bound via a dipyrrole cofactor (Hart et al., 1987; Jordan and Warren, 1987). In PBG deaminase from *E. coli*, the dipyrrole cofactor appears to attach to a cysteine group on the apoenzyme during formation of the protein, and remains permanently attached to the enzyme while the link between the cofactor and the nascent pyrrole chain is severed after the tetrapyrrole stage is reached. PBG deaminases from plant sources also contain the dipyrrole cofactor (Warren and Jordan, 1988).

Although PBG deaminase is a cytoplasmic enzyme in animal cells, it has been localized within the plastids in green and etiolated pea leaves and in *Arum* spadices (a nongreening tissue) (Smith, 1988) and has been shown to be associated with the stroma of developing pea leaf chloroplasts (Castelfranco et al., 1988). Earlier work had also suggested that a major proportion of activity in spinach leaves is associated with the chloroplasts (Bogorad, 1958).

3. Uroporphyrinogen III cosynthase. Uroporphyrinogen III cosynthase has been purified from *Euglena* (Hart and Battersby, 1985). The native enzyme is a monomer of 31,000 molecular weight and contains no reversibly bound cofactors or metal ions. The molecular weight value is similar to that of the rat liver enzyme (Kohashi et al., 1984) but contrasts with the value of 62,000 reported for the wheat germ enzyme (Higuchi and Bogorad, 1975). The insensitivity of the *Euglena* enzyme to diethyl pyrocarbonate (Hart and Battersby, 1985) suggests that it contains no essential histidine groups, in contrast to the human enzyme (Frydman and Feinstein, 1974).

PBG deaminase and uroporphyrinogen III cosynthase may form a complex that facilitates transfer of hydroxymethylbilane between the two enzymes. The presence of *Euglena* cosynthase influences the K_m of *Euglena* deaminase for PBG (Battersby et al., 1979c). The sedimentation velocity of wheat germ deaminase is also influenced by the presence of wheat germ cosynthase (Higuchi and Bogorad, 1975). The presence of *R. spheroides* cosynthase was reported to facilitate release of the tetrapyrrole product from PBG deaminase (Rosé et al., 1988).

4. Uroporphyrinogen decarboxylase. Uroporphyrinogen decarboxylase catalyzes the decarboxylation of all four of the acetate residues on uroporphyrinogen to yield coproporphyrinogen, which contains methyls in their place. There have been relatively few studies of this enzyme from photosynthetic organisms. Uroporphyrinogen decarboxylase activity was measured in leaf extracts of several plants and purified 72-fold from tobacco leaves (Chen and Miller, 1974). The highest activity was found in the soluble fraction of the leaf homogenate, and very little activity was found in the organelle fractions. No metal requirements were observed, and EDTA or other metal chelating agents enhanced activity. Uroporphyrinogen III was reported to be a much better substrate than uroporphyrinogen I for the tobacco enzyme.

5. Coproporphyrinogen oxidase. Although the ability of isolated cucumber plastids to form protoporphyrin from exogenous ALA indicates that plastids must contain coproporphyrinogen oxidase activity (Weinstein and Castelfranco, 1977; Castelfranco et al., 1979), the only reported extraction of this enzyme from higher plants indicated that in tobacco leaves coproporphyrinogen oxidase was associated with the mitochondria (Hsu and Miller, 1970).

Euglena coproporphyrinogen oxidase accepts ring A monovinyl porphyrinogen more readily than ring B monovinyl porphyrinogen as a substrate, suggesting that oxidative decarboxylation of the ring A propionate of coproporphyrinogen occurs before that of ring B (Cavaliero et al., 1974). Although O_2 is the electron acceptor in aerobic systems, extracts of anaerobic *R. spheroides* can carry out the reaction anaerobically in the presence of ATP, oxidized pyridine nucleotide, and methionine (Tait, 1972). These requirements are similar to those reported for anaerobic yeast extracts (Poulson and Polglase, 1974).

6. Protoporphyrinogen oxidase. Protoporphyrinogen oxidase activity has been detected in extracts of *R. spheroides* (Jacobs and Jacobs, 1981) and barley leaves (Jacobs et al., 1982; Jacobs and Jacobs, 1984a). The enzyme was found in both the plastid and mitochondrial fractions of etiolated barley leaves (Jacobs and Jacobs, 1987). The enzyme from the two organelles appeared to be identical. The approximately 210,000 molecular weight enzyme accepts both protoporphyrinogen and mesoporphyrinogen as a substrate, in contrast to the rat liver enzyme which accepts only protoporphyrinogen. Although the K_m of 5 μM for protoporphyrinogen was similar to the reported value for mammalian protoporphyrinogen oxidase, the pH optimum of 5 to 6 differed markedly from the optimum of 7.5 to 8.5 reported for the mammalian and yeast enzymes. Purified barley protoporphyrinogen oxidase ran as a single 36,000 molecular weight band on SDS-PAGE electrophoresis. Activity was stimulated by unsaturated fatty acids, suggesting that the plant enzyme may have a lipid requirement for activity (Jacobs and Jacobs, 1984b).

The electron acceptor in the reaction catalyzed by extracts of aerobically grown cells is O_2. However, nitrate or fumarate can function as the electron acceptor in the reaction in extracts of anaerobically grown *E. coli*, and presumably also in anaerobic photosynthetic bacteria.

C. Mg branch

1. Chlorophyll a formation

a. Chelation of Mg. Demonstration of the Mg-chelatase reaction in whole cells of *R. spheroides* was first achieved by Gorchein (1972). Protoporphyrin was incorporated into a mixture of lipids previously extracted from the bacteria and dispersed by sonication. This substrate mixture was administered to cells in the light under semi-anaerobic conditions (incubations were vigorously bubbled with N_2 and sealed with rubber stoppers). Aside from the cells and substrate mixture, the incubation contained only buffer and EGTA. Under these conditions, a typical 90-min incubation yielded approximately 20 nmol of Mg-protoporphyrin monomethyl ester. Independent formation of unesterified Mg-protoporphyrin could not be demonstrated. Incubation in the dark, aeration of the incubation mixture, or omission of the lipid resulted in drastically diminished (at least sixfold) recovery of product. Dialysis of the cells against distilled water for 16 h resulted in loss of half the activity, but this activity could be restored by inclusion of *S*-adenosyl-methionine or ATP plus methionine in the incubation mixture. Compounds which inhibit *S*-adenosyl-methionine formation also inhibited Mg-protoporphyrin monomethyl ester formation, although the unesterified form did not accumulate under conditions where formation of the methyl ester was prevented.

Attempts to demonstrate activity in cell-free extracts were unsuccessful even with gentle methods of cell breakage (Gorchein, 1973). Spheroplasts prepared by incubation with lysozyme retained much of the original activity, but this activity was lost even when the spheroplasts were lysed by osmotic shock. Activity was not restored by addition of hypothetical cofactors. Although activity was supported in the dark in an atmosphere containing 5% O_2, concentrations above 5% were inhibitory. Experiments with inhibitors of electron transport, uncouplers, and oligomycin suggested a need for ATP, which was not related to the methylation step. The experimental results of Gorchein (1972, 1973) suggest requirements for membrane intactness, low O_2 tension, ATP, and coupling of Mg insertion to methylation.

Although it is tempting to assume that Mg chelation in green plants occurs by the same process, the mechanisms may be as different as they are for ALA formation. Early attempts to measure Mg-chelatase activity in extracts of higher plants were not very successful or definitive. In the first partially successful attempt, unpurified homogenates of etiolated wheat seedlings formed very limited and nonreproducible amounts of Mg-protoporphyrin, as measured by incorporation of $^{28}Mg^{2+}$ (Ellsworth and Lawrence, 1973). ALA or protoporphyrinogen, but not protoporphyrin, could serve as a substrate for this reaction. Incubation of etioplasts or developing chloroplasts from cucumber cotyledons with protoporphyrin and a mixture of cofactors (ATP, NAD, CoA, GSH, and methanol) resulted in the accumulation of a mixture of components termed MPE-equivalents (Smith and Rebeiz, 1977). These components included Mg-protoporphyrin, Mg-protoporphyrin monomethyl ester, and other components that were presumed to be intermediates between Mg-protoporphyrin monomethyl ester and protochlorophyllide. Although the individual components were not resolved, the collection of products was detected and quantified by their fluorescence emission spectra.

A similar preparation of developing chloroplasts from cucumber cotyledons was further refined, in which only one (or two) major products accumulated, and the requirements and conditions for the reaction were examined in more detail (Castelfranco et al., 1979). Incubation of this chloroplast preparation with protoporphyrin, glutamate, and a cofactor mixture (ATP, NAD, and GSH) resulted in the accumulation of Mg-protoporphyrin and its monomethyl ester. The products were identified by their fluorescence excitation and emission spectra and by their retention times on reverse-phase HPLC. ATP and glutamate (or α-ketoglutarate) were absolutely required, but the requirement for protoporphyrin could be met by in situ generation from precursors. Essentially similar results were obtained using a radioactive assay and separating the fully methylated products by HPLC (Richter and Rienits, 1980). However, in contrast to the situation with plastids from cucumbers, the major product formed in incubations with plastids from dark-grown wheat was Zn-protoporphyrin.

The perplexing requirement for glutamate in Mg-protoporphyrin formation was subsequently explained by demonstrating that glutamate provided an indirect source of extra ATP by serving as a substrate for ATP generation via oxidative phosphorylation occurring in mitochondria which contaminated the chloroplast preparation (Pardo et al., 1980). High concentrations of ATP could be substituted for glutamate in developing plastids isolated by differential centrifugation, and plastids that were purified by density gradient centrifugation could not use glutamate to enhance Mg-protoporphyrin formation. Concentrations of

ATP as high as 10 mM did not saturate the reaction, and other nucleoside triphosphates could not substitute for ATP. AMP was strongly inhibitory; 50% inhibition was observed at 3.5 mM AMP in the presence of 10 mM ATP. Properties of the Mg-chelatase from developing cucumber chloroplasts were further defined by investigations of substrate concentration dependence (Fuesler et al., 1981) and methylation state of the product (Fuesler et al., 1982). Endogenous Mg^{2+} and Zn^{2+} were removed by repeated washings of the developing plastids in buffer containing 10 mM EDTA. Subsequent incubation of the washed plastids indicated an optimal Mg^{2+} concentration around 10 mM, with concentrations greater than 10 mM causing substantial inhibition. In plastids isolated from tissue that was greened for 20 h, the optimal ATP concentration was 10 mM, with slight inhibition occurring at higher concentrations, and half-maximal activity achieved at 3.5 mM. Half-maximal activity was achieved with 3.5 μM protoporphyrin, and saturation occurred at 10 μM. All of the concentration curves were sigmoidal in shape (Fuesler et al., 1981). The sigmoidal shape may reflect cooperative catalytic behavior of the enzyme, or it may reflect the barrier presented by the chloroplast envelope (however, see the information below on localization of the activity). The washed plastids were capable of forming Zn-protoporphyrin when 5 mM $ZnCl_2$ was added to the preparations, although half of this activity was nonenzymic.

Breakage of the developing chloroplasts by lysis in hypotonic media resulted in a drastic decrease in activity to a level less than 0.2% (on a pmol product h^{-1} mg^{-1} protein basis) of that in intact plastids (Richter and Rienits, 1982). Removal of the stromal components by centrifugation, and incubation of the membranes with substrates resulted in 2.5% of the activity of intact plastids. Under these conditions, protoporphyrin dependence was saturated at 0.1 μM, with half-maximal activity occurring at approximately 0.025 μM. The optimum concentration of added ATP was 3.0 mM, when an ATP-regenerating system was included. The concentration dependence curves for protoporphyrin and ATP were not sigmoidal.

Mg-chelatase activity was sensitive to the mercurial reagents, p-chloromercuribenzoate (PCMB) and p-chloromercuribenzoyl sulfonate (PCMBS), the latter being less capable of permeating biological membranes (Fuesler et al., 1984b). Pretreatment of plastids with PCMBS and recovery of the plastids after centrifugation through a pad of 45% Percoll, resulted in complete inhibition of Mg-chelatase activity upon subsequent incubation with substrates. A similar treatment had only minor effects on two PCMB-sensitive stromal enzymes. Intact chloroplasts formed equivalent amounts of Mg-protoporphyrin with 10 μM protoporphyrin or 6.0 mM ALA as the substrate (Fuesler et al., 1984a). The PCMBS inhibition of Mg-protoporphyrin accumulation was equivalent with either substrate. Thus, PCMBS was not acting via an effect on the entry of protoporphyrin into the plastid. It is difficult to explain these results in any way other than by postulating that the Mg-chelatase is localized in the chloroplast envelope (Fuesler et al., 1984b).

In the normal incubations, the major product was the unesterified form of Mg-protoporphyrin. When 1.0 mM S-adenosyl-methionine was included in the reaction mixture, the major product was Mg-proto-porphyrin monomethyl ester, and formation of the ester was dependent upon exogenous S-adenosyl-methionine (Fuesler et al., 1982). ATP plus methionine could not substitute for S-adenosyl-methionine. Thus, in developing chloroplasts from cucumber cotyledons, Mg chelation and methylation are not obligatorily coupled as they are in $R.$ $spheroides.$ In addition, the sequence of formation was confirmed as

$$\text{Protoporphyrin} \rightarrow \text{Mg-protoporphyrin}$$
$$\rightarrow \text{Mg-protoporphyrin monomethyl ester}$$

which is consistent with the earlier proposal of Radmer and Bogorad (1967).

b. Mg-protoporphyrin methyl transferase. The enzyme catalyzing the methylation of Mg-protoporphyrin, S-adenosyl-methionine-Mg-proto-porphyrin IX methyltransferase (EC 2.1.1.11), has been characterized from a number of sources, including $R.$ $spheroides$ (Gibson et al., 1963; Hinchigeri et al., 1984), wheat (Ellsworth et al., 1974; Ellsworth and St. Pierre, 1976; Hinchigeri et al., 1981), $Euglena$ (Ebbon and Tait, 1969; Hinchigeri et al., 1981), maize (Radmer and Bogorad, 1967), and barley and other plants (Shieh et al., 1978). This enzyme is relatively easy to assay and its kinetic mechanism has been the object of numerous studies.

The enzyme from $R.$ $spheroides$ was most active with Mg-proto-porphyrin, and very much less so with protoporphyrin, Ca- or Zn-proto-porphyrin, and not active at all with protoporphyrinogen, or heme (Gibson et al., 1963). The K_m values for Mg-protoporphyrin and S-adenosyl-methionine were 40 and 55 μM, respectively. The enzyme was tightly bound to membranous chromatophores, and was not present under conditions where bacteriochlorophyll is not formed (high aeration, in the dark). The enzyme from wheat is soluble in 0.5 M sucrose and 1.0 M NaCl, and has K_m values of 22 and 44 μM for Mg-protoporphyrin and S-adenosyl-methionine, respectively (Ellsworth et al., 1974). The wheat enzyme activity in extracts from etiolated and greening tissues did not differ significantly (Ellsworth and St. Pierre, 1976). Two forms of the enzyme were found in $Euglena$, one soluble (15 to 20% of the total) and the other bound to the chloroplast membranes. The bound form could be solubilized by Tween 80 (Ebbon and Tait, 1969). It was proposed that the soluble portion of the enzyme had not yet become incorporated into the membrane. The K_m for Mg-protoporphyrin was in the range of 10 to 34 μM, and the K_m for S-adenosyl-methionine varied between 20 to 160 μM, depending upon the fraction tested and the presence or absence of detergent in the assay. Cells grown in the light contained two to three times more activity than dark-grown cells.

The methyltransferase is a bisubstrate enzyme, and the kinetic mechanism has been investigated by classical initial velocity studies (Ellsworth et al., 1974) and by combining initial velocity studies with behavior on affinity columns (Hinchigeri et al., 1981, 1984; Richards et al., 1987a). The wheat enzyme has a ping-pong mechanism, with S-adenosyl-methionine binding first, followed by release of S-adenosyl-homocysteine before binding of the second substrate, Mg-protoporphyrin (Ellsworth et al., 1974; Hinchigeri et al., 1981; Richards et al., 1987a). This mechanism is consistent with the existence of a methylated enzyme intermediate. Treatment of the enzyme with [methyl-^{14}C]-S-adenosyl-methionine followed by exhaustive dialysis resulted in 60 times more radioactivity incorporated into the methyltransferase than into an equivalent amount of bovine serum albumen treated in a similar manner. More direct evidence for the methylated enzyme was not obtained (Hinchigeri et al., 1981). In contrast to the wheat enzyme, the enzyme from *Euglena* has a random mechanism (Hinchigeri et al., 1981), and the *R. spheroides* enzyme has an ordered mechanism, with Mg-protoporphyrin binding first (Hinchigeri et al., 1984).

The use of the affinity columns to gain insight into the kinetic mechanism is quite interesting, and the behavior of the wheat and *Euglena* enzymes on affinity columns will be described in more detail (Hinchigeri et al., 1981). In the case of the wheat enzyme, it was known that heme is an inhibitor that is competitive with Mg-protoporphyrin, and that there is a drastic decline in activity upon shifting from the optimum pH of 7.8 to 9 (Ellsworth et al., 1974). A column with covalently coupled heme was prepared and cell-free homogenates were passed through the column under a variety of conditions. The methyltransferase activity did not bind to the column unless S-adenosyl-methionine was included in the application buffer. Thus, the presence of S-adenosyl-methionine is required for binding to heme (or Mg-protoporphyrin). This behavior would be expected for an enzyme with a ping-pong mechanism or an ordered mechanism with S-adenosyl-methionine binding first. If the mechanism were ordered, it would be expected that the methyltransferase would be eluted simply by removing S-adenosyl-methionine from the elution buffer. However, removal of S-adenosyl-methionine was not sufficient for elution. Instead, elution required changing the pH. In contrast, the *Euglena* enzyme bound to columns having Mg-protoporphyrin or S-adenosyl-homocysteine ligands in the absence of the other substrate. This behavior is indicative of a random kinetic mechanism (Hinchigeri et al., 1981; Hinchigeri and Richards, 1982; Richards et al., 1987a). As would be expected, these affinity columns were also very useful for purification of the methyl-transferases. Purification factors for this step ranged from 460- to 2000-fold (Richards et al., 1987a).

c. Isocyclic ring formation. The formation of the isocyclic ring is a complex process in which one of the propionate side chains is converted to the fifth ring. In this series of reactions the methyl propionate side chain at position 6 of the macrocycle is joined to the γ-meso bridge of the metalloporphyrin ring, forming a five-membered ring between pyrrole ring C and the meso bridge (Fig. 7.6). The ring is substituted with a keto group on the β carbon, and the carboxyl group remains methylated. Attachment to the main ring is through the α carbon of the side chain. Formation of the ring creates a new asymmetric center in the R configuration on position 10 of the new macrocycle. The compound formed is called Mg-2,4-divinylpheoporphyrin a_5, and it has also been referred to

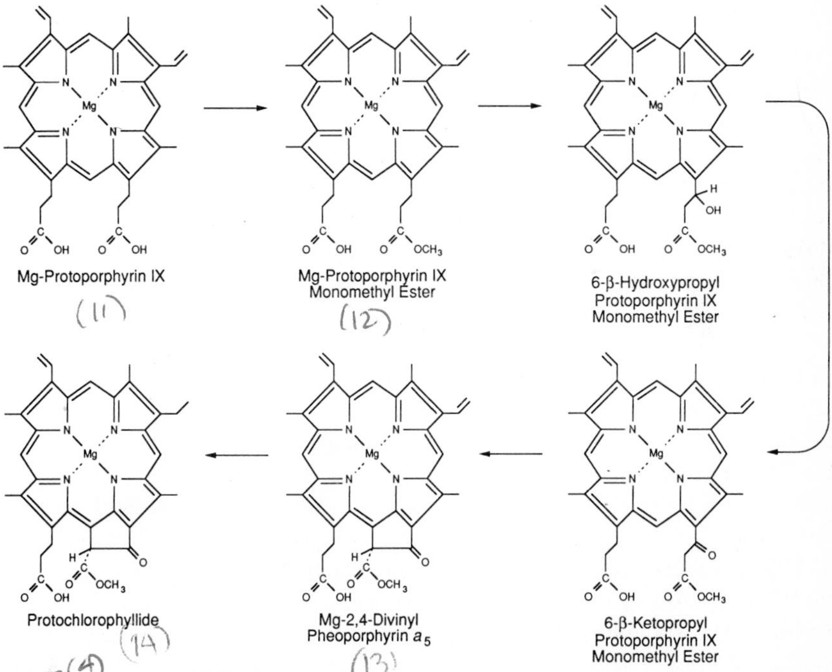

Figure 7.6 Proposed steps in the conversion of Mg-protoporphyrin IX to protochlorophyllide. The step where reduction of the B ring vinyl to ethyl occurs may vary with species and developmental conditions.

as divinylprotochlorophyllide. Reduction of the vinyl group at position 4 of the macrocycle yields protochlorophyllide. Formation of this product occurs in photosynthetic bacteria as well as in chloroplasts of eukaryotic organisms, but there is no assurance that the mechanisms are the same in these two very different classes of organisms. Information on the chemical nature of the intermediates has come from analysis of mutants which excrete or accumulate intermediates in the pathway beyond Mg-protoporphyrin. In other in vivo studies, the accumulation of putative intermediates has been caused by administration of inhibitors or by flooding the biosynthetic system with precursors. In each case, a sequence of steps has been inferred from the structures of the accumulated products and the chemistry required to proceed from Mg-protoporphyrin methyl ester to chlorophyllide. Those initial studies formed the basis of more recent investigations of the individual steps in cell-free systems.

Mg-divinylpheoporphyrin a_5 was identified in cultures of *R. spheroides* in which bacteriochlorophyll synthesis had been partially inhibited by treatment with 8-hydroxyquinoline (Jones, 1963a, b). This compound also accumulates, or is excreted, in some bacteriochlorophyll-deficient mutants of *R. spheroides* (Richards and Lascelles, 1969; Pradel and Clement-Metral, 1976). The Mg-divinylpheoporphyrin a_5 which accumulated in one of the above mutants was collected, purified, and administered to etioplast membranes from barley (Griffiths and Jones, 1975). When NADPH was added, the Mg-divinylpheoporphyrin a_5 was photoconverted to chlorophyllide. Thus, the Mg-divinylpheoporphyrin a_5 which accumulates in bacteriochlorophyll-deficient mutants of *R. spheroides* also served as a substrate for chlorophyllide biosynthesis in higher plants. The existence of Mg-divinylpheoporphyrin a_5 in the protochlorophyllide pool of etiolated cucumber cotyledons and other dark-grown higher plants was demonstrated by Rebeiz and co-workers (Belanger and Rebeiz, 1979, 1980a). They also demonstrated that both Mg-divinylpheoporphyrin a_5 and protochlorophyllide (monovinyl) are photoconverted to divinyl- and monovinylchlorophyllides after a brief flash of light (Belanger and Rebeiz, 1980b). Identification of the compound as Mg-divinylpheoporphyrin a_5 was made on the basis of its fluorescence emission and excitation spectra at 77 K and its behavior on thin layers of polyethylene. These properties were identical to those of a standard isolated from a *R. spheroides* mutant (Belanger and Rebeiz, 1980a).

Granick (1950) proposed that the formation of the isocyclic ring occurs via β oxidation of the 6-methyl propionate group to a 6-methyl β-keto-propionate side chain. The α-methylene group would then attach to the γ-meso bridge of the porphyrin in an oxidative cyclization. In the fatty acid β-oxidation model, the β-keto group is introduced by desaturation of the α-carbon–β-carbon bond, followed by hydration of the double bond to form a β-hydroxy substituent. The β-hydroxy is then oxidized to form the β-keto group. It has been proposed that the presence of the methylated ester prevents the spontaneous decarboxylation of what would otherwise be a β-ketoacid (Bogorad, 1966). Accumulated intermediates corresponding to the 6-methyl-, acrylate, β-hydroxy propionate, and β-ketopropionate derivatives of Mg-protoporphyrin were characterized in a series of chlorophyll-deficient mutants of *Chlorella* (Ellsworth and Aronoff, 1968, 1969).

Formation of protochlorophyllide from ^{3}H-labeled Mg-protoporphyrin monomethyl ester was demonstrated in crude extracts of etiolated wheat seedlings (Ellsworth and Hervish, 1975). Incorporation of label required a complex cofactor mixture including ATP, coenzyme A, *S*-adenosyl-methionine, and inorganic phosphate. Activities were not reported, nor was the product distinguished as being the mono- or divinyl form. A similar conversion was reported in developing cucumber chloroplasts (Mattheis and Rebeiz, 1977).

Formation of the isocyclic ring from exogenous porphyrins by developing cucumber chloroplasts has been investigated by Castelfranco and co-workers. Preliminary studies in intact tissue suggested that the conversion required O_2 and Fe (Spiller et al., 1982). A preparation of developing chloroplasts similar to that used for Mg-chelatase studies (above) converted added Mg-protoporphyrin to protochlorophyllide in the dark when either *S*-adenosyl-methionine or ATP plus methionine were included in the incubation mixture (Chereskin and Castelfranco, 1982). The conversion did not occur in an atmosphere of N_2. It was also found that the Mg-protoporphyrin substrate was unstable in the light in air. Even in the absence of plastids, a 1-h incubation in strong light (90 $\mu E \cdot m^{-2} \cdot s^{-1}$, PAR) caused almost complete disappearance of the Mg-protoporphyrin. The accumulated product was subsequently shown to be Mg-divinylpheoporphyrin a_5 by comparison of its fluorescence and chromatographic properties (Chereskin et al., 1982) to published properties and by detailed analysis of corrected fluorescence spectra at 77 K, nuclear magnetic resonance, and secondary-ion mass spectroscopy of the highly purified product of the incubation mixtures (Chereskin et al., 1983).

The optimal requirements for Mg-divinylpheoporphyrin a_5 formation from Mg-protoporphyrin and Mg-protoporphyrin monomethyl ester in intact chloroplasts were also reported (Chereskin et al., 1982). The optimal substrate concentration for either substrate was 10 μM, with activity declining at higher concentrations. The presence of 1 mM *S*-adenosyl-methionine stimulated activity with either substrate, although it was required only when Mg-protoporphyrin was the substrate. A separate experiment indicated that an active methyl esterase was present in the plastid preparation. Although not absolutely required, the presence of either NADP or NADPH at 0.6 mM stimulated activity. Dependence on O_2 was investigated by incubating samples in air/N_2, and air/CO mixtures. When activity was plotted vs. partial pressure of O_2 in the incubation, hyperbolic curves were obtained, with half-saturation occurring at 0.04 atm of O_2. Inhibitor studies did not support the involvement of a hemoprotein in a hydroxylation reaction to introduce the O_2, nor the involvement of a classical β-oxidation scheme. The location of the ring-forming enzyme(s) within the intact chloroplast was investigated by the use of permeant and nonpermeant mercurial reagents (Fuesler et al., 1984b). Unlike Mg-chelatase, the cyclase system in intact chloroplasts was insensitive to inhibition by PCMBS, but it was inhibited by PCMB, which is able to cross the membrane. Thus, the cyclase system is probably localized within the chloroplast.

Also unlike Mg-chelatase, the cyclase system was active in broken chloroplasts (Chereskin et al., 1982). This property was used to resolve the cyclase activity into two required enzymic fractions (Wong and Castelfranco, 1984). Developing chloroplasts were disrupted by sonication and fractionated into a high-speed supernatant and a membranous pellet. The enzymes in the supernatant were recovered by precipitation at 80% saturation of $(NH_4)_2SO_4$, followed by dialysis of the dissolved pellet. Reconstitution of cyclase activity required both membrane-bound and soluble protein fractions, plus Mg-porphyrin substrate, O_2, and reduced pyridine nucleotide. As with the intact system, activity with Mg-protoporphyrin methyl ester was stimulated by inclusion of S-adenosyl-methionine, and activity with Mg-protoporphyrin required S-adenosyl-methionine. The shape of the concentration curve for Mg-protoporphyrin methyl ester was hyperbolic to 10 μM, and activity declined at higher concentrations. Half-maximal activity was achieved with approximately 2 μM substrate. Unlike the intact plastid system, the requirement for a reduced pyridine nucleotide was absolute in the reconstituted cyclase system. The concentration curve with NADPH was hyperbolic, with a saturating concentration of approximately 5 mM and half-maximal activity achieved at approximately 0.9 mM. The NADH concentration dependence curve was slightly sigmoidal at lower concentrations, with half-maximal activity occurring at approximately 1.8 mM and saturation also at 5 mM. Activity with NADPH declined at concentrations greater than 5 mM, so that at higher concentrations, activity was equivalent with either cofactor. It must be noted that the activity measurements were for a 1-h incubation and were not initial-rate measurements. Thus, these values define the shape of the concentration dependence curves but cannot be considered to be kinetic constants.

The reconstituted cyclase system was used to test a variety of inhibitors and possible intermediates (Wong and Castelfranco, 1985; Wong et al., 1985; Walker et al., 1988). The cyclase was inhibited by mercurial sulfhydryl reagents and the sulfhydryl alkylating agent, N-ethylmaleimide. Both the membranous and soluble fractions of the cyclase system were susceptible to inhibition by the latter reagent. The sulfhydryl-containing compounds, dithiothreitol and mercaptoethanol, were also inhibitory, suggesting the presence of a sensitive disulfide. The Mg-porphyrin specificity of the cyclase system was tested by administration of synthetic derivatives of Mg-protoporphyrin IX monomethyl ester, in which the side chain at the 6 position of the macrocycle was modified. Both β-hydroxy and β-keto derivatives (Fig. 7.6) were effective substrates for Mg-divinylpheoporphyrin a_5 formation. However, the acrylate derivative was ineffective. Only one enantiomer of the β-hydroxy derivative was effective as a substrate. When Mg-protoporphyrin monomethyl ester was the substrate, a product from the incubation mixture having the transient kinetic behavior of an intermediate was isolated and identified as the β-hydroxy derivative (Wong et al., 1985). This intermediate was not detected when the β-keto derivative was used as a substrate. When the β-keto derivative was used as a substrate, formation of Mg-divinylpheoporphyrin a_5 still required the presence of O_2 and NADPH as well as both the soluble and membrane-bound portions of the reconstituted cyclase system. The monovinyl (2-vinyl, 4-ethyl) form of the β-keto derivative was four times more active than the divinyl, β-keto derivative in the cyclization reaction (Walker et al., 1988). When Mg-protoporphyrin was the substrate, the mono- and divinyl forms were equally effective.

A system catalyzing a similar reaction in isolated etioplasts of wheat has now been characterized by a continuous spectroscopic assay (Nasrulhaq-Boyce et al., 1987). While most of the properties of this preparation were similar to those of the cucumber preparation described above, there were some significant differences and additions. The wheat system has an absolute requirement for organelle intactness, and could be inhibited by lipophilic Fe chelators and anaerobiosis. The Zn-chelate could replace the Mg-chelate as substrate, but the Cu, Ni, and free porphyrins could not. Greening of etiolated tissue for 10 h did not increase or decrease the activity in subsequently isolated plastids.

In summary, formation of the isocyclic ring from Mg-protoporphyrin monomethyl ester requires O_2, NADPH, and enzyme(s) from the chloroplast stroma and membranes. Ring formation proceeds through 6-methyl-β-hydroxy- and 6-methyl-β-keto-propionate derivatives (Fig. 7.6), consistent with earlier proposals (Granick, 1950; Ellsworth and Aronoff, 1968, 1969). However, since the 6-methyl-acrylate derivative was ineffective as a substrate, the initial formation of the β-hydroxy derivative is probably not via hydration of a double bond as would be expected for a classical β-oxidation sequence. Instead, introduction of the O_2 may come about by a mixed-function oxidase reaction, as suggested by Castelfranco and co-workers (Chereskin et al., 1982; Wong and Castelfranco, 1984). The latter proposal is consistent with the O_2 and NADPH requirements for isocyclic ring formation, and with the recent finding that ^{18}O is incorporated into the product when ring formation occurs in the presence of $^{18}O_2$ (Walker et al., 1989).

d. Vinyl group reduction.   Although plants may contain some chlorophyll end products having vinyl groups in both the 2 and 4 positions of the macrocycle (reviewed in Rebeiz et al., 1983), the majority of chlorophyll end products have the 4 side chain reduced to an ethyl group. It appears likely that this reduction could occur at any number of points along the biosynthetic pathway, depending upon the nature of the plant and its growth history (Belanger and Rebeiz, 1980a–c, 1982; Rebeiz et al., 1983). Despite the relative importance of the vinyl reduction step to the branched pathway proposal (see below), there has not been very much work reported on the biochemistry of this step.

Ellsworth and Hsing (1973) used unpurified homogenates of etiolated wheat to catalyze incorporation of label from ^3H-NADH into the vinyl group. The original homogenization buffer had a relatively high salt concentration (0.2 M phosphate buffer) that might be expected to strip peripheral proteins off the membranes. Mg-protoporphyrin monomethyl ester was an effective porphyrin substrate, but protoporphyrin and Mg-divinylpheoporphyrin a_5 were not. NADPH was ineffective as a hydrogen donor. Incorporation of label into the 4 position rather than the 2 position was verified by analysis of the chromic acid oxidation products. Further analysis of this preparation indicated a pH optimum around 7.7 and a K_m for Mg-protoporphyrin monomethyl ester of 25 μM (Ellsworth and Hsing, 1974). The K_m for NADH could not be determined. In preliminary reports, Richards and co-workers (Kwan et al., 1986; Richards et al., 1987a) described the behavior of the 4-vinyl reductase on affinity columns. Most of the enzyme activity from a high-speed supernatant of etiolated wheat seedlings was retained on a column of Zn-protoporphyrin monomethyl ester, in the presence or absence of NAD. The enzyme was eluted by changing the pH from 7.7 to 9.0. A 70-fold purification was achieved compared to the activity of the applied extract.

The substrate specificity for the reduced pyridine nucleotide was also examined by enzymatic preparation of both 4-R and 4-S steriosomers of 4-[^3H]-NADH and 4-[^3H]-NADPH. Although insufficient detail was presented to allow comparison of their relative effectiveness, both Mg-protoporphyrin monomethyl ester and Mg-divinylpheoporphyrin a_5 were substrates for the reductase (Kwan et al., 1986; Richards et al., 1987a). With either porphyrin substrate, [4R-^3H]-NADPH was best able to transfer label to the reaction product. The specificity experiments were performed with whole or broken etioplast preparations, rather than unpurified extracts or purified enzyme, and both reported specificities conflict with the earlier results of Ellsworth and Hsing (1973).

e. Protochlorophyllide reduction. Plants, requiring light for greening, accumulate small amounts of protochlorophyllide when grown in the dark. Upon exposure to white light, the double bond between carbons 7 and 8 of ring D is reduced to form chlorophyllide (compare Figs. 7.2 and 7.6). Most algae and gymnosperms do not require light for greening, and the conversion of protochlorophyllide to chlorophyllide is independent of light. In this conversion, two new chiral centers are created and the molecule retains its aromaticity.

i. Light-requiring reduction catalyzed by protochlorophyllide oxidoreductase. The light-dependent transformation can be followed by observing the spectral changes associated with the protein-bound pigment. In situ, the protochlorophyllide of etiolated plants has an absorbance maximum near 650 nm, and a shoulder a 638 nm. Following a 10-s illumination, the absorbance maximum shifts to 678 nm and there is a corresponding decrease in the 650-nm absorbing form (Gassman et al., 1968). During the next 30 s in the dark, the wavelength shifts to 684 nm, and finally to 672 nm after about 20 min (Shibata, 1957). This last transformation is commonly referred to as the Shibata shift. An action spectrum indicated that the photoreceptor for these transformations is protochlorophyllide (Koski et al., 1951). When ALA was administered to the etiolated plants before illumination, another protochlorophyllide form, having a maximum at 630 nm, accumulated. This form was phototransformable only if the plants were given a series of flashes with intervening dark periods (Gassman, 1973). The physical state of protochlorophyllide in plant tissue has been reviewed (Virgin, 1981), as have some of the theories relating the photoreduction to developmental processes (Kasemir, 1983). The present discussion will focus on the biochemical explanation of these changes as well as some of the more rapid photochemical transformations.

Isolated etioplasts that are effective in phototransformation of protochlorophyllide have been studied (Horton and Leech, 1972) and used to identify the enzyme catalyzing the transformation as well as the required cofactors (Griffiths, 1974a, 1978; Oliver and Griffiths, 1980; reviewed in Griffiths and Oliver, 1984). The most effective preparations are from membranes that are recovered by centrifugation from lysed etioplasts. Supplementation of the membranes with an NADPH-regenerating system resulted in increased photoreduction activity (Griffiths, 1974a). Specific incorporation of ^{3}H-NADPH into chlorophyllide proved that NADPH was the source of reducing equivalents (Griffiths, 1981). Subsequently, it was shown that the hydride on the S face of NADPH was incorporated into the chlorophyllide (Richards et al., 1987a). Protochlorophyll was not an effective substrate in vitro (Griffiths, 1947b) and both the mono- and divinyl forms of protochlorophyllide were effective (Griffiths and Jones, 1975; Belanger and Rebeiz, 1980b) The formal name for the enzyme is NADPH : protochlorophyllide oxidoreductase (EC 1.6.99.1).

The polypeptide catalyzing the reaction was identified by labeling active membrane preparations with the sulfhydryl reagent, N-phenylmaleimide, while protected by substrates. Excess reagents were removed by gel filtration and the labeling was repeated in the light in the presence of ^{3}H-N-phenylmaleimide (Oliver and Griffiths, 1980). Light is required to photoreduce the bound protochlorophyllide and liberate the products, allowing the released products and the N-phenylmaleimide to compete for the site of the active thiol. The extent of photoconversion of the bound substrate was directly proportional to the extent of inhibition of activity upon subsequent reincubation of the modified membranes with fresh substrates (Griffiths and Oliver, 1984). The modified membrane proteins were electrophoresed on an SDS polyacrylamide gel and incorporation of label was detected by fluorography. Label incorporation into a 35,000 to 37,000 molecular weight band (perhaps a doublet) was proportional to the degree of photoconversion during the radioactive labeling period.

An active form of the enzyme could be solubilized from membranes with low concentrations of the nonionic detergent Triton X100 (Beer and Griffiths, 1981; Apel et al., 1980). The purified enzyme from etiolated oat seedlings is composed of 346 amino acids, contains one cysteine and no tryptophan residues, and has a molecular weight of 37,800 (Roper et al., 1987). An active enzyme could also be solubilized from membranes with the zwitterionic detergent, CHAPS (Richards et al., 1987b). In this case, the specific activity of the solubilized enzyme was greater than in the membranes. An affinity column with Mg- or Zn-divinylpheoporphyrin a_5 as the ligand could be used to enhance the purification of the CHAPS-solubilized enzyme. Although contaminating polypeptides were removed by this procedure, much of the activity was lost. The enzyme could be dissociated from the column by free ligand, but not by removal of NADP or by changing the pH. It can be concluded from these results that the enzyme does not require the presence of pyridine nucleotide for binding of the metalloporphyrin substrate. Enzyme activity was inhibited 50% by 20 μM of the flavin analogue, quinacrine, and the activity in various preparations was proportional to the amount of extractable FAD (Walker and Griffiths, 1988). However, more-definitive information is required before it can be concluded that the reductase is a flavoprotein.

The cell-free preparations have been used to analyze some of the spectral changes observed in situ. The photoactive complex from freshly isolated etioplasts has protochlorophyllide and NADPH tightly bound to it, and it absorbs at 628 and 650 nm. This form has been called protochlorophyllide holochrome and is now known to be the substrate-loaded reductase. When the preparation is exposed to light, the pro-tochlorophyllide is immediately photoconverted to chlorophyllide with an absorbance maximum at 678 nm. This form shifts to 672 nm upon further incubation in the dark. However, a 677-nm form can be stabilized in the dark if the preparation is supplemented with NADP. If the photoconversion is carried out in the presence of excess NADPH, or if an NADPH-regenerating system is added to a system containing the 677-nm form, the absorbance maximum shifts to 682-to-684 nm. Protochloro-phyllide alone in aqueous detergent suspension absorbs maximally at 628 to 630 nm, and is considered to be the nonphototransformable or un-bound form of the pigment observed in situ after ALA administration. Conversion to the 672-nm form is enhanced by the addition of free protochlorophyllide to the 682-to-684-nm form, or by addition of N-phenylmaleimide to either the 677- or 682-to-684-nm forms.

These results have been interpreted in terms of a ternary complex of the enzyme, the chromophore, and the reduced or oxidized form of the bound pyridine nucleotide (Oliver and Griffiths, 1982). The model is illustrated in Fig. 7.7. The 628-to-630-nm form is unbound protochloro-

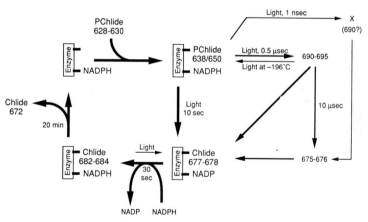

Figure 7.7 Light-dependent protochlorophyllide reduction cycle. The en-zyme is shown as a rectangle with binding sites for (proto)chlorophyllide and NADP(H). The pigment forms are designated by their light absorption maxima. The normal cycle, which occurs at room temperature in intact leaves or in reconstituted enzyme preparations, is shown on the left with heavy arrows. Intermediates in the light-dependent part of the cycle are shown in smaller letters and connected with lighter arrows. These intermedi-ates are observed at low temperatures and/or with rapidly responding optical equipment. Abbreviations: PChlide, protochlorophyllide; Chlide, chlorophyllide.

phyllide. The 638-to-650-nm form is the ternary complex between protochlorophyllide, enzyme, and NADPH. The 638-to-650-nm form is phototransformed by a brief flash of light to a 677-to-678-nm form which is the ternary complex of chlorophyllide, enzyme, and NADP. The NADP on the 677-to-678-nm form can be exchanged for fresh NADPH to form the 682-to-684-nm form. Finally, the chlorophyllide on the 684-nm ternary complex is slowly released (the Shibata shift) to become the 672-nm form, and to allow the binary complex of enzyme and NADPH to accept a new molecule of protochlorophyllide and repeat the cycle.

The dependence upon the NADP/NADPH ratio for the 678- to 682-to-684-nm shift was also shown independently by El Hamouri and Sironval (1980). In intact leaves, the 682-to-684-nm form (enzyme-chlorophyllide-NADPH) can be driven back to the 678-nm form (enzyme-chlorophyllide-NADP) by a brief intense flash of red light (Franck and Inoue, 1984). The light-driven back reaction is much slower at colder temperatures. If the 672-nm form was similarly illuminated, there was a substantial O_2 uptake by the etioplasts accompanied by photodestruction of the pigment. When the 682-to-684-nm form was illuminated, both the O_2 uptake and photodestruction were significantly diminished (Franck and Schmid, 1985). The authors concluded that the in situ formation of the 682-to-684-nm complex is a mechanism to protect the newly formed pigment from photodestruction.

Several other spectral shifts have been observed in situ or in vitro with rapid kinetic techniques and/or very low temperatures. An intermediate absorbing at 690 to 695 nm and formed from the 638-to-650-nm form was detected within 0.5 μs of a dye laser flash in crude extracts of bean leaves (Franck and Mathis, 1980). This intermediate was not fluorescent and partially decayed to a 675-to-676-nm form with a half-life of 7 to 10 μs. The half-life of the decay increased at temperatures below $-10°C$. A similar flash-induced and nonfluorescent intermediate forms at $-105°C$, and is stabilized at $-196°C$ (Dujardin et al., 1986). If the temperature is raised to $-20°C$, the intermediate decays to the 678-nm form. The 690-to-695-nm intermediate could be converted back to the photoactive protochlorophyllide by a subsequent laser flash of 695-nm light given at $-196°C$. Finally, when etioplast membranes were excited with a 35-ps pulse of light, the fluorescence at 657 nm due to the 638-to-650-nm-absorbing forms decayed within 1 ns (van Bochove et al., 1984). That the flash-induced fluorescence decay of 1 ns represented an initial step in photoconversion was supported by the following observations: Preillumination for 1 min eliminated the flash-induced fluorescence decay, presumably by photoconverting all the photoactive protochlorophyllide. Addition of NADPH after the preillumination restored the flash-induced fluorescence decay, presumably by allowing the reformation of phototransformable from endogenous nonphototransformable protochlorophyllide. The fluorescence decay was also temperature-dependent, increasing from 1 ns at 20°C to 3.5 ns at -196°C. It is not clear whether the fluorescence decay represents the formation of the 690-to-695-nm-absorbing intermediate. However, when repetitive pulses were given at -196°C, fluorescence decay was still observed, but no product accumulated, suggesting that flash-induced formation of an intermediate is reversible at that temperature. This observation is consistent with the flash-induced reversibility of the 690-to-695-nm form at -196°C.

ii. Dark protochlorophyllide reduction. Some plants, including gymnosperms and algae, do not require light for chlorophyll formation, although protochlorophyllide is an intermediate in the pathway (Bogard, 1950; Bogdanović, 1973). These organisms must have a light-independent mode of protochlorophyllide reduction. Some progress in analyzing such a system in extracts of the blue-green alga *Anabaena* has been reported (Adamson et al., 1987). The cells were lysed by osmotic adjustment, supplemented with protochlorophyllide and an NADPH-regenerating system, and incubated in complete darkness. A linear relationship between protochlorophyllide consumed and chlorophyllide formed was observed, and the rate was temperature-dependent. It should be noted that these organisms, as well as all others where the question has been examined, also have a light-dependent mode of protochlorophyllide reduction (Selstam et al., 1987; Senger and Brinkmann, 1986).

If plants and algae that are capable of forming chlorophyll in the dark have two mechanisms for protochlorophyllide reduction, it might be asked whether the angiosperms also have a light-independent as well as a light-dependent pathway. The question becomes even more compelling when the phenomenon of the light-induced breakdown of the light-dependent reductase is considered (see section titled Regulation of Protochlorophyllide Photoreduction). A number of investigators have observed increases in chlorophyll accumulation in the dark when greening plants were transferred from the light to the dark. In some plants such as *Zostera* (Adamson and Packer, 1987) and *Tradescantia* (Adamson et al., 1980), dark accumulation can be quite substantial. Smaller dark increases have also been observed in green barley (Adamson et al., 1985).

Attempts to correlate these increases with the dark synthesis and incorporation of newly formed tetrapyrroles into chlorophyll(ide) have had conflicting results. In one experiment, barley was germinated in the dark for 5 days, the intact plants were illuminated for various periods of time, and then the shoots were excised and incubated for 2 h in the dark with ^{14}C-ALA (Apel et al., 1984). At this point, the shoots were either ground in liquid N_2 and the pigments extracted or the shoots were exposed to light for 10 min before extraction. Incorporation of label into protochlorophyllide, chlorophyllide, and chlorophyll were determined after separation of the pigments by reverse-phase HPLC. It was concluded that of the total incorporation into the three pigments, no more than 1.2% was incorporated into chlorophyllide in the dark, under conditions where preillumination ranged from 0 to 72 h. Similar experiments were performed by Packer and Adamson (1986), except that in this case, the shoots were not excised from the seed and the dark incubation with label was for 18 h. After a more-rigorous purification and degradation of the chlorophyll to the tetrapyrrole-derived portions, substantial dark incorporation into chlorophylls a and b was measured. When incorporation in intact seedlings was compared to that of excised shoots, no incorporation of label was detected in the chlorophylls from the excised shoots. On the contrary, the amount of chlorophyll present in the leaves decreased by more than 50% during the dark incubation. When incorporation of label into chlorophylls and protochlorophyllide was compared, the label in the chlorophyll was only 5% of the label in protochlorophyllide. Finally, both ^{14}C-ALA and ^{14}C-glutamate were incorporated into chlorophyll in the dark in intact barley leaves and isolated developing chloroplasts (Tripathy and Rebeiz, 1987). Again, the dark label incorporation into chlorophyll was minor compared to incorporation into protochlorophyllide. While it seems safe to conclude that some dark reduction of protochlorophyllide may occur in green barley, the extent is small compared to the light-dependent reduction.

f. Esterification of the ring D propionate. All naturally occurring chlorophylls (with the exception of the c-type chlorophylls discussed below) are found with the ring D propionate esterified to a long-chain alcohol. With rare exceptions, the alcohol is a polyisoprene. Chlorophylls a and b in plants and green algae are normally esterified only with the C-20 alcohol 2-E, 7-R, 11-R-phytol. The photosynthetic bacterial chlorophylls, on the other hand, can be found esterified with phytol, geranylgeraniol, tetrahydrogeranylgeraniol, farnesol, and stearol (see below).

Chlorophyllase, a ubiquitous plastid enzyme, can catalyze hydrolysis of the phytyl ester, transesterification (e.g., replacement of phytol with methanol), and esterification under some conditions in vitro (Ellsworth, 1971). At one time chlorophyllase was considered to have a biosynthetic role in phytylation. However, this enzyme is now generally believed to function only hydrolytically in vivo.

Chlorophyll synthetase from maize shoots or oat etioplast membranes catalyzes the esterification of chlorophyllide a with geranylgeranyl-pyrophosphate, but not with free geranylgeraniol (Rüdiger et al., 1977, 1980). Chlorophyllide is also esterified with geranylgeraniol and its monophosphate if ATP is added to the incubations. In addition to geranylgeranyl-pyrophosphate, the pyrophosphates of phytol and farnesol can also serve as substrates, but those of geraniol or pentadecanol cannot (Rüdiger et al., 1980). Acceptable pigment substrates were chlorophyllides a and b, but not protochlorophyllide or bacteriochlorophyllide (Benz and Rüdiger, 1981).

In the esterification of bacteriochlorophyllide a in *R. spheroides* and *Rhodospirillum rubrum*, both the bridge and the nonbridge oxygen atoms of the ester were found to be derived from the propionic acid of the chlorophyllide (Emery and Akhtar, 1985; Ajaz et al., 1985).

In the early stages of greening of etiolated tissues, chlorophyll a appears to be initially esterified with all-trans geranylgeraniol, and the conversion of the geranylgeranyl group to phytol occurs after esterification (Schoch et al., 1977). Geranylgeraniol has double bonds at positions 2, 6, 10, and 14, whereas phytol retains only the one at position 2 (Schoch and Schäfer, 1978). The double bond in geranylgeraniol at position 6 is the first to be hydrogenated (Fig. 7.8), followed by that at position 10, and the double bond at position 14 is the last to be hydrogenated (Schoch and Schäfer, 1978). Illuminated etioplast fragments are able to esterify endogenous chlorophyllide a with exogenous geranylgeraniol-pyrophosphate, and then carry out the hydrogenations (Benz et al., 1980). The hydrogenation reactions require the pyridine nucleotide NADPH. Certain herbicides interfere with the hydrogenation

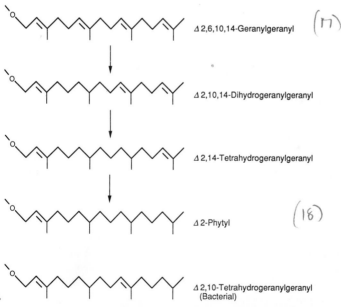

Figure 7.8 Sequence of dehydrogenation steps in the conversion of the geranylgeranyl group to phytyl in plants. Also illustrated is the tetrahydrogeranylgeranyl group found in some bacteriochlorophylls.

of geranylgeraniol and cause the accumulation of chlorophyll molecules containing geranylgeraniol and dihydrogeranylgeraniol instead of phytol (Rüdiger et al., 1976). Anaerobiosis appears to interfere with the hydrogenation of geranylgeraniol-chlorophyllide, but not with protochlorophyllide photoreduction or esterification with geranylgeraniol (Schoch et al., 1980). There exists a mutant strain of *Scenedesmus* that is deficient in vitamin E because it cannot form the phytol moiety of the vitamin (Bishop and Wong, 1974). Cells of this strain also are unable to complete chlorophyll synthesis, and instead accumulate near-normal amounts of chlorophylls a and b that contain geranylgeraniol instead of phytol (Henry et al., 1986).

Minor amounts of bacteriochlorophyll a esterified with geranylgeraniol, dihydrogeranylgeraniol, and tetrahydrogeranylgeraniol were detected in purple photosynthetic bacteria (Shioi and Sasa, 1984). These results suggest that, like greening etiolated plant tissues, those photosynthetic bacteria which form phytylated bacteriochlorophylls begin with the pigment esterified with geranylgeraniol.

Contrary to the case in greening etiolated tissues and photosynthetic bacteria, in green plants chlorophyllide appears to be esterified directly with phytol (Rüdiger, 1987). This direct phytylation may be able to occur in green plants because the plastids of these tissues contain a larger pool of phytyl-pyrophosphate than those of etiolated tissues.

2. Chlorophyll b.   Higher plants and green algae contain, in addition to chlorophyll a, generally smaller amounts of chlorophyll b, which differs from chlorophyll a only by the presence of a formyl group in place of the methyl on ring B of the tetrapyrrole ring (Fig. 7.9). Chlorophyll b typically comprises close to 25% of the total chlorophyll present in green plant tissues.

a. In vivo studies.   Early work suggested that the immediate precursor of chlorophyll b is chlorophyll a. Godnev et al. (1960) reported that label from exogenous ^{14}C-chlorophyll a was transferred to chlorophyll b in greening onion leaves. The reverse transfer of label from chlorophyll b to chlorophyll a was not observed. In these experiments, the pigments were dissolved in vegetable oil for introduction into the tissue.

Akoyunoglou et al. (1967) generated ^{14}C-labeled chlorophyll a in situ by incubating excised etiolated barley leaves with ^{14}C-ALA and exposing the leaves to a series of light flashes separated by 15-min dark periods. Under the flashing-light regime, very little chlorophyll b was formed, although considerable chlorophyll a appeared during 24 cycles extending to a total of 6 h (Akoyunoglou et al., 1966). The leaves were next washed free of exogenous ^{14}C-ALA, then exposed to 100 more flash cycles to use up any ^{14}C-ALA remaining within the leaves, and then the leaves were transferred to continuous light. During the continuous-light phase the total radioactivity of the chlorophyll a pool decreased, while the total radioactivity of newly formed chlorophyll b increased. The specific radioactivity of both chlorophylls decreased during the continuous-light phase, that of chlorophyll b decreasing faster than chlorophyll a. The investigators concluded from these results that chlorophyll b is formed from a subpopulation of newly formed chlorophyll a molecules.

Shlyk and Prudnikova (1967) allowed greening barley leaves to assimilate $^{14}CO_2$ and form radioactive chlorophyll. The leaves were then homogenized and incubated in the dark. Chlorophyll b became labeled during the dark incubation. Added unlabeled chlorophyll a lessened the degree of labeling of chlorophyll b. Light had no effect on the transfer of label (Shlyk et al., 1975). The action spectrum for chlorophyll b formation in etiolated wheat leaves was found to be identical to the action spectrum for chlorophyll a formation, and both were similar to the absorption spectrum of protochlorophyllide (Ogawa et al., 1973). Thus, although light was not specifically required for chlorophyll b formation, it was thought to stimulate the conversion by supplying a pool of newly synthesized chlorophyll a molecules.

The prevailing hypothesis that chlorophyll b is made from chlorophyll a has been challenged by a number of investigators. Oelze-Karow et al. (1978) and Oelze-Karow and Mohr (1978) observed that chlorophyllide a and chlorophyll b accumulation are both more sensitive to inhibition by far-red light than is chlorophyll a accumulation, and it was postulated that the precursor of chlorophyll b might be chlorophyllide a rather than chlorophyll a, with conversion of the 3-methyl moiety to a formyl group

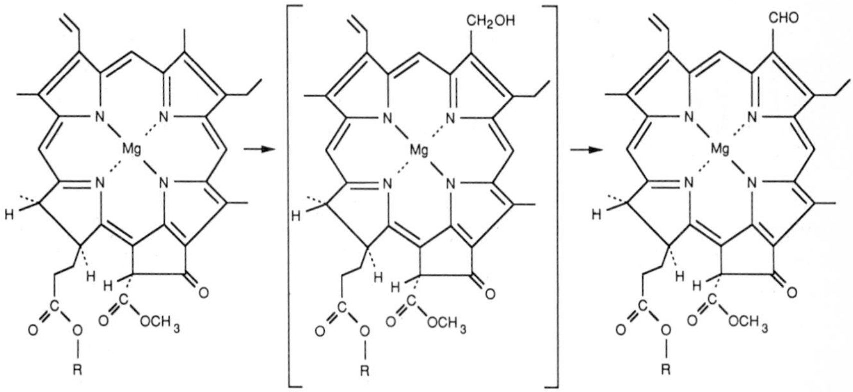

Chlorophyll *a* Hypothetical Intermediate Hydroxymethyl Chlorophyll Chlorophyll *b*

Figure 7.9 Structures of chlorophylls a and b, and a hypothetical intermediate hydroxymethyl chlorophyll. It is uncertain at which stage in the phytylation process the conversion of the B ring methyl to formyl occurs.

occurring before the phytylation step. This scheme is consistent with the observation that in broken etioplast preparations from dark-grown oat seedlings, chlorophyllide b undergoes enzymatic esterification with geranylgeranyl pyrophosphate as readily as chlorophyllide a (Benz and Rüdiger, 1981).

Duggan and Rebeiz (1982) detected chlorophyllide b by fluorescence spectroscopy in extracts from greening and photoperiodically grown cucumber cotyledons, and confirmed the identification by synthesizing the oxime and the methyl ester, which had the expected spectrofluorometric and chromatographic properties. ^{14}C-chlorophyll b synthesized in vivo from ^{14}C-ALA and purified by thin-layer chromatography was used to check how much of the observed chlorophyllide b could have arisen by chlorophyllase activity during pigment extraction. This approach indicated that no more than 13% of the chlorophyllide b detected spectrofluorometrically could have been an artifact of in vitro hydrolysis.

Although these findings suggest that chlorophyllide b may be a biosynthetic intermediate on the route to chlorophyll b, an alternative explanation for the occurrence of chlorophyllide b in greening tissues is that chlorophylls and chlorophyll-protein complexes are subject to turnover before they become established at stable sites within the thylakoid membranes. It is known that chlorophylls do turn over. Chlorophyll b turns over to a greater extent than chlorophyll a in seedlings greening under intermittent illumination (Thorne and Boardman, 1971) or after transfer to the dark following a period of continuous light (Bennett, 1981). Both the protein and pigment components of newly formed light-harvesting chlorophyll-protein complexes are subject to degradation in the dark (Bennett, 1981) or when chlorophyll b synthesis is blocked by mutation (Bellemare et al., 1982). During the early stages of greening, chlorophyll a may not be made at a rate sufficient to saturate the requirements of the simultaneously forming light-harvesting complexes, and incomplete complexes might then be degraded, along with any attached molecules of chlorophyll b. The first step of chlorophyll b degradation is likely to be dephytylation to chlorophyllide b. In vitro chlorophyllase activity may not be an accurate measure of the potential for in vivo chlorophyll dephytylation, which could be accelerated by factors such as pigment association with unstable proteins.

Results from Rüduger's laboratory suggest that the immediate precursor of the formyl-containing pigment may be neither chlorophyllide a nor chlorophyll a, but rather the geranylgeranyl ester of chlorophyllide a (Benz et al., 1984). Growing suspension cultures of tobacco cells can incorporate exogenous labeled monophosphate and pyrophosphate esters of geranylgeraniol, and also the pyrophosphate ester of phytol, into chlorophylls. With either of the geranylgeranyl compounds, label was incorporated at equal specific activity into chlorophylls a and b. However, phytol pyrophosphate was incorporated significantly better into chlorophyll a as compared to chlorophyll b. The investigators concluded from their results that the cells cannot convert phytylated chlorophyll a into chlorophyll b, but that chlorophyllide a esterified with geranyl-geraniol can undergo the conversion. This implies that the natural biosynthetic sequence may be esterification with geranylgeraniol, then formyl group formation, and finally reduction of the geranylgeranyl group to phytol. Since the phytylation process lags behind and occurs at a slower rate than protochlorophyllide reduction, the proposed chloro-phyll b biosynthetic sequence also explains the observed need for "young" chlorophyll a molecules, since the young molecules would be newly esterified with geranylgeraniol, but not yet reduced to the phytyl level.

Shioi and Sasa (1983b) had earlier reported the existence in greening cucumber cotyledons of chlorophyll b species having all possible degrees of polyisoprene group hydrogenation between geranylgeranyl and phytyl, suggesting that the a-to-b transformation may occur before phytylation, or at least before the process is completed. However, these workers also detected protochlorophyllide pools having the same range of polyiso-prene group hydrogenation (Shioi and Sasa, 1983a), making interpreta-tion of their results difficult.

In summary, it is presently not certain whether oxidative conversion of the ring B methyl group occurs before or after phytylation, or if parts of the phytylation process take place both before and after the a-to-b conversion. If phytylation comes first, then chlorophyll a would be a biosynthetic intermediate. If the opposite is true, the reaction sequence would be chlorophyllide a to chlorophyllide b to chlorophyll b. If the last possibility occurs, the true conversion substrate would be geranylgeranyl chlorophyllide a or a chlorophyllide a with a partially reduced iso-prenoid.

b. In vitro studies. Ellsworth et al. (1970) reported that transfer of ^{14}C from exogenous chlorophyll a to chlorophyll b in soybean leaf ho-mogenates occurred in all parts of the molecule, that is, the phytyl chain, the methyl ester group on the cyclopentenone ring, and the tetrapyrrole portion. This result indicates that a true conversion had taken place, rather than transfer of methyl or phytyl groups from ^{14}C-chlorophyll a to newly formed chlorophyll b. These workers also reported that $NADP^+$ stimulated the reaction. This latter observation was confirmed by Shlyk and co-workers (Shlyk et al., 1971), who additionally showed that con-version of exogenous chlorophyll a to chlorophyll b can occur in leaves of barley, rye, and maize even without prior light exposure. In contrast to these, results, Rebeiz and Castelfranco (1971) reported that upon incuba-tion with ^{14}C-ALA, homogenates of cucumber cotyledons incorporated ^{14}C into both chlorophyll a and chlorophyll b only if the cotyledons had been preilluminated for 4.5 h, while preillumination for 2.5 h resulted in label incorporation into chlorophyll a only.

Chlamydomonas reinhardtii strain *y*-1 requires light for chlorophyll accumulation but can be grown heterotrophically in the dark. Bednarik and Hoober (1985, 1986) have made the interesting observation that when degreened cells of strain *y*-1 are incubated in the dark at elevated temperatures (38°C) with *o*- or *m*-phenanthroline a pigment rapidly accumulates and is excreted into the medium. The pigment was characterized as chlorophyllide b. The conversion required the presence of O_2. Green cells treated the same way excreted a slightly different pigment that was characterized as divinylchlorophyllide b. Cells incubated in the dark at elevated temperature without phenanthroline excreted protochlorophyllide. A membrane fraction was isolated from degreened cells which, when supplemented with phenanthroline, converted exogenous protochlorophyllide to chlorophyllide b. These results are consistent with the possibility that protochlorophyll(ide), rather than chlorophyll(ide) a, is the precursor to chlorophyll b, and that the reason why the presence of chlorophyll a is normally required for the formation of chlorophyll b is that chlorophyll a plays some regulatory role. It was suggested by the authors that phenanthroline stimulates chlorophyllide b formation by mimicking chlorophyll a at some regulatory site in the chlorophyllide-b-forming system. It will be of great interest to attempt to exploit this apparent breakthrough in the in vitro biosynthesis of chlorophyll b, toward understanding the mechanism of chlorophyll b formation and its regulation.

3. Possible existence of multiple forms of chlorophylls a and b.   A mutant strain of maize exists in which the ring B ethyl groups are replaced by vinyls on both chlorophylls a and b (Bazzaz et al., 1982; Brereton et al., 1983). The divinyl structure of the variant chlorophyll b was confirmed (Wu and Rebeiz, 1985). The mutant (Olive Necrotic 8147) is necrotic, its leaves contain 70% less chlorophyll than wild-type leaves and its chlorophyll a-to-b ratio is three times higher, but is can carry out photosynthesis (Bazzaz et al., 1974). It is probable that the mutant lacks the enzyme that catalyzes the vinyl-reduction step in the biosynthesis of chlorophyll a, and chlorophyll b is formed from the variant chlorophyll a. A pigment having the properties of divinylchlorophyll a was also found in a free-living unicellular marine prochlorophyte (Chisholm et al., 1988). This organism also contains apparently normal chlorophyll b, in approximately equal abundance as the novel chlorophyll a.

Several other novel chlorophyll types have been reported in greening barley leaves and cucumber cotyledons (Belanger and Rebeiz, 1979, 1980a–c; Rebeiz et al., 1980, 1983). These pigments have different low-temperature fluorescence excitation and emission maxima, and are partially separable by HPLC. The investigators have proposed that the chemical differences among the different species of chlorophylls include different states of oxidation at positions 2, 4, and 10, and different substitutions for phytol at position 7 (Rebeiz et al., 1980, 1983). As many as 16 chemically and spectroscopically unique species of chlorophyll a, and perhaps the same number of chlorophyll b species, have now been reported by Rebeiz et al. (1980, 1983). In addition, these investigators have postulated that the ratio of end products and sequence of biosynthetic reactions is dependent upon the individual plant species and its growth history (Tripathy and Rebeiz, 1986, 1988). It will be interesting to learn the precise structure of each chlorophyll type, and to possibly correlate these with different functional pools of chlorophyll and different chlorophyll-protein complexes. After the structures of the novel chlorophylls have been determined, it will still remain to be established whether the pigments are functionally significant in photosynthesis.

Four chlorophyll a species having different HPLC mobilities were detected by Eskins and Harris (1981). The separated chlorophylls might be molecules having varying degrees of polyisoprene chain hydrogenation, that is, the intermediates between geranylgeranyl chlorophyllide a and chlorophyll a, as described by Schoch et al. (1977, 1980) and Rüdiger et al. (1977, 1980). A study by Shioi and Sasa (1983b) also identified four HPLC-separable chlorophyll species in extracts of spinach leaves as the intermediates between geranylgeranyl chlorophyllide a and chlorophyll a. No other anomalous pigments were detected, even though many chlorophyll breakdown products and derivatives were characterized.

4. Chlorophylls c. Chlorophylls c are accessory light-harvesting pigments found in many groups of eukaryotic algae that do not contain chlorophyll b, including diatoms, dinoflagellates, brown macrophytic algae, and cryptophytes (the latter also contain phycobiliprotein accessory pigments). There is also one report of a species that contains both chlorophyll b and chlorophyll c (Wilhelm, 1987). The chlorophyll c macrocycle is structurally not a chlorin, but a porphyrin, since there are no reduced pyrrole rings. Two c-type chlorophylls have been described, c_1 and c_2 (Fig. 7.10). A distinguishing feature of both of these pigments is that in place of the phytylated propionic acid group on ring D, there is a free, unesterified acrylic acid, which has a trans dehydrogenated structure. Chlorophyll c_1 has an ethyl group on ring B, like protochlorophyllide, and on chlorophyll c_2 the ethyl is replaced by vinyl, as on the precursor of protochlorophyllide, Mg-divinylpheoporphyrin a_5 (Dougherty et al., 1966 1970; Budzikiewicz and Taraz, 1971). Algae containing either chlorophyll c_1 or c_2 alone, or both, have been described (Anderson and Mulkey, 1983). In addition, species have been found

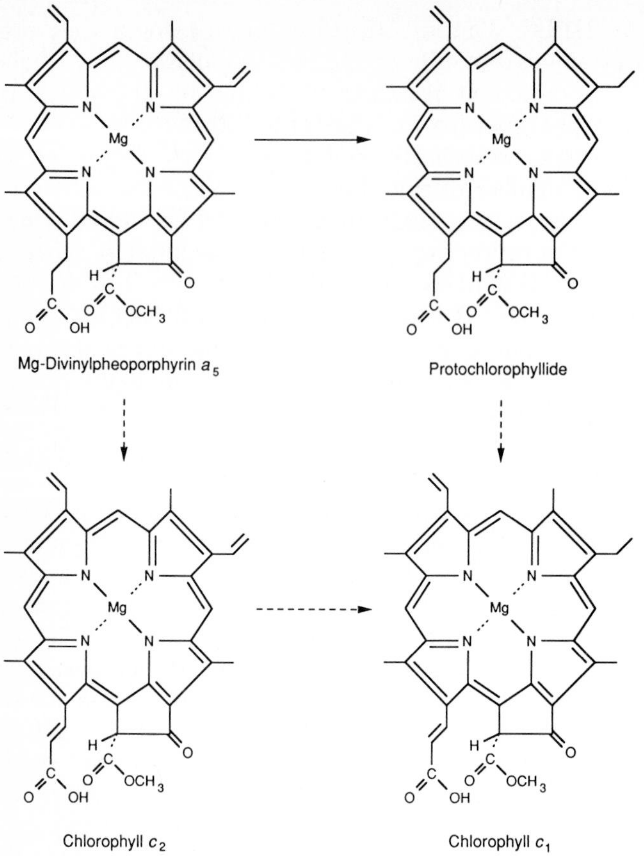

Figure 7.10   Structures of chlorophylls c and their possible biosynthetic relationships. Broken arrows indicate hypothetical steps which have not been experimentally demonstrated.

which apparently use the structurally similar Mg-divinylpheoporphyrin a_5 (Brown, 1985), or a closely related molecule named chlorophyll c_3 (Jeffrey and Wright, 1987), as an accessory pigment.

The close structural resemblance of chlorophylls c to Mg-divinylpheoporphyrin a_5 and protochlorophyllide suggests that chlorophylls c derive directly from these precursors (Fig. 7.10), rather than from chlorophyll a.

5. Bacteriochlorophylls. The photosynthetic bacteria contain a large number of tetrapyrrole pigments which are employed to capture a large portion of the visible and near-infrared light spectrum. Three of these pigments, bacteriochlorophylls a, b, and g, are also found in the bacterial photosynthetic reaction centers.

a. Bacteriochlorophyll a. This pigment was the first chlorophyll described in photosynthetic bacteria. It differs from chlorophyll a in two ways: Instead of a single reduced pyrrole ring at position D, the bacteriochlorin macrocycle contains two reduced rings at opposite corners, rings B and D; and instead of a vinyl on ring A, there is an acetyl group. While the esterifying alcohol on the ring D propionate is often phytol, in other cases it is geranylgeraniol (Katz et al., 1972; Brockmann et al., 1973).

b. Bacteriochlorophyll b. This pigment (Fig. 7.11) is found in some nonsulfur purple bacteria (Eimhjellen et al., 1963; Gloe and Pfennig, 1974). Bacteriochlorophyll b differs from bacteriochlorophyll a in having an ethylidine group in place of an ethyl on ring B (Scheer et al., 1974). The esterifying alcohol can be phytol, geranylgeraniol, or Δ2,10-phytadienol (tetrahydrogeranylgeraniol) (Gloe and Pfennig, 1974; Steiner et al., 1981). The existence of the last esterifying alcohol suggests that in the conversion of geranylgeraniol to phytol, the sequence of double-bond hydrogeranylgeraniol to phytol that occurs in plants does not involve this tetrahydrogeranylgeraniol isomer (see Fig. 7.8) (Schoch and Schäfer, 1978).

c. Bacteriochlorophyll g. This pigment (Fig. 7.11) has been reported in several strictly anaerobic photosynthetic bacteria (Gest and Favinger, 1983; Berr-Romero and Gest, 1987; J.G. Ormerod, personal communication). Bacteriochlorophyll g shares with bacteriochlorophyll b the ethylidine group on ring B, but unlike either bacteriochlorophylls a or b, and like chlorophyll a, ring A contains a vinyl group (Brockmann and

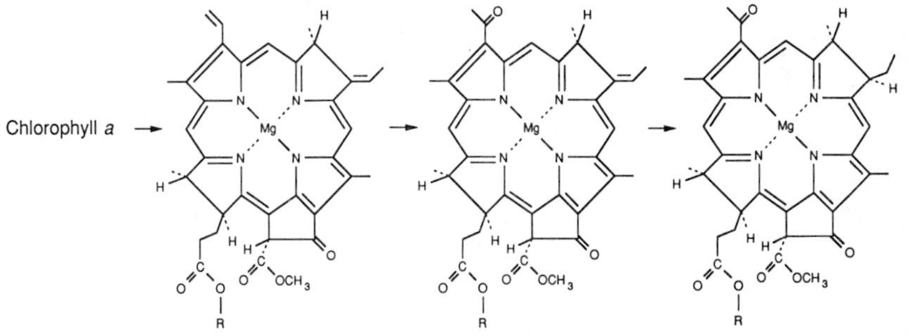

Chlorophyll a →

Bacteriochlorophyll g   Bacteriochlorophyll b   Bacteriochlorophyll a

Figure 7.11 Structures of bacteriochlorophylls a, b, and g, and a hypothetical biosynthetic relationship.

Lipinski, 1983). The esterifying alcohol of bacteriochlorophyll g is geranylgeraniol (Brockmann and Lipinski, 1983) or farnesol (Michalski et al., 1987). The macrocycle of bacteriochlorophyll g is isomeric with that of chlorophyll a, and bacteriochlorophyll g readily isomerizes to this pigment in vitro and in aging cells (Beer-Romero and Gest, 1987).

d. Bacteriochlorophylls c, d, and e. These pigments (Fig. 7.12) are also known as *Chlorobium* chlorophylls and are found in strictly anaerobic green photosynthetic bacteria and in the facultatively aerobic *Chloroflexus* group. The pigments are employed primarily as light-harvesting accessory pigments within subcellular vesicles, called chlorosomes, that are attached to the photosynthetically active plasma membrane. Bacteriochlorophylls c, d, and e have only one reduced pyrrole ring and are, therefore, chlorins likes chlorophylls a and b, rather than bacteriochlorins like bacteriochlorophylls a, b, and g. Two other features shared by all *Chlorobium* chlorophylls are the absence of a methoxycarbonyl group on the isocyclic ring and the presence of an α-hydroxyethyl instead of a vinyl group on ring B. The α-hydroxyethyl group can be of either the S or R configuration (Smith and Goff, 1985; Simpson and Smith, 1988). Bacteriochlorophylls c and e contain a methyl group on the δ-meso bridge of the macrocycle. Bacteriochlorophyll e differs from bacterio-

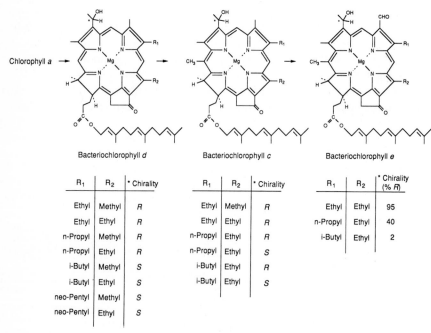

R_1	R_2	* Chirality		R_1	R_2	* Chirality		R_1	R_2	* Chirality (% R)
Ethyl	Methyl	R		Ethyl	Methyl	R		Ethyl	Ethyl	95
Ethyl	Ethyl	R		Ethyl	Ethyl	R		n-Propyl	Ethyl	40
n-Propyl	Methyl	R		n-Propyl	Ethyl	R		i-Butyl	Ethyl	2
n-Propyl	Ethyl	R		n-Propyl	Ethyl	S				
i-Butyl	Methyl	S		i-Butyl	Ethyl	R				
i-Butyl	Ethyl	S		i-Butyl	Ethyl	S				
neo-Pentyl	Methyl	S								
neo-Pentyl	Ethyl	S								

Figure 7.12 Structures of bacteriochlorophylls c, d, and e, and a hypothetical biosynthetic relationship.

chlorophyll c in having the ring B methyl replaced by a formyl group (Gloe et al., 1975). [A pigment having the ring B formyl group but lacking the δ-meso-bridge methyl has been chemically synthesized and characterized (Risch et al., 1988). The pigment, which was named bacteriochlorophyll f, has not yet been reported to occur naturally.] Varying numbers of additional methyl groups are found added to the ring B ethyl and ring C methyl groups of the *Chlorobium* chlorophylls, so that the ring B ethyl is converted progressively to *n*-propyl, isobutyl, and neopentyl, and ring C methyl to ethyl (Smith and Goff, 1985). These extra methyl groups, as well as the one found on the δ-meso-bridge carbon of bacteriochlorophylls d and e, are derived from methionine (Smith and Huster, 1987). Finally, the esterifying alcohol group on the ring D propionate of *Chlorobium* chlorophylls is usually *E,E*-farnesyl (Rapoport and Hamlow, 1961; Jensen et al., 1964; Gloe et al., 1975), although fractions of bacteriochlorophyll c isolated from *Chloroflexus aurantiacus* were reported to be esterified with phytol, geranylgeraniol, and stearyl alcohol (Risch et al., 1979). Bacteriochlorophyll c esterified with phytol has been implicated as the primary acceptor pigment in the photosynthetic reaction center of the green sulfur bacterium *Prosthecochloris aestuardii* (Braumann et al., 1986). The reaction center of *Heliobacterium chlorum* may also contain bacteriochlorophyll c as the primary acceptor, while the donor is bacteriochlorophyll g (Nuijs et al., 1985).

Usually, only one series of *Chlorobium* chlorophyll is present in a given strain of cells. However, under laboratory culture conditions, a slow change appears to take place where, for example, a *Chlorobium* strain initially producing bacteriochlorophylls d at some point begins to accumulate bacteriochlorophylls c instead (Broch-Due and Ormerod, 1978; Smith and Bobe, 1987).

e. Possible biosynthetic relationships among the bacteriochlorophylls. In the absence of direct information on the biosynthesis of bacteriochlorophylls, it is possible to devise a plausible biosynthetic scheme relating the macrocyclic structures of the known bacteriochlorophylls (Figs. 7.11 and 7.12). The starting point is chlorophyll(ide) a, which is presumed to be a precursor because it, and also protochlorophyllide and Mg-divinylpheophyrin a_5, accumulate in mutant strains (Sistrom et al., 1956; Richards and Lascelles, 1969; Drews et al., 1971) and inhibitor-treated (Jones, 1963a, b; Wong, 1978) wild-type photosynthetic bacterial cells. Moving one electron from the ring B ethyl group into the ring results in reduction of the ring and conversion of the ethyl to an ethylidine group, thus forming bacteriochlorophyll g. Hydration of the ring A vinyl bacteriochlorophyll g to an α-hydroxyethyl group, followed by oxidation of the α-hydroxyethyl to an acetyl group produces the structure of bacteriochlorophyll b. Reduction of the ethylidine of bacteriochlorophyll b back to an ethyl group produces bacteriochlorophyll a. Bacteriochlorophylls g and b are extremely unstable in light and O_2 (Scheer et al., 1974; Brockmann and Lipinski, 1983) and would not have been seen in cell extracts examined for bacteriochlorophyll a precursors using conventional techniques. Along another branch starting from chlorophyll a, removal of the methoxycarbonyl group on the isocyclic ring and hydration of the ring B vinyl to an α-hydroxyethyl group produces bacteriochlorophyll d. Methylation of the δ-meso-bridge carbon of bacteriochlorophyll d yields bacteriochlorophyll c. Finally, oxidation of the ring B methyl to a formyl group produces bacteriochlorophyll e.

Various pigments which accumulate in certain mutant strains suggest other biosynthetic sequences. For example, a strain of *R. spheroides* was reported to excrete 2-desacetyl-2-vinylbacteriopheophytin (Pudek and Richards, 1975), which suggests (assuming that the pheophytin arises by loss of Mg upon excretion) that ring B reduction may precede the oxidation of the ring A vinyl group. Another mutant strain of *R. spheroides* accumulates 2-desvinyl-2-(1-hydroxyethyl) chlorophyllide a (Houghton et al., 1983), which suggests that the vinyl-to-acetyl conversion begins before the reduction of ring B occurs. The conflicting conclusions derivable from these results indicate that caution is warranted in the interpretation of studies with mutants that accumulate putative intermediates.

6. Reaction center chlorophylls.   The most abundant of the tetrapyrroles found in photosynthetic organisms is chlorophyll a, or one of its common derivatives. Functionally, most of this chlorophyll is used for light harvesting and transfer of the absorbed energy to specialized reaction centers where photochemistry occurs. Although they make up only a small percentage of the total, chlorophylls also occur in the reaction centers. Attempts have been made to explain the unique properties of the reaction centers in terms of modifications to the chlorophyll prosthetic groups, and/or by interactions of chlorophyll a (or bacteriochlorophyll a) with the specialized proteins which constitute the reaction center. This dilemma has been approached in two ways. Measured physical properties of the reaction center have been correlated with the measured physical properties of synthesized model compounds. In addition, the reaction center pigments have been extracted and examined for the presence of small, but consistent, amounts of modified pigment.

Various chlorophyll a derivatives have been suggested as the primary electron donor pigment of photosystem I (P_{700}). One proposed pigment, called chlorophyll RC I, is 13(S)-hydroxy-20-chloro-chlorophyll a (Dörnemann and Senger, 1982, 1986). The structure of the chromophore was confirmed by a variety of physical techniques (nmr, infrared, mass spectrometry, etc.), and by partial synthesis from chlorophyll a (Scheer et al., 1986). The same pigment was isolated from *Spirulina* whether or not chlorinated substances were used in the extraction procedure (Scheer et al., 1986). Dörnemann and Senger did not specify whether the RC I might be the chromophore for P_{700} or the first primary acceptor. Comparison of the redox and optical properties of RC I and chlorophyll a provided no basis for assuming that RC I was any better than chlorophyll a in satisfying the requirements for the reaction center. In both cases additional aggregation states and interactions with proteins are required (Fajer et al., 1987). Other results suggest that there are insufficient amounts of this compound in purified reaction centers to account for P_{700} (Katoh and Yasuda, 1987), and the RC I derivative may arise as an artifact of purification. Another P_{700} candidate is chlorophyll a', the C-10 epimer of chlorophyll a (Watanabe et al., 1985). This pigment was reported to exist in approximately equimolar amounts as P_{700} in various plant and algal preparations (Watanabe et al., 1987). Watanabe et al. (1987) found that the ratio increased with harsher isolation treatments, but under mild conditions the ratio was always 1. This group also detected a chlorophyll derivative, designated as "component X", and tentatively identified as RC I on the basis of visible absorbance and fluorescence spectra. They found that component X is absent in fresh plant material and increased with time in dead material, and during fractionation. Redox- and spectral-induced P_{700}-like spectral changes were observed when chlorophyll *a'* was added to a 65,000 molecular weight photosystem I apoprotein (Watanabe et al., 1987). However, because epimerization about C-10 is known to occur spontaneously in chlorophyll solutions, further work is required to establish whether chlorophyll *a'* is the natural P_{700} pigment.

7. Reaction center pheophytins. In the reaction centers of some groups of photosynthetic bacteria (but not others), Mg-free bacteriopheophytins serve as the primary electron acceptor (Amesz, 1987; Glazer and Melis, 1987). Similarly, photosystem II (but not photosystem I) reaction centers of oxygenic plants and algae contain pheophytin a as the primary acceptor. Although the only pheophytin found in photosystem II reaction centers is pheophytin a, bacterial reaction center bacteriopheophytin structures generally follow those of the corresponding reaction center bacteriochlorophylls, and can be of the a, b, or g type.

It has generally been assumed that the pheophytins are derived from the corresponding chlorophylls by loss of Mg accompanying incorporation into the reaction center proteins. However, it should be noted that the reaction center bacteriopheophytin a of *R. rubrum* is esterified with phytol, while the bacteriochlorophyll a molecules in the same reaction centers are esterified with geranylgeraniol (Walter et al., 1979). This finding suggests that the pheophytin is formed by removal of Mg from newly esterified pigment molecules, before hydrogenation of the polyisoprene to phytol has begun.

D. Fe branch

1. Ferrochelatase and protoheme formation. Ferrochelatase (protoheme ferrolyase, EC 4.99.1.1), the enzyme responsible for insertion of Fe into the porphyrin macrocycle, is described elsewhere in this volume. Membrane-bound ferrochelatase from the photosynthetic bacterium, *R. spheroides*, has been purified and characterized (Dailey, 1982; Dailey et al., 1986). The enzyme is a single polypeptide of molecular weight 115,000. The apparent K_m values for protoporphyrin and Fe^{2+} are 18 and 22 μM, respectively. Although the enzyme has not been purified to homogeneity from any plant source, its activity has been measured in cell-free extracts of plant material (Goldin and Little, 1969; Little and Jones, 1976; Porra and Lascelles, 1968; Jones, 1967, 1968) and it has been partially purified from etiolated barley (Goldin and Little, 1969). Unlike preparations from bacteria and animals, in the barley preparation, 50% of the activity appeared to be in the soluble fraction after a 20,000 $\times$ g centrifugation. Ferrochelatase activity copurified with Zn chelatase activity through ammonium sulfate fractionation and gel filtration chromatography on Sephadex G-150. The estimated molecular weight, by gel filtration, was 55,000-to-65,000. Mesoporphyrin, hematoporphyrin, and deuteroporphyrin were all better substrates than protoporphyrin in the ferrochelatase assay. Ferrochelatase activity has also been characterized from spinach chloroplasts that were stripped of their outer envelope membranes (Jones, 1968). The preparation was free of mitochondrial contamination, as judged by phase contrast microscopy. The K_m for Fe^{2+} in the presence of 25 μM protoporphyrin or mesoporphyrin was 8 or 36 μM, respectively. The K_m values for protoporphyrin and mesoporphyrin were 0.2 and 0.4 μM, respectively (at nonsaturating Fe^{2+} concentration). Like most ferrochelatase preparations from other sources, the enzyme was membrane-bound.

Because chloroplasts and mitochondria have independent needs for hemes, it is logical to assume that each organelle has its own independent machinery for heme biosynthesis. A more-detailed discussion of this premise will be presented in the section on regulation. Porra and Lascelles (1968) prepared chloroplasts, proplastids, and mitochondria from a variety of plant tissues by differential centrifugation. Spinach chloroplasts had ferrochelatase activity, as did chloroplasts and proplastids from greening bean cotyledons and oat seedlings. Microscopic exami-

nation of the above preparations indicated little contamination by mitochondria. Because the specific activity did not change upon washing, the
authors concluded that the activity was not due to mitochondrial contamination. Mitochondria from the above tissues also had ferrochelatase
activity, but the preparations were obviously contaminated with chloroplast fragments. Mitochondria, slightly contaminated with leucoplasts,
were prepared from potato tubers. These mitochondria had ferrochelatase activity and cytochrome oxidase activity. When the mitochondria were washed, the ratios of the two activities remained the
same. No ferrochelatase activity was detected in the leucoplast fraction.
The authors concluded that ferrochelatase is localized in both mitochondria and chloroplasts of plant cells.

The subcellular localization of ferrochelatase in both chloroplasts and
mitochondria of plant cells was put on more firm foundation by the
studies of Little and Jones (1976). These investigators prepared washed
etioplasts and washed mitochondrial fractions from etiolated barley by
differential centrifugation. These fractions were then subjected to su-
crose-density gradient centrifugation. The density-gradient-purified
etioplasts had ferrochelatase activity and no detectable cytochrome
oxidase activity. Upon density gradient centrifugation, the washed mitochondria yielded two bands of ferrochelatase activity, one coinciding
with cytochrome oxidase and succinate dehydrogenase activity, and
other having a density corresponding to the etioplasts. Even with density gradient centrifugation, it was not possible to free completely the
mitochondria from contamination with chloroplast fragments. Ferrochelatase in the washed etioplast preparation had optimum activity at
pH 7.3, while the activity in the gradient-purified mitochondrial fraction
had an optimum at pH 8.0. The ferrochelatase activity from both
organelles was inhibited 50% or more by Fe-, Mg-, or Zn-protoporphyrin
at concentrations between 3.0 and 7.0 μM.

Brown et al. (1984) measured ferrochelatase activity in extracts of
C. caldarium, by using Co^{2+} and deuteroporphyrin IX in place of the
physiological substrates Fe^{2+} and protoporphyrin IX. In wild-type cells,
which do not normally form pigment in the dark, the in vitro ferrochelatase level increased severalfold within 72 h after the cells were
exposed to light. The increase in ferrochelatase activity paralleled the
accumulation of phycocyanin, which suggests that the level of this
enzyme may be an important rate-controlling factor in phycobilin synthesis. The intracellular localization of the measured ferrochelatase activity was not reported.

N-Methylporphyrins apparently inhibit plant ferrochelatase, as they
do the animal enzyme. Administration of N-methylprotoporphyrin or
N-methylmesoporphyrin to growing Cyanidium cells caused protopor-

phyrin accumulation and inhibited phycobilin formation (Brown et al., 1982; Beale and Chen, 1983). This result supported other evidence that heme is a precursor to the phycobilins (see below).

2. Bilin formation

a. **Heme as a phycobilin precursor.** The participation of heme in phycobilin formation is suggested by similarities of the phycobilins to the tetrapyrrole macrocycle ring-opening reaction products appearing in animal heme catabolism. Also, mechanistic studies have indicated the necessity of the central Fe atom in the ring-opening reaction.

Direct evidence for the participation of heme was reported by Brown et al. (1981) and Schuster et al. (1983b), who showed that exogenous ^{14}C-heme could contribute label to phycocyanobilin in greening *C. caldarium* cells. The specificity of heme incorporation was indicated by the fact that unlabeled chlorophyll was formed simultaneously with the labeled phycocyanobilin when greening cells were incubated with ^{14}C-heme. Further evidence supporting a role for heme was provided by the observation that nonradioactive heme was able to decrease the incorporation of ^{14}C-labeled ALA into phycocyanobilin (Brown et al., 1981).

b. **Biliverdin as a phycobilin precursor.** Biliverdin was reported to accumulate in the culture medium of *C. caldarium* cells grown in the dark with exogenous ALA (Köst and Benedikt, 1982). Although this result was interpreted as evidence that biliverdin is a precursor of phycocyanobilin, the biliverdin accumulation could also have resulted from degradation of excess heme that might have been formed as a result of ALA administration.

Beale and Cornejo (1983) found that the phycocyanin chromophore became labeled when purified ^{14}C-biliverdin IXα was administered to *C. caldarium* cells growing in the dark in the presence N-methylmesoporphyrin IX to block endogenous heme formation. The strain of cells used in these experiments was capable of forming phycocyanin in the dark. Dark growth was used to eliminate possible phototoxic effects of administered N-methylmesoporphyrin or biliverdin. Cellular protoheme remained unlabeled during the incubations with ^{14}C-biliverdin, indicating that the conversion of biliverdin to phycocyanobilin was direct, rather than via degradation of the administered labeled compound and subsequent reutilization of the [14]C. The ability of exogenous ^{14}C-biliverdin to label the phycocyanin chromophore in vivo was confirmed (Brown et al., 1984; Holroyd et al., 1985).

c. **Algal heme oxygenase.** Several key features of the heme oxygenase reaction occur in phycobilin formation in vivo. When intact *C. caldarium* cells were allowed to form phycocyanin in the presence of

[^{14}C-5]ALA, ^{14}CO and ^{14}C-phycocyanobilin were formed in equimolar amounts (Troxler, 1972). Also, each of the lactam oxygen atoms of phycocyanobilin is derived from a different O_2 molecule (Brown et al., 1980; Troxler et al., 1979).

Beale and Cornejo (1984b) detected heme oxygenase activity in extracts of *C. caldarium*. Originally, it was necessary to utilize mesoheme in place of the physiological substrate protoheme. The advantage of mesoheme is that the reaction product mesobiliverdin is more stable than biliverdin in the cell extract and, thus, accumulates to detectable levels during the incubation. Using optimized incubation conditions, conversion of protoheme to biliverdin was also detected in these cell extracts (Cornejo and Beale, 1988).

Cyanidium heme oxygenase differs from the animal cell-derived microsomal system in that it is soluble, with virtually all of the activity appearing in the high-speed supernatant. This finding is not too surprising in view of the fact that the reaction is thought to occur in the plastids, and also presumably occurs in prokaryotic blue-green algae. Neither plastids nor prokaryotes have microsomes.

Like the animal system, *Cyanidium* heme oxygenase requires reduced pyridine nucleotide (NADPH is about twice as effective as NADH), as well as O_2. In addition to the reduced pyridine nucleotide, isoascorbate or another moderately strong reductant stimulates the reaction in unpurified cell extracts, and is required in more purified preparations. Perhaps the isoascorbate serves to reduce heme to the ferrous state, or otherwise supplies reducing power in the incompletely purified system. Like the microsomal enzyme (Drummond and Kappas, 1981), the algal heme oxygenase is powerfully inhibited by Sn-protoporphyrin IX.

Algal heme oxygenase was fractionated into three required protein components, having molecular weights of 22,000, 37,000, and 38,000 (Cornejo and Beale, 1988). The small 22,000 molecular weight protein contains an Fe/S cluster, as is the case with other nonmicrosomal monooxygenases, and can be replaced by commercial ferredoxin (Cornejo and Beale, 1988). The 37,000 molecular weight protein fraction binds NADPH and has ferredoxin-linked cytochrome c reductase activity. The 38,000 molecular weight fraction is inactivated by diethyl pyrocarbonate and the inactivation is blocked by heme, indicating that this fraction is the one that binds heme. The proposed roles of the three *Cyanidium* protein fractions that reconstitute heme oxygenase activity are illustrated in Fig. 7.13.

d. Biliverdin reduction to phycocyanobilin.   All of the phycobilins that have been described (Fig. 7.14) contain four more hydrogen atoms than biliverdin. Beale and Cornejo (1984a) measured enzymatic conversion of biliverdin to free phycocyanobilin in cell-free extracts of *C. caldarium*.

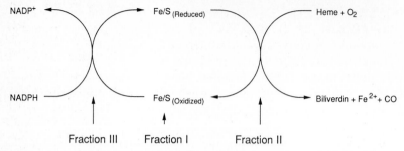

NADP⁺ ← ... → Fe/S (Reduced) ... → Heme + O₂

NADPH → ... Fe/S (Oxidized) ← ... → Biliverdin + Fe²⁺+ CO

Fraction III   Fraction I   Fraction II

Figure 7.13 Proposed roles for the three protein components of the algal heme oxygenase system from *C. caldarium*. In this system, fraction III accepts electrons from NADPH and reduces fraction I, which is a ferredoxin-like protein. Electrons are passed from fraction I to fraction II, which binds heme and catalyzes the macrocycle ring opening reaction.

In addition to biliverdin IXα, the reaction required a reduced pyridine nucleotide; NADPH being more effective than NADH. Activity was retained in the high-speed supernatant fraction and eluted with the protein fraction on gel filtration. Product identification was by comparative absorption spectroscopy, reverse-phase HPLC, and chemical derivatization. Products of the reaction included both the *Z*- and *E*-ethylidine

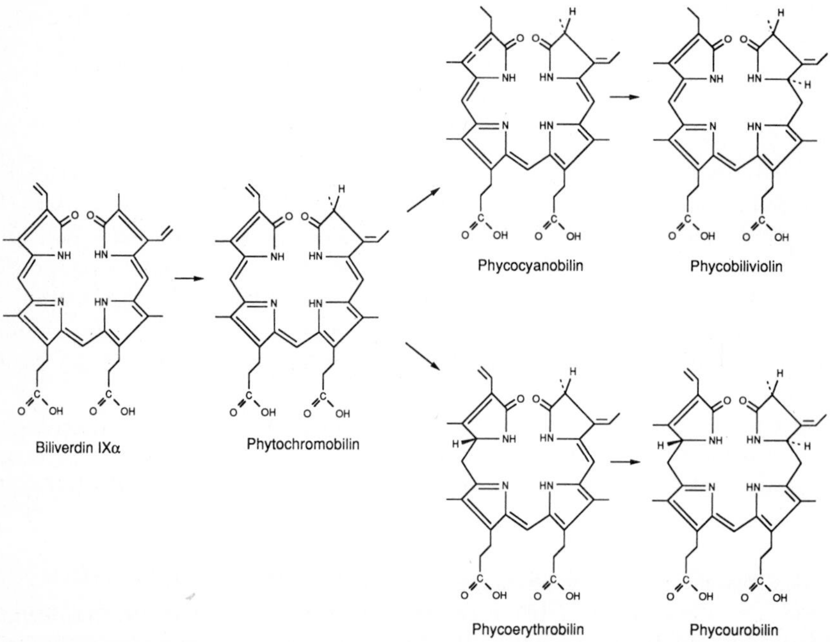

Biliverdin IXα   Phytochromobilin

Phycocyanobilin

Phycobiliviolin

Phycoerythrobilin

Phycourobilin

Figure 7.14 Structures of the free phycobilin chromophores and hypothetical biosynthetic relationship.

isomers of phycocyanobilin. At early reaction times, the less stable Z isomer was the predominant reaction product (Beale and Cornejo, 1984a). The time course for the appearance of the two isomers suggests a precursor-product relationship between the Z and E forms. Preliminary evidence indicates that enzymatic isomerization is catalyzed by cell extract in the presence of reduced glutathione (Beale and Cornejo, unpublished). Several other cis-trans isomerases have been reported that required reduced glutathione for activity (Knox, 1960; Seltzer, 1972).

Interestingly, both phycocyanobilin ethylidine isomers are also formed upon methanolytic cleavage of the phycocyanin chromophore from the protein moiety (Fu et al., 1979), but the Z isomer, being less stable (Weller and Gossauer, 1980), isomerizes rapidly at the elevated temperatures employed for methanolysis, and the equilibrium isomer ratio strongly favors the E form.

α-Hydroxymesobiliverdin IXα was reported to be excreted, in addition to biliverdin and free phycocyanobilin, when ALA is administered to *C. caldarium* cells in the dark (Benedikt and Köst, 1985). Although the authors suggested that the compound might arise as a degradation product of phycocyanobilin, another interpretation is possible: If the initial two-electron reduction step, acting on biliverdin, is reduction of the pyrrole ring, then the resulting product will contain a vinyl group that is no longer conjugated to the rest of the tetrapyrrole double-bond system. This molecule, with its relatively unstable vinyl group, could be the activated substrate for ligation to the apoprotein. In the absence of a suitable acceptor apoprotein, the vinyl double bond would shift toward the pyrrole ring, to form the free ethylidine and reestablish conjugation. This scenario would also explain the generation of free phycocyanobilin isomers having both E- and Z-ethylidine configurations in the in vitro conversion of biliverdin to phycocyanobilin (Beale and Cornejo, 1984a). An alternative fate of the reactive vinyl-containing intermediate, in the absence of apoprotein, would be for water to be added across the vinyl group, forming α-hydroxymesobiliverdin.

e. Biosynthesis of other phycobilins. Phycocyanobilin and phycoerythrobilin were the first phycobiliprotein chromophores to be chemically characterized (Siegelman et al., 1968). Other chromophores with mesobiliverdin, urobilin, and violin-like spectral characteristics have been detected in some phycobiliproteins, where they coexist with the two major phycobilins (Glazer and Hixson, 1977; O'Carra et al., 1980). Several of these chromophores have been characterized structurally (Bishop et al., 1987; Killilea and O'Carra, 1985; Nagy et al., 1985).

All of the algae that contain phycobilins also contain phycocyanobilin, but there are some species that contain only phycocyanobilin. This distribution suggests the possibility that phycocyanobilin may be a precursor to other phycobilins. However, it should be noted that in the absence of phycocyanobilin, excitation energy probably cannot be transferred from the other chromophores to chlorophyll. Therefore, the distribution of the phycobilin types among algal species may reflect the functional dependence on phycocyanobilin, rather than indicate a biosynthetic relationship.

The possibility exists that some phycobilins are formed from protein-linked precursors. However, when *C. caldarium* cells (even mutant cells that do not accumulate phycocyanin) are incubated with exogenous ALA, they excrete a blue pigment that is identical to the free chromophore that is cleaved from phycocyanin by methanolysis (Troxler and Bogorad, 1966; Troxler and Lester, 1967). In this instance, it is unlikely that the excreted bilin is derived from cleavage of phycocyanin. This observation, and the ability of cell-free extracts of *C. caldarium* to catalyze free-phycocyanobilin formation from biliverdin, strongly suggest that, in vivo, at least this phycobilin can be synthesized as the free chromophore, with an ethylidine group present, and that a free bilin is the precursor of the bound pigment.

Although all four of the phycobilin chromophores thus far described are isomeric (Bishop et al., 1987), they may not be derived one from another. Instead, all might be derived independently from biliverdin or from a precursor with a reduced pyrrole ring, the different products being determined by the site of the second two-electron reduction step. A hypothetical biosynthetic sequence for phytochromobilin and all of the known phycobilins is shown in Fig. 7.14.

f. Ligation of phycobilins to apoproteins. The phycobilins exist, in their photosynthetically functional state, as covalently attached chromophores of the phycobiliproteins. A clearer picture of the bilin-to-apoprotein attachment modes is beginning to emerge from work with defined bilipeptides derived from the larger phycobiliproteins by proteolytic cleavage. The most frequently encountered linkage is a thioether bond between an apoprotein cysteine and the 3′ position (the α- carbon of what originated as the ring B vinyl group of protoheme). It is noteworthy that the linkage of heme to the apoprotein of cytochrome c is also by attachment of both, or occasionally one, of the tetrapyrrole vinyl groups to cysteinyl residues (Paul, 1951). Stereochemical investigations (Brockmann and Knobloch, 1973; Gossauer, 1983; Klein and Rüdiger, 1978; Schoenleber et al., 1983) have revealed that the absolute configuration about the 3′ carbon that is attached to cysteine sulfur in the phycobiliproteins examined, as well as both of the chiral centers in the attached ring, are all *R*. Spectral differences among the individual chromophores have been interpreted to indicate that some phycocyanobilin (Bishop et al., 1986) and phycoerythrobilin (Klotz et al., 1986) groups are linked to the apoprotein by the 18' position (the α- carbon of what originated as the ring A vinyl group of protoheme) instead of the 3' position. Also, in some cases, phycoerythrobilin (Schoenleber et al., 1984) and phycourobilin (Klotz and Glazer, 1985) chromophores may be doubly linked to the apoprotein, by thioether links at both the 3' and 18' positions. However, some of these conclusions regarding different linkage modes have been challenged, and the data reinterpreted in terms of different conformations of the bilins on the biliproteins leading to different bilin meso-bridge carbon configurations upon denaturation of the proteins (Schmidt et al., 1987). Finally, some evidence has been interpreted to indicate the existence of an ester bond between an apoprotein serine group and one of the propionate carboxyl groups of the bilin (Killilea and O'Carra, 1985).

There is little direct information concerning the mechanism by which the bilin chromophore is ligated to the cysteine sulfhydryl group(s) of the apo-phycobiliproteins. The bilin could be activated for apoprotein ligation by reduction of the pyrrole ring, leaving a vinyl group that is not conjugated with the rest of the tetrapyrrole double-bond system. The existence of such an intermediate is consistent with the production of α-hydroxymesobiliverdin (Benedikt and Köst, 1985) and both E- and Z-ethylidine phycocyanobilin isomers (Beale and Cornejo, 1984a) in the absence of apoprotein acceptor molecules.

Although in vitro ligation of phycobilins to apo-phycobiliproteins has not been reported, Elich et al. (1989) were able to measure incorporation of exogenous biliverdin and phycocyanobilin into phytochrome in etiolated oat leaves that had been prevented from synthesizing endogenous bilins by administration of the inhibitor of ALA formation, gabaculine. After incubation of the gabaculine-treated leaves with exogenous bilins, the phytochrome was isolated and found to undergo photoreversible spectral changes. In the case of phycocyanobilin administration, the isolated phytochrome had its absorption maxima shifted as a result of incorporation of a bilin other than the natural one, phytochromobilin.

g. Possible biosynthetic relationship of the phytochrome chromophore to phyco-bilins. The structure of the phytochrome chromophore resembles very closely those of the phycobilins (Smith and Kendrick, 1976). Phytochrome is present in higher and lower plants and at least some algae, including several green algae and the rhodophyte *Porphyra tenera* (Dring, 1974). Elich and Lagarias (1987) obtained evidence that the phytochrome chromophore, like phycocyanobilin, can be synthesized in vivo from exogenously supplied biliverdin. These workers found that phytochrome levels are substantially reduced in oat seedlings germinated in the presence of gabaculine, a specific inhibitor of ALA formation via the five-carbon pathway. If either ALA or biliverdin was administered to the gabaculine-grown seedlings, there was a rapid increase in spectrophotometrically-detected phytochrome. Finally ^{14}C-labeled exogenous biliverdin was shown to be specifically incorporated into the phytochrome chromophore in oat leaves establishing a clear biosynthetic link between this chromophore and the phycobilins (Elich et al., 1989).

It is interesting to note that a hypothetical partially reduced intermediate between biliverdin and the phycobilins, having the reduced pyrrole ring but still retaining both the *exo*-vinyl group and a fully conjugated ring system, is chemically equivalent to the free form of the phytochrome chromophore (Fig. 7.14). Thus, it could be proposed that the phytochrome chromophore originated in nature as a precursor to the phycobilin chromophores.

III. Regulation

A. Environmental and physiological modulation of pigment composition

1. Physiology of greening in plants and algae. When seeds of flowering plants are germinated in the dark, the seedlings are etiolated, that is, they are tall and yellow in color. Hemes are present in these tissues, and although chlorophyll is absent, small amounts of protochlorophyll(ide) are present. The plastids, termed etioplasts, do not have the characteristic stromal and granal thylakoid system, nor do they have photosynthetic capacity. Instead, the etioplasts have a prolamellar body which appears "paracrystalline" in electron micrographs, and has as its main protein constituent protochlorophyllide reductase (Ikeuchi and Murakami, 1983; Dehesh and Ryberg, 1985). Upon exposure to light, the protochlorophyll(ide) is immediately photoconverted to chlorophyll(ide), the prolamellar bodies begin to break down and are replaced by thylakoids, and, after a lag period, a phase of rapid chlorophyll accumulation begins. The length of the lag period appears dependent upon the age of the etiolated seedling; the longer the plant was in the dark, the longer the lag period (Sisler and Klein, 1963). Chlorophyll accumulation is complete after 24 to 36 h. If the plants are returned to the dark during greening, chlorophyll accumulation stops, small amounts of protochlorophyllide build up again, and prolamellar bodies reform (Fluhr et al., 1975; Minkov et al., 1988). Thus continuous chlorophyll accumulation requires light.

Similar studies, in which levulinic acid was included to prevent ALA utilization, demonstrated that ALA accumulation parallels chlorophyll accumulation in the absence of inhibitors (Beale and Castelfranco, 1974a; Klein et al., 1975). If ALA is administered in the dark to the dark-grown seedlings, protochlorophyllide and several porphyrin and

Mg-porphyrin intermediates accumulate (Nadler and Granick, 1970). Even though ALA can be transformed to protochlorophyll(ide) in plants that have never been exposed to light, formation of ALA, and hence, chlorophyll, requires continuous light. Dark-grown seedlings exposed to light for a short period and then returned to the dark for several hours, no longer exhibit the lag period in ALA or chlorophyll accumulation when the plants are subsequently brought back into the light (Fluhr et al., 1975).

The light effect upon chlorophyll accumulation can be divided into two components. There is an obvious and immediate effect upon the photoreduction of protochlorophyll(ide) to chlorophyll(ide), which may have indirect regulatory consequences (see below). In addition, it has been proposed that the enzymes responsible for ALA formation are induced by the phytochrome response. Red light can be substituted for white light and the effect of red light can, sometimes, be reversed by far-red light (Klein et al., 1977; Masoner and Kasemir, 1975). It has been shown that, although extractable ALA-forming activity is present in dark-grown tissue, the extractable activity increases severalfold during the first few hours of greening (Weinstein and Beale, 1985a; Weinstein, 1979; Kannangara and Gough, 1979; Harel and Ne'eman, 1983). Presumably, at least one of the enzymic components increases in response to light, because the RNA component does not increase in response to greening in these systems (Weinstein et al., 1986a; Berry-Lowe, 1987). Light quality was not investigated in the above reports.

The mRNA for the apoprotein of the nuclear-encoded chlorophyll a/b light-harvesting complex is also under phytochrome control (Mösinger et al., 1985; Silverthorne and Tobin, 1984). The presence of the chlorophyll-binding proteins is required for stabilization of the newly synthesized chlorophyll in the membrane. The light requirement for the phytochrome-mediated elimination of the lag phase in chlorophyll accumulation and the induction of transcription of the light-harvesting protein gene have been investigated in considerable detail (Briggs et al., 1988; Horwitz et al., 1988). Both the kinetics and the fluence response for chlorophyll accumulation were different from those influencing the appearance of mRNA coding for the light-harvesting protein. These results suggested to the authors that availability of apoprotein is not the limiting factor during the early stages of greening.

Treatment of cotyledons in the dark with cytokinins can mimic the effect of light pretreatment with respect to overcoming the lag phase in chlorophyll and ALA accumulation (Fletcher et al., 1973; Arnold and Fletcher, 1986). Cytokinin treatment increased the level of the mRNA for the light-harvesting complex apoprotein as well (Teyssendier de la Serve et al., 1985). Pretreatment of cotyledons with cytokinins and/or gibberellic acid in the dark also stimulated the capacity of subsequently isolated plastids to convert exogenous ALA to protochlorophyllide

(Daniell and Rebeiz, 1982; Daniell and Rebeiz, 1986). Both cytokinin and phytochrome pretreatment are time-dependent with respect to whether the pretreatments will shorten or lengthen the lag period. Pretreatment within 24 h before continuous illumination eliminates or shortens the lag period, while pretreatment 72 h before continuous light lengthens the lag period (Cohen et al., 1988). The mechanism of these effects has not been established.

Etiolated tissues have been used for the investigation of greening and chloroplast development, because exposing the dark-grown tissue to light provides a means of initiating and synchronizing the myriad steps required for the developmental process. Under normal conditions, plants grow from seed in a diurnal light/dark cycle. The plastids begin as proplastids, which are capable of several developmental fates, including chromoplasts, amyloplasts, mature chloroplasts, and so forth. In plant tissues that normally develop above the ground, such as grass leaves, etioplasts are formed only under highly artificial conditions. It is reasonable to expect that the regulatory aspects of tetrapyrrole biosynthesis observed in the transformation of etioplasts to chloroplasts may not be applicable to "normal" chloroplast development. On the other hand, in tissues such as cucumber cotyledons, which carry out a considerable part of their development underground before emerging into the light, etioplasts may be a normal developmental stage of plastid development.

Unlike the angiosperms, most gymnosperms and algae do not require light for chlorophyll formation. However, several algal strains or mutants have been isolated that do require light for greening, and these have been used as convenient model systems for greening in the angiosperms. These include the C-10 mutant of *Chlorella vulgaris* (Weinstein and Beale, 1985a), the *y*-1 mutant of *Chlamydomonas reinhardtii* (Bednarik and Hoober, 1985), and the C-2A′ mutant of *S. obliquus* (Oh-hama and Hase, 1980). In addition, the phytoflagellate, *Euglena*, requires light for chlorophyll formation and chloroplast development (Schiff, 1974). These strains that require light for plastid development have been useful experimental models for studying light effects on plastid development. It is not known whether the nonlight-requiring wild-type algal strains contain two separate protochlorophyllide-reducing systems, one light-requiring and the other light-independent, or if, instead, they contain an additional component that confers the ability of a universal light-requiring system to function in the dark.

2. Effects of Fe chelators and anaerobiosis on greening in intact tissue and chloroplasts. When etiolated bean leaves were treated in the dark with bidentate aromatic Fe chelators, such as α,α'-dipyridyl or *o*-phenanthroline, a doubling of protochlorophyllide accumulation was observed over a 21-h period (Duggan and Gassman, 1974). During this treatment Mg-protoporphyrin methyl ester increased from an undetectable level to a level nearly three times the protochlorophyllide level in untreated tissue. Smaller amounts of other porphyrin intermediates were also detected. Accumulation of Mg-porphyrins was linear during the treatment period, and similar responses were observed with maize coleoptiles, cucumber cotyledons, and pea leaves. If the tissue was also treated with levulinic acid, chelator treatment caused a doubling of ALA accumulation. The ability of the chelators to enhance Mg-porphyrin and ALA accumulation were greatest in greening tissue, compared to etiolated or fully greened tissue (Gassman and Duggan, 1974; Vlcek and Gassman, 1979). In addition to raising the level of Mg-porphyrins accumulated, chelator treatment diminished by 38% the amount of extractable heme present in the tissue (Gassman and Duggan, 1974). Finally, treatment of the leaves with salts of Fe^{2+}, Zn^{2+}, or Co^{2+} overcame the effects of chelator treatment. When the metal salts were added, Mg-protoporphyrin methyl ester disappeared in a time-dependent manner. In the light, the disappearance was accompanied by an increase in protochlorophyllide, but in the dark, the decline in Mg-porphyrin was apparently enzyme-mediated, because the loss was slower in the cold and inhibited by protein synthesis inhibitors (Vlcek and Gassman, 1979). It was postulated that the chelators have a twofold effect on the pathway. First, chelation of Fe stimulates the synthesis of ALA, probably by removing an Fe-containing inhibitor such as heme. Second, chelation of Fe inhibits the conversion of Mg-protoporphyrin methyl ester to protochlorophyllide, perhaps at a specific step. These effects can be reversed by the above-mentioned transition metals.

Anaerobiosis can be expected to have a wide variety of effects on plant growth and development. Some of these effects can be localized to the tetrapyrrole biosynthetic pathway. In the early part of the pathway, O_2 is required for coproporphyrinogen oxidase. In the above experiments with α,α'-dipyridyl, O_2 was required for the conversion of Mg-protoporphyrin methyl ester to protochlorophyllide in the light when the metal salts were added (Vlcek and Gassman, 1979). In addition, anaerobiosis or Fe deficiency caused a decrease in chlorophyll, concomitant with an accumulation of small amounts of Mg-protoporphyrin. The same conditions inhibited the conversion of exogenously supplied ALA to protochlorophyllide (Spiller et al., 1982).

Treatment of isolated chloroplasts with α,α'-dipyridyl resulted in an increase (20 to 30%) in the conversion of glutamate to ALA (Weinstein and Castelfranco, 1978; Chereskin and Castelfranco, 1982). Anaerobiosis was also shown to have an inhibitory effect on the process (Huang and Castelfranco, 1988). In this case, ALA synthesis in isolated chloroplasts could be supported in the dark with exogenous ATP and an

NADPH-regenerating system, or in the light with no exogenous cofactors. The light-driven synthesis was sensitive to DCMU, indicating a requirement for photosynthetic electron transport. Anaerobiosis caused a 26% inhibition of the dark reaction and a 90% inhibition of the light-driven reaction. When ATP and reducing power were added to the anaerobic incubation in the light, ALA synthesis was restored to 70% of the light control value. Addition of 5 mM oxaloacetic acid could replace the O_2 requirement in the light-driven reaction. It was proposed that O_2 or oxaloacetic acid is required as an electron acceptor in the regeneration of ATP, by an unexplained mechanism. As noted before, O_2 was absolutely required for the cyclase reaction in intact chloroplasts (Chereskin and Castelfranco, 1982; Chereskin et al., 1982; Nasrulhaq-Boyce et al., 1987).

3. Chlorophyll and heme turnover.   The subject of tetrapyrrole degradation in plants has recently been reviewed (Hendry et al., 1987). Aspects of degradation which are related to senescence will not be discussed in this chapter. When dark-grown barley is exposed to light for 12 h, chlorophyll accumulation increases to an amount 100 times greater than the original amount of protochlorophyllide present in the tissue before illumination (Castelfranco and Jones, 1975). During this period there is only a very minor increase in the amount of extractable, noncovalently bound protoheme (Stillman and Gassman, 1978). If ^{14}C-ALA is administered to the plants during a 5-h illumination period, the specific radioactivities of purified protoheme and pheophorbide (chlorophyll derivative) are almost identical (Castelfranco and Jones, 1975). Since new protoheme is synthesized but does not accumulate, it must turn over at a rate comparable to its rate of synthesis. Supplying ALA to etiolated shoots increased the amount of extractable protochlorophyllide, but not that of heme (Nasrulhaq-Boyce and Jones, 1981). When $^{55}Fe^{2+}$ was administered to the shoots along with the ALA, the specific radioactivity of the extracted heme was 30% higher than that from the incubation without added ALA. Similarly, in rapidly dividing cultures of *Euglena*, the relative specific radioactivities of newly formed chlorophyll and heme indicated that heme must be subject to metabolic turnover (Weinstein and Beale, 1983). If etiolated barley shoots are administered high, nonphysiological concentrations of heme through the cut base, the plant material takes up a portion of the heme, and the subsequent disappearance of the heme from the tissue can be monitored (Hendry and Stobart, 1978). Under these conditions, the exogenous heme was degraded faster in the dark than in the light, and the half-life of heme in the dark was estimated to be between 8 and 9 h. Although the conditions of the experiment are artificial, and the half-life calculations may not reflect physiological conditions, the experiment clearly shows the capacity of the tissue to eliminate unnecessary hemes.

The question of chlorophyll turnover is somewhat more complex. Turnover of newly formed chlorophyll in greening leaves of barley and wheat has been reported to be quite substantial (Hendry and Stobart, 1986; Stobart and Hendry, 1984). The method was based on the observation that after preillumination of levulinic acid-treated shoots (which are blocked from forming new chlorophyll) for 2 to 62 h, a further illumination (3600–4000 lux ≈ 50–55 $\mu E \cdot m^{-2} \cdot s^{-1}$, assuming similar light qualities) resulted in a decrease in the amount of chlorophyll present. In wheat, the half-life of chlorophyll during the first 6 h of greening was calculated to be 6.5 to 8.2 h. The half-life increased to 33 to 36 h after 2 days of greening (Stobart and Hendry, 1984). These chlorophyll losses were not observed in the dark. Examination of chlorophyll levels in untreated greening barley revealed an increase from 37 nmol/leaf after 24 h in the light to 65 nmol/leaf after 48 h in the light (Hendry and Stobart, 1986). Yet the calculated degradation rate constant was equivalent to or greater than the biosynthetic rate constant at 24 h, and the degradation rate was twice the biosynthetic rate at 48 h, suggesting that the total chlorophyll should decrease between 24 and 48 h. It therefore, seems likely that levulinic acid treatment indirectly promoted chlorophyll breakdown. During the early phase of greening, when both apoprotein and pigments are being synthesized, there may be a mechanism to prevent the accumulation of incomplete complexes as might occur when chlorophyll synthesis is artificially blocked.

When kidney bean cotyledons were returned to the dark after 8.5 h of greening, chlorophyll a remained constant while chlorophyll b decreased by 80% in 50 h (Argyroudi-Akoyunoglou et al., 1982). If the cotyledons were greened for 50 h before returning to darkness, chlorophyll b decreased only about 20%, while chlorophyll a again remained constant. During the dark period, the amount of light-harvesting complex decreased while the number of photosystem II reaction centers increased. It was suggested that the chlorophyll a from the light-harvesting complexes was recycled and the chlorophyll b degraded. Treatment of etiolated barley segments for 5 min with ^{14}C-ALA of high specific radioactivity allowed the formation of protochlorophyllide in the dark and chlorophyll in the light to be monitored (Manetas and Akoyunoglou, 1981). The specific radioactivity and total radioactivity of the isolated protochlorophyllide did not change over a period of 3 h in the dark, indicating no turnover. When the segments were brought into light of low intensity (13 $\mu E \cdot m^{-2} \cdot s^{-1}$), the total radioactivity remained constant until the end of the experiment at 4 h. The specific radioactivity began to decline after 1.5 h as new chlorophyll was made. At a higher light intensity (36 $\mu E \cdot m^{-2} \cdot s^{-1}$), there was a time-dependent decline to 40% of the original total radioactivity of the chlorophyllide. The decline leveled off in 45 min and the total radioactivity remained constant during the next 4 h of greening. The specific radioactivity declined after the onset of new chlorophyll biosynthesis. Thus, the stability of newly formed chlorophyll(ide) is dependent upon time and light intensity. The results of the pulse-labeling experiments indicate that chlorophyll does not turn over rapidly during greening in barley shoots.

In summary, we know that flowering plants require light for the massive chlorophyll build-up that is necessary for the formation of mature chloroplasts. Without light, the only intermediate that accumulates is a small amount of protochlorophyll(ide) which is immediately photoconverted to chlorophyll(ide) when the plants are exposed to light. Even in the dark all enzymes are present that are necessary for formation of chlorophyll(ide) and hemes from ALA. Despite the massive ALA formation during greening, heme levels do not build up, and there is strong evidence that heme is turned over rapidly. Although there is conflicting evidence, it appears that the turnover of newly formed chlorophyll is minor unless the developmental process is interrupted by darkness or inhibitors. Before the enzymatic properties that may give rise to these developmental features are discussed, the demand for nonplastid hemes and the subcellular compartmentation of the enzymes will be considered.

4. Nonplastid heme synthesis and turnover.   Mitochondrial development in plants has been studied mostly in nongreen tissues, such as germinating seeds, root tips, and cauliflower buds. As is the case in chloroplasts, the mitochondria require hemes for their cytochromes. In mitochondria isolated from germinating peanut cotyledons, the absorbancies due to cytochromes increased severalfold between 2 and 10 days after germination (Breidenbach et al., 1967). Similarly, the mitochondrial cytochrome content of germinating mung beans also increased severalfold between 2 and 8 days of germination (Hendry et al., 1981a). However, microsomal cytochrome b_5 rose to a peak at 4 days and fell drastically thereafter, while the level of microsomal cytochrome P450 declined in the light but recovered in the dark (Hendry et al., 1981a, b).

When sliced Jerusalem artichokes (tubers without chlorophyll) are aged in the dark, cytochromes b_5 and P450 are induced (Benveniste et al., 1977). Induction of these cytochromes, as well as other oxygenases, is enhanced by inclusion of $MnCl_2$, herbicides, or various xenobiotic materials (Reichart et al., 1980; Fonne-Pfister et al., 1988). The total induced levels can be 10 times greater than the basal level present in freshly cut tissues. The Mn-enhanced induction of these microsomal hemoproteins was effectively blocked by gabaculine, the inhibitor of ALA formation from glutamate (Werck-Reichhart et al., 1988). Inclusion of 100 μM gabaculine in the aging medium also prevented the wound-induced buildup of cytochrome P450 and guaiacol peroxidase, and caused a 10-fold decrease in the extractable heme content. The decrease in heme content in response to gabaculine inhibition of ALA formation occurred in the light or dark and indicates a substantial capacity for heme turnover. Although hemes appeared to turn over with gabaculine treatment, the respiratory capacity (as measured by O_2 consumption) was unaffected. Three possible reasons may be advanced. First, consumption of O_2 may occur by a mechanism which does not require cytochromes (alternate oxidase). Second, the hemes for the respiratory cytochromes may be formed through a pathway that is insensitive to gabaculine. Third, respiratory cytochromes may not be subject to the same turnover rates as other cellular hemes. The last reason is consistent with the evidence of Hendry et al. (1981a) which suggests that mitochondrial cytochromes are more stable than microsomal cytochromes. Labeling of the heme a moiety of cytochrome oxidase by glutamate in etiolated maize coleoptiles indicated that respiratory hemes are formed primarily or entirely via the five-carbon pathway (Schneegurt and Beale, 1986), although the possible existence of a minor gabaculine-insensitive pathway cannot be ruled out.

It is clear from the foregoing discussion that a general model for the regulation of tetrapyrrole biosynthesis in plants must take into account the substantial pools of both mitochondrial cytochromes and cytosolic hemoproteins in addition to the chloroplast cytochromes and chlorophyll-protein complexes. Cytosolic hemoproteins can be induced and turned over independently of chloroplast development. In tubers and germinating seeds, mitochondrial cytochromes appear to be stable, although this question has not been directly addressed for mature tissue or tissue undergoing the transition from heterotrophic to autotrophic growth conditions. Finally, a general regulatory model must address the subcellular localization of the biosynthetic and regulatory processes.

5. Regulation of phycobilin content by light and nutritional status

a. Light effects. Wild-type cells of *C. caldarium* form neither chlorophyll nor phycocyanin in the dark, although the cells are capable of vigorous dark growth in glucose-supplemented medium. When cells are transferred to the light, both bilin and apoprotein moieties of phycocyanin are synthesized de novo in stoichiometric amounts, rather than being assembled from preexisting components (Troxler and Brown, 1970).

Administration of exogenous ALA in the dark causes the cells to synthesize and excrete free phycocyanobilin (Troxler and Bogorad, 1966), indicating that there is no light-requiring step in bilin biosynthesis from ALA. Nevertheless, the normal inhibition of phycobilin formation by darkness does indicate some sort of photoregulation of the process. Mutant strains which normally are unable to form phycobiliproteins in the light or dark accumulate the phycobilin moiety, but not the apoprotein, if supplied with exogenous ALA. On the other hand, if levulinic acid is administered to wild-type cells in vivo to block pigment formation, apoprotein is still synthesized to some extent (Schuster et al., 1983a). These results imply that apoprotein formation is not linked directly to bilin formation. However, neither bilin nor apoprotein normally accumulates in cells undergoing wide changes in phycobiliprotein level. Therefore, some sort of indirect coregulation must occur to keep the components in approximate stoichiometric ratio.

In cells that are accumulating both hemes and phycobilins, the first biosynthetic step unique to the phycobilin branch would be the heme oxygenase reaction. This reaction therefore is a logical candidate for a physiological control point, regulating the cellular level of phycobilins.

Nichols and Bogorad (1962) examined the action spectrum for phycobilin formation in a nonphotosynthetic, chlorophyll-less mutant of *C. caldarium*. Light of 420-nm wavelength was most effective in promoting bilin formation. A second peak in the action spectrum occurred at about 580 nm. The authors proposed that the photoreceptor may be a heme compound. They also reported that dark phycocyanin synthesis could be induced by unidentified factors present in some culture medium components.

Another mutant strain of *C. caldarium* accumulates chlorophyll a but not phycocyanin. The action spectrum for chlorophyll synthesis corresponds to the absorption spectrum of protochlorophyllide (Schneider and Bogorad, 1978). Wild-type cells, which contain both chlorophyll and phycocyanin, have a single action spectrum for synthesis of both pigments, and this resembles the sum of the action spectra exhibited by the two mutant strains.

Many algae have been reported to change both their absolute phycobilin content and the relative abundances of phycocyanin and phycoerythrin in response to variations in the light regime. Marine intertidal red macroalgae contain increasing amounts of phycobilin pigments when grown at decreasing average light levels which occur at increasing water depths (Ramus et al., 1976). In blue-green algae, at least three mechanisms are known to operate in bringing about changes in phycobilin pigment composition. In some species, the ratio of phycoerythrin to phycocyanin changes during chromatic adaptation (Bennett and Bogorad, 1973). Other species also vary the subunit number and composition in phycocyanin (Bryant and Cohen-Bazire, 1981). Still other organisms have been reported to incorporate different bilins into apoprotein subunits under different growth conditions (Yu et al., 1981).

Among cyanophytes that exhibit complementary chromatic adaptation, cells growing in red light contain little or no phycoerythrin, but this becomes the major phycobiliprotein during growth in green light. A search for pigments that might mediate the response to variations in spectral light distribution has resulted in the detection of several photochromic species, both in vivo and in vitro (Björn and Björn, 1980). Isolated photochromic pigments appear to be similar or identical to some phycobiliprotein subunits. They undergo photoreversible transformations, with peak positions that are close to the peaks of the action spectra for the chromatic adaptation responses, that is, 520 to 550 nm for the green-light effects and 640 to 660 nm for the red-light effects (Vogelman and Scheibe, 1978). The photochromic species were named phycochromes by Björn and Björn (1976). There is no agreement yet on which of the isolated photochromic pigments (at least four have been described) correspond(s) to the physiologically active light quality-sensing pigment(s) in vivo. One report indicates that the photoreversible pigments of *Tolypothrix tenuis* are chromoproteins that are derived from phycobiliproteins upon photobleaching (Okhi and Fujita, 1979). Because of their close structural and functional resemblance to phytochrome, the phycochromes are attractive candidates for its evolutionary predecessors.

Since phycobiliproteins differ from each other in the protein moieties as well as in their phycobilin complement, differential synthesis or breakdown of proteins must be a requirement for complementary chromatic adaptation. Gendel et al. (1979) have shown that the induction of phycoerythrin synthesis by green light in the blue-green alga *Fremyella diplosiphon* is blocked by rifamycin, indicating a requirement for gene transcription in the response. Transfer from green light to darkness slowed, but did not stop, phycoerythrin synthesis, indicating that differential phycobiliprotein synthesis is induced by green light, but that continuous irradiation is not required for the response to occur. Cells that were transferred from green to red light stopped synthesizing phycoerythrin within 45 min. The same time course for cessation of phycoerythrin synthesis was observed when rifamycin was administered to cells growing in green light, suggesting that the chromatic adaptation response is mediated at the transcriptional level (Gendel et al., 1979). Green light was shown to induce specifically the transcription of a phycoerythrin operon containing the gene coding for both the α and β subunits of phycoerythrin (Mazel et al., 1986).

Egelhoff and Grossman (1983) reported that in eukaryotic algae, the phycobilin apoproteins are synthesized on plastid ribosomes. This conclusion was based on differential sensitivity to inhibitors of protein synthesis. The same conclusion is supported by the results of Belford et al. (1983), who found that cell-free synthesis of *C. caldarium* phycocyanin subunits occurred when a reticulocyte lysate translation system was supplied with the non-poly(A) fraction of mRNAs isolated from the algae.

Other evidence suggests that in eukaryotic cells the rate-limiting steps of phycobilin synthesis are catalyzed by enzymes synthesized on cytoplasmic ribosomes. For example, it is known from exogenous feeding experiments that ALA availability is rate-limiting for phycobilin synthesis and excretion. ALA formation is rapidly inhibited in the algae by the administration of cycloheximide, which blocks cytoplasmic protein synthesis.

Yu et al. (1981) reported that the red alga *Callithamnion roseum*, when grown under different light intensities, acquires phycoerythrin with different ratios of phycoerythrobilin to phycourobilin, while the protein subunit composition remains constant. The mechanism responsible for the substitution of bilins is not yet known.

Beguin et al. (1985) described a mutant strain of *F. diplosiphon* that does not accumulate phycoerythrin under any light regime. In red light, the cells are phenotypically indistinguishable from the wild type. In green light, some of the phycocyanin subunits contain a bilin of unknown structure, that has a distinctive violinlike visible absorption spectrum. These interesting observations have been interpreted as supporting the hypothesis that bilins other than phycocyanobilin are derived from protein-bound phycocyanobilin, either by enzymatic isomerization or nonenzymatically as a result of protein folding (Beguin et al., 1985). However, a clearer understanding of these results may have to await determination of the structure of the novel bilin and the nature of the defect in the mutant cells.

Successful cloning of a DNA fragment from the blue-green alga *Synechococcus* sp. PCC 7002 (*Agmenellum quadruplicatum*) containing the genes for both the a and b subunits of phycocyanin has been reported (de Lorimier et al., 1984). The cloned genes will make possible the study of the regulation of expression of the genes for the apoproteins (Elich and Lagarias, 1987). Also, the expression of these genes in *E. coli* may make it possible to obtain substrate quantities of apoprotein for in vitro studies of the chromophore ligation reactions (Bryant et al., 1985).

One important result has already emerged from a study using the cloned phycocyanin genes. When the cloned genes were reintroduced into *Synechococcus* at higher multiplicity, overexpression of the genes resulted. The cells accumulated correspondingly greater than normal amounts of chromophore-containing phycocyanin (de Lorimier et al., 1988). Apparently, the cells were able to synthesize sufficient phycobilins to accommodate the increased demand for pigment. This result suggests that bilin formation does not limit the rate of phycocyanin accumulation, but that, instead, the bilin biosynthetic rate may respond to the availability of apo-biliprotein.

At present, the only study at the enzyme level to reveal regulation of a specific step of phycobilin synthesis is that of Brown et al. (1984), which reported a large increase in the activity of ferrochelatase paralleling the rise in phycocyanin accumulation when dark-grown wild-type *C. caldarium* cells are transferred from the dark to the light.

b. Responses to nitrogen status. Phycobiliproteins comprise a significant proportion of total cellular proteins of cyanobacteria when the cells are grown in medium containing nonlimiting amounts of nitrogen. When the cells are shifted to growth on limiting nitrogen, they specifically degrade much of their phycobiliproteins (Allen and Smith, 1969). Foulds and Carr (1977) have described a proteolytic enzyme activity in extracts of *Anabaena cylindrica* that is specific for phycocyanin. Enzyme activity was associated with both the $100,000 \times g$ pellet and supernatant fractions. Activity was severalfold higher in extracts of cells harvested during heterocyst development in response to growth at low nitrogen than in extracts of cells grown on nonlimiting nitrogen. It was suggested that the in vitro proteolytic activity is physiologically related to in vivo phycocyanin degradation, and the enzyme responsible for the activity was named phycocyaninase. The fate of the bilin chromophores was not reported.

6. Regulation of bacteriochlorophyll formation by light and O_2 in facultative photosynthetic bacteria

a. Physiological responses to light and O_2. Certain purple nonsulfur facultative photosynthetic bacteria (e.g., *R. spheroides* and *R. capsulatus*, *Rhodospirillum rubrum*) can grow heterotrophically in the dark when supplied with a reduced carbon source and an aerobic environment. These organisms also grow phototrophically under anaerobic conditions, and synthesis and accumulation of bacteriochlorophyll are controlled by O_2 and light (Cohen-Bazire et al., 1957). Thus, cultures growing anaerobically in the light experience an immediate cessation of bacteriochlorophyll synthesis upon introduction of O_2 into the culture. In light-grown anaerobic cultures, the accumulation of bacteriochlorophyll is inversely proportional to light intensity, although light is, of course, required for photosynthetic growth. Finally, dark-grown aerobic cultures are not pigmented, but form bacteriochlorophyll in the dark if O_2 is depleted. Although synthesis of bacteriochlorophyll is dependent upon light and O_2, heme and corrinoid synthesis are relatively unaffected by changes in the growth conditions.

It was originally assumed that the inverse relationship of bacteriochlorophyll synthesis to light intensity and O_2 tension was modulated through a single mechanism related to the redox state of the cell. However, in experiments in which O_2 tension and light intensity could be carefully controlled by maintaining a constant cell density under continuous culture conditions, it was demonstrated that light and O_2 acted by essentially different mechanisms (Arnheim and Oelze, 1983). When the effects of cell growth were eliminated, it was found that bacteriochlorophyll content decreased in a hyperbolic fashion with increasing O_2 tension, whether the cells were grown in the light or dark. In contrast, when cells were maintained in either anaerobic conditions or in 3% of air-saturated O_2 tension, bacteriochlorophyll content decreased sigmoidally with increasing light intensity. Thus, the two effects could be manipulated independently, were additive, and followed different kinetics. Light was shown to affect the accumulation of bacteriochlorophyll rather than synthesis (Biel, 1986). Incubation of cells (*R. capsulatus*) with radioactively labeled ALA in the dark resulted in accumulation of bacteriochlorophyll, which could be separated by thin-layer chromatography and quantified spectrophotometrically or by label incorporation. When the same experiment was repeated in bright light, label incorporation into a colorless compound, which migrated with the same R_f as bacteriochlorophyll in three different solvent systems, increased with time in the same manner as bacteriochlorophyll did in dark-grown cultures. Although the colorless compound was not identified, a compound with identical chromatographic behavior was obtained by illumination of a methanolic extract of the bacteria. It was suggested that in bright light bacteriochlorophyll synthesis proceeds normally but accumulation is prevented, possibly by photodestruction of the pigment. However, these experiments do not rule out the possibility of additional light regulation at the level of ALA synthesis.

b. Effectors of enzyme activity.   Addition of exogenous ALA to normally growing *R. spheroides* cells resulted in the accumulation of several intermediates of the biosynthetic pathway (Lascelles, 1966). Thus, tetrapyrrole formation is regulated primarily at the level of ALA formation. ALA synthase purified from *R. spheroides* was reversibly inhibited more than 50% by 5 μM heme (Warnick and Burnham, 1971), and to a lesser extent by protoporphyrin and Mg-protoporphyrin (Yubisui and Yoneyama, 1972). Evidence suggesting that heme inhibition operates in vivo has been reviewed by Lascelles (1978). In one set of experiments, incubation of cells with the ferrochelatase inhibitor, N-methylprotoporphyrin, resulted in a decrease in cytochrome content and an increase in excreted Mg-porphyrins when cells with a genetic block in the bacteriochlorophyll pathway were used (Houghton et al., 1982). It was suggested that the inhibitor decreased the cellular heme concentration, which removed the inhibition of ALA synthase, resulting in overproduction of porphyrins. In addition to the sensitivity of the enzyme to feedback inhibition by end products, activity was also inhibited as much as 90% by 1.0 mM ATP (Fanica-Gaignier and Clement-Metral, 1973).

When ALA synthase was purified from cell extracts, two forms, active and inactive, could be separated from each other by DEAE-Sephadex chromatography (Sandy et al., 1975). The purified inactive form was converted to the active form by incubation with cystine- or glutathione-trisulfides, R-S-S-S-R. Two proteins were reported to be involved in the conversion of the inactive form to the active form in cell extracts incubated with disulfides such as cystine (Inoue et al., 1979; Oyama and Tuboi, 1979). In the presence of the enzyme cystathionase, the sulfur of cystine was incorporated into to a "regulatory protein" forming a trisulfide with two cysteine residues in the regulatory protein. The modified regulatory protein then was able to activate the inactive form of ALA synthase. ALA synthase activity in vitro was also modulated by thioredoxin (Clement-Metral, 1979), which has now been purified and characterized from these cells (Clement-Metral et al., 1986). Although the intracellular concentration of trisulfides fell during aeration of *Rhodobacter* cultures (Sandy et al., 1975), bacteriochlorophyll synthesis was arrested and the percentage of active ALA synthase was decreased 50% by treating the cells with a 10% v/v O_2/N_2 mixture, even though the intracellular trisulfide concentration was unaffected (Wider de Xifra et al., 1976). Thus, a mechanism relating aeration of cultures with a decrease in trisulfides and inactivation of ALA synthase is still speculative at this point.

Beyond the steps catalyzing formation of ALA, the only enzyme before the branch point that has shown regulatory properties is ALA dehydratase. The enzyme from *R. spheroides* (Nandi et al., 1968), but not *R. capsulatus* (Nandi and Shemin, 1973), was inhibited by heme. Of the enzymes beyond protoporphyrin, only ferrochelatase has been purified and characterized (Dailey, 1982; Dailey et al., 1986). Although this enzyme is much larger than eukaryotic ferrochelatase enzymes, no regulatory properties could be ascribed to the *R. spheroides* enzyme. Mg-chelatase activity was reported to be highly sensitive to O_2 (Gorchein, 1972, 1973), but, because the experiments were performed in whole cells, it was not possible to ascertain if the O_2 had a direct effect on enzyme activity.

c. **Molecular genetics of bacteriochlorophyll formation.** Only limited information is available on regulation of enzyme synthesis. The O_2 sensitivity and the complex role of trisulfides in regulating ALA synthase, and the inability to measure directly the activities of enzymes in the Mg branch of the pathway, limit the reliability of experiments that attempt to follow enzyme synthesis by activity measurements alone. Fortunately, progress has been made using a molecular genetic approach to this problem. Photosynthetic membrane biosynthesis, including bacteriochlorophyll formation, in *Rhodobacter* has recently been reviewed by Kiley and Kaplan (1988).

The structural genes for many of the enzymes of the bacteriochlorophyll pathway have been identified on the basis of mutation and restoration of a functional pathway by complementation with plasmids containing DNA sequences from wild-type cells (Marrs, 1981; Yen and Marrs, 1976; Youvan et al., 1983). The identification of these genes has facilitated the study of their expression, even in the absence of having correlated enzyme activities with the genes. In an interesting variation on the molecular approach, the Mu d1 phage was used to create fusions of the *lacZ* gene (β-galactosidase structural gene) with various bacteriochlorophyll genes so that the *lacZ* gene was under the control of the promoters of the bacteriochlorophyll genes (Biel and Marrs, 1983). The interrupted genes were identified by the products which accumulated. The activity of the promoters could then be followed under different environmental conditions by measuring the β-galactosidase activity. Using this approach, it was found that in *R. capsulatus*, genes *bch* A, B, C, G, and H increased their expression two- to fourfold when cells were switched from 20% O_2 to 2% O_2. Mutation of these genes resulted in the accumulation of chlorophyllide, Mg-divinylpheoporphyrin a_5, 2-hydroxyethyl-bacteriochlorophyllide a, bacteriochlorophyllide a, and protoporphyrin, respectively. There was no evidence for these genes being under the control of a single operon. Using as probes DNA from genes that were identified by their ability to restore bacteriochlorophyll formation to mutants, dot blot analysis of mRNA demonstrated increased transcription of several bacteriochlorophyll genes within 1 h of lowering the O_2 content of *R. spheroides* cultures (Hunter and Coomber, 1988).

In addition to bacteriochlorophyll formation, the synthesis of pigment-binding protein components of the light-harvesting and reaction center complexes is also under regulatory control by O_2 (Kiley and Kaplan, 1988), and the two processes are tightly coupled (Takemoto and Lascelles, 1973). Marrs and co-workers have studied the O_2-regulated expression of the *puf* operon, which encodes several pigment-binding proteins of the light-harvesting and reaction center complexes (Bauer et al., 1988). They discovered an additional open reading frame (*pufQ*) which, when fused with a β-galactosidase structural gene, was transcribed and translated in a manner similar to that of the light-harvesting and reaction center polypeptides. If a part of the operon including *pufQ*, was deleted, then bacteriochlorophyll accumulation was severely depleted. Bacteriochlorophyll accumulation could be restored if *pufQ* was restored in trans on a plasmid (Bauer and Marrs, 1988). When fused with the *lacZ* gene, the expression could be monitored and was found to be directly proportional to bacteriochlorophyll accumulation. Introduction of *puf* operon deletions into bacteriochlorophyll mutant strains which accumulate specific Mg-porphyrin intermediates results in the lack of intermediate accumulation in the new constructs. Introduction of *pufQ*, in trans, resulted in renewed accumulation of intermediate. Thus, the expression of an unidentified gene product of the *puf* operon is necessary for the synthesis of bacteriochlorophyll intermediates beyond protoporphyrin. It was proposed that this small hydrophobic protein (deduced by sequence analysis) is a porphyrin "carrier polypeptide" which regulates and is necessary for synthesis of intermediates in the Mg branch of the pathway. The existence of such a carrier was postulated by Lascelles on the basis of excretion of protein-bound intermediates in certain mutants (Rebeiz and Lascelles, 1982).

B. Regulation of biosynthetic steps

1. Subcellular compartmentation of tetrapyrrole biosynthesis. Isolated chloroplasts are capable of converting exogenously supplied glutamate to chlorophyll(ide) (Fuesler et al., 1984a; Gomez-Silva et al., 1985; Tripathy and Rebeiz, 1987). By inference the chloroplasts must contain all the enzymes necessary for those transformations. Isolated etioplasts and mature chloroplasts also have ferrochelatase activity (Porra and Lascelles, 1968; Jones, 1968; Little and Jones, 1976). Thus, chloroplasts are theoretically capable of providing either hemes or heme precursors for all cellular tetrapyrroles. It is not clear to what extent, if any, mitochondria provide heme precursors or hemes for nonplastid hemoproteins. As indicated above, mitochondrial hemes in plants are formed via the five-carbon path of ALA biosynthesis. The same is true for cytosolic hemes, as was indicated by the gabaculine inhibition studies (above) and by direct labeling studies of the heme moiety of cationic peroxidase in peanut suspension cultures (Chibbar and van Huystee, 1983). Thus, it is not possible to determine the origin of the heme for specific cytosolic hemoproteins by differential labeling with precursors for either the five-carbon pathway or for ALA synthase. This approach is possible in *Euglena* (Weinstein and Beale, 1983), but for phylogenetic reasons the results would not be applicable to higher plants or other algae.

In contrast to the situation for chloroplasts, it is not known if plant mitochondria are capable of independent tetrapyrrole biosynthesis. Three enzymes, coproporphyrinogen oxidase (Hsu and Miller, 1970), protoporphyrinogen oxidase (Jacobs et al., 1982; Jacobs and Jacobs, 1987), and ferrochelatase (Little and Jones, 1976; Porra and Lascelles, 1968) have been detected in both mitochondria and chloroplasts of plants. In studies of the latter two enzymes, the organelles were purified by sucrose density gradient centrifugation, and the putative mitochondrial activity coincided in the gradients with cytochrome oxidase activity (Little and Jones, 1976; Jacobs et al., 1982). However, none of the above studies established conclusively that the mitochondrial membranes were totally free of chloroplast or etioplast contamination. In the most detailed of the studies (in terms of subcellular localization), a washed mitochondrial pellet from etiolated barley was subjected to equilibrium density centrifugation (Little and Jones, 1976). Ferrochelatase exhibited two bands of activity. The low-density band (1.18 to 1.19 g/mL) also contained symmetrical bands of two mitochondrial markers, cytochrome oxidase and succinic dehydrogenase. However, when washed mitochondria were prepared from 4-h greened barley and subjected to the same centrifugation, chlorophyll was observed "...as a single broad peak between the densities of 1.18 and 1.24 g/ml..." (Little and Jones, 1976), indicating that the mitochondrial peak may have had some chloroplast membrane contamination. Fortunately, the ferrochelatase in the etioplast-enriched membranes had a different pH optimum than the one in the mitochondrial-enriched membranes, supporting the notion that each organelle has its own ferrochelatase.

Distribution of two soluble tetrapyrrole biosynthetic enzymes, ALA dehydratase and porphobilinogen deaminase, was investigated in green and etiolated leaves of peas, and in spadices of *Arum* (Smith, 1988). The latter tissue is not green and undergoes a major increase in the activity of several Krebs cycle enzymes at the stage when they are harvested. The distribution of the dehydratase and deaminase in all three tissues most closely followed the markers for two soluble chloroplast enzymes, ADP-glucose pyrophosphorylase and alkaline pyrophosphatase. Even in etiolated peas and *Arum* spadices, the tetrapyrrole biosynthetic enzymes did not cosediment with the mitochondrial marker (NAD-dependent malic enzyme) on density gradients. In addition, the tetrapyrrole biosynthetic enzymes did not behave as cytosolic enzymes. Although some activity always sedimented with a pellet, the percentage in the pellet corresponded to the percentage of soluble chloroplast marker in the pellet. Both ALA dehydratase and porphobilinogen deaminase are cytosolic enzymes in animal cells (Granick and Beale, 1978). The refractory cell walls of most plant tissues preclude the isolation of intact organelles without breaking a substantial fraction of the organelles. Thus, it would be impossible to differentiate between large amounts of activity released from broken organelles (in this case the plastids) and a small amount of activity that may normally be localized in the cytosol. If a cytosolic fraction could be prepared that is free of enzymes originating from broken organelles (e.g., by gentle lysis of protoplasts), activity measured in the cytosol may be due to enzyme synthesized on cytoplasmic ribosomes and in the process of being transported to the organelle. The activity of this fraction, measured in vitro, may not have a physiological role.

In an attempt to determine the subcellular origin of the heme moiety of cationic peroxidase in cultured peanut cells, the cells were labeled with ^{14}C-ALA and the radioactivity of the hemes in various subcellular fractions was compared (Chibbar and van Huystee, 1986). The hemes extracted from the mitochondrial fraction had 15 times more total radioactivity than those from the amyloplast fraction. However, no indication was given of the specific radioactivity of the hemes, nor was there an estimation of the purity of the subcellular fractions based on marker enzymes. While the results suggest a mitochondrial origin of the heme moiety of peroxidase, this conclusion is tentative. If the preceding results are accepted, it should also be determined whether the mitochondria supply heme for the peroxidase under conditions where the chloroplasts are actively synthesizing new tetrapyrroles.

2. Regulation of metabolic activity. A model for the regulation of the flux of precursors through the tetrapyrrole pathway in the chloroplast must account for many of the aspects of greening and turnover which occur after the lag phase. Most of these changes occur on a more rapid time scale than changes that would result from enzyme turnover. Briefly, these aspects include: (1) Porphyrin and Mg-porphyrin intermediates, except for protochlorophyllide, do not normally accumulate in the dark or the light. (2) Administration of ALA to isolated plastids or intact tissue causes the accumulation of several porphyrin and Mg-porphyrin intermediates, including protochlorophyllide. In the light, some of the accumulated protochlorophyllide is converted to chlorophyllide. The amount of extractable heme does not increase when exogenous precursors are administered. (3) During greening of etiolated barley, the ratio of extractable Mg-porphyrins to Fe-porphyrins increases from 1.7 to almost 70 after 24 h in the light (Castelfranco and Jones, 1975; Stillman and Gassman, 1978). During this change there is only a marginal increase in heme content, so that the increase in chlorophyll content accounts for most of the change in the ratio. (4) Newly synthesized protochlorophyllide and chlorophyll are relatively stable, while hemes undergo substantial turnover. (5) Transfer of greening material to the dark results in an almost complete cessation of chlorophyll accumulation, and only a small amount of protochlorophyllide accumulates. (6) During light/dark transitions, ALA accumulation in levulinic-acid- or dioxoheptanoic-acid-treated tissue parallels chlorophyll accumulation in untreated tissue. Many of these observations can be explained in terms of effector-mediated control of individual enzymes and/or conversion of the effectors to noninhibitory compounds. The following discussion of effector-mediated control of enzyme activity refers only to plants which require light for greening, and which have proceeded beyond the initial lag phase in the greening curve.

3. Effector-mediated regulation of ALA-forming activity. A model for regulation has been proposed by Castelfranco and Jones (1975) and, in an expanded form, by Chereskin and Castelfranco (1982) and Castelfranco and Beale (1983). The model accounts for regulation of chlorophyll synthesis during greening after a dark/light transition. In this model the primary point of regulation is the formation of ALA from glutamate. Heme is a potent inhibitor of this step in intact plastids (Chereskin and Castelfranco, 1982) and most of the soluble enzyme systems which have been characterized (Gough and Kannangara, 1979; Wang et al., 1984; Weinstein and Beale, 1985a; Rieble and Beale, 1988; Rieble et al., 1988). There is a substantial body of evidence that heme directly inhibits ALA formation in vivo as well.

Exogenous heme administered to intact barley shoots (Hendry and Stobart, 1978) and to cultures of *Chlamydomonas* (Hoober and Stegeman, 1973) inhibited the formation of chlorophyll in vivo, although in both cases the concentration of exogenous heme was extremely high. It is likely that the increased ALA accumulation noted in intact tissue treated with aromatic Fe chelators (Duggan and Gassman, 1974) was due to interference with heme formation, causing a decrease in the concentration of this feedback inhibitor. Similar effects were observed in intact plastids, where the Fe chelator eliminated the inhibition caused by added protoporphyrin (Chereskin and Castelfranco, 1982). It has been shown that chloroplasts are capable of heme biosynthesis (Jones, 1968; Little and Jones, 1976), and that hemes undergo significant turnover in vivo (Castelfranco and Jones, 1975; Hendry and Stobart, 1978). If heme breakdown is an aerobic (Cornejo and Beale, 1988; Hendry et al., 1981a) and ongoing process, then anaerobic conditions might be expected to prevent normal heme breakdown and thereby inhibit ALA biosynthesis. This effect has been observed in isolated plastids. Light-driven ALA formation in isolated plastids requires O_2. Although most of the O_2 requirement could be overcome by the addition of ATP and NADPH, there was still a 30% inhibition of ALA formation under anaerobic conditions in the light or the dark (Huang and Castelfranco, 1988). It is possible that anaerobic conditions prevented O_2-dependent heme breakdown, allowing the buildup of inhibitory concentrations of heme.

Genetic evidence also supports the role of heme in regulating ALA formation in vivo. A light-brown mutant of *Chlamydomonas* that is deficient in chlorophyll synthesis accumulated small amounts of protoporphyrin (Huang and Wang, 1986b). Introduction of a second mutation resulted in a dark-brown phenotype in which the organism accumulated

15 times more protoporphyrin than the first mutant. The specific activity of the ALA-forming enzymes in the unpurified extract of the first mutant was about 16% of the wild type, while the double mutant had 64% of the activity of the wild type. Because both extracts were equally sensitive to heme, the authors proposed that the phenotype of the original mutation was caused by a block at a step that utilizes protoporphyrin. In the original mutant, accumulation of a small amount of protoporphyrin results in repression of the ALA-forming enzyme system. A defective regulatory gene in the double mutant allows higher expression of the enzymes. The authors further suggested that heme is the corepressor in this system, although no direct evidence was presented to support this view. Introduction of a different second mutation, nonallelic with the first, also resulted in a dark-brown phenotype with elevated protoporphyrin accumulation. However, in this case, the enzyme activity was much less sensitive to heme. Thus, in *Chlamydomonas*, heme appears to regulate both the activity and expression of ALA-synthesizing enzymes.

Heme concentrations which inhibit in vitro activity by 50% ranged from 0.05 μM in partially purified *Chlamydomonas* extracts (Huang and Wang, 1986b) to 1.2 μM in *Chlorella* extracts (Weinstein and Beale, 1985a). In contrast to most of the organisms examined, very high concentrations (25 μM) of heme were required for 50% inhibition in *Euglena* (Mayer et al., 1987). It is not likely that heme plays a significant role in regulating ALA formation from glutamate in this organism. Except for the special case of intact plastids, the heme concentrations required for 50% inhibition appear to be higher in the more highly purified preparations. Although Mg-protoporphyrin was inhibitory in intact plastids (Chereskin and Castelfranco, 1982), relatively high concentrations were required for 50% inhibition in the solubilized systems (Weinstein and Beale, 1985a; Huang and Wang, 1986b). Other potential feedback inhibitors (protoporphyrin, protochlorophyllide, and chlorophyllide) were not effective, except at very high concentrations. In experiments designed to test for a possible in vivo regulatory role of protochlorophyllide, the dark accumulation of ALA in levulinic-acid-treated barley leaves was found to be inversely proportional to the level of protochlorophyllide bound in the ternary complex with the reductase enzyme (Stobart and Ameen-Bukhari, 1984, 1986). However, ALA accumulation could still take place in leaves that were artificially manipulated to have relatively high levels of free reductase and free protochlorophyllide. To explain these results, the authors proposed an indirect relationship between protochlorophyllide reduction and ALA synthesis via a common supply of NADPH, whereby photoreduction of the ternary protochlorophyllide complex would release bound NADP, which could then be reduced and used for ALA biosynthesis from glutamate. It should be noted that these experiments did not take into account variations in the level of free heme. In addition, experiments comparing the pool sizes of NADP(H) and protochlorophyllide reductase were not reported.

It was reported that of the three enzyme activities required for ALA formation in vitro, heme exerts its effect only on the enzyme responsible for reduction of the glutamyl-tRNA adduct (Huang and W.-Y. Wang, 1986a). However, more recent work with separated fractions from *Chlamydomonas* revealed that both the glutamyl-tRNA synthetase and the dehydrogenase activities were inhibited by heme, with 50% inhibition occurring at 2 and 10 μM, for the synthetase and dehydrogenase steps, respectively (Wang, personal communication). Finally, it was reported that preincubation of partially purified extracts with ATP stimulated ALA formation upon subsequent addition of the remaining substrates and cofactors (Weinstein and Beale, 1985a). Although the behavior was consistent with a protein kinase phosphoprotein phosphatase modulation of activity, no direct evidence was obtained to support that hypothesis.

4. Expression and turnover of ALA-forming enzymes.   Direct measurement of synthesis and turnover of the proteins catalyzing ALA synthesis has not yet been accomplished. The most reliable method for determining the level of enzyme protein is by immunochemical techniques which require purified protein to elicit the antibodies. Although antibodies to the glutamyl-tRNA synthetase from barley chloroplasts and *Chlamydomonas* (Bruyant and Kannangara, 1987; Chang et al., 1988) have now been prepared, they have not yet been used for turnover studies. However, there have been several studies based on the effects of inhibitors of protein synthesis on ALA accumulation in vivo, or the levels of extractable ALA synthesis activity during greening, which have been interpreted in terms of expression and turnover of enzyme protein. It should be emphasized that with either of these approaches, changes in ALA accumulated in vivo or changes in extractable activity in vitro can be the result of processes other than the turnover of new enzyme (e.g., changes in substrate supply or effector concentration in vivo, or covalent modification in vitro).

Levulinic-acid-dependent accumulation of ALA in *Chlorella* was inhibited by treatment with the protein synthesis inhibitor, cycloheximide (Beale, 1971). Inhibition was complete after 30 min, suggesting that continuous synthesis of enzyme is required in this organism. The phytochrome-mediated elimination of the lag phase in chlorophyll synthesis is also thought to involve new enzyme synthesis. Thus, the normally rapid accumulation of ALA that occurs upon illumination in levulinic-acid-treated, dark-germinated maize or beans is prevented by application of cycloheximide 2 h prior to light treatment (Klein et al., 1975). Application of cycloheximide to intact plants at the same time as illumination, or later, did not significantly affect ALA accumulation for another 4 or 6 h. The interpretation was that cycloheximide treatment prior to illumination prevented the synthesis of ALA biosynthetic enzymes during the normal lag phase. Cycloheximide treatment during the lag phase allowed enzyme synthesis to continue while the inhibitor was penetrating and reaching the sites of protein synthesis. The plants could then accumulate ALA until the newly synthesized enzyme turned over. A half-life of 80 min for the activity was estimated by returning greening leaves to the dark and relating the length of the dark period to the level of ALA accumulation when the plants were subsequently brought back into the light (Fluhr et al., 1975).

The plant and algal systems which require light for greening, and from which active cell-free ALA-synthesizing systems have been obtained, had a basal amount of activity even in dark-grown cells or plants. The level of activity in relatively unpurified extracts increased three- to fourfold when the plants or algae were exposed to light for 2 to 4 h prior to extraction. This phenomenon was observed in barley (Kannangara and Gough, 1979), cucumber plastids (Weinstein, 1979), maize (Harel and Ne'eman, 1983), and *Chlorella* (Weinstein and Beale, 1985a). It is not clear which of the enzyme components increase(s) upon light exposure, but in *Chlorella* (Weinstein et al., 1986a) and barley (Berry-Lowe, 1987), the tRNA component does not increase during greening.

Regulation of ALA synthesis in *Euglena* is a particularly perplexing problem. It is the only organism known in which both routes to ALA exist and operate simultaneously, albeit in separate compartments. In the dark, the level of ALA synthase was relatively high and decreased drastically when cells were brought into the light (Foley et al., 1982). Light-grown cells had low ALA synthase activity which increased four-fold after 4 h in the dark. Activity of the five-carbon route was absent in dark-grown cells and high in light-grown cells (Mayer et al., 1987). The interplay between the two biosynthetic routes was demonstrated by treatment of light-grown cells with gabaculine, the inhibitor of the glutamate pathway. The gabaculine treatment caused a twofold increase in extractable ALA synthase activity in the light (Corriveau and Beale, 1986). Pretreatment with gabaculine also prevented the decrease in extractable ALA synthase activity which normally occurs upon transfer of dark-grown cells to the light. Thus, it is clear that the cells have some mechanism to maintain a supply of porphyrin precursors and that this mechanism is not solely a light-dependent phenomenon. To complicate the matter further, both ALA synthase (Foley et al., 1982) and the five-carbon route to ALA (Mayer et al., 1987) are insensitive to heme inhibition in vitro.

As yet, no physiological effectors have been characterized which modulate the level of activity of the enzymes that catalyze the reactions between ALA and protoporphyrin. However, enzymatic activities of ALA dehydratase, porphobilinogen deaminase, and uroporphyrinogen III cosynthase were present in etiolated peas, and increased three- to fourfold during 60 h of greening (Smith, 1986). In the case of ALA dehydratase and porphobilinogen deaminase, there was a corresponding increase in enzyme protein, as detected by immunochemical techniques.

5. Branch point regulation.   Insertion of the central metal ion into protoporphyrin is the step that controls the flux of porphyrins to either hemes or chlorophylls. As such it is a branch point in the metabolic pathway, and it would be expected that the activities of the two enzymes are highly regulated. However, activities of ferrochelatase and Mg-chelatase have never been compared in the same tissue under similar conditions. Nor has either enzyme been systematically investigated with respect to changes in activity during greening.

The membrane-bound ferrochelatase requires only its substrates and no other cofactors. Both its reaction product, heme, and Mg-protoporphyrin are inhibitory in the micromolar concentration range (Little and Jones, 1976). In contrast, Mg-chelatase requires ATP as a cosubstrate. Mg-chelatase activity in intact plastids was effectively inhibited by exogenous protochlorophyllide and chlorophyllide, with 50% inhibition occurring at 1.0 and 3.0 μM, respectively (Fuesler, 1984). A role for protochlorophyllide acting as a feedback inhibitor of Mg-chelatase is also supported by mutant analysis in *Chlamydomonas* (Wang et al., 1977). In addition, Mg-chelatase was inhibited by AMP; 50% inhibition at 3.5 mM AMP in the presence of 10 mM ATP, suggesting that the energy charge of the cell may have some effect in regulating chlorophyll biosynthesis (Pardo et al., 1980). Thus, it is possible to account for the shutdown of chlorophyll biosynthesis and continued heme production for nonplastid hemoproteins, by postulating a buildup of protochlorophyllide (see below) and/or ATP depletion. However, it is still difficult to explain the high ratio of chlorophyll to heme accumulation which occurs during greening.

The argument that the lower K_m for protoporphyrin of Mg-chelatase compared to ferrochelatase (0.025 μM vs. 0.2 μM) in plastid membranes can account for the preferential synthesis of Mg-porphyrins during greening is deficient. The catalytic rate and molar amount of each enzyme present must also be considered. Moreover, it is still not certain that Mg-porphyrins are synthesized at a higher rate than hemes during greening. It is possible that the preferential accumulation of Mg-porphyrins is due solely to the turnover of hemes.

No information is available on the regulation of the steps between Mg-protoporphyrin and protochlorophyllide. However, it is known that S-adenosyl-methionine, which is required for the methylation step, is not made in the plastid, and must originate in the cytosol (Wallsgrove et al., 1983).

6. Regulation of protochlorophyllide photoreduction. In plants that require light for chlorophyll biosynthesis, the photoreduction of protochlorophyllide is the signal that initiates the biosynthetic process. This is the only step that has a direct light requirement. NADPH : protochlorophyllide oxidoreductase is present in etiolated tissue and is localized in the etioplast membranes. The enzyme behaves in a peculiar manner in response to light. Upon exposure to light, the enzyme activity (Mapelston and Griffiths, 1980; Santel and Apel, 1981), the amount of enzyme protein (Santel and Apel, 1981; Dehesh et al., 1987), and the amount of poly-A mRNA from which the protein is translated (Apel, 1981; Batschauer and Apel, 1984) all decrease dramatically and continuously. The proteolysis of the reductase was also observed when isolated etioplasts or etioplast membranes obtained from dark-grown barley were exposed to continuous light (Kay and Griffiths, 1983; Hauser et al., 1984). The protease is membrane-bound and apparently specific for the reductase, and other plastid proteins are not degraded in a similar light-dependent manner. In the experiments with etioplasts and etioplast membranes, the light-dependent proteolysis was prevented by inclusion of exogenous substrates, and promoted (in the dark) by inclusion of an inhibitor which prevented substrate binding (Walker and Griffiths, 1986). The authors suggested that proteolysis can occur equally well in the dark or light, whereas in the dark, proteolysis is prevented by the binding of substrate to the free enzyme. The reductase could be localized by immunoblotting of specific fractions and immunogold labeling of leaf slices (Shaw et al., 1985; Dehesh et al., 1986a, b; Dehesh et al., 1987). As expected, the reductase was mostly localized to the etioplast membranes. However, a significant portion was also observed in the cytoplasmic membranes. The reductase in developing plastid membranes was more susceptible to light-induced breakdown than the cytoplasmic enzyme. After a 72-h illumination almost 90% of the immunoreactive reductase was no longer detectable, and the 10% remaining was mostly, but not entirely, localized in the cytoplasm (Dehesh et al., 1987). If the plants were placed on a 12-h light/12-h dark cycle for 72 h, the level of reductase in the plastids was 20% of that in dark-grown tissue. Thus, even in fully greened young tissue the amount of reductase remaining would be sufficient to account for the amount of chlorophyll synthesis at this stage.

A double role can be postulated for the large amount of protochlorophyllide reductase present in etiolated tissue and its subsequent proteolysis in the light. Relatively large amounts of the enzyme in the etioplast are required to prevent the accumulation of free protochlorophyllide, since the free pigment would be phototoxic when the seedlings emerge into the light. The rapid photoreduction of the large amount of bound protochlorophyllide can supply pigment for the immediate assembly of reaction centers to get photosynthesis underway. The bulk of the enzyme can then serve as a plastid-localized source of free amino acids as it undergoes proteolysis in the absence of substrate. The remaining activity will be sufficient to catalyze steady-state chlorophyll synthesis during greening.

A model for the regulatory steps which account for the rapid response of chlorophyll and ALA synthesis to light while accommodating the need for heme in both photosynthetic and nonphotosynthetic processes is presented in Fig. 7.15. This model does not include phytochrome- and/or phytohormone-mediated responses on de novo synthesis of enzymes. In the model, ALA synthesis is controlled by substrate supply and feedback inhibition by heme at possibly two enzymatic steps, the formation and subsequent reduction of glutamyl-tRNA. There appears to be no regulatory restriction on protoporphyrin formation from ALA. Ferrochelatase is probably subject to product inhibition by heme and possibly by Mg-protoporphyrin as well. In the dark, modulation of ALA synthesis is

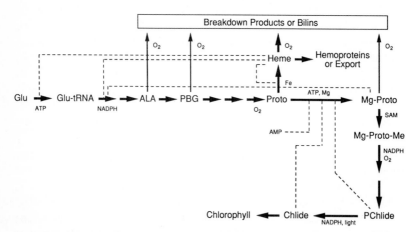

Figure 7.15 Model for the regulation of chlorophyll and heme synthesis in the chloroplast during greening. The predominant flux of intermediates is indicated by heavy arrows, and minor fluxes by lighter arrows. Each feedback inhibition is indicated by a broken line connecting the inhibitor to the arrow representing the step that is inhibited. Abbreviations: Chlide, chlorophyllide; Proto, protoporphyrin; Mg-Proto, Mg-protoporphyrin; Mg-Proto-Me, Mg-protoporphyrin monomethyl este;, PChilde, protochlorophyllide; SAM, S-adenosyl-methionine.

controlled by the level of a heme pool which constantly turns over. Thus, an increased demand for cytosolic heme could probably be supplied by the plastid even in the dark, simply by depletion of the pool. (The mechanism by which heme might be transported out of the plastid is unknown; see Chap. 9 in this volume for a review of heme transport from mitochondria in animals and fungi.) Protochlorophyllide also accumulates in the dark. Most of it will be bound to the reductase, but there is both in vitro and genetic evidence to suggest that some of it serves as a feedback inhibitor to inhibit Mg-chelatase. Inhibition of Mg-chelatase by protochlorophyllide forces the flux of protoporphyrin through the Fe branch, thus contributing to a constant supply of heme. In contrast to heme, protochlorophyllide probably does not turn over in the dark. In the light, the bound protochlorophyllide is immediately photoreduced, thus freeing up sites on the reductase for free protochlorophyllide, and the lowering of free protochlorophyllide concentration in turn relieves the inhibition of Mg-chelatase. Activation of Mg-chelatase diminishes the flux of protoporphyrin through the Fe branch, causing a depletion of the heme pool, thereby relieving the inhibition of ALA synthesis.

In this model, ALA formation is modulated by light indirectly through the effect of protochlorophyllide on Mg-chelatase and the heme pool. The model also allows for modulation of ALA synthesis in a light-independent manner. It predicts that there will be a competition for heme between apoproteins and heme-degrading systems. It is not known if the system responsible for heme degradation is localized in the plastid or cytosol or both. Nor is it known if it functions in a manner similar to the heme oxygenase of red and blue-green algae, where it is a biosynthetic enzyme system.

C. Enzymes catalyzing degradation of chlorophylls and precursors

A key feature of the above regulatory model is that it relies on a heme pool and the constant breakdown and resynthesis of hemes. In contrast to hemes, a pool of free porphyrins or Mg-porphyrins would be phototoxic in the presence of O_2 due to the generation of oxygen radicals. It is this phenomenon which is responsible for the light-induced lesions and disfigurements of some porphyria diseases. It is also the basis of action of certain herbicides which have now been dubbed "photodynamic herbicides" (Witkowski and Halling, 1988; Rebeiz et al., 1987). It is likely that plants have scavenging systems to prevent the buildup of these potentially toxic intermediates, and the possibility cannot be excluded that such degradative systems are an integral part of regulation.

An activity which catalyzes the O_2-dependent breakdown of Mg-protoporphyrin and its monomethyl ester has been detected and partially characterized in germinating kidney beans and etiolated barley (Hougen et al., 1982; Gassman and Ramanujam, 1986). The reaction was monitored by the disappearance of substrate, although the substrate specificity and the product(s) of the reaction have not yet been reported. The activity increased up to 12-fold over 4 days when greening seedlings were returned to the dark, and decreased when the plants were reilluminated. The soluble enzyme was partially purified on DEAE-cellulose, and the appearance of the activity upon return to darkness coincided with the appearance of a 49,000 molecular weight glycoprotein on SDS polyacrylamide gels.

When ^{14}C-porphobilinogen was administered to barley segments for 4 h, less than 1% of the label that was taken up was incorporated into stable tetrapyrroles. The rest was incorporated into various biochemical fractions or released as CO_2 (Duggan et al., 1982a). Similar results were obtained when ^{14}C-ALA was administered (Duggan et al., 1982b). The enzymes responsible for catabolism of these tetrapyrrole precursors have not yet been characterized, and it is not known if they are specific for these substrates. Other intermediates may be degraded nonspecifically through the generation of oxygen radicals by lipoxygenase. The reader is referred to a recent review on chlorophyll degradation (Hendry et al., 1987) for a more detailed discussion of the dimensions and processes involved in chlorophyll breakdown during senescence.

ACKNOWLEDGMENTS

We thank the many investigators who made their results available to us before publication, and Y. J. Avissar and P. A. Castelfranco for critical comments on the manuscript.

REFERENCES

Abboud, M. M., and Akhtar, M. (1976). Sterochemistry of hydrogen elimination in the enzymatic formation of the C-2–C-3 double bond of porphobilinogen, *J. Chem. Soc. Chem. Comm.* 1007–1008.

Abboud, M. M., Jordan, P. M., and Akhtar, M. (1974). Biosynthesis of 5-aminolevulinic acid: Involvement of a retention-reversion mechanism, *J. Chem. Soc. Chem. Comm.* 643–644.

Adamson, H., Griffiths, T., Packer, N., and Sutherland, M. (1985). Light-independent accumulation of chlorophyll a and b and protochlorophyllide in green barley (*Hordeum vulgare*), *Physiol. Plant.* **64**:345–352.

Adamson, H., and Packer, N. (1987). Chlorophyll labelling patterns in *Zostera* transferred to darkness, *Photosynthetica* **21**:472–481.

Adamson, H., Walker, C., Bees, A., and Griffiths, T. (1987). Protochlorophyllide reduction in *Anabaena*, *Progress in Photosynthesis Research* (J. Biggins, Ed.), Martinus Nijhoff, Boston, Vol. IV, pp. 483–486.

Adamson, H. Y., Hiller, R. G., and Vesk, M. (1980). Chloroplast development and the synthesis of chlorophyll a and b and chlorophyll protein complexes I and II in the dark in *Tradescantia albiflora* (Kunth), *Planta* **150**:269–274.

Ajaz, A. A., Corina, D. L., and Akhtar, M. (1985). The mechanism of the C-13[3] esterification step in the biosynthesis of bacteriochlorophyll a, *Eur. J. Biochem.* **150**:309–312.

Akoyunoglou, G., Argyroudi-Akoyunoglou, J. H., Michel-Wolwertz, M. R., and Sironval, C. (1966). Effect of intermittent and continuous light on chlorophyll formation in etiolated plants, *Physiol. Plant.* **19**:1101–1104.

Akoyunoglou, G., Argyroudi-Akoyunoglou, J. H., Michel-Wolwertz, M. R., and Sironval, C. (1967). Chlorophyll a as a precursor for chlorophyll b. Synthesis in barley leaves, *Chim. Chron.* **32**:5–8.

Allen, M. M., and Smith, A. J. (1969). Nitrogen chlorosis in blue-green algae, *Arch. Mikrobiol.* **69**:114–120.

Amesz, J. (1987). Primary electron transport and related processes in green photosynthetic bacteria, *Photosynthetica* **21**:225–235.

Anderson, R. A., and Mulkey, T. J. (1983). The occurrence of chlorophylls c_1 and c_2 in the Chrysophyceae, *J. Phycol.* **19**:289–294.

Apel, K. (1981). The protochlorophyllide holochrome of barley (*Hordeum vulgare* L.): Phytochrome induced decrease of translatable mRNA coding for the NADPH : protochlorophyllide oxidoreductase, *Eur. J. Biochem.* **89**:89–93.

Apel, K., Motzkus, M., and Dehesh, K. (1984). The biosynthesis of chlorophyll in greening barley (*Hordeum vulgare*). Is there a light-independent protochlorophyllide reductase?, *Planta* **161**:550–554.

Apel, K., Santel, H.-J., Redlinger, T. E., and Falk, K. (1980). The protochlorophyllide holochrome of barley (*Hordeum vulgare* L.). Isolation and characterization of the NADPH : protochlorophyllide oxidoreductase, *Eur. J. Biochem.* **111**:251–258.

Argyroudi-Akoyunoglou, J. H., Akoyunoglou, A., Kalosakas, K., and Akoyunoglou, G. (1982). Reorganization of the photosystem II unit in developing thylakoids of higher plants after transfer to darkness, *Plant Physiol.* **70**:1242–1248.

Arnheim, K., and Oelze, J. (1983). Differences in the control of bacteriochlorophyll formation by light and oxygen, *Arch. Microbiol.* **135**:299–304.

Arnold, V., and Fletcher, R. A. (1986). Stimulation of chlorophyll synthesis by benzyladenine and potassium in excised and intact cucumber cotyledons, *Physiol. Plant.* **68**:169–174.

Avissar, Y. J. (1980). Biosynthesis of 5-aminolevulinate from glutamate in *Anabaena variabilis*, *Biochim. Biophys. Acta* **613**:220–228.

Avissar, Y. J., and Beale, S. I. (1988). Biosynthesis of tetrapyrrole pigment precursors: Formation and utilization of glutamyl-tRNA for δ-aminolevulinic acid synthesis by isolated enzyme fractions from *Chlorella vulgaris*, *Plant Physiol.* **88**:879–886.

Avissar, Y. J., and Beale, S. I. (1989). Biosynthesis of tetrapyrrole pigment precursors: Pyridoxal requirement of the aminotransferase step in the formation of δ-aminolevulinate from glutamate in extracts of *Chlorella vulgaris*. *Plant Physiol.* **89**:852–859.

Avissar, Y. J., Ormerod, J. G., and Beale, S. I. (1989). Distribution of δ-aminolevulinic acid biosynthetic pathways among phototrophic bacterial groups, *Arch. Microbiol.*, **151**:513–519.

Barreiro, O. L. C. de (1975). Effect of pyridoxal phosphate and cysteine on δ-aminolaevulinate synthetase and dehydratase in soya, *Phytochemistry* **14**:2165–2168.

Batlle, A. M. del C., Llambias, E. B. C., Wider de Xifra, E., and Tigier, H. A. (1975). Porphyrin biosynthesis in the soybean callus tissue system. XV. The effect of growth conditions, *Int. J. Biochem.* **6**:591–606.

Batschauer, A., and Apel, K. (1984). An inverse control by phytochrome of the expression of two nuclear genes in barley, *Eur. J. Biochem.* **143**:593–597.

Battersby, A. R., Fookes, C. J. R., Gustafson-Potter, K. E., Matcham, G. W. J., and McDonald, E. (1979a). Proof by synthesis that unrearranged hydroxymethylbilane is the product from deaminase and the substrate for cosynthetase in the biosynthesis of Uro'gen-III, *J. Chem. Soc. Chem. Comm.* 1155–1158.

Battersby, A. R., Fookes, C. J. R., Matcham, G. W. J., and McDonald, E. (1979b). Order of assembly of the four pyrrole rings during biosynthesis of the natural porphyrins, *J. Chem. Soc. Chem. Comm.* 539–541.

Battersby, A. R., Fookes, C. J. R., Matcham, G. W. J., McDonald, E., and Gustafson-Potter, K. E. (1979c). Biosynthesis of the natural porphyrins: Experiments on the ring-closure steps with the hydroxy-analogue of porphobilinogen, *J. Chem. Soc. Chem. Comm.* 316–319.

Battersby, A. R., Fookes, C. J. R., Matcham, G. W. J., McDonald, E., and Hollenstein, R. (1983). Biosynthesis of porphyrins and related molecules. 20. Purification of deaminase and studies on its mode of action, *J. Chem. Soc. Perkin Trans. I* 3031–3040.

Bauer, C. E., and Marrs, B. L. (1988). The *Rhodobacter capsulatus puf* operon encodes a regulatory protein (*pufQ*) for bacteriochlorophyll biosynthesis, *Proc. Nat. Acad. Sci. (U.S.A.)*, **85**:7074–7078.

Bauer, C. E., Young, D. A., and Marrs, B. L. (1988). Analysis of the *Rhodobacter capsulatus puf* operon. Location of the oxygen-regulated promoter region and the identification of an additional *puf*-encoded gene, *J. Biol. Chem.* **263**:4820–4827.

Bazzaz, M. B., Bradley, C. V., and Brereton, R. G. (1982). 4-Vinyl-4-desethyl chlorophyll a: Characterization of a new naturally occurring chlorophyll using fast atom bombardment, field desorption and "in beam" electron impact mass spectroscopy, *Tet. Lett.* **23**:1211–1214.

Bazzaz, M. B., Govindjee, and Paolillo, D. J., Jr. (1974). Biochemical, spectral and structural study of Olive Necrotic 8147 mutant of *Zea mays* L., *Z. Pflanzenphysiol.* **72**:181–192.

Beale, S. I. (1971). Studies on the biosynthesis and metabolism of δ-aminolevulinic acid in *Chlorella*, *Plant Physiol.* **48**:316–319.

Beale, S. I. (1984). Biosynthesis of photosynthetic pigments, *Chloroplast Biogenesis* (N. R. Baker and J. Barber, Eds.), Elsevier, Amsterdam, pp. 133–205.

Beale, S. I., and Castelfranco, P. A. (1974a). The biosynthesis of δ-aminolevulinic acid in higher plants. I. Accumulation of δ-aminolevulinic acid in greening plant tissues, *Plant Physiol.* **53**:291–296.

Beale, S. I., and Castelfranco, P. A. (1974b). The biosynthesis of δ-aminolevulinic acid in higher plants. II. Formation of ^{14}C-δ-aminolevulinic acid from labeled precursors in greening plant tissues, *Plant Physiol.* **53**:297–303.

Beale, S. I., and Chen, N. C. (1983). N-Methyl mesoporphyrin IX inhibits phycocyanin, but not chlorophyll synthesis in *Cyanidium caldarium*, *Plant Physiol.* **71**:263–268.

Beale, S. I., and Cornejo, J. (1983). Biosynthesis of phycocyanobilin from exogenous labeled biliverdin in *Cyanidium caldarium*, *Arch. Biochem. Biophys.* **227**:279–286.

Beale, S. I., and Cornejo, J. (1984a). Enzymatic heme oxygenase activity in soluble extracts of the unicellular red alga, *Cyanidium caldarium*, *Arch. Biochem. Biophys.* **235**:371–384.

Beale, S. I., and Cornejo, J. (1984b). Enzymic transformation of biliverdin to phycocyanobilin by extracts of the unicellular red alga, *Cyanidium caldarium*, *Plant Physiol.* **76**:7–15.

Beale, S. I., and Foley, T. (1982). Induction of δ-aminolevulinic acid synthase and inhibition of heme synthesis in *Euglena gracilis* by N-methyl mesoporphyrin IX, *Plant Physiol.* **69**:1331–1333.

Beale, S. I., Foley, T., and Dzelzkalns, V. (1981). δ-Aminolevulinic acid synthase from *Euglena gracilis*, *Proc. Nat. Acad. Sci. (U.S.A.)* **78**:1666–1669.

Beale, S. I., Gough, S. P., and Granick, S. (1975). The biosynthesis of δ-aminolevulinic acid from the intact carbon skeleton of glutamic acid in greening barley, *Proc. Nat. Acad. Sci. (U.S.A.)* **72**:2719–2723.

Bednarik, D. P., and Hoober, J. K. (1985). Synthesis of chlorophyllide b from protochlorophyllide in *Chlamydomonas reinhardtii y*-1, *Science* **230**:450–453.

Bednarik, D. P., and Hoober, J. K. (1986). Chlorophyllide b synthesis in phenanthroline-treated *Chlamydomonas reinhardtii y*-1 in the dark, *Regulation of Chloroplast Differentiation* (G. Akoyunoglou and H. Senger, Eds.), Alan R. Liss, New York, pp. 105–114.

Beer, N. S., and Griffiths, W. T. (1981). Purification of the enzyme NADPH : protochlorophyllide oxidoreductase, *Biochem. J.* **195**:83–92.

Beer-Romero, P., and Gest, H. (1987). *Heliobacillus mobilis*, a peritrichously flagellated anoxyphototroph containing bacteriochlorophyll g, *FEMS Microbiol. Lett.* **41**:109–114.

Beguin, S., Guglielmi, G., Rippka, R., and Cohen-Bazire, G. (1985). Chromatic adaptation in a mutant of *Fremyella diplosiphon* incapable of phycoerythrin synthesis, *Biochemie* **67**:109–117.

Belanger, F. C., and Rebeiz, C. A. (1979). Chloroplast biogenesis. XXVII. Detection of novel chlorophyll and chlorophyll precursors in higher plants, *Biochem. Biophys. Res. Comm.* **88**:365–372.

Belanger, F. C., and Rebeiz, C. A. (1980a). Chloroplast biogenesis: Detection of divinyl protochlorophyllide in higher plants, *J. Biol. Chem.* **255**:1266–1272.

Belanger, F. C., and Rebeiz, C. A. (1980b). Chloroplast biogenesis. 30. Chlorophyll(ide) (E459F675) and chlorophyll(ide) (E449F675) the first detectable products of divinyl and monovinyl protochlorophyll photoreduction, *Plant Sci. Lett.* **18**:343–350.

Belanger, F. C., and Rebeiz, C. A. (1980c). Chloroplast biogenesis: Detection of divinylprotochlorophyllide ester in higher plants, *Biochemistry* **19**:4875–4883.

Belanger, F. C., and Rebeiz, C. A. (1982). Chloroplast biogenesis: Detection of monovinyl magnesium protoporphyrin monoester and other monovinyl magnesium-porphyrins in higher plants, *J. Biol. Chem.* **257**:1360–1371.

Belford, H. S., Offner, G. D., and Troxler, R. F. (1983). Phycobiliprotein synthesis in the unicellular Rhodophyte, *Cyanidium caldarium*. Cell-free translation of the mRNAs for the α and β subunit polypeptides of phycocyanin, *J. Biol. Chem.* **258**:4503–4510.

Bellemare, G., Bartlett, S. G., and Chua, N.-H. (1982). Biosynthesis of chlorophyll a/b-binding polypeptides in wild type and the Chlorina f2 mutant of barley, *J. Biol. Chem.* **257**:7762–7767.

Benedikt, E., and Köst, H.-P. (1985). A-α-Hydroxymesobiliverdin, a new bile pigment, *Z. Naturforsch.* **40c**:755–759.

Bennett, A., and Bogorad, L. (1973). Complementary chromatic adaptation in a filamentous blue-green alga, *J. Cell Biol.* **58**:419–435.

Bennett, J. (1981). Biosynthesis of the light-harvesting chlorophyll a/b protein. Polypeptide turnover in darkness, *Eur. J. Biochem.* **118**:61–70.

Benveniste, I., Salaun, J. P., and Durst (1977). Wounding-induced cinnamic acid hydroxylase in Jerusalum artichoke tuber. *Phytochemistry* **16**:69–73.

Benz, J., Lempert, U., and Rüdiger, W. (1984). Incorporation of phytol precursors into chlorophylls of tobacco cell cultures, *Planta* **162**:215–219.

Benz, J., and Rüdiger, W. (1981). Chlorophyll biosynthesis: Various chlorophyllides as exogenous substrates for chlorophyll synthetase, *Z. Naturforsch.* **36c**:51–57.

Benz, J., Wolf, C., and Rüdiger, W. (1980). Chlorophyll biosynthesis: Hydrogenation of geranylgeraniol, *Plant Sci. Lett.* **19**:225–230.

Berry-Lowe, S. (1987). The chloroplast glutamate tRNA gene required for δ-aminolevulinate synthesis, *Carlsberg Res. Comm.* **52**:197–210.

Biel, A. J. (1986). Control of bacteriochlorophyll accumulation by light in *Rhodobacter capsulatus*, *J. Bacteriol.* **168**:655–659.

Biel, A. J., and Marrs, B. L. (1983). Transcriptional regulation of several genes for bacteriochlorophyll biosynthesis in *Rhodopseudomonas capsulata* in response to oxygen, *J. Bacteriol.* **156**:686–694.

Bishop, J. E., Lagarias, J. C., Nagy, J. O., Schoenleber, R. W., Rapoport, H., Klotz, A. V., and Glazer, A. N. (1986). Phycobiliprotein-bilin linkage diversity. I. Structural studies on A- and D-ring-linked phycocyanobilins, *J. Biol. Chem.* **261**:6790–6796.

Bishop, J. E., Rapoport, H., Klotz, A. V., Chan, C. F., Glazer, A. N., Füglistaller, P., and Zuber, H. (1987). Chromopeptides from phycoerythrocyanin. Structure and linkage of the three bilin groups, *J. Amer. Chem. Soc.* **109**:875–881.

Bishop, N. I., and Wong, J. (1974). Photochemical characteristics of a vitamin E deficient mutant of *Scenedesmus obliquus*, *Ber. Deutsch. Bot. Gaz.* **87**:359–371.

Björn, G. S., and Björn, L. O. (1976). Photochromic pigments from blue-green algae: Phycochromes a, b, and c, *Physiol. Plant.* **36**:297–304.

Björn, L. O., and Björn, G. S. (1980). Photochromic pigments and photoregulation in blue-green algae, *Photochem. Photobiol.* **32**:849–852.

Bogdanović, M. (1973). Chlorophyll formation in the dark. I. Chlorophyll in pine seedlings, *Physiol. Plant.* **29**:17–18.

Bogorad, L. (1950). Factors associated with the synthesis of chlorophyll in the dark in seedlings of *Pinus jeffreyi*, *Bot. Gaz.* **111**:221–241.

Bogorad, L. (1958). The enzymatic synthesis of porphyrins from porphobilinogen. I. Uroporphyrin I, *J. Biol. Chem.* **233**:501–509.

Bogorad, L. (1966). The biosynthesis of chlorophylls, *The Chlorophylls* (L. P. Vernon and G. R. Seeley, Eds.), Academic, New York, pp. 481–510.

Braumann, T., Vasmil, H., Grimme, L. H., and Amesz, J. (1986). Pigment composition of the photosynthetic membrane and reaction center of the green bacterium *Prosthecochloris aestuarii*, *Biochim. Biophys. Acta* **848**:83–91.

Breidenbach, R. W., Castelfranco, P. A., and Criddle, R. S. (1967). Biogenesis of mitochondria in germinating peanut cotyledons. II. Changes in cytochromes and mitochondrial DNA, *Plant Physiol.* **42**:1035–1041.

Brereton, R. G., Bazzaz, M. B., Santikarn, S., and Williams, D. H. (1983). Positive and negative ion fast atom bombardment mass spectrometric studies on chlorophylls: Structure of 4-vinyl-4-desethyl chlorophyll b, *Tet. Lett.* **24**:5775–5778.

Briggs, W. R., Mosinger, E., and Schäfer, E. (1988). Phytochrome regulation of greening in barley: Effects on chlorophyll accumulation, *Plant Physiol.* **86**:435–440.

Broch-Due, M., and Ormerod, J. G. (1978). Isolation of a Bchl c mutant from *Chlorobium* with Bchl d by cultivation at low intensity, *FEMS Microbiol. Lett.* **3**:305–308.

Brockmann, H. J., and Lipinski, A. (1983). Bacteriochlorophyll g. A new bacteriochlorophyll from *Heliobacterium chlorum*, *Arch. Microbiol.* **136**:17–19.

Brockmann, H., Jr., and Knobloch, G. (1973). Substituierte Bernsteinsäuren. V. Die absolute Konfiguration des 2E-Äthyliden-3-methyl-succinimids. Ein Beitrag zur Bestimmung der absoluten Konfiguration von Phycobilinen und Phytochrom, *Chem. Ber.* **106**:803–811.

Brockmann, H., Jr., Knobloch, G., Schweer, I., and Trowitzsch, W. (1973). Die Alkoholkomponente des Bacteriochlorophyll a aus *Rhodospirillum rubrum*, *Arch. Mikrobiol.* **90**:161–164.

Brown, J. S. (1985). Three photosynthetic antenna porphyrins in a primitive green alga, *Biochim. Biophys. Acta* **807**:143–146.

Brown, S. B., Holroyd, J. A., and Troxler, R. F. (1980). Mechanism of bile-pigment synthesis in algae. ^{18}O Incorporation into phycocyanobilin in the unicellular Rhodophyte, *Cyanidium caldarium*, *Biochem. J.* **190**:445–449.

Brown, S. B., Holroyd, J. A., Troxler, R. F., and Offner, G. D. (1981). The effect of N-methylprotoporphyrin IX on the synthesis of photosynthetic pigments in *Cyanidium caldarium*. Further evidence for the role of haem in the biosynthesis of plant bilins, *Biochem. J.* **191**:137–147.

Brown, S. B., Holroyd, J. A., Vernon, D. I., and Jones, O. T. G. (1984). Ferrochelatase activity in the photosynthetic alga *Cyanidium caldarium*. Development of the enzyme during biosynthesis of photosynthetic pigments, *Biochem. J.* **220**:861–863.

Brown, S. B., Holroyd, J. A., Vernon, D. I., Troxler, R. F., and Smith, K. M. (1982). The effect of N-methylprotoporphyrin IX on the synthesis of photosynthetic pigments in *Cyanidium caldarium*. Further evidence for the role of haem in the biosynthesis of plant bilins, *Biochem. J.* **208**:487–491.

Bruyant, P., and Kannangara, C. G. (1987). Biosynthesis of δ-aminolevulinate in greening barley leaves. VIII. Purification and characterization of the glutamate-tRNA ligase, *Carlsberg Res. Comm.* **52**:99–109.

Bryant, D. A., and Cohen-Bazire, G. (1981). Effects of chromatic illumination on cyanobacterial phycobilisomes. Evidence for the specific induction of a second pair of phycocyanin subunits in *Pseudanabaena* 7409 grown in red light, *Eur. J. Biochem.* **119**:415–424.

Bryant, D. A., Dubbs, J. M., Fields, P. I., Porter, R. D., and de Lorimier, R. (1985). Expression of phycobiliprotein genes in *Escherichia coli*, *FEMS Microbiol. Lett.* **29**:343–349.

\udzikiewicz, H., and Taraz, K. (1971). Chlorophyll c, *Tetrahedron* **27**:1447–1460.

\stelfranco, P. A., and Beale, S. I. (1983). Chlorophyll biosynthesis: Recent advances and areas of current interest, *Annu. Rev. Plant Physiol.* **34**:241–278.

telfranco, P. A., and Jones, O. T. G. (1975). Protoheme turnover and chlorophyll synthesis in greening barley tissue, *Plant Physiol.* **55**:485–490.

\lfranco, P. A. Thayer, S. S., Wilkinson, J. Q., and Bonner, B. A. (1988). Labeling of phobilinogen deaminase by radioactive 5-aminolevulinic acid in isolated developing chloroplasts, *Arch. Biochem. Biophys.* **266**:219–226.

Castelfranco, P. A., Weinstein, J. D., Schwarcz, S., Pardo, A. D., and Wezelman, B. E. (1979). The Mg insertion step in chlorophyll biosynthesis, *Arch. Biochem. Biophys.* **192**:592–598.

Cavaleiro, J. A. S., Kenner, G. W., and Smith, K. M. (1974). Pyrroles and related compounds. XXXII. Biosynthesis of protoporphyrin-IX from coproporphyrinogen-III, *J. Chem. Soc. Perkin Trans. I* 1188–1194.

Chang, T.-E., Wang, W.-Y., and Wegmann, B. (1988). Purification of the first enzyme in the chlorophyll biosynthetic pathway from *Chlamydomonas reinhardtii, Plant Physiol.* **86S**:60.

Chen, T. C., and Miller, G. W. (1974). Purification and characterization of uroporphyrinogen decarboxylase from tobacco leaves, *Plant Cell Physiol.* **15**:993–1005.

Chereskin, B. A., and Castelfranco, P. A. (1982). Effects of iron and oxygen on chlorophyll biosynthesis. II. Observations on the biosynthetic pathway in isolated etiochloroplasts, *Plant Physiol.* **69**:112–116.

Chereskin, B. A., Castelfranco, P. A., Dallas, J. L., and Straub, K. M. (1983). Mg-2,4-divinyl pheoporphyrin a_5: The product of a reaction catalyzed in vitro by developing chloroplasts, *Arch. Biochem. Biophys.* **226**:10–18.

Chereskin, B. A., Wong, Y.-S., and Castelfranco, P. A. (1982). In vitro synthesis of the chlorophyll isocyclic ring: Transformation of magnesium-protoporphyrin IX and magnesium-protoporphyrin IX monomethyl ester into magnesium-2,4-divinyl pheoporphyrin a_5, *Plant Physiol.* **70**:987–993.

Chibbar, R. N., and van Huystee, R. B. (1983). Glutamic acid is the haem precursor for peroxidase synthesized by peanut cells in suspension culture, *Phytochemistry* **22**:1721–1723.

Chibbar, R. N., and van Huystee, R. B. (1986). Site of haem synthesis in cultured peanut cells, *Phytochemistry* **25**:585–587.

Chisholm, S. W., Olson, R. J., Zettler, E. R., Goericke, R., Waterbury, J. B., and Welschmeyer, N. A. (1988). A novel free-living prochlorophyte abundant in the oceanic euphotic zone, *Nature* **334**:340–343.

Clement-Metral, J. D. (1979). Activation of ALA synthetase by reduced thioredoxin in *Rhodopseudomonas spheroides* Y, *FEBS Lett.* **101**:116–120.

Clement-Metral, J. D., Hoog, J.-O., and Holmgren, A. (1986). Characterization of the thioredoxin system in the facultative phototroph *Rhodobacter sphaeriodes* Y. *Eur. J. Biochem.* **161**:119–126.

Cohen, L., Arzee, T., and Zilberstein, A. (1988). Mimicry by cytokinin of phytochrome-regulated inhibition of chloroplast development in etiolated cucumber cotyledon, *Physiol. Plant.* **72**:57–64.

Cohen-Bazire, G., Sistrom, W. R., and Stanier, R. Y. M. (1957). Kinetic studies of pigment synthesis by non-sulfur purple bacteria, *J. Cell. Comp. Physiol.* **49**:25–68.

Cornejo, J., and Beale, S. I. (1988). Algal heme oxygenase from *Cyanidium caldarium*: Partial purification and fractionation into three required protein components, *J. Biol. Chem.* **263**:11915–11921.

Corriveau, J. L., and Beale, S. I. (1986). Influence of gabaculine on growth, chlorophyll synthesis, and δ-aminolevulinic acid synthase activity in *Euglena gracilis, Plant Sci.* **45**:9–17.

Dailey, H. A. (1982). Purification and characterization of membrane bound ferrochelatase from *Rhodopseudomonas sphaeroides, J. Biol. Chem.* **257**:14714–14718.

Dailey, H. A., Fleming, J. E., and Harbin, B. M. (1986). Ferrochelatase from *Rhodopseudomonas sphaeroides*: Substrate specificity and role of sulfhydryl and arginyl residues, *J. Bacteriol.* **165**:1–5.

Daniell, H., and Rebeiz, C. A. (1982). Chloroplast culture. VIII. A new effect of kinetin in enhancing the synthesis and accumulation of protochlorophyllide in vitro, *Biochem. Biophys. Res. Comm.* **104**:837–843.

Daniell, H., and Rebeiz, C. A. (1986). Chloroplast culture. XI. Involvement of phytohormones in the greening plants, *Regulation of Chloroplast Differentiation* (G. Akoyunoglou and H. Senger, Eds.), Alan R. Liss, New York, pp. 63–70.

Dehesh, K., Klaus, M., Hauser, I., and Apel, K. (1986a). Light-induced changes in the distribution of the $36\,000$-M_r polypeptide of NADPH-protochlorophyllide oxidoreductase within different cellular compartments of barley (*Hordeum vulgare* L.). I. Localization by immunoblotting in isolated plastids and total leaf extracts, *Planta* **169**:162–171.

Dehesh, K., Kreuz, K., and Apel, K. (1987). Chlorophyll synthesis in green leaves and isolated chloroplasts of barley (*Hordeum vulgare*), *Physiol. Plant.* **69**:173–181.

Dehesh, K., and Ryberg, M. (1985). The NADPH-protochlorophyllide oxidoreductase is the major protein constituent of prolamellar bodies in wheat (*Triticum aestivum* L.), *Planta* **164**:396–399.

Dehesh, K., van Cleve, B., Ryberg, M., and Apel, K. (1986b). Light-induced changes in the distribution of the 36 000-M_r polypeptide of NADPH-protochlorophyllide oxidoreductase within different cellular compartments of barley (*Hordeum vulgare* L.). II. Localization by immunogold labelling in ultrathin sections, *Planta* **169**:172–183.

de Lorimier, R., Bryant, D. A., Porter, R. D., Liu, W.-Y., Jay, E., and Stevens, S. E., Jr. (1984). Genes for the α and β subunits of phycocyanin, *Proc. Nat. Acad. Sci. (U.S.A.)* **81**:7946–7950.

de Lorimier, R., Wang, Y.-J., and Yeh, M.-L. (1988). Overexpression of phycocyanin with attendant alteration of phycobilisome structure, *Proc. Third Ann. Penn. State Symp. Plant Physiol.*, pp. 332–336.

Dörnemann, D., and Senger, H. (1982). Physical and chemical properties of chlorophyll RC I extracted from photosystem I of spinach leaves and from green algae, *Photochem. Photobiol.* **35**:821–826.

Dörnemann, D., and Senger, H. (1986). The structure of chlorophyll RC I, a chromophore of the reaction center of photosystem I, *Photochem. Photobiol.* **43**:573–581.

Dougherty, R. C., Strain, H. H., Svec, W. A., Uphaus, R. A., and Katz, J. J. (1966). Structure of chlorophyll c, *J. Amer. Chem. Soc.* **88**:5037–5038.

Dougherty, R. C., Strain, H. H., Svec, W. A., Uphaus, R. A., and Katz, J. J. (1970). The structure, properties, and distribution of chlorophyll c, *J. Amer. Chem. Soc.* **92**:2826–2833.

Drews, G., Leutiger, I., and Ladwig, R. (1971). Production of protochlorophyll, protopheophytin, and bacteriochlorophyll by the mutant A1a of *Rhodopseudomonas capsulata*, *Arch. Mikrobiol.* **76**:349–363.

Dring, M. J. (1974). Reproduction, *Algal Physiology and Biochemistry* (W. D. P. Stewart, Ed.), University of California Press, Berkeley, pp. 814–837.

Drummond, G. S., and Kappas, A. (1981). Prevention of neonatal hyperbilirubinemia by tin protoporphyrin IX, a potent competitive inhibitor of heme oxidation, *Proc. Nat. Acad. Sci. (U.S.A.)* **78**:6466–6470.

Duggan, J., and Gassman, M. (1974). Induction of porphyrin synthesis in etiolated bean leaves by chelators of iron, *Plant Physiol.* **53**:206–215.

Duggan, J. X., Meller, E., and Gassman, M. L. (1982a). Catabolism of porphobilinogen by etiolated barley leaves, *Plant Physiol.* **69**:602–608.

Duggan, J. X., Meller, E., and Gassman, M. L. (1982b). Catabolism of 5-aminolevulinic acid to CO_2 by etiolated barley leaves, *Plant Physiol.* **69**:19–22.

Duggan, J. X., and Rebeiz, C. A. (1982). Chloroplast biogenesis 38. Quantitative detection of a chlorophyllide b pool in higher plants, *Biochim. Biophys. Acta* **714**:248–260.

Dujardin, E., Franck, F., Gysemberg, R., and Sironval, C. (1986). The protochlorophyllide-chlorophyllide cycle and photosynthesis, *Photobiochem. Photobiophys.* **12**:97–105.

Dunlap, J. C., Hastings, J. W., and Shimomura, O. (1981). Dinoflagellate luciferin is structurally related to chlorophyll, *FEBS Lett.* **135**:273–276.

Dzelzkalns, V., Foley, T., and Beale, S. I. (1982). δ-Aminolevulinic acid synthase of *Euglena gracilis*: Physical and kinetic properties, *Arch. Biochem. Biophys.* **216**:196–203.

Ebbon, J. G., and Tait, G. H. (1969). Studies on S-adenosylmethionine-magnesium protoporphyrin methyltransferase in *Euglena gracilis* strain Z, *Biochem. J.* **111**:573–582.

Egelhoff, T., and Grossman, A. (1983). Cytoplasmic and chloroplast synthesis of phycobilisome polypeptides, *Proc. Nat. Acad. Sci. (U.S.A.)* **80**:3339–3343.

Eimhjellen, K. E., Aasmundrud, O., and Jensen, A. (1963). A new bacterial chlorophyll, *Biochem. Biophys. Res. Comm.* **10**:232–236.

El Hamouri, B., and Sironval, C. (1980). NADP$^+$/NADPH control of the protochlorophyllide-chlorophyllide-proteins in cucumber etioplasts, *Photobiochem. Photobiophys.* 1:219–223.

Elich, T. D., and Lagarias, J. C. (1987). Phytochrome chromophore biosynthesis. Both 5-aminolevulinic acid and biliverdin overcome inhibition by gabaculine in etiolated *Avena sativa* L. seedlings, *Plant Physiol.* 84:304–310.

Elich, T. D., McDonagh, A. F., Palma, L. A., and Lagarias, J. C. (1989). Phytochrome chromophore biosynthesis. Treatment of tetrapyrrole-deficient *Avena* explants with natural and non-natural bilatrienes leads to formation of spectrally active holoproteins, *J. Biol. Chem.* 264:183–189.

Ellsworth, R. K. (1971). Studies on chlorophyllase. I. Hydrolytic and esterification activities of chlorophyllase from wheat seedlings, *Photosynthetica* 5:226–232.

Ellsworth, R. K., and Aronoff, S. (1968). Investigation on the biogenesis of chlorophyll. III. Biosynthesis of Mg-vinyl-phaeoporphine a$_5$ methylester from Mg-protoporphine IX monomethyl ester as observed in *Chlorella* mutants, *Arch. Biochem. Biophys.* 125:269–277.

Ellsworth, R. K., and Aronoff, S. (1969). Investigation on the biogenesis of chlorophyll a. IV. Isolation and partial characterization of some biosynthetic intermediates between Mg-protoporphine IX monomethyl ester and Mg-vinyl-phaeoporphine a$_5$ methylester, obtained from *Chlorella* mutants, *Arch. Biochem. Biophys.* 130:374–383.

Ellsworth, R. K., Dullaghan, J. P., and St. Pierre, M. E. (1974). The reaction of *S*-adenosyl-L-methionine : magnesium-protoporphyrin IX methyltransferase of wheat, *Photosynthetica* 8:375–384.

Ellsworth, R. K., and Hervish, P. V. (1975). Biosynthesis of protochlorophyllide a from Mg-protoporphyrin IX in vitro, *Photosynthetica* 9:125–139.

Ellsworth, R. K., and Hsing, A. S. (1973). The reduction of vinyl side-chains of Mg-protoporphyrin IX monomethyl ester in vitro, *Biochim. Biophys. Acta* 313:119–129.

Ellsworth, R. K., and Hsing, A. S. (1974). Activity and some properties of Mg-4-ethyl-(4-desvinyl)-protoporphyrin IX monomethyl ester : NAD$^+$ oxidoreductase in crude homogenates from etiolated wheat seedlings, *Photosynthetica* 8:228–234.

Ellsworth, R. K., and Lawrence, G. D. (1973). Synthesis of magnesium protoporphyrin IX in vitro, *Photosynthetica* 7:73–86.

Ellsworth, R. K., Perkins, H. J., Detwiller, J. P., and Liu, K. (1970). On the enzymatic conversion of ^{14}C-labeled chlorophyll a to ^{14}C-labeled chlorophyll b, *Biochim. Biophys. Acta* 223:275–280.

Ellsworth, R. K., and St. Pierre, M. E. (1976). Biosynthesis and inhibition of (−)-*S*-adenosyl-L-methionine : magnesium-protoporphyrin methyltransferase of wheat, *Photosynthetica* 10:291–301.

Emery, V. C., and Akhtar, M. (1985). Mechanistic studies on the phytylation step in bacteriochlorophyll a biosynthesis: an application of the ^{18}O induced isotope effect in ^{13}C N.M.R. spectroscopy, *J. Chem. Soc. Chem. Comm.* 600–601.

Eskins, K., and Harris, L. (1981). High-performance liquid chromatography of etioplast pigments in red kidney leaves, *Photochem. Photobiol.* 33:131–133.

Fajer, J., Fujita, E., Frank, H. A., Chadwick, B., Simpson, D., and Smith, K. M. (1987). Are chlorinated chlorophylls components of photosystem I reaction centers?, *Progress in Photosynthesis Research* (J. Biggins, Ed.), Martinus Nijhoff, Boston, Vol. I, pp. 307–310.

Fanica-Gaignier, M., and Clement-Metral, J. D. (1973). 5-Aminolevulinic acid synthetase of *Rhodopseudomonas spheroides* Y. Kinetic mechanism and inhibition by ATP, *Eur. J. Biochem.* 40:19–24.

Fleischmann, D., Evans, W. R., Shanmugasundaram, S., and Shanmugasundaram, S. (1988). Induction of photosynthetic capability in a *Rhizobium, Plant Physiol.* 86S:21.

Fletcher, R. A., Teo, C., and Ali, A. (1973). Stimulation of chlorophyll synthesis in cucumber cotyledons by benzyladenine, *Canad. J. Bot.* 51:937–939.

Fluhr, R., Harel, E., Klein, S., and Meller, E. (1975). Control of δ-aminolevulinic acid and chlorophyll accumulation in greening maize leaves upon light-dark transitions, *Plant Physiol.* 56:497–501.

Foley, T., Dzelzkalns, V., and Beale, S. I. (1982). δ-Aminolevulinic acid synthase of *Euglena gracilis*: Regulation of activity, *Plant Physiol.* 70:219–226.

Fonne-Pfister, R., Simon, A., Salaun, J.-P., and Durst, F. (1988). Xenobiotic metabolism in higher plants. Involvement of microsomal cytochrome P-450 in aminopyrine N-demethylation, *Plant Sci.* **55**:9–20.

Foulds, I. J., and Carr, N. G. (1977). A proteolytic enzyme degrading phycocyanin in the cyanobacterium *Anabaena cylindrica*, *FEMS Microbiol. Lett.* **2**:117–119.

Franck, F., and Inoue, Y. (1984). Light-driven reversible transformation of chlorophyllide $P_{696,682}$ into chlorophyllide $P_{688,678}$ in illuminated etiolated bean leaves, *Photobiochem. Photobiophys.* **8**:85–96.

Franck, F., and Mathis, P. (1980). A short-lived intermediate in the photoenzymatic reduction of protochlorophyll(ide) into chlorophyll(ide) at a physiological temperature, *Photochem. Photobiol.* **32**:799–803.

Franck, F., and Schmid, G. H. (1985). On the correlation between oxygen uptake in plastids of greening etiolated oat leaves and pigment photooxidation, *Z. Naturforsch.* **40c**:699–704.

Friedmann, H. C., and Thauer, R. K. (1986). Ribonuclease-sensitive δ-aminolevulinic acid formation from glutamate in cell extracts of *Methanobacterium thermoautotrophicum*, *FEBS Lett.* **207**:84–88.

Friedmann, H. C., Thauer, R. K., Gough, S. P., and Kannangara, C. G. (1987). δ-Aminolevulinic acid formation in the archaebacterium *Methanobacterium thermoautotrophicum* requires tRNA^{Glu}, *Carlsberg Res. Comm.* **52**:363–371.

Frydman, R. B., and Feinstein, G. (1974). Studies on porphobilinogen deaminase and uroporphyrinogen III cosynthase from human erythrocytes, *Biochim. Biophys. Acta* **350**:358–373.

Fu, E., Friedman, L., and Siegelman, H. W. (1979). Mass-spectral identification and purification of phycoerythrobilin and phycocyanobilin, *Biochem. J.* **179**:1–6.

Fuesler, T. P. (1984). The biosynthesis of magnesium protoporphyrin IX and related pigments in developing cucumber chloroplasts, Ph.D. Dissertation, University of California, Davis, 123 pp.

Fuesler, T. P., Castelfranco, P. A., and Wong, Y.-S. (1984a). Formation of Mg-containing chlorophyll precursors from protoporphyrin IX, δ-aminolevulinic acid, and glutamate in isolated, photosynthetically competent, developing chloroplasts, *Plant Physiol.* **74**:928–933.

Fuesler, T. P., Hanamoto, C. M., and Castelfranco, P. A. (1982). Separation of Mg-protoporphyrin IX and Mg-protoporphyrin IX monomethyl ester synthesized de novo by developing cucumber etioplasts, *Plant Physiol.* **69**:421–423.

Fuesler, T. P., Wong, Y.-S., and Castelfranco, P. A. (1984b). Localizaton of Mg-chelatase and Mg-protoporphyrin IX monomethyl ester (oxidative) cyclase activities within isolated, developing cucumber chloroplasts, *Plant Physiol.* **75**:662–664.

Fuesler, T. P., Wright, L. A., Jr., and Castelfranco, P. A. (1981). Properties of magnesium chelatase in greening etioplasts: Metal ion specificity and effect of substrate concentrations, *Plant Physiol.* **67**:246–249.

Gassman, M. L. (1973). The conversion of photoactive protochlorophyllide to phototransformable protochlorophyllide in etiolated bean leaves treated with 5-aminolevulinic acid, *Plant Physiol.* **52**:295–300.

Gassman, M., and Duggan, J. (1974). Chemical induction of porphyrin synthesis in higher plants, *Proc. Third International Congress on Photosynthesis* (M. Avron, Ed.), Elsevier, Amsterdam, pp. 2105–2113.

Gassman, M., and Ramanujam, P. (1986). Relation between enzymatic destruction of magnesium porphyrins and chloroplast development, *Regulation of Chloroplast Differentiation* (G. Akoyunoglou and H. Senger, Eds.) Alan R. Liss, New York, pp. 115–123.

Gassman, M. L., Granick, S., and Mauzerall, D. (1968). A rapid spectral change in etiolated kidney bean leaves following phototransformation of protochlorophyllide, *Biochem. Biophys. Res. Comm.* **32**:295–309.

Gendel, S., Ohad, I., and Bogorad, L. (1979). Control of phycoerythrin synthesis during chromatic adaptation, *Plant Physiol.* **64**:786–790.

Gest, H., and Favinger, J. L. (1983). *Heliobacterium chlorum*, an anoxygenic brownish-green photosynthetic bacterium containing a "new" form of chlorophyll, *Arch. Microbiol.* **136**:11–16.

Gibson, K. D., Neuberger, A., and Tait, G.H. (1963). Studies on the biosynthesis of porphyrin and bacteriochlorophyll by *Rhodopseudomonas spheroides*. 4. S-Adenosyl-methionine-magnesium protoporphyrin methyltransferase, *Biochem. J.* **88**:325–334.

Glazer, A. N., and Hixson, C. S. (1977). Subunit structure and chromophore composition of Rhodophytan phycoerythrins. *Porphyridium cruentum* B-phycoerythrin and b-phycoerythrin, *J. Biol. Chem.* **252**:32–42.

Glazer, A. N., and Melis, A. (1987). Photochemical reaction centers: Structure, organization, and function, *Annu. Rev. Plant Physiol.* **38**:11–45.

Gloe, A., and Pfennig, N. (1974). Das Vorkommen von Phytol und Geranylgeraniol in den Bacteriochlorophyllen roter und grüner Schwefelbakterien, *Arch. Microbiol.* **96**:93–101.

Gloe, A., Pfennig, N., Brockmann, H., and Trowitzsch, W. (1975). A new bacteriochlorophyll from brown-colored Chlorobiaceae, *Arch. Microbiol.* **102**:103–109.

Godnev, T. N., Rotfarb, R. M., and Shlyk, A. A. (1960). On the possibility of transformation of chlorophyll a into chlorophyll b during the biosynthetic process, *Dokl. Akad. Nauk. USSR* **130**:663–666.

Goldin, B. R., and Little, H. N. (1969). Metalloporphyrin chelatase activity from barley, *Biochim. Biophys. Acta* **171**:321–332.

Gomez-Silva, B., Timko, M. P., and Schiff, J. A. (1985). Chlorophyll biosynthesis from glutamate or 5-aminolevulinate in intact *Euglena* chloroplasts, *Planta* **165**:12–22.

Gorchein, A. (1972). Magnesium protoporphyrin chelatase activity in *Rhodopseudomonas spheroides*: Studies with whole cells, *Biochem. J.* **127**:97–106.

Gorchein, A. (1973). Control of magnesium-protoporphyrin chelatase activity in *Rhodopseudomonas spheroides*: Role of light, oxygen, and electron and energy transfer, *Biochem. J.* **134**:833–845.

Gossauer, A. (1983). Studies on the stereochemistry of biliprotein chromophores and related model compounds. *Tetrahedron* **39**:1933–1941.

Gough, S. P., and Kannangara, C. G. (1977). Synthesis of δ-aminolevulinate by a chloroplast stroma preparation from greening barley leaves, *Carlsberg Res. Comm.* **42**:459–464.

Gough, S. P., and Kannangara, C. G. (1979). Biosynthesis of δ-aminolevulinate in greening barley leaves. III. The formation of δ-aminolevulinate in *tigrina* mutants of barley, *Carlsberg Res. Comm.* **44**:403–416.

Granick, S. (1950). The structural and functional relationships between heme and chlorophyll, *Harvey Lectures* **44**:220–245.

Granick, S., and Beale, S. I. (1978). Hemes, chlorophylls and related compounds: Biosynthesis and metabolic regulation, *Adv. Enzymol.* **46**:33–203.

Griffiths, W. T. (1974a). Source of reducing equivalents for the in vitro synthesis of chlorophyll from protochlorophyll, *FEBS Lett.* **46**:301–304.

Griffiths, W. T. (1974b). Protochlorophyll and protochlorophyllide as precursors for chlorophyll synthesis in vitro, *FEBS Lett.* **49**:196–200.

Griffiths, W. T. (1978). Reconstitution of chlorophyllide formation by isolated etioplast membranes, *Biochem. J.* **174**:681–692.

Griffiths, W. T. (1981). Role of NADPH in chlorophyll synthesis by protochlorophyllide reductase, *Photosynthesis* (G. Akoyunoglou, Ed.), Balaban, Philadelphia, Vol. V, pp. 65–71.

Griffiths, W. T., and Jones, O. T. G. (1975). Magnesium 2,4-divinyl phaeoporphyrin a_5 as a substrate for chlorophyll biosynthesis in vitro, *FEBS Lett.* **50**:355–358.

Griffiths, W. T., and Oliver, R. P. (1984). Protochlorophyllide reductase—structure, function and regulation, *Chloroplast Biogenesis* (R. J. Ellis, Ed.), Cambridge University Press, Cambridge, pp. 245–258.

Harashima, K., Shiba, T., Totsuka, T., Shimidu, U., and Taga, N. (1978). Occurrence of bacteriochlorophyll a in a strain of an aerobic heterotrophic bacterium, *Agric. Biol. Chem.* **42**:1627–1628.

Harel, E. (1978). Initial steps in chlorophyll synthesis—problems and open questions, *Chloroplast Development* (G. Akoyunoglou and J. H. Argyroudi-Akoyunoglou, Eds.), Elsevier, Amsterdam, pp. 33–44.

Harel, E., and Ne'eman, E. (1983). Alternate routes for the synthesis of 5-aminolevulinic acid in maize leaves. II. Formation from glutamate, *Plant Physiol.* **72**:1062–1067.

Hart, G. J., and Battersby, A. R. (1985). Purification and properties of uroporphyrinogen III synthase (co-synthase) from *Euglena gracilis, Biochem. J.* **232**:151–160.

Hart, G. J., Miller, A. D., Leeper, F. J., and Battersby, A. R. (1987). Biosynthesis of natural porphyrins: Proof that hydroxymethylbilane synthase (porphobilinogen deaminase) uses a novel binding group in its catalytic action, *J. Chem. Soc. Chem. Comm.* 1762–1765.

Hauser, I., Dehesh, K., and Apel, K. (1984). The proteolytic degradation in vitro of NADPH : protochlorophyllide oxidoreductase of barley (*Hordeum vulgare* L.), *Arch. Biochem. Biophys.* **228**:577–586.

Hendry, G. A. F., Houghton, J. D., and Brown, S. B. (1987). The degradation of chlorophyll —a biological enigma, *N. Phytol.* **107**:255–302.

Hendry, G. A. F., Houghton, J. D., and Jones, O. T. G. (1981a). The cytochromes in microsomal fractions of germinating mung beans, *Biochem. J.* **194**:743–751.

Hendry, G. A. F., Houghton, J. D., and Jones, O. T. G. (1981b). Light-dependent cytochrome P-450 changes in mung beans (*Phaseolus aureus*), *Biochem. J.* **196**:825–829.

Hendry, G. A. F., and Stobart, A. K. (1978). The effect of haem on chlorophyll synthesis in barley leaves, *Phytochemistry* **17**:73–77.

Hendry, G. A. F., and Stobart, A. K. (1986). Chlorophyll turnover in greening barley, *Phytochemistry* **25**:2735–2737.

Henry, A., Powls, R., and Pennock, J. F. (1986). *Scenedesmus obliquus* PS28: A tocopherol-free mutant which cannot form phytol, *Biochem. Soc. Trans.* **14**:958–959.

Higuchi, M., and Bogorad, L. (1975). The purification and properties of uroporphyrinogen I synthases and uroporphyrinogen III cosynthase. Interactions between the enzymes, *Ann. N.Y. Acad. Sci.* **244**:401–418.

Hinchigeri, S. B., Chan, J. C.-S., and Richards, W. R. (1981). Purification of S-adenosyl-L-methionine : magnesium protoporphyrin methyltransferase by affinity chromatography, *Photosynthetica* **15**:351–359.

Hinchigeri, S. B., Nelson, D. W., and Richards, W. R. (1984). The purification and reaction mechanism of S-adenosyl-L-methionine : magnesium protoporphyrin methyltransferase from *Rhodopseudomonas spheroides, Photosynthetica* **18**:168–178.

Hinchigeri, S. B., and Richards, W. R. (1982). The reaction mechanism of S-adenosyl-L-methionine : magnesium protoporphyrin methyltransferase from *Euglena gracilis, Photosynthetica* **16**:554–560.

Holroyd, J. A., Vernon, D. I., and Brown, S. B. (1985). Biliverdin, an intermediate in the biosynthesis of plant pigments, *Biochem. Soc. Trans.* **13**:209–210.

Hoober, J. K., Kahn, A., Ash, D., Gough, S., and Kannangara, C. G. (1988). Biosynthesis of δ-aminolevulinate in greening barley leaves. IX. Structure of the substrate, mode of gabaculine inhibition, and the catalytic mechanism of glutamate 1-semialdehyde aminotransferase, *Carlsberg Res. Comm.* **53**:11–25.

Hoober, J. K., and Stegeman, W. J. (1973). Control of the synthesis of a major polypeptide of chloroplast membranes in *Chlamydomonas reinhardi, J. Cell Biol.* **56**:1–12.

Horton, P., and Leech, R. M. (1972). The effect of ATP on photoconversion of protochlorophyllide in isolated etioplasts, *FEBS Lett.* **26**:277–280.

Horwitz, B. A., Thompson, W. F., and Briggs, W. R. (1988). Phytochrome regulation of greening in *Pisum*: Chlorophyll accumulation and abundance of mRNA for the light-harvesting chlorophyll a/b binding proteins, *Plant Physiol.* **86**:299–305.

Houen, G., Gough, S. P., and Kannangara, C. G. (1983). δ-Aminolevulinate synthesis in greening barley. V. The structure of glutamate 1-semialdehyde, *Carlsberg Res. Comm.* **48**:567–572.

Hougen, C. L., Meller, E., and Gassman, M. L. (1982). Magnesium protoporphyrin monoester destruction by extracts of etiolated red kidney bean leaves, *Plant Sci. Lett.* **24**:289–294.

Houghton, J. D., Honeybourne, C. L., Smith, K. M., Tabba, H. D., and Jones, O. T. G. (1982). The use of N-methylprotoporphyrin dimethyl ester to inhibit ferrochelatase in *Rhodopseudomonas spheroides* and its effect in promoting biosynthesis of magnesium tetrapyrroles, *Biochem. J.* **208**:479–486.

Houghton, J. D., Jones, O. T. G., Quirke, J. M. E., Murray, M., and Honeybourne, C. L. (1983). 2-(1-hydroxyethyl)-2-desvinyl chlorophyllide a: Characterization by nuclear over-hauser enhancement proton magnetic resonance of a novel pigment obtained from mutants of *Rhodopseudomonas sphaeroides*, *Tet. Lett.* **24**:5703–5706.

Hsu, W. P., and Miller, G. W. (1970). Coproporphyrinogenase in tobacco (*Nictiana tabacum* L.), *Biochem. J.* **117**:215–220.

Huang, L., and Castelfranco, P. A. (1986). Regeneration of magnesium-2,4-divinylpheoporphyrin a_5 (divinyl protochlorophyllide) in isolated developing chlorophlasts, *Plant Physiol.* **82**:285–288.

Huang, D.-D., and Wang, W.-Y. (1986a). Chlorophyll synthesis in *Chlamydomonas* starts with the formation of glutamyl-tRNA, *J. Biol. Chem.* **261**:13451–13455.

Huang, D.-D., and Wang, W.-Y. (1986b). Genetic control of chlorophyll biosynthesis: Regulation of delta aminolevulinate synthesis in *Chlamydomonas*, *Mol. Gen. Genet.* **205**:217–220.

Huang, D.-D., Wang, W.-Y., Gough, S. P., and Kannangara, C. G. (1984). δ-Aminolevulinic acid-synthesizing enzymes need an RNA moiety for activity, *Science* **225**:1482–1484.

Huang, L., and Castelfranco, P. A. (1988). A re-examination of 5-aminolevulinic acid synthesis by isolated, intact, developing chloroplasts: The O_2 requirement in the light, *Plant Sci.* **54**:185–192.

Hucklesby, D. P., James, D. M., Banwell, M. J., and Hewitt, E. J. (1976). Properties of nitrite reductase from *Cucurbita pepo*, *Phytochemistry* **15**:599–603.

Humbeck, K., and Senger, H. (1981). Chlorophyll formation and ALA biosynthesis via two different pathways during the cell cycle of wild type cells of *Scenedesmus*, *Photosynthesis* (G. Akoyunoglou, Ed.), Balaban, Philadelphia, Vol. V, pp. 161–170.

Hunter, C. N., and Coomber, S. A. (1988). Cloning and oxygen-regulated expression of the bacteriochlorophyll biosynthesis genes *bch E*, *B*, *A*, and *C* of *Rhodobacter sphaeroides*, *J. Gen. Microbiol.* **134**:1491–1497.

Ikeuchi, M., and Murakami, S. (1983). Separation and characterization of prolamellar bodies and prothylakoids from squash etioplasts, *Plant Cell Physiol.* **24**:71–80.

Inoue, I., Oyama, H., and Tuboi, S. (1979). On the nature of the activating enzyme of the inactive form of δ-aminolevulinate synthetase in *Rhodopseudomonas spheroides*, *J. Biochem.* (*Tokyo*) **86**:477–482.

Jacobs, J. M., and Jacobs, N. J. (1981). Protoporphyrinogen oxidation in *Rhodopseudomonas spheroides*, a step in heme and bacteriochlorophyll synthesis, *Arch. Biochem. Biophys.* **211**:305–311.

Jacobs, J. M., and Jacobs, N. J. (1984a). Protoporphyrinogen oxidation, an enzymatic step in heme and chlorophyll synthesis: Partial characterization of the reaction in plant organelles and comparison with mammalian and bacterial systems, *Arch. Biochem. Biophys.* **229**:312–319.

Jacobs, J. M., and Jacobs, N. J. (1984b). Effect of unsaturated fatty acids on protoporphyrinogen oxidation, a step in heme and chlorophyll synthesis in plant organelles, *Biochem. Biophys. Res. Comm.* **123**:1157–1164.

Jacobs, J. M., and Jacobs, N. J. (1987). Oxidation of protoporphyrinogen to protoporphyrin, a step in chlorophyll and haem biosynthesis, *Biochem. J.* **244**:219–224.

Jacobs, J. M., Jacobs, N. J., and De Maggio, A. E. (1982). Protoporphyrinogen oxidation in chloroplasts and plant mitochondria, a step in heme and chlorophyll synthesis, *Arch. Biochem. Biophys.* **218**:233–239.

Jeffrey, S. W., and Wright, S. W. (1987). A new spectrally distinct component of chlorophyll c from the micro-alga *Emiliania huxleyi* (Prymnesiophyceae), *Biochim. Biophys. Acta* **894**:180–188.

Jensen, A., Aasmundrud, O., and Eimhjellen, K. E. (1964). Chlorophylls of the photosynthetic bacteria, *Biochim. Biophys. Acta* **88**:466–479.

Jones, M. S., and Jones, O. T. G. (1969). The structural organization of haem synthesis in rat liver mitochondria, *Biochem. J.* **113**:507–514.

Jones, O. T. G. (1963a). The inhibition of bacteriochlorophyll biosynthesis in *Rhodopseudomonas spheroides* by 8-hydroxyquinoline, *Biochem. J.* **88**:335–343.

Jones, O. T. G. (1963b). Magnesium 2,4-divinylphaeoporphyrin a_5 monomethyl ester, a protochlorophyll-like pigment produced by *Rhodopseudomonas spheroides*, *Biochem. J.* **89**:182–189.

Jones, O. T. G. (1967). Haem synthesis by isolated chloroplasts, *Biochem. Biophys. Res. Comm.* **28**:671–674.

Jones, O. T. G. (1968). Ferrochelatase of spinach chloroplasts, *Biochem. J.* **107**:113–119.

Jordan, P. M., and Berry, A. (1981). Mechanism of action of porphobilinogen deaminase. The participation of stable enzyme substrate covalent intermediates between porphobilinogen and the porphobilinogen deaminase from *Rhodopseudomonas spheroides*, *Biochem. J.* **195**:177–181.

Jordan, P. M., and Seehra, J. S. (1979). The biosynthesis of uroporphyrinogen III: Order of assembly of the four porphobilinogen molecules in the formation of the tetrapyrrole ring, *FEBS Lett.* **104**:364–366.

Jordan, P. M., and Seehra, J. S. (1980). Mechanism of action of 5-aminolevulinic acid dehydratase: Stepwise order of addition of the two molecules of 5-aminolevulinic acid in the enzymic synthesis of porphobilinogen, *J. Chem. Soc. Chem. Comm.* 240–242.

Jordan, P. M., Sharma, R. P., and Warren, M. J. (1988). A cyclic intermediate, hydroxy amino tetrahydropyran-1-one, as the precursor for 5-aminolevulinic acid biosynthesis in greening barley, *Tet. Lett*, to appear.

Jordan, P. M., and Shemin, D. (1973). Purification and properties of uroporphyrinogen I synthetase from *Rhodopseudomonas spheroides*, *J. Biol. Chem.* **248**:1019–1024.

Jordan, P. M., and Warren, M. J. (1987). Evidence for a dipyrromethane cofactor at the catalytic site of *E. coli* porphobilinogen deaminase, *FEBS Lett.* **225**:87–92.

Juknat, A. A., Dörnemann, D., and Senger, H. (1988a). Biosynthesis of porphyrinogens in etiolated *Euglena gracilis* Z. I. Isolation and purification of an endogenous factor stimulating the formation of porphyrinogens, *Z. Naturforsch.* **43c**:351–356.

Juknat, A. A., Dörnemann, D., and Senger, H. (1988b). Biosynthesis of porphyrinogens in etiolated *Euglena gracilis* Z. II. Identification of a regulatory pteridine, *Z. Naturforsch.* **43c**:357–362.

Jurgenson, J. E., Beale, S. I., and Troxler, R. F. (1976). Biosynthesis of δ-aminolevulinic acid in a unicellular Rhodophyte, *Cyanidium caldarium*, *Biochem. Biophys. Res. Comm.* **69**:149–157.

Kah, A., Dörnemann, D., Ruhl, D., and Senger, H. (1981). The influence of light and levulinic acid on the regulation of enzymes for ALA-biosynthesis in two pigment mutants of *Scenedesmus obliquus*, *Photosynthesis* (G. Akoyunoglou, Ed.), Balaban, Philadelphia, Vol. V, pp. 137–144.

Kahn, A., and Kannangara, C. G. (1987). Gabaculine-resistant mutants of *Chlamydomonas reinhardtii* with elevated glutamate 1-semialdehyde aminotransferase activity, *Carlsberg Res. Comm.* **52**:73–81.

Kannangara, C. G., and Gough, S. P. (1978). Biosynthesis of δ-aminolevulinate in greening barley leaves: Glutamate 1-semialdehyde aminotransferase, *Carlsberg Res. Comm.* **43**:185–194.

Kannangara, C. G., and Gough, S. P. (1979). Biosynthesis of δ-aminolevulinate in greening barley leaves. II. Induction of enzyme synthesis by light, *Carlsberg Res. Comm.* **44**:11–20.

Kannangara, C. G., Gough, S. P., Bruyant, P., Hoober, J. K., Kahn, A., and von Wettstein, D. (1988). tRNA^{Glu} as a cofactor in δ-aminolevulinate biosynthesis: Steps that regulate chlorophyll synthesis, *Trends Biochem. Sci.* **13**:139–143.

Kannangara, C. G., Gough, S. P., and Girnth, C. (1981). δ-Aminolevulinate synthesis in greening barley. 2. Purification of enzymes, *Proc. Fifth International Photosynthesis Congress* (G. Akoyunoglou, Ed.), Balaban, Philadelphia, pp. 117–127.

Kannangara, C. G., Gough, S. P., Oliver, R. P., and Rasmussen, S. K. (1984). Biosynthesis of δ-aminolevulinate in greening barley leaves. VI. Activation of glutamate by ligation to RNA, *Carlsberg Res. Comm.* **49**:417–437.

Kannangara, C. G., and Schouboe, A. (1985). Biosynthesis of δ-aminolevulinate in greening barley leaves. VII. Glutamate 1-semialdehyde accumulation in gabaculine treated leaves, *Carlsberg Res. Comm.* **50**:179–191.

Kasemir, H. (1983). Action of light of chlorophyll(ide) appearance, *Photochem. Photobiol.* **37**:701–708.

Katoh, T., and Yasuda, K. (1987). Separation of Cl-containing chlorophylls by column chromatography, *Plant Cell Physiol.* **28**:1529–1536.

Katz, J. J., Strain, H. H., Harkness, A. L., Studier, M. H., Svec, W. A., Janson, T. R., and Cope, B. T. (1972). Esterifying alcohols in the chlorophylls of purple photosynthetic bacteria. A new chlorophyll, bacteriochlorophyll (gg), *all-trans*-geranylgeranyl bacteriochlorophyllide a, *J. Amer. Chem. Soc.* **94**:7938–7939.

Kay, S. A., and Griffiths, W. T. (1983). Light-induced breakdown of NADPH : protochlorophyllide oxidoreductase in vitro, *Plant Physiol.* **72**:229–236.

Kikuchi, G., Kumar, A., Talmage, P., and Shemin, D. (1958). The enzymatic synthesis of δ-aminolevulinic acid, *J. Biol. Chem.* **233**:1214–1219.

Kiley, P. J., and Kaplan, S. (1988). Molecular genetics of photosynthetic membrane biosynthesis in *Rhodobacter sphaeroides*, *Microbiol. Rev.* **52**:50–69.

Killilea, S. D., and O'Carra, P. (1985). Structure and apoprotein linkages of phycourobilin, *Biochem. J.* **226**:723–731.

Kipe-Nolt, J. A., and Stevens, S. E., Jr. (1980). Biosynthesis of δ-aminolevulinic acid from glutamate in *Agmenellum quadruplicatum*, *Plant Physiol.* **65**:126–128.

Klein, G., and Rüdiger, W. (1978). Über die Bindungen zwischen Chromophor und Protein in Biliproteiden, V. Stereochemie von Modell-Imiden, *Liebigs Ann. Chem.* 267–279.

Klein, O., and Senger, H. (1978a). Biosynthetic pathways to δ-aminolevulinic acid induced by blue light in the pigment mutant C-2A′ of *Scenedesmus obliquus*, *Photochem. Photobiol.* **27**:203–208.

Klein, O., and Senger, H. (1978b). Two biosynthetic pathways to δ-aminolevulinic acid in a pigment mutant of the green alga, *Scenedesmus obliquus*, *Plant Physiol.* **62**:10–13.

Klein, S., Harel, E. Ne'eman, E., Katz, E., and Meller, E. (1975). Accumulation of δ-aminolevulinic acid and its relation to chlorophyll synthesis and development of plastid structure in greening leaves, *Plant Physiol.* **56**:486–496.

Klein, S., Katz, E., and Ne'eman, E. (1977). Induction of δ-aminolevulinic acid formation in etiolated maize leaves controlled by two light systems, *Plant Physiol.* **60**:335–338.

Klotz, A. V., and Glazer, A. N. (1985). Characterization of the bilin attachment sites in R-phycoerythrin, *J. Biol. Chem.* **260**:4856–4863.

Klotz, A. V., Glazer, A. N., Bishop, J. E., Nagy, J. O., and Rapoport, H. (1986). Phycobiliprotein-bilin linkage diversity. II. Structural studies on A- and D-ring-linked phycoerythrobilins, *J. Biol. Chem.* **261**:6797–6805.

Knox, W. E. (1960). Glutathione, *The Enzymes* (P. D. Boyer, H. Lardy, and K. Myrback, Eds.), Academic, New York, Vol. 2, pp. 253–294.

Kohashi, M., Clement, R. P., Tse, J., and Piper, W. N. (1984). Rat hepatic uroporphyrinogen III co-synthase. Purification and evidence for a bound folate coenzyme participating in the biosynthesis of uroporphyrinogen III, *Biochem. J.* **220**:755–765.

Koski, V. M., French, C. S., and Smith, J. H. C. (1951). The action spectrum for the transformation of protochlorophyll to chlorophyll a in normal and albino corn seedlings, *Arch. Biochem. Biophys.* **31**:1–17.

Köst, H.-P., and Benedikt, E. (1982). Biliverdin IXα, intermediate and end product of tetrapyrrole biosynthesis, *Z. Naturforsch.* **37c**:1057–1063.

Kotler, M. L., Fumagalli, S. A., Juknat, A. A., and Batlle, A. M. del C. (1987). Porphyrin biosynthesis in *Rhodopseudomonas palustris*. VIII. Purification and properties of deaminase, *Comp. Biochem. Physiol.* **87B**:601–606.

Kwan, L. Y.-M., Darling, D. L., and Richards, W. R. (1986). Affinity chromatography of two enzymes of the latter stages of chlorophyll synthesis, *Regulation of Chloroplast Differentiation* (G. Akoyunoglou and H. Senger, Eds.) Alan R. Liss, New York, pp. 57–62.

Laghai, A., and Jordan, P. M. (1976). A partial reaction of δ-aminolaevulinate synthetase from *Rhodopseudomonas spheroides*, *Biochem. Soc. Trans.* **4**:52–53.

Laghai, A., and Jordan, P. M. (1977). An exchange reaction catalysed by δ-aminolaevulinate synthase from *Rhodopseudomonas spheroides*, *Biochem. Soc. Trans.* **5**:299–300.

Lapointe, J., Duplain, L., and Proulx, M. (1986). A single glutamyl-tRNA synthetase aminoacylates tRNA^{Glu} and tRNA^{Gln} in *Bacillus subtilis* and efficiently misacylates *Escherichia coli* tRNA$_1^{Gln}$ in vitro, *J. Bacteriol.* **165**:88–93.

Lascelles, J. (1966). The accumulation of bacteriochlorophyll precursors by mutant and wild type strains of *Rhodopseudomonas spheroides*, *Biochem. J.* **100**:175–183.

Lascelles, J. (1978). Regulation of pyrrole synthesis, *The Photosynthetic Bacteria* (R. K. Clayton and W. R. Sistrom, Eds.), Plenum, New York, pp. 795–808.

Laycock, M. V., and Wright, J. C. C. (1981). The biosynthesis of phycocyanobilin in *Anacystis nidulans, Phytochemistry* **20**:1265–1268.

Liedgens, W., Grützmann, R., and Schneider, H. A. W. (1980). Highly efficient purification of the labile plant enzyme 5-aminolevulinate dehydratase (EC 4.2.1.24) by means of monoclonal antibodies, *Z. Naturforsch.* **35c**:958–962.

Little, H. N., and Jones, O. T. G. (1976). The subcellular localization and properties of the ferrochelatase of etiolated barley, *Biochem. J.* **156**:309–314.

Manetas, Y., and Akoyunoglou, G. (1981). Turnover of chlorophyllous pigments during the dark and the early stages of greening, *Photosynthetica* **15**:534–539.

Mapleston, E. R., and Griffiths, W. T. (1980). Light modulation of the activity of protochlorophyllide reductase, *Biochem. J.* **189**:125–133.

Marrs, B. (1981). Mobilization of the genes for photosynthesis from *Rhodopseudomonas capsulata* by a promiscuous plasmid, *J. Bacteriol.* **146**:1003–1012.

Masoner, M., and Kasemir, H. (1975). Control of chlorophyll synthesis by phytochrome. I. The effect of phytochrome on the formation of 5-aminolevulinate in mustard seedlings, *Planta* **126**:111–117.

Mattheis, J. R., and Rebeiz, C. A. (1977). Chloroplast biogenesis: Net synthesis of protochlorophyllide from magnesium protoporphyrin monester by developing chloroplasts, *J. Biol. Chem.* **252**:4022–4024.

Mau, Y.-H. L., and Wang, W.-Y. (1988). Biosynthesis of δ-aminolevulinic acid in *Chlamydomonas reinhardtii*. Study of the transamination mechanism using specifically labeled glutamate, *Plant Physiol.* **86**:793–797.

Mayer, S. M., Weinstein, J. D., and Beale, S. I. (1987). Enzymatic conversion of glutamate to δ-aminolevulinate in soluble extracts of *Euglena gracilis, J. Biol. Chem.* **262**:12541–12549.

Mazel, D. Guglielmi, G., Houmard, J., Sidler, W., Bryant, D. A., and Tandaeu de Marsac, N. (1986). Green light induces transcription of the phycoerythrin operon in the cyanobacterium *Calothrix* 7601, *Nucl. Acids Res.* **14**:8279–8290.

McKie, J., Lucas, C., and Smith, A. (1981). δ-Aminolaevulinate biosynthesis in the cyanobacterium *Synechococcus* 6301, *Phytochemistry* **20**:1547–1549.

Meisch, H.-U., and Maus, R. (1983). Untersuchungen zur Synthese und biologischen Bedeutung von Glutaminsäure-1-semialdehyd als Vorstufe der Chlorophylle, *Z. Naturforsch.* **38c**:563–570.

Meller, E., Belkin, S., and Harel, E. (1975). The biosynthesis of δ-aminolevulinic acid in greening maize leaves, *Phytochemistry* **14**:2399–2402.

Meller, E., and Gassman, M. L. (1982). Biosynthesis of 5-aminolevulinic acid: Two pathways in higher plants, *Plant Sci. Lett.* **26**:23–29.

Meller, E., and Harel, E. (1978). The pathway of 5-aminolevulinic acid synthesis in *Chlorella vulgaris* and in *Fremyella diplosiphon, Chloroplast Development* (G. Akoyunoglou and J. H. Argyroudi-Akoyunoglou, Eds.), Elsevier, Amsterdam, pp. 51–57.

Michalski, T. J., Hunt, J. E., Bowman, M. K., Smith, U., Bardeen, K., Gest, H., Norris, J. R., and Katz, J. J. (1987). Bacteriopheophytin g: Properties and some speculations on a possible role for bacteriochlorophylls b and g in the biosynthesis of chlorophylls, *Proc. Nat. Acad. Sci. (U.S.A.)* **84**:2570–2574.

Miller, J. W., and Teng, D. (1967). The purification and kinetics of aminolevulinic acid synthetase from higher plants, *Proc. Seventh International Congress of Biochemistry Tokyo*, p. 1059.

Minkov, I. N., Ryberg, M., and Sundqvist, C. (1988). Properties of reformed prolamellar bodies from illuminated and redarkened wheat plants, *Physiol. Plant.* **72**:725–732.

Mösinger, E., Batschauer, A., Schäfer, E., and Apel, K. (1985). Phytochrome control of in vitro transcription of specific genes in isolated nuclei from barley (*Hordeum vulgare*), *Eur. J. Biochem.* **147**:137–142.

Murphy, M. J., Siegel, L. M., Tove, S. R., and Kamen, H. (1974). Siroheme: A new prosthetic group participating in six-electron reduction reactions catalyzed by both sulfite and nitrite reductases, *Proc. Nat. Acad. Sci. (U.S.A.)* **71**:612–616.

Nadler, K., and Granick, S. (1970). Controls on chlorophyll synthesis in barley, *Plant Physiol.* **46**:240–246.

Nagy, J. O., Bishop, J. E., Klotz, A. V., Glazer, A. N., and Rapoport, H. (1985). Bilin attachment sites in the α, β, and γ subunits of R-phycoerythrin. Structural studies on singly and doubly linked phycourobilins, *J. Biol. Chem.* **260**:4864–4868.

Nandi, D. L., Baker-Cohen, K. F., and Shemin, D. (1968). δ-Aminolaevulinic acid dehydratase of *Rhodopseudomonas spheroides*. Isolation and properties, *J. Biol. Chem.* **243**:1224–1230.

Nandi, D. L., and Shemin, D. (1973). δ-Aminolevulinic acid dehydratase of *Rhodopseudomonas capsulata*, *Arch. Biochem. Biophys.* **158**:305–311.

Nandi, D. L., and Shemin, D. (1977). Quaternary structure of δ-aminolevulinic acid synthase from *Rhodopseudomonas spheroides*, *J. Biol. Chem.* **252**:2278–2280.

Nandi, D. L., and Waygood, E. R. (1967). Biosynthesis of porphyrins in wheat leaves. II. 5-Aminolaevulinate hydro-lyase, *Canad. J. Biochem.* **45**:327–336.

Nasri, F., Huault, C., and Belangé, A. P. (1988). 5-Aminolevulinate dehydrastase activity in thylakoid-related structures of etiochloroplasts from radish cotyledons, *Phytochemistry* **27**:1289–1295.

Nasrulhaq-Boyce, A., Griffiths, W. T., and Jones, O. T. G. (1987). The use of continuous assays to characterize the oxidative cyclase that synthesizes the chlorophyll isocyclic ring, *Biochem. J.* **243**:23–29.

Nasrulhaq-Boyce, A., and Jones, O. T. G. (1981). Tetrapyrrole biosynthesis in greening etiolated barley seedlings, *Phytochemistry* **20**:1005–1009.

Nichols, K. E., and Bogorad, L. (1962). Action spectra studies of phycocyanin formation in a mutant of *Cyanidium caldarium*, *Bot. Gaz.* **124**:85–93.

Nuijs, A. M., van Dorssen, R. J., Duysens, L. N. M., and Amesz, J. (1985). Excited states and primary photochemical reactions in the photosynthetic bacterium *Heliobacterium chlorum*, *Proc. Nat. Acad. Sci. (U.S.A.)* **82**:6865–6868.

O'Carra, P., Murphy, R. F., and Killilea, S. D. (1980). The native forms of the phycobilin chromophores of algal biliproteins. A clarification, *Biochem. J.* **187**:303–309.

Oelze-Karow, H., Kasemir, H., and Mohr, H. (1978). Control of chlorophyll b formation by phytochrome and a threshold level of chlorophyllide a, *Chloroplast Development* (G. Akoyunoglou and J. H. Argyroudi-Akoyunoglou, Eds.), Elsevier, Amsterdam, pp. 787–792.

Oelze-Karow, H., and Mohr, H. (1978). Control of chlorophyll b biosynthesis by phytochrome, *Photochem. Photobiol.* **27**:189–193.

Ogawa, T., Inoue, Y., Kitajima, M., and Shibata, K. (1973). Action spectra for biosynthesis of chlorophylls a and b and β-carotene, *Photochem. Photobiol.* **18**:229–235.

Oh-hama, T., and Hase, E. (1980). Formation of protochlorophyll(ide) in wild type and mutant C-2A′ cells of *Scenedesmus obliquus*, *Plant Cell Physiol.* **21**:1263–1272.

Oh-hama, T., Seto, H., Otake, N., and Miyachi, S. (1982). ^{13}C-NMR evidence for the pathway of chlorophyll biosynthesis in green algae, *Biochem. Biophys. Res. Comm.* **105**:647–652.

Oh-hama, T., Seto, H., and Miyachi, S. (1986a). ^{13}C-NMR evidence of bacteriochlorophyll a formation by the C_5 pathway in *Chromatium*, *Arch. Biochem. Biophys.* **246**:192–198.

Oh-hama, T., Seto, H., and Miyachi, S. (1986b). ^{13}C-NMR evidence for bacteriochlorophyll c formation by the C_5 pathway in green sulfur bacterium, *Prosthecochloris*, *Eur. J. Biochem.* **159**:189–194.

Oh-hama, T., Stolowich, N. J., and Scott, A. I. (1988). 5-Aminolevulinic acid formation from glutamate via the C_5 pathway in *Clostridium thermoaceticum*, *FEBS Lett.* **228**:89–93.

Ohki, K., and Fujita, Y. (1979). In vivo transformation of phycobiliproteins during photobleaching of *Tolypothrix tenuis* to forms active in photoreversible absorption changes, *Plant Cell Physiol.* **20**:1341–1347.

Oliver, R. P., and Griffiths, W. T. (1980). Identification of the polypeptides of NADPH : protochlorophyllide oxidoreductase, *Biochem. J.* **191**:277–280.

Oliver, R. P., and Griffiths, W. T. (1982). Pigment-protein complexes of illuminated etiolated leaves, *Plant Physiol.* **70**:1019–1025.

O'Neill, G. P., Peterson, D. M., Schön, A., Chen, M.-W., and Söll, D. (1988). Formation of the chlorophyll precursor δ-aminolevulinic acid in cyanobacteria requires aminoacylation of a tRNA^{Glu} species, *J. Bacteriol.* **170**:3810–3816.

Oyama, H., and Tuboi, S. (1979). Occurrence of a novel high molecular weight activator of δ-aminolevulinate synthetase in *Rhodopseudomonas spheroides*, *J. Biochem. (Tokyo)* **86**:483–489.

Packer, N., and Adamson, H. (1986). Incorporation of 5-aminolevulinic acid into chlorophyll in darkness in barley, *Physiol. Plant.* **68**:220–230.

Pardo, A. D., Chereskin, B. M., Castelfranco, P. A., Franceschi, V. R., and Wezelman, B. E. (1980). ATP requirement for Mg chelatase in developing chloroplasts, *Plant Physiol.* **65**:956–960.

Paul, K. G. (1951). The porphyrin component of cytochrome c and its linkage to the protein, *Acta Chem. Scand.* **5**:389–405.

Pierson, B. K., and Castenholz, R. W. (1971). Bacteriochlorophylls in gliding filamentous prokaryotes from hot springs, *Nature* **233**:25–27.

Porra, R. J., and Grimme, L. H. (1974). Chlorophyll synthesis and intracellular fluctuations of 5-aminolaevulinate formation during the regreening of nitrogen-deficient *Chlorella fusca*, *Arch. Biochem. Biophys.* **164**:312–321.

Porra, R. J., Klein, O., and Wright, P. E. (1983). The proof by ^{13}C-NMR spectroscopy of the predominance of the C$_5$ pathway over the Shemin pathway in chlorophyll biosynthesis in higher plants and the formation of the methyl ester group of chlorophyll from glycine, *Eur. J. Biochem.* **130**:509–516.

Porra, R. J., and Lascelles, J. (1968). Studies on ferrochelatase: The enzymic formation of haem in proplastids, chloroplasts and plant mitochondria, *Biochem. J.* **108**:343–348.

Poulson, R., and Polglase, W. J. (1974). Aerobic and anaerobic coproporphyrinogenase activities in extracts from *Saccharomyces cerevisiae*, *J. Biol. Chem.* **249**:6367–6371.

Pradel, J., and Clement-Metral, J. D. (1976). A 4-vinyl protochlorophyllide complex accumulated by "Phofil" mutant of *Rhodopseudomonas spheroides*. An authentic intermediate in the development of the photosynthetic apparatus, *Biochim. Biophys. Acta* **430**:253–264.

Pudek, M. R., and Richards, W. R. (1975). A possible alternate pathway of bacteriochlorophyll biosynthesis in a mutant of *Rhodopseudomonas spheroides*, *Biochemistry (U.S.A)* **14**:3132–3137.

Radmer, R. J., and Bogorad, L. (1967). (−)S-adenosyl-L-methionine-magnesium protoporphyrin methyltransferase, an enzyme in the biosynthetic pathway of chlorophyll in *Zea mays*, *Plant Physiol.* **42**:463–465.

Ramaswamy, N. K., and Nair, P. M. (1973). δ-Aminolevulinic acid synthetase from cold-stored potatoes, *Biochim. Biophys. Acta* **293**:269–277.

Ramaswamy, N. K., and Nair, P. M. (1974). Temperature and light dependency of chlorophyll synthesis in potatoes, *Plant Sci. Lett.* **2**:249–256.

Ramaswamy, N. K., and Nair, P. M. (1976). Pathway for the biosynthesis of delta-aminolevulinic acid in greening potatoes, *Indian J. Biochem. Biophys.* **13**:394–397.

Ramus, J., Beale, S. I., Mauzerall, D., and Howard, K. L. (1976). Changes in photosynthetic pigment concentration in seaweeds as a function of water depth, *Mar. Biol.* **37**:223–229.

Rapoport, H., and Hamlow, H. P. (1961). *Chlorobium* chlorophyll-660. The esterifying alcohol, *Biochem. Biophys. Res. Comm.* **6**:134–137.

Rebeiz, C. A., Belanger, F. C., Freyssinet, G., and Saab, D. G. (1980). Chloroplast biogenesis. XXIX. The occurrence of several novel chlorophyll a and b chromophores in higher plants, *Biochim. Biophys. Acta* **590**:234–247.

Rebeiz, C. A., and Castelfranco, P. A. (1971). Chlorophyll biosynthesis in a cell-free system from higher plants, *Plant Physiol.* **47**:33–37.

Rebeiz, C. A., and Lascelles, J. (1982). Biosynthesis of pigments in plants and bacteria, *Photosynthesis: Energy Conversion by Plants and Bacteria* (Govindjee, Ed.), Vol. I, pp. 699–780.

Rebeiz, C. A., Montazer-Zouhoor, A., Mayasich, J. M., Tripathy, B. C., Wu, S. M., and Rebeiz, C. C. (1987). Photodynamic herbicides and chlorophyll biosynthesis modulators, *Light Activated Pesticides*, ACS Symposium Series (J. R. Heitz and K. R. Downum, Eds.), American Chemical Society, Washington, D.C., No. 339, pp. 295–328.

Rebeiz, C. A., Smith, B. B., Mattheis, J. R., Rebeiz, C. C., and Dayton, D. F. (1975). Chloroplast biogenesis: Biosynthesis and accumulation of Mg-protoporphyrin-IX monoester and other metalloporphyrins by isolated etioplasts and developing chloroplasts, *Arch. Biochem. Biophys.* **167**:351–365.

Rebeiz, C. A., Wu, S. M., Kuhadja, M., Daniell, H., and Perkins, E. J. (1983). Chlorophyll a biosynthetic routes and chlorophyll a chemical heterogeneity in plants, *Mol. Cell. Biochem.* **57**:97–125.

Reichhart, D., Salaun, J. P., Benveniste, I., and Durst, F. (1980). Time course of induction of cytochrome P-450, NADPH-cytochrome c reductase, and cinnamic acid hydroxylase by phenobarbital, ethanol, herbicides, and manganese in higher plant microsomes, *Plant Physiol.* **66**:600–604.

Richards, W. R., Fung, M., Wessler, A. N., and Hinchigeri, S. B. (1987a). The purification and properties of three later-stage enzymes of chlorophyll synthesis, *Progress in Photosynthesis Research* (J. Biggins, Ed.), Martinus Nijhoff, Boston, Vol. IV, pp. 475–482.

Richards, W. R., and Lascelles, J. (1969). The biosynthesis of bacteriochlorophyll: The characterization of the latter stage intermediates from mutants of *Rhodopseudomonas spheroides*, *Biochemistry* **8**:3473–3482.

Richards, W. R., Walker, C. J., and Griffiths, W. T. (1987b). The affinity chromatographic purification of NADPH : protochlorophyllide oxidoreductase from etiolated wheat, *Photosynthetica* **21**:462–471.

Richter, M. L., and Rienits, K. G. (1980). The synthesis of magnesium and zinc protoporphyrin and their methyl esters in etioplast preparations studied by high pressure liquid chromatography, *FEBS Lett.* **116**:211–216.

Richter, M. L., and Rienits, K. G. (1982). The synthesis of magnesium-protoporphyrin IX by etiochloroplast membrane preparations, *Biochim. Biophys. Acta* **717**:255–264.

Rieble, S., and Beale, S. I. (1988). Enzymatic transformation of glutamate to δ-aminolevulinic acid by soluble extracts of *Synechocystis* sp. 6803 and other oxygenic prokaryotes, *J. Biol. Chem.* **263**:8864–8871.

Rieble, S., Ormerod, J. G., and Beale, S. I. (1988). Cell-free extracts from the obligately anaerobic photosynthetic bacterium *Chlorobium limicola* 8327 catalyze conversion of glutamate to δ-aminolevulinic acid, *Plant Physiol.* **86S**:60.

Risch, N., Brockmann, H., Jr., and Gloe, A. (1979). Strukturaufklärung von neuartigen Bacteriochlorophyllen aus *Chloroflexus aurantiacus*, *Liebigs Ann. Chem.* 408–418.

Risch, N., Köster, B., Schormann, A., Siemens, T., and Brockmann, H. (1988). Bacteriochlorophyll f. Partialsynthese und Eigenschaften eineger Derivate, *Liebigs Ann. Chem.* 343–347.

Roper, U., Prinz, H., and Lutz, C. (1987). Amino acid composition of the enzyme NADPH : protochlorophyllide oxidoreductase, *Plant Sci.* **52**:15–19.

Rosé, S., Frydman, R. B., de los Santos, C., Sburlati, A., Valasinas, A., and Frydman, B. (1988). Spectroscopic evidence for a porphobilinogen deaminase-tetrapyrrole complex that is an intermediate in the biosynthesis of uroporphyrinogen III, *Biochemistry* (*U.S.A.*) **27**:4871–4879.

Rüdiger, W. (1987). Chlorophyll synthetase and its implication for regulation of chlorophyll biosynthesis, *Progress in Photosynthesis Research* (J. Biggins, Ed.), Martinus Nijhoff, Boston, Vol. IV, pp. 461–467.

Rüdiger, W., Benz, J., and Guthoff, C. (1980). Detection and partial characterization of activity of chlorophyll synthetase in etioplast membranes, *Eur. J. Biochem.* **109**:193–200.

Rüdiger, W., Benz, J., Lempert, U., and Steffens, D. (1976). Inhibition of phytol accumulation with herbicides. Geranylgeraniol and dihydrogeranylgeraniol-containing chlorophyll from wheat seedlings, *Z. Pflanzenphysiol.* **80**:131–143.

Rüdiger, W., Hedden, P., Köst, H.-P., and Chapman, D. J. (1977). Esterification of chlorophyllide by geranylgeranyl pyrophosphate in a cell-free system from maize shoots, *Biochem. Biophys. Res. Comm.* **74**:1268–1272.

Sandy, J. D., Davies, R. C., and Neuberger, A. (1975). Control of 5-aminolevulinate synthetase activity in *Rhodopseudomonas spheroides*: A role for trisulphides, *Biochem. J.* **150**:245–257.

Santel, H.-J., and Apel, K. (1981). The protochlorophyllide holochrome of barley (*Hordeum vulgare* L.): The effect of light on the NADPH : protochlorophyllide oxidoreductase, *Eur. J. Biochem.* **120**:95–103.

Sato, K. (1978). Bacteriochlorophyll formation by facultative methylotrophs *Protaminobacter ruber* and *Psudomonas* AM-1, *FEBS Lett.* **85**:207–210.

Sawyer, E., and Smith, R. A. (1958). δ-Aminolevulinate synthesis in *Rhodopseudomonas spheroides*, *Bacteriol. Proc.* 111.

Scheer, H., Gross, E., Nitsche, B., Cmiel, E., Schneider, S., Schäfer, W., Schiebel, H.-M., and Schulten, H.-R. (1986). Structure of Methylpheophorbide-RCI, *Photochem. Photobiol.* **43**:559–571.

Scheer, H., Svec, W. A., Cope, B. T., Studier, M. H., Scott, R. G., and Katz, J. J. (1974). Structure of bacteriochlorophyll b, *J. Amer. Chem. Soc.* **96**:3714–3716.

Schiff, J. A. (1974). The control of chloroplast differentiation in *Euglena*, *Proc. Third International Congress on Photosynthesis* (M. Avron, Ed.), Elsevier, Amsterdam, pp. 1691–1717.

Schmidt, G., Siebzehnrübl, S., Fischer, R., Rüdiger, W., Scheer, H., Schirmer, T., Bode, W., and Huber, R. (1987). ZZE-Configuration of chromophore β-153 in C-phycocyanin from *Mastigocladus laminosus*, *Z. Naturforsch.* **42c**:845–848.

Schneegurt, M. A., and Beale, S. I. (1986). Biosynthesis of protoheme and heme a from glutamate in maize, *Plant Physiol.* **81**:965–971.

Schneegurt, M. A., and Beale, S. I. (1988). Characterization of the RNA required for biosynthesis of δ-aminolevulinic acid from glutamate. Purification by anticodon-based affinity chromatography and determination that the UUC glutamate anticodon is a general requirement for function in ALA biosynthesis, *Plant Physiol.* **86**:497–504.

Schneegurt, M. A., Rieble, S., and Beale, S. I. (1988). tRNA$^{\text{Glu(UUC)}}$ of plants and algae: HPLC separation into two subfractions, and determination of their relative effectiveness in homologous in vitro translation and ALA-forming systems, *Plant Physiol.* **86S**:61.

Schneider, H. A. W., and Bogorad, L. (1978). On the regulation of phycobiliprotein accumulation in relation to chlorophyll and ALA formation in *Cyanidium caldarium*, *Chloroplast Development* (G. Akoyunoglou and J. H. Argyoudi-Akoyunoglou, Eds.), Elsevier, Amsterdam, pp. 823–826.

Schoch, S., Hehlein, C., and Rüdiger, W. (1980). Influence of anaerobiosis on chlorophyll biosynthesis in greening oat seedlings *Avena sativa* L., *Plant Physiol.* **66**:576–579.

Schoch, S., Lempert, U., and Rüdiger, W. (1977). On the last steps of chlorophyll biosynthesis. Intermediates between chlorophyllide and phytol-containing chlorophyll, *Z. Pflanzenphysiol.* **83**:427–436.

Schoch, S., and Schäfer, W. (1978). Tetrahydrogeranylgeraniol, a precursor of phytol in the biosynthesis of chlorophyll a—localization of the double bonds, *Z. Naturforsch.* **33c**:408–412.

Schoenleber, R. W., Leung, S.-L., Lundell, D. J., Glazer, A. N., and Rapoport, H. (1983). Chromopeptides from phycoerythrins. Structure and linkage of a phycoerythrobilin tryptic tripeptide derived from a B-phycoerythrin, *J. Amer. Chem. Soc.* **105**:4072–4076.

Schön, A., Kannangara, C. G., Gough, S., and Söll, D. (1988). Protein biosynthesis in organelles requires misaminoacylation of tRNA, *Nature* **331**:187–190.

Schön, A., Krupp, G., Gough, S., Berry-Lowe, S., Kannangara, C. G., and Söll, D. (1986). The RNA required in the first step of chlorophyll biosynthesis is a chloroplast glutamate tRNA, *Nature* **322**:281–284.

Schuster, A., Köst, H.-P., Rüdiger, W., and Eder, J. (1983a). Investigations on the apoprotein of phycocyanin from *Cyanidium caldarium*, *Arch. Microbiol.* **135**:30–35.

Schuster, A., Köst, H.-P., Rüdiger, W., Holroyd, J. A., and Brown, S. B. (1983b). Incorporation of haem into phycocyanobilin in levulinic acid treated *Cyanidium caldarium*, *Plant Cell Rep.* **2**:85–87.

Scott, A. I., Burton, G., Jordan, P. M., Matsumoto, H., Fagerness, P. E., and Pryde, L. M. (1980). N.M.R. spectroscopy as a probe for the study of enzyme-catalysed reactions. Further observations of preuroporphyrinogen, a substrate for uroporphyrinogen III cosynthetase, *J. Chem. Soc. Chem. Comm.* 384–387.

Seehra, J. S., and Jordan, P. M. (1980). Mechanism of action of porphobilinogen deaminase: Ordered addition of the four porphobilinogen molecules in the formation of preuroporphyrinogen, *J. Amer. Chem. Soc.* **102**:6841–6846.

Selstam, E., Widell, A., and Johansson, L. B.-Å. (1987). A comparison of prolamellar bodies from wheat, Scots pine and Jeffrey pine. Pigment spectra and properties of protochlorophyllide oxidoreductase, *Physiol. Plant.* **70**:209–214.

Seltzer, S. (1972). Cis-trans isomerization, *The Enzymes* (P. D. Boyer, Ed.), 3rd ed., Academic, New York, Vol. VI, pp. 381–406.

Senger, H., and Brinkmann, G. (1986). Protochlorophyll(ide) accumulation and degradation in the dark and photoconversion to chlorophyll in the light in pigment mutant C-2A' of *Scenedesmus obliquus*, *Physiol. Plant.* **68**:119–124.

Shaw, P., Henwood, J., Oliver, R., and Griffiths, T. (1985). Immunogold localisation of protochlorophyllide oxidoreductase in barley etioplasts, *Eur. J. Cell Biol.* **39**:50–55.

Shetty, A. S., and Miller, G. W. (1969). Purification and general properties of δ-aminolaevulate dehydratase from *Nicotiana tabacum* L., *Biochem. J.* **114**:331–337.

Shibata, H., and Ochiai, H. (1977). Purification and properties of δ-aminolevulinic acid dehydratase from radish cotyledons, *Plant Cell Physiol.* **18**:421–429.

Shibata, K. (1957). Spectroscopic studies of chlorophyll formation in intact leaves, *J. Biochem. (Tokyo)* **44**:147–173.

Shieh, J., Miller, G. W., and Psenak, M. (1978). Properties of S-adenosyl-L-methionine-magnesium protoporphyrin IX methyltransferase from barley, *Plant Cell Physiol.* **19**:1051–1059.

Shioi, Y., Nagamine, M., Kuroki, M., and Sasa, T. (1980). Purification by affinity chromatography and properties of uroporphyrinogen I synthetase from *Chlorella regularis*, *Biochim. Biophys. Acta* **616**:300–309.

Shioi, Y., and Sasa, T. (1983a). Compositional heterogeneity of protochlorophyllide ester in etiolated leaves of higher plants, *Arch. Biochem. Biophys.* **220**:286–292.

Shioi, Y., and Sasa, T. (1983b). Esterification of chlorophyllide b in higher plants, *Biochim. Biophys. Acta* **756**:127–131.

Shioi, Y., and Sasa, T. (1984). Terminal steps of bacteriochlorophyll a phytol formation in purple photosynthetic bacteria, *J. Bacteriol.* **158**:340–343.

Shlyk, A. A., and Prudnikova, I. V. (1967). Dark biosynthesis of chlorophyll b by fractions of barley chloroplasts, *Photosynthetica* **1**:157–170.

Shlyk, A. A., Prudnikova, I. V., and Malashevich, A. V. (1971). Dark conversion of externally introduced chlorophyll a to chlorophyll b in a homogenate of etiolated corn seedlings, *Dokl. Akad. Nauk. SSSR* **201**:1481–1484.

Shlyk, A. A., Vlasenok, L. I., Akhramovich, N. I., Vrubel, S. V., and Akulovich, E. M. (1975). Biosynthesis of chlorophyll b in a homogenate of green leaves in the dark and under light, *Dokl. Akad. Nauk. SSSR* **221**:1234–1236.

Siegelman, H. W., Chapman, D. J., and Cole, W. J. (1968). The bile pigments of plants, *Porphyrins and Related Compounds* (T. W. Goodwin, Ed.), Academic, New York, pp. 107–120.

Silverthorne, J., and Tobin, E. M. (1984). Demonstration of transcriptional regulation of specific genes by phytochrome action, *Proc. Nat. Acad. Sci. (U.S.A.)* **81**:1112–1116.

Simpson, D. J., and Smith, K. M. (1988). Structures and transformations of the bacteriochlorophylls e and their bacteriopheophorbides, *J. Amer. Chem. Soc.* **110**:1753–1758.

Sisler, E. C., and Klein, W. H. (1963). The effect of age and various chemicals on the lag phase of chlorophyll synthesis in dark grown bean seedlings, *Physiol. Plant.* **16**:315–322.

Sistrom, W. R., Griffiths, M., and Stanier, R. Y. (1956). A note on the porphyrins excreted by the blue-green mutant of *Rhodopseudomonas spheroides*, *J. Cell. Comp. Physiol.* **48**:459–472.

Smith, A. G. (1986). Enzymes for chlorophyll synthesis in developing peas, *Regulation of Chloroplast Differentiation* (G. Akoyunoglou and H. Senger, Eds.), Alan R. Liss, New York, pp. 49–54.

Smith, A. G. (1988). Subcellular localization of two porphyrin-synthesis enzymes in *Pisum sativum* (pea) and *Arum* (cuckoo-pint) species, *Biochem. J.* **249**:423–428.

Smith, B. B., and Rebeiz, C. A. (1977). Chloroplast biogenesis: Detection of Mg-protoporphyrin chelatase in vitro, *Arch. Biochem. Biophys.* **180**:178–185.

Smith, H., and Kendrick, R. E. (1976). The structure and properties of phytochrome, *Chemistry and Biochemistry of Plant Pigments* (T. W. Goodwin, Ed.), 2nd ed., Academic, New York, Vol. 1, pp. 377–424.

Smith, K. M., and Bobe, F. W. (1987). Light adaptation of bacteriochlorophyll-d producing bacteria by enzymic methylation of their antenna pigments, *J. Chem. Soc. Chem. Comm.* 276–277.

Smith, K. M., and Goff, D. A. (1985). Bacteriochlorophylls-d from *Chlorobium vibrioforme*: Chromatographic separations and structural assignments of the methyl bacteriopheophorbides, *J. Chem. Soc. Perkin Trans I* 1099–1113.

Smith, K. M., and Huster, M. S. (1987). Bacteriochlorophyll-c formation via the glutamate C-5 pathway in *Chlorobium* bacteria, *J. Chem. Soc. Chem. Comm.* 14–16.

Spiller, S. C., Castelfranco, A. M., and Castelfranco, P. A. (1982). Effects of iron and oxygen of chlorophyll biosynthesis. I. In vivo observations on iron and oxygen-deficient plants, *Plant Physiol.* **69**:107–111.

Steiner, R., Schäfer, W., Blos, I., Wieschhoff, H., and Scheer, H. (1981). Δ2,10-Phytadienol as esterifying alcohol of bacteriochlorophyll b from *Ectothiorhodospira halochloris*, *Z. Naturforsch.* **36c**:417–420.

Stillman, L. C., and Gassman, M. L. (1978). Characterization of protoheme levels in etiolated and greening plant tissues, *Plant Physiol.* **62**:182–184.

Stobart, A. K., and Ameen-Bukhari, I. (1984). Regulation of δ-aminolaevulinic acid synthesis and protochlorophyllide regeneration in the leaves of dark-grown barley (*Hordeum vulgare*) seedlings, *Biochem. J.* **222**:419–426.

Stobart, A. K., and Ameen-Bukhari, I. (1986). Photoreduction of protochlorophyllide and its relationship to δ-aminolaevulinic acid synthesis in the leaves of dark-grown barley (*Hordeum vulgare*) seedlings, *Biochem. J.* **236**:741–748.

Stobart, A. K., and Hendry, G. A. F. (1984). The turnover of chlorophyll in greening wheat leaves, *Phytochemistry* **23**:27–30.

Tait, G. H. (1972). Coproporphyrinogenase activities in extracts of *Rhodopseudomonas spheroides* and *Chromatium* strain D, *Biochem. J.* **128**:1159–1169.

Takemoto, J., and Lascelles, J. (1973). Coupling between bacteriochlorophyll and membrane protein synthesis in *Rhodopseudomonas spheroides*, *Proc. Nat. Acad. Sci.* (*U.S.A.*) **70**:799–803.

Tamai, H., Shioi, Y., and Sasa, T. (1979). Purification and characterization of δ-aminolevulinic acid dehydratase from *Chlorella regularis*, *Plant Cell Physiol.* **20**:435–444.

Teyssendier de la Serve, B., Axelos, M., and Peaud-Lenoel, C. (1985). Cytokinins modulate the expression of genes encoding the protein of the light-harvesting chlorophyll a/b complex, *Plant Mol. Biol.* **5**:155–163.

Thorne, S. W., and Boardman, N. K. (1971). Formation of chlorophyll b, and the fluorescence properties and photochemical activities of isolated phastids from greening pea seedlings, *Plant Physiol.* **47**:252–261.

Tigier, H. A., Batlle, A. M. del C., and Locascio, G. A. (1970). Porphyrin biosynthesis in the soybean callus tissue system. II. Improved purification and some properties of delta amino-laevulic acid dehydratase, *Enzymologia* **38**:43–56.

Tripathy, B. C., and Rebeiz, C. A. (1986). Chloroplast biogenesis. Demonstration of the monovinyl and divinyl monocarboxylic routes of chlorophyll biosynthesis in higher plants, *J. Biol. Chem.* **261**:13556–13564.

Tripathy, B. C., and Rebeiz, C. A. (1987). Non-equivalence of glutamic and δ-aminolevulinic acids as substrates for protochlorophyllide and chlorophyll biosynthesis in darkness, *Progress in Photosynthesis Research* (J. Biggins, Ed.), Martinus Nijhoff, Boston, Vol. IV, pp. 439–443.

Tripathy, B. C., and Rebeiz, C. A. (1988). Chlorophlast biogenesis. 60. Conversion of divinyl protochlorophyllide to monovinyl protochlorophyllide in green(ing) barley, a dark monovinyl/light divinyl plant species, *Plant Physiol.* **87**:89–94.

Troxler, R. F. (1972). Synthesis of bile pigments in plants. Formation of carbon monoxide and phycocyanobilin in wild-type and mutant strains of the alga, *Cyanidium caldarium*, *Biochemistry* **11**:4235–4242.

Troxler, R. F., and Bogorad, L. (1966). Studies of the formation of phycocyanin, porphyrins, and a blue phycobilin by wild-type and mutant strains of *Cyanidium caldarium*, *Plant Physiol.* 41:491–499.

Troxler, R. F., and Brown, A. (1970). Biosynthesis of phycocyanin in vivo, *Biochim. Biophys. Acta* 215:503–511.

Troxler, R. F., Brown, A. S., and Brown, S. B. (1979). Bile pigment synthesis in plants. Mechanism of ^{18}O incorporation into phycocyanobilin in the unicellular Rhodophyte, *Cyanidium caldarium*, *J. Biol. Chem.* 254:3411–3418.

Troxler, R. F., and Lester, R. (1967). Biosynthesis of phycocyanobilin, *Biochemistry* 6:3840–3846.

van Bochove, A. C., Griffiths, W. T., and van Grondelle, R. (1984). The primary reaction in the photoreduction of protochlorophyllide monitored by nanosecond fluorescence measurements, *Photochem. Photobiol.* 39:101–106.

van Heyningen, S., and Shemin, D. (1971). Quaternary structure of δ-aminolevulinate dehydratase from *Rhodopseudomonas spheroides*, *Biochemistry* 10:4676–4682.

Viale, A. A., Wider, E. A., and Batlle, A. M. del C. (1987). Porphyrin biosynthesis in *Rhodopseudomonas palustris*. XI. Extraction and characterization of δ-aminolevulinate synthetase, *Comp. Biochem. Physiol.* 87B:607–613.

Virgin, H. I. (1981). The physical state of protochlorophyll(ide) in plants, *Annu. Rev. Plant Physiol.* 32:451–463.

Vlcek, L. M., and Gassman, M. L. (1979). Reversal of α,α'-dipyridyl-induced porphyrin synthesis in etiolated and greening red kidney bean leaves, *Plant Physiol.* 64:393–397.

Vogelmann, T. C., and Scheibe, J. (1978). Action spectra for chromatic adaptation in the blue-green alga *Fremyella diplosiphon*, *Planta* 143:233–239.

Walker, C. J., and Griffiths, W. T. (1986). Light independent proteolysis of protochlorophyllide reductase, *Regulation of Chloroplast Differentiation* (G. Akoyunoglou and H. Senger, Eds.), Alan R. Liss, New York, pp. 99–104.

Walker, C. J., and Griffiths, W. T. (1988). Protochlorophyllide reductase: a flavoprotein?, *FEBS Lett.* 239:259–262.

Walker, C. J., Mansfield, K. E., Rezzano, I. N., Hanamoto, C. H., Smith, K. M., and Castelfranco, P. A. (1988). The magnesium-protoporphyrin IX (oxidative) cyclase system. Studies on the mechanism and specificity of the reaction sequence, *Biochem. J.* 255:685–692.

Walker, C. J., Mansfield, K. E., Smith, K. M., and Castelfranco, P. A. (1989). Incorporation of atmospheric oxygen into the carbonyl functionality of the protochlorophyllide isocyclic ring, *Biochem. J.* 257:599–602.

Wallsgrove, R. M., Lea, P. J., and Miflin, B. J. (1983). Intracellular localization of aspartate kinase and the enzymes of threonine and methionine biosynthesis in green leaves, *Plant Physiol.* 71:780–784.

Walter, E., Schreiber, J., Zass, E., and Eschenmoser, A. (1979). Bakteriochlorophyll a_{Gg} und Bakteriophäophytin a_P in den ptotosynthetischen Reaktionszentren von *Rhodospirillum rubrum* G-9$^+$, *Helv. Chim. Acta* 62:899–920.

Wang, W.-Y., Boynton, J. E., and Gillham, N. W. (1977). Genetic control of chlorophyll biosynthesis: Effect of increased δ-aminolevulinic acid synthesis on the phenotype of the *y*-1 mutant of *Chlamydomonas*, *Mol. Gen. Genet.* 152:7–12.

Wang, W.-Y., Gough, S. P., and Kannangara, C. G. (1981). Biosynthesis of δ-aminolevulinate in greening barley leaves. IV. Isolation of three soluble enzymes required for the conversion of glutamate to δ-aminolevulinate, *Carlsberg Res. Comm.* 46:243–257.

Wang, W.-Y., Huang, D.-D., Stachon, D., Gough, S. P., and Kannangara, C. G. (1984). Purification, characterization, and fractionation of the δ-aminolevulinic acid synthesizing enzymes from light-grown *Chlamydomonas reinhardtii* cells, *Plant Physiol.* 74:569–575.

Warnick, G. R., and Burnham, B. F. (1971). Regulation of porphyrin biosynthesis: Purification and characterization of δ-aminolevulinic acid synthase, *J. Biol. Chem.* 246:6880–6885.

Warren, M. J., and Jordan, P. M. (1988). Further evidence for the involvement of a dipyrromethene cofactor at the active site of porphobilinogen deaminase, *Biochem. Soc. Trans.* 16:963–965.

Watanabe, T., Kobayashi, M., Nakazato, M., Ikegami, I., and Hiyama, T. (1987). Chlorophyll a' in photosynthetic apparatus: Reinvestigation, *Progress in Photosynthesis Research* (J. Biggins, Ed.), Martinus Nijhoff, Boston, Vol. I, pp. 303–306.

Watanabe, T., Nakazato, M., Mazaki, H., Hongu, A., Konno, M., Saitoh, S., and Honda, K. (1985). Chlorophyll a epimer and pheophytin a in green leaves, *Biochim. Biophys. Acta* **807:**110–117.

Weinstein, J. D. (1979). Ph.D. Dissertation, University of California, Davis, 123 pp.

Weinstein, J. D., and Beale, S. I. (1983). Separate physiological roles and subcellular compartments for two tetrapyrrole biosynthetic pathways in *Euglena gracilis, J. Biol. Chem.* **258:**6799–6807.

Weinstein, J. D., and Beale, S. I. (1984). Biosynthesis of protoheme and heme a precursors solely from glutamate in the unicellular red alga, *Cyanidium caldarium, Plant Physiol.* **74:**146–151.

Weinstein, J. D., and Beale, S. I. (1985a). Enzymatic conversion of glutamate to δ-aminolevulinate in soluble extracts of the unicellular green alga, *Chlorella vulgaris, Arch. Biochem. Biophys.* **237:**454–464.

Weinstein, J. D., and Beale, S. I. (1985b). RNA is required for enzymatic conversion of glutamate to δ-aminolevulinic acid by extracts of *Chlorella vulgaris, Arch. Biochem. Biophys.* **239:**87–93.

Weinstein, J. D., and Castelfranco, P. A. (1977). Protoporphyrin IX biosynthesis from glutamate in isolated greening chloroplasts, *Arch. Biochem. Biophys.* **178:**671–673.

Weinstein, J. D., and Castelfranco, P. A. (1978). Mg-protoporphyrin-IX and δ-aminolevulinic acid synthesis from glutamate in isolated greening chloroplasts. δ-Aminolevulinic acid synthesis, *Arch. Biochem. Biophys.* **186:**376–382.

Weinstein, J. D., Mayer, S. M., and Beale, S. I. (1986a). RNA is required for enzymatic conversion of glutamate to δ-aminolevulinic acid by algal extracts, *Regulation of Chloroplast Differentiation* (G. Akoyunoglou and H. Senger, Eds.), Alan R. Liss, New York, pp. 43–48.

Weinstein, J. D., Mayer, S. M., and Beale, S. I. (1986b). Stimulation of δ-aminolevulinic acid formation in algal extracts by heterologous RNA, *Plant Rhysiol.* **82:**1096–1101.

Weinstein, J. D., Mayer, S. M., and Beale, S. I. (1987). Formation of δ-aminolevulinic acid from glutamic acid in algal extracts. Separation into an RNA and three required enzyme components by serial affinity chromatography. *Plant Physiol.* **84:**244–250.

Weller, J.-P., and Gossauer, A. (1980). Synthesen von Gallenfarbstoffen. X. Synthese und Photoisomerisierung des *racem.* Phytochromobilin-dimethylesters, *Chem. Ber.* **113:**1603–1611.

Werck-Reichhart, D., Jones, O. T. G., and Durst, F. (1988). Haem synthesis during cytochrome P-450 induction in higher plants. 5-Aminolaevulinic acid synthesis through a five-carbon pathway in *Helianthus tuberosus* tuber tissues aged in the dark, *Biochem. J.* **249:**473–480.

Wider de Xifra, E. A., Batlle, A. M. del C., and Tigier, H. (1971). δ-Aminolaevulinate synthestase in extracts of cultured soybean cells, *Biochim. Biophys. Acta* **235:**511–517.

Wider de Xifra, E. A., Sandy, J. D., Davies, R. C., and Neuberger, A. (1976). Control of 5-aminolaevulinate synthetase activity in *Rhodopseudomonas spheroides, Philos. Trans. Roy. Soc. Lond. Ser. B* **273:**79–98.

Wider de Xifra, E. A., Stella, A. M., and Batlle, A. M. del C. (1978). Porphyrin biosynthesis—immobilized enzymes and ligands. IX. Studies on δ-aminolaevulinate synthetase from cultured soybean cells, *Plant Sci. Lett.* **11:**93–98.

Wilhelm, C. (1987). Purification and identification of chlorophyll c_1 from the green alga *Mantoniella squamata, Biochim. Biophys. Acta* **892:**23–29.

Williams, D. C., Morgan, G. S., McDonald, E., and Battersby, A. R. (1981). Purification of porphobilinogen deaminase from *Euglena gracilis* and studies of its kinetics, *Biochem. J.* **193:**301–310.

Witkowski, D. A., and Halling, B. P. (1988). Accumulation of photodynamic tetrapyrroles induced by acifluoren-methyl, *Plant Physiol.* **87:**632–637.

Wong, K. K. (1978). 4-Vinyl protochlorophyllide excretion by *Rhodopseudomonas gelatinosa* in nicotinamide-enriched medium, *Plant Sci. Lett.* **13:**269–273.

Wong, Y.-S., and Castelfranco, P. A. (1984). Resolution and reconstitution of the Mg-proto-porphyrin IX monomethyl ester (oxidative) cyclase, the enzyme system responsible for the formation of the chlorophyll isocyclic ring, *Plant Physiol.* **75**:658–661.

Wong, Y.-S., and Castelfranco, P. A. (1985). Properties of the Mg-protoporphyrin IX monomethyl ester (oxidative) cyclase system, *Plant Physiol.* **79**:730–733.

Wong, Y.-S., Castelfranco, P. A., Goff, D. A., and Smith, K. M. (1985). Intermediates in the formation of the chlorophyll isocyclic ring, *Plant Physiol.* **79**:725–729.

Wu, S.-M., and Rebeiz, C. A. (1985). Chlorophyll biogenesis. Molecular structure of chlorophyll b (E489F666), *J. Biol. Chem.* **260**:3632–3634.

Yen, H.-C., and Marrs, B. L. (1976). Maps of genes for carotenoid and bacteriochlorophyll biosynthesis in *Rhodopseudomonas capsulata*, *J. Bacteriol.* **126**:619–629.

Youvan, D. C., Hearst, J. E., and Marrs, B. L. (1983). Isolation and characterization of enhanced fluorescence mutants of *Rhodopseudomonas capsulata*, *J. Bacteriol.* **154**:748–755.

Yu, M.-H., Glazer, A. N., Spencer, K. G., and West, J. A. (1981). Phycoerythrins of the red alga *Callithamnion*. Variation in phycoerythrobilin and phycourobilin content, *Plant Physiol.* **68**:482–488.

Yubisui, T., and Yoneyama, Y. (1972). δ-Aminolevulinic acid synthetase of *Rhodopseu-domonas spheroides*: Purification and properties of the enzyme, *Arch. Biochem. Bio-phys.* **150**:77–85.

Zaman, Z., Jordan, P. M., and Akhtar, M. (1973). Mechanism and stereochemistry of the 5-aminolaevulinate synthetase reaction, *Biochem. J.* **135**:257–263.

Zumft, W. G. (1972). Ferredoxin : nitrite oxidoreductase from *Chlorella*. Purification and properties, *Biochim. Biophys. Acta* **276**:363–375.

Iron Metabolism in Relation to Heme Synthesis

Prem Ponka

Herbert M. Schulman

Timothy M. Cox

I. Introduction

Iron is indispensable for life, being essential for such processes as oxygen transfer, electron transfer, nitrogen fixation, and DNA synthesis (Wrigglesworth and Baum, 1980). Iron functions either in the form of nonheme-iron-containing proteins, which will not be discussed here, or when inserted into protoporphyrin as the prosthetic group of various hemoproteins. In solution, iron exists in two oxidation states, ferrous [Fe(II)] and ferric [Fe(III)], which, respectively, can donate or accept electrons relatively easily. These redox actions, which are so important for the biochemical functions of iron, may, however, become hazardous for the organism. At physiological pH and oxygen tension Fe(II) is readily oxidized to Fe(III), which is prone to hydrolysis forming essentially insoluble ferric hydroxide and oxohydroxide polymers (Aisen, 1977). In addition, unless appropriately chelated, iron, due to its catalytic action in one-electron redox reactions, plays a key role in the formation of harmful oxygen radicals which ultimately cause peroxidative damage to vital cell structures. Because of this virtual insolubility and potential toxicity, specialized mechanisms and molecules for the acquisition, transport, and storage of iron in a soluble nontoxic form have evolved to meet cellular and organismal iron requirements. Thus, these physiological iron-complexing agents leave body fluids and cells with extremely low concentrations of "free" iron.

Unicellular organisms produce low molecular weight iron-chelating compounds, siderophores, that facilitate iron uptake (Neilands, 1981). In vertebrates, iron is transported within the body between sites of absorption, storage, and utilization by the plasma glycoprotein transferrin, which binds iron very tightly but reversibly. Transferrin is recognized by specific cell membrane receptors which are crucial for cellular iron acquisition. Following its intracellular release from transferrin-receptor complexes, iron enters functional compartments or is stored in ferritin. These three proteins involved in iron transport and storage, that is, transferrin, transferrin receptors, and ferritin will be discussed later in this chapter. Iron, the most important essential trace element, represents 55 and 45 mg per kilogram of body weight in adult men and women, respectively. Normally, about 60 to 70% of total body iron is present in hemoglobin in circulating erythrocytes. Myoglobin, cytochromes, and other iron-containing enzymes comprise a further 10% and the remaining 20 to 30% is stored in ferritin. Although iron bound to transferrin is less than 0.1% ($\sim$ 3 mg) of the total body iron, dynamically it is the most important iron pool with the highest rate of turnover.

The turnover of plasma (or transferrin) iron is on the order of 30 mg/24 h. Normally about 80% of this iron is transported to the bone marrow in humans and also to the spleen in rodents for hemoglobin synthesis in developing erythroid cells. From these sites reticulocytes are released into the circulation where, within about 24 h, they lose transferrin receptors, mitochondria, ribosomes, and all the other components of hemoglobin synthesis and develop into mature erythrocytes which circulate in the blood for about 120 days (in humans). Senescent erythrocytes are phagocytized by the cells of the reticuloendothelial system where the heme moiety is split from hemoglobin and catabolized. The liberated iron is released back to plasma transferrin at a rate which normally matches the rate of iron transport for erythropoiesis. Although the ingoing branch of this well-maintained dynamic equilibrium of transferrin iron is reasonably well understood, the mechanisms and controls involved in the release of iron from reticuloendothelial cells have not been defined.

The remaining approximately 5 mg of the daily plasma iron turnover is exchanged with nonerythroid tissues, namely the liver. About 1 mg of dietary iron is absorbed per 24 h, and the total organismal iron balance is maintained by a daily loss of approximately 1 mg via nonspecific mechanisms (mostly cell desquamations). In summary, there are two important features in organismal iron metabolism. First, iron turnover is virtually an internal event in the body, and, second, most of the iron turning over is used for the synthesis of heme in erythroid cells.

There are two additional important aspects of erythroid cell iron metabolism which should be mentioned before discussing detailed intracellular iron pathways. First, as indicated by both in vivo and in vitro studies, transferrin is the only physiological source of iron for erythroid cell heme synthesis. Normally, all plasma iron is associated with transferrin and ferrokinetic studies provided clear evidence that all iron utilized for hemoglobin synthesis passes through plasma (Pollycove and Mortimer, 1961; Hosain and Finch, 1964; Najean et al., 1967). An absolute requirement for transferrin by erythroid precursors is demonstrated by the observations that both humans (Heilmayer, 1966; Goya et al., 1972) and mice (Bernstein, 1987) with hereditary atransferrinemia have severe hypochromic and microcytic anemias which can be explained only by the requirement of transferrin for hemoglobin synthesis. Furthermore, in vitro studies, mostly with reticulocytes, show that the only physiological chelator which can provide iron for hemoglobin synthesis is transferrin. Second, in general, the iron content of normal nonerythroid cells is infinitesimal compared to the amount of heme iron in mature erythrocytes (about 12×10^8 Fe atoms per cell). In our experience, reticulocytes take up about 10 pmol $Fe/10^6$ cells/h from transferrin corresponding to 6×10^6 atoms Fe/cell/h which gives 200 h (or 8.3 days) for iron to accumulate in the total erythrocyte hemoglobin. This interval is slightly longer than the average erythroid cell maturation time (about 6 to 7 days) but, since iron uptake by reticulocytes is probably lower than in bone marrow erythroblasts, the agreement is remarkably close. The fact that all hemoglobin iron is transported from transferrin and that this delivery system operates so efficiently, leaving mature erythrocytes with negligible amounts of nonheme iron, suggests to us that the iron transport machinery in erythroid cells is an integral part of the heme biosynthesis pathway.

There are no data available about the proportion of freshly delivered transferrin iron, as compared to intracellular iron, used for heme synthesis in nonerythroid cells. However, there is one important distinction between erythroid and nonerythroid cells. While hemoglobin does not turn over within erythrocytes, but only in the reticuloendothelial system after destruction of senescent cells, generally nonhemoglobin hemoproteins turn over relatively rapidly in nonerythroid cells without cell destruction. Although there are no experimental data available, it is reasonable to assume that, within a single nonerythroid cell, hemeoxygenase-liberated iron, as well as intracellular stored iron, may be the major sources for de novo heme synthesis. If this proves to be the case, then the involvement of transferrin iron in nonerythroid cell heme synthesis is much less stringent than in those which synthesize hemoglobin. It, thus, appears that in nonerythroid cells iron may be relatively readily available to meet the low requirements of the metal for heme synthesis. On the other hand, erythroid cells, in order to obtain and utilize iron, must be equipped with a complex and efficient machinery for recognizing, binding, and processing transferrin, for liberating iron from its tight bond with the carrier, and for transporting the metal to protoporphyrin within the mitochondria.

A. Model systems for studies of iron metabolism and heme synthesis

1. Hemoglobin synthesizing cells

a. Reticulocytes are immature red blood cells formed in the bone marrow when orthochromatic erythroblasts eject their nuclei. Therefore, they do not contain DNA but still contain mitochondria, ribosomes, and remnants of Golgi bodies. Ehrlich was probably the first investigator to describe them in 1881 but only the advent of isotopes, together with pivotal experiments of several groups in the late 1940s and 1950s, made them an indispensable tool for studying hemoglobin synthesis. Using ^{15}N-glycine, Shemin and Rittenberg (1946) were the first to demonstrate heme synthesis in reticulocytes and the uptake of transferrin-bound iron by reticulocytes was first reported by Walsh et al. (1949). In 1959 Jandl and co-workers showed that treatment of reticulocytes with trypsin abolished iron uptake from transferrin and inferred the existence of membrane receptors for transferrin. The advantage of reticulocytes, which have been widely used ever since, is that they are the only system of pure erythroid cells available and they are easily obtained from the peripheral blood of anemic individuals. However, since they are enucleated, they can only be used to investigate the posttranscriptional aspects of heme synthesis and iron transport. Nevertheless, reticulocytes, where over 90% of the iron taken up from transferrin is used for heme synthesis (Martinez-Medellin and Schulman, 1972; Ponka et al. 1982b), are extremely valuable for investigating mechanisms and controls operating in fully induced hemoglobin-synthesizing cells.

b. Friend murine erythroleukemia (MEL) cells are virus-transformed erythroid cells blocked in a relatively early stage of differentiation which are derived from mice infected with the Friend virus complex (Friend, 1957). Friend and her co-workers (1966) successfully established a number of cell lines from the spleens of infected mice, which when grown in culture display a low level of erythroid differentiation ($\leq 1\%$), the extent of which can be enormously enhanced by dimethylsulfoxide

(Friend et al., 1971) or numerous other chemical inducers (Marks and Rifkind, 1978). MEL differentiation is characterized by (1) an increase in the enzymes of the heme biosynthetic pathway (Ebert and Ikawa, 1974; Sassa, 1976; Grandchamp et al., 1985; Fadigan and Dailey, 1987), (2) an increase in transferrin receptor expression and iron uptake (Hu et al., 1977; Glass et al., 1978; Yeoh and Morgan, 1979; Wilczynska and Schulman, 1980; Wilczynska et al., 1984; Laskey et al., 1986), and (3) an increase in globin mRNA (Ross et al., 1972), all of which lead to the accumulation of large amounts of hemoglobin. This differentiation process, which is accompanied by the onset of terminal cell division (i.e., the loss of capacity for proliferation), in many ways parallels that of normal erythroid development and, therefore, provides a model system to investigate transcription aspects of iron transport and heme synthesis during terminal erythroid differentiation.

More recently, Koury et al. (1984) developed a procedure to procure a large number of developmentally synchronized, relatively pure erythroid cells from the spleens of mice infected with the anemia strain of Friend virus. Unlike the previously described cell lines, these are responsive to the physiological regulator of erythropoiesis, erythropoietin, which induces the synthesis of hemoglobin, red cell specific membrane proteins (Koury et al., 1984, 1987), and transferrin receptors (Sawyer and Krantz, 1986).

However, there is a serious limitation in the use of MEL as a model of normal erythroid differentiation. There is an abundance of recent literature suggesting that, in nonerythroid cells, transferrin receptors are correlated with cell proliferation (Larrick and Creswell, 1979; Sutherland et al., 1981; Trowbridge and Omary, 1981) and that cultured transformed cells (Neckers, 1984) as well as malignant cells in vivo (Faulk et al., 1980; Aulbert et al., 1980) have high numbers of transferrin receptors. Moreover, malignant cells have also been shown to contain higher than average levels of ferritin (Drysdale et al., 1977) which probably results from an increase in transferrin-receptor-mediated iron uptake. Therefore, the basal level of iron transport and the amount of iron stored in uninduced Friend cells, which are virus-transformed cells, may be considerably higher than what would be found in the normal physiological equivalent, the pronormoblast.

2. Nonerythroid cells

a. Hepatocytes.   About 10 to 20% of plasma iron turnover in humans is directed to the liver (Pollycove and Mortimer, 1961). The uptake of transferrin-bound iron by perfused liver or liver slices has been demonstrated by Gardiner and Morgan (1974). However, the demonstration of transferrin interaction with hepatocytes required preparations which, unlike total liver tissue, were free of Kupffer cells and sinusoidal endothelial cells. Some investigators used transformed cell lines derived from either rat (Beamish et al., 1975) or human (White and Jacobs, 1978; Dautry-Varsat et al., 1983) hepatocytes but, as explained above, the use of cell lines has severe limitations.

In other studies hepatocytes isolated from mature (Grohlich et al., 1977, 1979; Young and Aisen, 1980, 1981) or fetal (Trinder et al., 1986) rat or mouse (Cole and Glass, 1983) were used to examine various aspects of iron or transferrin uptake.

b. Established cell lines.   Recently, there have been numerous studies dealing with transferrin receptors and/or the transferrin cycle in established cell lines such as mouse teratocarcinoma cells (Karin and Mintz, 1981), B- or T-lymphoblastoid cell lines (Schulman et al., 1981), HeLa cells (Ward et al., 1982a), HL-60 cells (Trepel et al., 1987), and K562 cells (Schulman et al., 1981; Frazier et al, 1982; Klausner et al., 1983). The bulk of the iron taken up by these cells is incorporated into ferritin and only up to 10% of the iron is recovered in heme (Schulman et al., 1981). This is the case also with K562 cells, which are sometimes referred to as a human equivalent of Friend cells. Although K562 cells are inducible for hemoglobin synthesis by hemin and some other inducers, they are ill-defined cells originating from a patient with chronic myeloid leukemia (Lozzio and Lozzio, 1975). Moreover, hemoglobin produced upon heme addition is entirely of embryonic or fetal types (Rutherford et al., 1979) and δ-aminolevulinic acid dehydratase induced in K562 cells following butyric acid treatment is immunologically distinct from the enzyme of normal adult or fetal erythrocytes (Chang and Sassa, 1985). Thus, K562 cells would seem to be inappropriate as a model of normal erythroid differentiation with regard to the regulation of heme synthesis.

None of the studies with hepatocyte or established cell lines was aimed at investigating the intracellular iron pathways for heme synthesis. Such studies are needed to characterize iron pathways for heme synthesis in nonerythroid cells and to enable comparison with the relatively well-characterized pathway in erythroid cells.

II. Proteins of Iron Transport and Storage

A. Transferrin

Plasma transferrin belongs to a family of related iron binding proteins which include the lactoferrins, found both intracellularly and in fluids such as milk, tears, and semen, and ovotransferrin which is present in avian egg white. Together these proteins, which have molecular weights around 80,000 and a high degree of sequence homology (Metz-Boutique et al., 1984), are referred to as the transferrins. Their discovery is generally credited to Schade and Caroline (1944) who observed that raw egg white inhibited bacterial growth but that the bacteriostatic activity could be reversed by iron. The active component in egg white was shown to be ovotransferrin (previously termed conalbumin) by Alderton et al. (1946). Schade and Caroline (1946) were the first to prepare transferrin from human plasma and demonstrate that it too had bacteriostatic activity. Although it became evident that plasma transferrin (hereafter referred to as transferrin) acts as a carrier of iron for erythroid heme synthesis both in vivo [e.g., Pollycove and Mortimer (1961)] and in vitro (Jandl et al., 1959), the significance of transferrin and lactoferrin as antibacterial agents is still being investigated (Bullen and Griffiths, 1987). Transferrin is an essential ingredient for culturing mammalian cells in serum-free media (Bernes and Sato, 1980) and it functions in this context solely as a transporter of iron into the cells (Landschultz et al., 1984; Brock and Stevenson, 1987; Tsao et al., 1987; Laskey et al., 1988).

The transferrins are monomeric glycoproteins consisting of two homologous domains each of which contains one high-affinity Fe(III) binding site. Concomitant binding of a suitable anion is obligatory for Fe(III) binding with the physiologically relevant anion being bicarbonate. When iron and anion are bound to transferrin a typical salmon-pink color develops with an absorption maximum at 460 nm. Three protons are released per iron atom and bound anion, causing the protein to be more acidic than in its iron-free state.

The two-domain structure of the transferrins was first indicated by fragmentation of the proteins by limited proteolysis, which yielded half-molecules containing single iron binding sites [reviewed by Bezkorovainy (1980, 1987)]. Recently, the bilobal structure has been established by the elucidation of the three-dimensional conformation of human lactoferrin at a 3.2-Å resolution (Anderson et al., 1987). It is now clear that the N- and C-terminal halves of the protein form separate globular lobes having one iron binding site each. At each site the iron atom is coordinated by four protein ligands (two tyrosines, one histidine, and one asparagine) and the bound anion (Anderson et al., 1987; Schlabach and Bates, 1975).

Although it has long been believed that the two iron binding sites of transferrins are equivalent and independent, this is not the case. Electron spin resonance [e.g., Keung et al. (1982) and Zak et al. (1983)] and absorption spectroscopy studies (Yamamura et al., 1984) comparing the iron binding sites of the N- and C-terminal domians provide convincing evidence that the two iron binding sites are not identical. Furthermore, the two sites exhibit differences with respect to the effect of pH on the stability of iron binding (Princiotto and Zapolski, 1975) and in their affinity for iron at a constant pH (Aisen et al., 1978). Iron binding to the site in the N-terminal domain is both more acid labile and of a lower affinity than the binding to the site in the C-terminal domain (association constants of 6.8×10^{19} and 4×10^{20}, respectively, for human transferrin at pH 7.4).

Since transferrin in serum is only about 30% saturated with iron, it would be predicted from the thermodynamics and kinetics of iron binding (Aisen et al., 1978) that all four species of transferrin would be present, that is, iron-free apotransferrin, fully saturated diferric transferrin, and the two monoferric transferrins containing iron in either the N-terminal or C-terminal domain binding sites [reviewed by Baldwin and Egan (1987)]. The four forms of transferrin can be separated and quantitated by gel electrophoresis in the presence of 6 M urea (Makey and Seal, 1976). Using this technique, Leibman and Aisen (1979) and Williams and Moreton (1980) found all four species of transferrin in normal human serum in the following order of abundance: apotransferrin > monoferric transferrin with iron occupying the N-terminal site > diferric transferrin > monoferric transferrin with iron occupying the C-terminal site. The predominance of iron in the weaker binding N-terminal site is puzzling; however, dialysis of normal human serum elicits a redistribution of iron to the C-terminal site, suggesting that a low molecular weight serum substance causes the preferential binding of iron to the N-terminal site (Williams and Moreton, 1980). There is no evidence which would suggest a functional significance for the differences in the two iron binding sites of transferrin or for the distribution of iron between the sites in normal human serum. Reticulocytes [e.g., Huebers et al. (1981)] and hepatocytes (Young, 1982) in vitro remove iron equally well from either of the transferrin iron binding sites.

The two-sited nature of the transferrins and early evidence of internal amino acid sequence homology led Greene and Feeney (1968) to propose that present-day vertebrate transferrins evolved by duplication of an ancestral gene. Apparent support of this concept was reported by Martin et al. (1984) who isolated and partially characterized an iron binding protein from urochordate plasma having some properties in common with vertebrate transferrin but possessing only one iron binding site and a molecular weight of around 40,000.

B. Transferrin receptors

1. Characterization of transferrin receptors. Based on their experiments showing that trypsin virtually abolished reticulocyte uptake of iron from transferrin, Jandl and co-workers (1959) were the first to suggest the existence of specific receptors for transferrin on the reticulocyte membrane. In the late 1970s several laboratories reported the successful isolation of transferrin receptors from reticulocyte membranes (Hu and Aisen, 1978; Witt and Woodworth, 1978; Ecarot-Charrier et al., 1980) and subsequently from placenta (Enns and Sussman, 1981) and from cultured cell lines [e.g., Sutherland et al. (1981) and Trowbridge and Omary (1981)].

The transferrin receptor is a disulfide-linked transmembrane glycoprotein with a molecular weight of about 180,000, each receptor binding one or two molecules of transferrin (Hu and Aisen, 1978; Schneider et al., 1982). Each subunit contains at least three N-asparagine-linked oligosaccharides probably composed of two high-mannose chains and one complex-type oligosaccharide (Omary and Trowbridge, 1981a, b; Schneider et al., 1982). The transferrin receptor is also modified posttranslationally by the addition of fatty acid residues as shown by labeling experiments with [^{3}H]palmitate (Omary and Trowbridge, 1981a, b). The major part of the transferrin receptor is a 70,000-dalton fragment facing the extracellular environment which can be proteolytically cleaved from cells by trypsin while retaining its transferrin binding ability. That portion of the receptor which is exposed on the cytoplasmic face of the plasma membrane has an estimated molecular weight of 5000 and a phosphorylated serine residue (Schneider et al., 1982). Hemin stimulates the phosphorylation of reticulocyte transferrin receptors (Cox et al., 1985a) but the functional significance of this is unknown.

The reported association constants of transferrin for the receptor vary greatly (10^{-7} to $10^{-9} M$), probably depending on conditions of measurement and cells used. The iron status of transferrin has an important effect on the affinity of transferrin for its receptor; diferric transferrin having the greatest affinity, monoferric transferrins intermediate affinities and apotransferrin very low (Young et al., 1984). Normal plasma transferrin concentration is about $5 \times 10^{-5} M$ of which diferric transferrin is approximately 10% or around $5 \times 10^{-6} M$. Since the association constant of diferric transferrin is 30- and 500-fold higher than those of monoferric and apotransferrin, respectively (Young et al., 1984), the delivery of iron to cells is predominantly by diferric transferrin. The concentration of diferric transferrin in normal plasma is adequate for saturating all cellular transferrin receptors with the ligand. The structural features of transferrin which are required for the interaction of transferrin with the receptor have not yet been established.

2. Transferrin receptor gene.   Recently cDNA and genomic clones of the human (Schneider et al., 1983, 1984; McClelland et al., 1984; Kühn et al., 1984) and mouse (Stearne et al., 1985) transferrin receptors have been isolated and sequenced.

Ruddle and co-workers identified a group of uncharacterized proteins that bind to the promoter region of the transferrin receptor gene (Miskimins et al., 1985). More recently, they sequenced the 5' region of the human transferrin gene containing the promoter which is highly GC rich and shares regions of homology with other mitogen responsive genes (Miskimins et al., 1986). It seems clear that these sequences in the 5' flanking region as well as in the 3' noncoding region (Casey et al., 1988; Müllner and Kühn, 1988) of the transferrin receptor gene may play an important role in the control of transferrin receptor expression.

3. Distribution and regulation of transferrin receptors.   With the exception of mature erythrocytes, transferrin receptors are probably expressed on all cells but their levels vary greatly. Cells and tissues with the highest densities of transferrin receptors include hemoglobin-synthesizing cells, placental tissue, and rapidly dividing cells. High expression of transferrin receptors on erythroid cells is not surprising since these cells have the greatest requirement for iron because the iron in hemoglobin can account for as much as 70% of the total iron content of a normal adult.

One of the systems about which the most is known with respect to the functional interaction between cells and transferrin is developing erythroid cells. One striking feature of erythroid transferrin receptor regulation should be emphasized. While receptor numbers are positively correlated with proliferation in nonerythroid cells, in the case of erythroid cells their numbers increase during differentiation and, therefore, are negatively correlated with proliferation, but related to an increased iron demand for hemoglobin synthesis.

The early erythroid precursor cell has only a few transferrin receptors, while the precursor cell committed to erythroid differentiation clearly contains identifiable transferrin receptors (Sieff et al., 1982; Lesley et al., 1984). Following erythropoietin-induced differentiation (Iacopetta et al., 1982; Sawyer and Krantz, 1986), there is a gradual increase in receptor expression with a maximum of about 800,000 transferrin receptors per cell on the intermediate normoblast, followed by a slight decrease with further maturation. There are still very high numbers of receptors on orthochromatic normoblasts and reticulocytes (100,000 to 500,000 per cell, probably depending on their maturity), none of which is capable of cell division. During the maturation of reticulocytes to erythrocytes, the cells lose all activities of the components of the hemoglobin-synthesizing system (Schulman, 1968; Rapoport et al., 1974), including transferrin receptors (Jandl et al., 1959). Transferrin receptors may be released from reticulocytes by "shedding" (Pan et al., 1983) but it is not known whether this is the only mechanism involved in their disappearance. Recent evidence obtained by two of us (HMS and PP) indicates that the decline in transferrin-receptor-mediated iron uptake during maturation results in decreasing rates of heme and, secondarily, globin synthesis which can be partially reversed by utilizable, but nontransferrin, forms of iron. Thus, the disappearance of transferrin receptors and the loss in the capacity to take up iron from transferrin may be the primary event in the cessation of hemoglobin synthesis.

Myocytes (Fava et al., 1981) and spermatocytes (Holmes et al., 1983) are both also rich in transferrin receptors. This may reflect their high rates of heme synthesis required for their large content of myoglobin and cytochromes, respectively.

Although the detailed mechanisms leading to the increased expression of transferrin receptors on hemoglobin-synthesizing or proliferating cells are unknown, some factors modulating their expression have been defined. Ward and his colleagues were the first to demonstrate that if HeLa cells (1982a) or fibroblasts (1982b) are incubated with iron salts, the numbers of transferrin receptors decrease. The mechanism responsible for turning down transferrin receptor numbers does not appear to monitor intracellular ferritin iron levels (Ward et al., 1982b), but probably iron levels in an ill-defined "transit iron pool." Conversely, sequestration of iron from this pool by iron-chelating agents such as desferrioxamine or picolinic acid leads to an increase in transferrin receptor numbers on K562 cells (Mattia et al., 1984; Testa et al., 1985). Further studies with K562 cells suggested that intracellular levels of iron influence the transcription of the transferrin receptor gene (Rao et al., 1985). However, Owen and Kühn (1987), using mouse L cells transfected with human transferrin receptor cDNA, showed that iron-dependent regulation could not be attributed to effects on initiation of transcription. They demonstrated that a large deletion in the 3' nontranslated region of the cDNA abolished the response to changes in iron concentration. More recently, Müllner and Kühn (1988) showed that this 3' region is sufficient for conferring iron-dependent regulation to an mRNA transcribed from a human gene totally unrelated to the transferrin receptor.

No data are available to indicate whether iron has a similar effect in modulating transferrin receptor expression in hemoglobin-synthesizing cells. Such a mechanism might not be expected to operate in erythroid cells since they maintain high levels of transferrin receptors in spite of their high rates of iron uptake. However, since the iron taken up by erythroid cells is rapidly used for heme synthesis, it is possible that it is never present in a form which is recognized by the element(s) controlling transferrin receptor levels.

Nevertheless, the idea that there is an erythroid-specific regulatory mechanism for the transferrin receptor which is distinct from that operating in non-erythroid cells is intriguing and has recently been supported experimentally. Chan et al. (1989) showed that the murine erythroleukemia cells induced into erythroid differentiation did not respond to either DNA synthesis inhibitors (e.g. hydroxyurea) or iron chelating agents which both stimulate transferrin receptor expression in proliferating non-erythroid cells. The lack of responsiveness to these stimuli suggests that there is a distinct regulatory mechanism for transferrin receptor expression in hemoglobin synthesizing cells. Alternatively, erythroid cells may express a unique transferrin receptor isoform (Cotner et al., 1989) subjected to different control mechanism.

In addition to iron, hemin also causes a decrease in transferrin receptor numbers (Pelicci et al., 1982). Furthermore, decreasing intracellular heme by inhibiting δ-aminolevulinic acid dehydratase with succinylacetone heads to an increase in transferrin receptor numbers (Ward et al., 1984). A similar decrease in transferrin receptor number caused by hemin was also described in hemoglobin-synthesizing Friend erythroleukemia cells (Wilczynska et al., 1984) and this may represent a transcriptional component of a feedback control of iron uptake and, consequently, erythroid cell heme synthesis. The effect of hemin per se was questioned and it was suggested that the iron released from heme intracellularly is responsible for the effect (Rouault et al., 1985). However, no data regarding the quantities and rates of iron liberated from exogenous hemin are available. Moreover, in K562 cells, which were mostly used in these studies, hemin significantly inhibits heme oxygenase (Hoffman et al., 1980; Trakshel et al., 1987), the enzyme responsible for liberating iron from heme. It is conceivable that iron and heme operate independently and the elimination of heme-induced decline in receptor numbers by desferrioxamine may mean that deprivation of iron represents a much stronger signal than the presence of heme in terms of transferrin receptor regulation. It should be emphasized that the heme-induced decrease in transferrin receptor synthesis is distinct from another effect of heme which occurs specifically in hemoglobin-synthesizing cells where heme feedback inhibits the uptake of iron from transferrin (see pg. 418).

Somewhat paradoxically, heme was shown to be essential for maintaining a normal rate of transferrin receptor synthesis in reticulocytes. Cox et al. (1985b) demonstrated that inhibition of heme synthesis by succinylacetone depresses receptor synthesis which can be restored by the addition of heme. It is conceivable that heme has opposite effects on the transcription and translation of the transferrin receptor mRNA.

It is generally believed that those factors which modulate transferrin receptor expression ultimately control iron entry into cells. As will be discussed in more detail later, this is probably true in hemoglobin-synthesizing cells where heme controls both receptor synthesis and the efficiency of iron extraction from transferrin. However, such a regulatory role of heme in nonerythroid cells is less obvious, and although the modulatory role of iron in nonerythroid transferrin receptor synthesis is well documented, this mechanism clearly fails to prevent excessive iron uptakes by cells in iron overloaded individuals.

C. Ferritin

Ferritin, first isolated and crystallized by Laufberger (1934, 1937) is a ubiquitous protein whose only clearly defined function is the sequestration and storage of iron. It has been detected in almost all animal and plant tissues and also in fungi and bacteria (Theil, 1987). Mammalian ferritin consists of a protein shell having a molecular weight of around 450,000 and composed of 24 subunits. Ferritin shells can contain up to approximately 4500 Fe atoms per molecule (Harrison et al., 1980). Thus, the molecule consists of a paracrystalline iron core surrounded by a protein shell which confers solubility on the complex and also protects against potential Fe(III) mediated oxidative damage to cell constituents. The biochemical mechanisms involved in the loading and unloading of iron in cellular ferritin have not been defined, although some progress has been made in accomplishing this in vitro. Assembled ferritin molecules contain six channels with a fourfold axis of symmetry that passes through the shell. These channels probably function to enable iron, and other molecules involved in its storage and mobilization, to enter or leave the shell's interior. In vitro evidence indicates that relatively soluble ferrous iron, which is incorporated into the shell much more efficiently than ferric iron, is oxidized and deposited following its association with the inner surface of the subunits. Reduced flavins or various other reducing agents (cysteine, glutathione, or ascorbic acid) facilitate iron release from ferritin in vitro which may further be stimulated by chelating agents (Harrison et al., 1980). However, there are no data indicating that these mechanisms operate in intact cells.

There are two major sources of ferritin heterogeneity; polydispersity caused by differing amounts of iron within the protein shells, and charge heterogeneity caused by differences in the subunit composition of the protein shells. Normally, most mammalian ferritin is composed of two different kinds of subunits—H subunits with a molecular weight of 21,000 which are more acidic than L subunits that have a molecular weight of 19,000. Different proportions of H and L subunits in the protein shell, all composed of 24 subunits, give rise to populations of "isoferritins" such that H-rich ferritins have a pI of 4.8 to 5.2 and L-rich ferritins have a pI of 5.3 to 5.8 (Arosio et al., 1978). The genes for human (Santoro et al., 1986; Costanzo et al., 1986) and rat (Leibold and Munro, 1987; Murray et al., 1987) H and L subunits have been cloned and sequenced.

Ferritin synthesis is inducible by iron by a mechanism in which iron recruits ferritin mRNA from an inactive pool (Zahringer et al., 1976; Aziz and Munro, 1986). Recently, sequences in the 5' untranslated region of apoferritin mRNA have been identified which may be involved in this iron-regulated translational control mechanism (Leibold and Munro, 1988). There also is some evidence for transcriptional regulation by iron of ferritin gene expression (Cairo et al., 1985; White and Munro, 1988).

III. Mechanism of Iron Supply for Heme Synthesis

Our understanding of the mechanism of cellular iron uptake and intracellular iron pathways is incomplete but is most advanced in hemoglobin-synthesizing cells. Although this is undoubtedly due to efforts in numerous laboratories, the pivotal work of some investigators, whose experiments have represented significant contributions to the field, should be emphasized. Walsh et al. (1949) first showed that reticulocytes can take up iron from plasma and incorporate it into hemoglobin in vitro. Paoletti et al. (1958) showed that reticulocytes remove iron from transferrin without catabolizing the protein. This finding, which indicated that transferrin was not consumed during iron delivery, was further elaborated by Katz (1961) who found that in vivo iron is cleared from plasma at approximately 10 times the rate of transferrin. The affinity of transferrin for iron is so high that a spontaneous dissociation of iron cannot occur at a significant rate (Aisen and Leibman, 1968), thus, cells must possess special mechanisms for releasing iron from transferrin. The observation of Jandl and co-workers (1959) that following trypsin treatment reticulocytes lost the ability to take up iron from transferrin, first suggested the existence of a membrane transferrin receptor. Somewhat later Morgan and his colleagues obtained the first evidence for the internalization of transferrin by cells, probably via endocytic vesicles, and suggested that this may be a prerequisite for iron uptake from transferrin (Morgan and Appleton, 1969; Appleton et al., 1971). Later Schulman and co-workers demonstrated that (apo)transferrin-receptor complexes remained stable at pH 5.0 (Ecarot-Charrier et al., 1977, 1980), and Morgan (1981) found that methylamine and ammonium chloride, which inhibited intravesicular acidification, decreased the release of iron from transferrin within reticulocytes. This clearly suggested that acidification may be involved in intracellular iron acquisition from transferrin, thus giving a physiological relevance to the old observation that at acid pH iron is readily released from transferrin (Surgenor et al., 1949). When the concept of transferrin endocytosis was still highly controversial, support for internalization and movement to an acidic intracellular compartment came from studies with cell lines that did not synthesize hemoglobin (van Resnowoude et al., 1982; Dautry-Varsat et al., 1983). The central role of mitochondria in iron movement to heme in reticulocytes was recognized by Borova et al. (1973) who demonstrated that upon inhibition of protoporphyrin synthesis, mitochondria become overloaded with nonheme iron which can, however, still be used for heme synthesis.

A. Iron transferrin cycle

In the last several years a generally accepted scheme of how cells acquire iron from transferrin has emerged: (1) Transferrin attaches to specific receptors on the cell surface by a physicochemical interaction, not requiring temperature and energy. (2) By a temperature- and energy-dependent process the transferrin-receptor complexes are internalized by the cells enclosed within endocytic vesicles. (3) Iron and carbonate are concomitantly released from the transferrin within the endocytic vesicles by a temperature- and energy-dependent process which probably involves intravesicular acidification (pH ~ 5.5). Lysosomes are not involved in this process. (4) Iron is transported to intracellular sites of utilization and/or storage. (5) The iron-free apotransferrin attached to the receptor, returns to the cell surface where at pH 7.4, the apotransferrin is released from the cell functionally intact and the receptor is reutilized for another cycle of iron acquisition.

1. Erythroid cells. In hemoglobin-synthesizing cells, which physiologically have the greatest requirement for iron, the acquisition of iron from transferrin is controlled and tightly coordinated to the synthesis of hemoglobin. As discussed elsewhere, there is evidence that the removal of iron from transferrin limits the overall rate of heme synthesis in the erythroid cells of some species.

The initial hypothesis that transferrin iron was released at the erythroid cell membrane (Jandl et al., 1959) was challenged by Morgan and Appleton in 1969. These authors employed electron microscopic autoradiography of reticulocytes which had been incubated with ^{125}I-transferrin and demonstrated that transferrin enters reticulocytes during incubation at 37°C but does not do so when the cells are incubated at 4°C. Later, ferritin (Appleton et al., 1971; Sullivan et al., 1976; Hemmaplardh and Morgan, 1977), horseradish peroxidase (Hemmaplardh and Morgan, 1977), and colloidal gold (Light and Morgan, 1982) were used to label transferrin for electron microscope investigations of the cellular localization of the protein. All of these experiments showed that the localization of tagged transferrin is largely confined to intracellular vesicles and suggested that the entry of transferrin into the cells occurs via endocytosis. Internalization of transferrin was confirmed by fractionation of lysed reticulocytes following their incubation with radioiodinated transferrin (Martinez-Medellin and Schulman, 1972; Borova et al., 1973) and more importantly by experiments which employed lactoperoxidase catalyzed radioiodination. Martinez-Medellin et al. (1977) demonstrated that transferrin which was taken up by reticulocytes at 37°C was largely protected from subsequent labeling at 4°C by ^{125}I under the action of lactoperoxidase, while transferrin taken up by the cells at 4°C was labeled with ^{125}I. More recent investigations have shown that a large proportion of transferrin receptors are protected from the action of proteolytic enzymes (Schulman et al., 1983) and suggested that receptors are internalized with the transferrin during endocytosis.

Evidence that transferrin endocytosis is a prerequisite for iron uptake came from experiments with inhibitors of microtubule function. Several of these agents (colchicine, vinblastine, vincristine, and deuterium oxide) were shown to block not only transferrin but also iron uptake by reticulocytes and bone marrow cells (Hemmaplardh et al., 1974; Hemmaplardh and Morgan, 1977).

Internalized transferrin can be distinguished from surface-bound transferrin by its resistance to digestion with pronase and this allows the quantification of transferrin endocytosis. Endocytosis of Fe(III) transferrin occurs at the same rate as exocytosis of apotransferrin and the rate constant of the process, which is 0.45 min^{-1} at 37°C, decreases with lower temperatures. The maximum rate of transferrin endocytosis (at 37°C) by reticulocytes is approximately 500 molecules/cell/s and the recycling time for the transferrin-receptor complex is about 3 min (Iacopetta and Morgan, 1983). Immature erythroid cells remove iron from transferrin with very high efficiency so that transferrin released from them contains only very little iron (Morgan et al., 1966; Hradilek and Neuwirt, 1987). The efficiency of iron extraction from transferrin is decreased, and the whole transferrin cycle is slowed down, when the level of an intracellular controlling "heme pool" in reticulocytes is increased (Ponka et al., 1988). The efficiency of iron removal from transferrin is also much lower in, and the release of transferrin is slower from, uninduced as compared to induced Friend cells (Hradilek and Neuwirt, 1987).

The molecular mechanisms underlying the transferrin cycle are poorly understood. There is controversy as to whether (Klausner et al., 1983) or not (Watts, 1985) triggering of transferrin receptors into the cycle occurs only in the presence of transferrin. In the experience of two of us (HMS and PP) ^{125}I-transferrin-labeled reticulocytes release only about 60% of labeled ligand if the cells are incubated in the absence of transferrin, while upon addition of transferrin virtually all cell-associated ^{125}I-transferrin is released from the cells. This would seem to indicate that transferrin is essential for the cycling of transferrin receptors.

As mentioned previously, the transferrin receptor is a phosphoprotein and, therefore, phosphorylation or dephosphorylation may be considered as a potential signal for transferrin receptor internalization. However,

Kühn and his co-workers recently excluded a role for receptor phosphorylation in transferrin receptor endocytosis. In their experiments mutation of serine-24 completely abolished transferrin receptor phosphorylation but the mutated receptor was internalized with the same efficiency as the wild-type transferrin receptor (Rothenberger et al., 1987).

Except for endosome acidification, our knowledge of the intracellular metabolism of iron and transferrin is rather obscure. A recent report on the isolation from reticulocytes of coated vesicles bearing the transferrin–transferrin-receptor complex (Choe et al., 1987) may provide an important tool for elucidating the mechanism and carrier(s) involved in the release of iron from transferrin. The purified vesicles had the expected appearance on electron microscopic examination and contained transferrin, transferrin receptors, clathrin (180,000 daltons), and "coated vesicle assembly factor proteins" (100,000 daltons) as determined by SDS-PAGE and Western blot analyses. In addition, the vesicles had a Mg^{2+}-dependent ATPase and some evidence was provided that this ATPase could acidify the interior of the vesicle. Another group succeeded in isolation of endosomes from K562 cells preincubated with ^{59}Fe-^{125}I-transferrin (Bakkeren et al., 1987) and demonstrated that the endosomes were capable of internal acidification upon ATP addition. ATP itself was not sufficient to induce ^{59}Fe release from endosomes which, however, did occur upon the addition of the lipophilic iron chelator pyridoxal isonicotinoyl hydrazone (PIH). This indicates that acidification itself is insufficient for iron release from endosomes. More importantly, the spontaneous release of iron from transferrin at pH 5.5 (i.e., pH within endosomes) requires many minutes to hours (Theil and Aisen, 1987), while transferrin-bound iron appears in reticulocyte heme within 30 seconds (Ponka et al., 1988). These observations clearly suggest the necessity for an iron acceptor that would facilitate iron release from transferrin and probably also serve to transport iron through endosomal membranes.

In spite of the convincing evidence for transferrin internalization, there are some reports that internalization is not essential for erythroid cell iron acquisition. However, none of these reports, which generally conclude that iron is released from transferrin at the plasma membrane, can withstand critical analysis. Some investigators reported that membrane preparations from reticulocytes, preincubated with double-labeled transferrin, contained relatively more ^{59}Fe than ^{125}I-transferrin (Fielding and Speyer, 1974; Glass et al., 1980). However, the presence of mitochondria, which would always contain some ^{59}Fe, can easily explain these observations since it is extremely difficult to obtain mitochondria-free membranes from rabbit reticulocytes (Ponka et al., 1977). The finding that reticulocytes can take up some iron from transferrin bound to a solid matrix (Glass et al., 1977; Loh et al., 1977; Zaman et al., 1980) is also insufficient since the rate of iron exchange was extremely low (3 to 10% of the rate from free transferrin) and could have been mediated by reticulocyte-associated transferrin.

a. Iron uptake and utilization from ferric acyl hydrazones. Although transferrin is the only physiological source of iron for hemoglobin synthesis, iron complexed to a recently described new group of acyl hydrazones (Ponka et al., 1979) can be taken up by erythroid cells and used for heme synthesis by a process not requiring transferrin or transferrin receptors. The most efficient of these chelates are ferric complexes of pyridoxal isonicotinoyl hydrazone (PIH, Ponka et al., 1982a), pyridoxal benzoyl hydrazone (PBH, Ponka et al., 1985a), and salicylaldehyde isonicotinoyl hydrazone (SIH, Ponka et al., 1985b; Laskey et al., 1986). These chelators and their iron complexes are highly lipophilic and probably cross the erythroid cell membrane by diffusion. It is not known whether the iron complexed to acyl hydrazones is exchanged to a physiological intracellular carrier or, following reduction, is a direct substrate for ferrochelatase.

2. Hepatocytes. Iron metabolism in liver parenchymal cells is a highly versatile process and pathways of iron transport through the hepatocyte membrane are more complex and diverse than in any other cell in the body. Hepatocytes have mechanisms for iron uptake via several unrelated routes from different iron-bearing compounds and also for iron release to plasma transferrin. Hepatocytes take up iron from nonheme iron sources (i.e., transferrin, ferritin, and some low molecular weight iron compounds) as well as from heme (heme-hemopexin and hemoglobin-haptoglobin complexes (see Chap. 9)). Under physiological conditions the bulk of hepatocyte iron is derived from transferrin.

a. Uptake of transferrin-bound iron. Hepatocytes possess saturable high-affinity transferrin binding sites (Young and Aisen, 1980; Cole and Glass, 1983; Morley and Bezkorovainy, 1983; Thorstensen and Romslo, 1984a; Trinder et al., 1986) which probably mediate the uptake of transferrin-bound iron. In addition, hepatocytes take up transferrin by a nonsaturable low-affinity process which also leads to net iron accumulation. There is some controversy as to whether albumin does (Thorstensen and Romslo, 1984b) or does not (Cole and Glass, 1983; Trinder et al., 1986) eliminate the uptake of transferrin and iron by the low-affinity process. More recent study by Trinder et al. (1988) showed that at high transferrin concentration, when the nonsaturable uptake process predominates, albumin reduces transferrin uptake. However, the intracellular accumulation of iron was not significantly affected indicating the unimportance of the low-affinity process in hepatocyte iron acquisition.

It has been estimated that each hepatocyte has 37,000 to 60,000 transferrin receptors (Young and Aisen, 1980; Cole and Glass, 1983) and it is believed that the transferrin-to-cell cycle in iron uptake by hepatocytes is identical or very similar to the one described above for erythroid cells. Experiments with hepatoma cells showed that the pH dependence of apotransferrin and iron transferrin binding to transferrin receptors in these cells is virtually identical to that in erythroid cells (van Renswoude et al., 1982; Dautry-Varsat et al., 1983) but no such study has so far been performed using fresh hepatocyte suspensions. It is reasonable to suppose that the receptor-dependent acquisition of iron by hepatocytes and erythroid cells is similar but at transferrin concentrations above those needed to saturate the transferrin receptors (0.1 to 0.5 μM), hepatocytes take up iron from transferrin predominantly by a plasma membrane reduction process (Thorstensen and Romslo, 1988). These authors demonstrated that hepatocyte iron uptake does not require endocytosis or endosomal acidification of transferrin when transferrin is added at 1 μM concentration. However, contrary to reticulocytes, the uptake of iron from transferrin by isolated rat hepatocytes varies in parallel with plasma membrane NADH : ferricyanide oxidoreductase activity and is inhibited by ferricyanide (Thorstensen and Romslo, 1988). The quantitative importance of reductive-vs. receptor-mediated iron uptake by hepatocytes in vivo remains to be established. Further experimentation is also needed to elucidate the cellular destination of iron provided by transferrin, either via endocytosis or reductive release. Although it has been determined that within 15 min of incubation with ^{59}Fe-transferrin, 60 to 70% of cell-associated iron is found in cytosolic ferritin and the rest in mitochondria (Thorstensen and Romslo, 1987), the cellular pathways involved are unknown.

b. Uptake of ferritin. Although ferritin is the iron storage protein localized predominantly in tissues, small amounts of ferritin of unknown origin are present in blood plasma. The iron content of plasma ferritin is very low, even in iron overloaded patients with very high plasma ferritin levels (Worwood et al., 1976) and, thus, plasma ferritin is an unlikely source of transport iron. Therefore, the physiological significance of a specific membrane receptor for ferritin (Mack et al., 1983) is not obvious in relation to plasma ferritin. However, studies of Aisen and his co-workers may suggest a physiological role for hepatocyte ferritin receptors. Kondo et al. (1988) showed that, following phagocytosis of ^{59}Fe-labeled erythrocytes, Kupffer cells release iron, about half of which is in iron-rich ferritin. The released ferritin is rapidly taken up when reincubated with isolated hepatocytes which may accumulate iron efficiently via this pathway (> 60,000 Fe atoms/cell/min). The ingested ferritin is rapidly degraded, probably within lysosomes, and the released iron is stored in newly synthesized hepatocyte ferritin (Sibille et al., 1988). The possibility that the ferritin is "leaking" from Kupffer cells damaged by erythrophagocytosis cannot be ruled out and if such a ferritin-mediated transfer of iron from Kupffer cells to hepatocytes occurs in vivo, the generally accepted views on organismal iron transport as described in the Introduction will need to be revised. Moreover, this mechanism might account for the difference in sensitivity of bone marrow and liver to iron lack. To the best of our knowledge, the synthesis of heme in hepatocytes, as contrasted to bone marrow, is never deficient in animals lacking iron. For example, it is well known that cytochrome P450 levels are not affected by iron deficiency (Catz et al., 1970; Bailey-Wood et al., 1975).

   c. Iron uptake from low molecular weight complexes. Plasma transferrin is normally 30% saturated with iron but it may become fully saturated in individuals with iron overload. These include patients with idiopathic hemochromatosis or thalassemia. Iron added to the plasma of such patients cannot be bound to transferrin and becomes nonspecifically associated with albumin and complexed with low molecular weight chelators such as citrate, ascorbate, certain amino acids, carbohydrates, and so forth (Hershko et al., 1978; Brissot et al., 1985; Wright et al., 1986). Similar iron-carrying nontransferrin substances must exist in vivo in humans (Heilmayer, 1966; Goya et al., 1972) and in mice (Bernstein, 1987) with hereditary hypo- or atransferrinemia. Affected individuals have a hypochromic microcytic anemia together with parenchymal iron overload with massive iron deposition in the liver and pancreas. This demonstrates the existence of an uptake system for nontransferrin-bound iron in hepatocytes and also in other parenchymal cells. Further evidence for the existence of such a system comes from reports showing a more rapid clearance of iron from plasma when the iron binding capacity of transferrin is exceeded (Laurell, 1947; Wheby and Jones, 1963; Craven et al., 1987).

   The transport of nontransferrin-bound iron into liver seems to be carrier-mediated, as demonstrated by saturation, competitive inhibition by other transition metal ions, and temperature dependence. Moreover, the uptake of iron is strongly calcium-dependent and is relatively insensitive to inhibitors of cellular energy metabolism (Wright et al., 1986). The recent findings of Wright and her co-workers (1988) are consistent with an electrogenic transport mechanism for uptake of nontransferrin-bound iron that is driven by the transmembrane potential difference. The intracellular destiny of iron taken up by this transport mechanism and whether or not it is available for heme synthesis are not known.

   d. Uptake of hemoglobin-haptoglobin and heme-hemopexin complexes. These uptake systems are described in considerable detail in Chap. 9 and here are touched on only briefly to complete the total picture of iron uptake mechanisms. Normally, only a small proportion of erythrocytes break down intravascularly but in some hemolytic diseases, such as sickle cell anemia, intravascular hemolysis increases, resulting in increased free hemoglobin in the circulation. Here hemoglobin binds to haptoglobin but when this protein's binding capacity is exceeded, hemoglobin is oxidized to methemoglobin, the heme moiety of which is then transferred to hemopexin. The uptake of both hemoglobin-haptoglobin and heme-hemopexin complexes involves binding to specific receptors, followed by endocytosis with release of heme to the microsomal heme oxygenase degradation site. By the action of heme oxygenase iron is released from heme and the iron most probably enters an intracellular pool common to that derived from transferrin.

B. Intracellular iron pathways for heme synthesis

While the overall cellular transferrin cycle is understood in considerable detail, identification of the ligands which may be involved in the intracellular transport of iron after its release from transferrin has been elusive. There are no definitive physiological descriptions of iron-containing intermediates between transferrin-bound iron and intracellular iron-containing components such as heme, ferritin, and nonheme iron proteins. However, an intermediate pool of possibly low molecular weight iron ligands has been inferred from observations that newly incorporated iron in cells and tissues can be readily chelated (Jacobs, 1977).

Although there have been suggestions that ferritin iron is an intermediate for heme synthesis in erythroid cells (Mazur and Carleton, 1963; Speyer and Fielding, 1979), there is convincing evidence that the iron incorporated into ferritin in reticulocytes has the kinetic properties of an end product rather than an intermediate and cannot be used for heme synthesis (Ponka et al., 1982b). Some studies show indirectly that ferritin iron may be involved in heme synthesis in liver. Isolated rat liver mitochondria contain specific ferritin binding sites (Ulvik, 1982) and can mobilize iron from ferritin and incorporate it into heme (Ulvik and Romslo, 1978, 1979), but evidence that this happens in intact cells is lacking. It would be important to perform similar experiments with mitochondria from erythroid cells; however, to the best of our knowledge, these have not yet been done.

The existence of an intramitochondrial iron-containing intermediate in the heme pathway in erythroid cells is suggested by the accumulation of iron in erythroblast mitochondria of patients with sideroblastic anemia (May et al., 1982) which is caused by impaired heme synthesis (Bottomley, 1982; Kushner and Cartwright, 1977). Furthermore, when heme synthesis is inhibited in reticulocytes in vitro, iron which can subsequently be utilized for heme synthesis accumulates in mitochondria (Borova et al., 1973; Ponka et al., 1982b; Adams et al., 1989).

Endogenous mitochondrial iron has also been implicated as an inter-mediate in heme synthesis in liver mitochondria. Camadro et al. (1984) found that protoporphyrin stimulated heme synthesis by isolated human liver mitochondria without the addition of iron. About 40% of the iron in rat liver mitochondria is not associated with cytochromes or iron-sulfur proteins (Tangeras et al., 1980) and some of this "non-heme non-FeS iron" is available for heme synthesis by mitochondria in vitro (Tangeras, 1985). That the size of this iron pool is tightly regulated is suggested by the finding that it is not increased in liver mitochondria of mice with porphyria induced by griseofulvin; a condition in which ferrochelatase activity is inhibited by almost 90% and mitochondrial protoporphyrin accumulates (Tangeras, 1986). However, this is in contrast to mitochon-drial iron accumulation when erythroid cell heme synthesis is inhibited as discussed above. This, together with the clinical observations that only erythroid but not other mitochondria become iron overloaded, (Ghadially, 1988) indicates that hemoglobin-synthesizing cells possess a unique mitochondrial iron uptake system.

There are reports that isolated rat liver mitochondria can take up iron directly from transferrin (Konopka, 1978) and incorporate some of it into heme in the presence of a suitable porphyrin substrate (Nilsen and Romslo, 1985). However, it would be difficult to reconcile a mechanism involving the direct interaction of transferrin and mitochondria with the release of iron from transferrin within acidified endosomes.

Many candidates for a low molecular weight transporter of iron from endosomes to intracellular sites of utilization and storage have been suggested because of the ability of so many physiological compounds such as sugars, amino acids, and nucleotides to chelate iron. However, recently, attention has been focused on pyrophosphate as the active low molecular weight intracellular iron ligand. Egyed (1975) was the first to report that pyrophosphate could directly remove iron from transferrin, possibly by first substituting for transferrin-bound bicarbonate, followed by formation of ferric pyrophosphate. It has also been demonstrated that pyrophosphate can mediate the transfer of iron from transferrin to ferritin (Konopka et al., 1981) and stimulate the utilization of transferrin iron for heme synthesis by isolated mitochondria (Konopka, 1978; Konopka and Romslo, 1981; Nilsen and Romslo, 1984, 1985). Neverthe-less, a physiological role for pyrophosphate in intracellular iron metabolism remains to be demonstrated.

From the results of pulse-chase experiments with ^{59}Fe-labeled trans-ferrin guinea pig reticulocytes are reported to contain a low molecular weight iron ligand with the kinetic properties of an intermediate in heme synthesis (Pollack and Campana, 1980). This low molecular weight ligand is distinguishable from pyrophosphate by thin-layer chromatogra-phy (Pollack et al., 1985) but it has not yet been fully characterized and there are no reports of its existence in reticulocytes from other species or in other types of cells.

When iron reaches the outer mitochondrial membrane, it is trapped by ill-defined iron binding ligands and transferred across the inner membrane to ferrochelatase (see Chap. 3). Ferrochelatase, which inserts Fe(II) into protoporphyrin IX, spans the inner mitochondrial bilayer, its active site facing the mitochondrial matrix (Harbin and Dailey, 1985). Since only the reduced form of iron can be processed by ferrochelatase (Porra and Jones, 1963), reduction of iron must occur at some point following its release from transferrin. Recent kinetic data obtained with solubilized mitochondrial membrane-bound and vesicle-reconstituted enzymes provided evidence for substrate channeling between protoporphyrinogen oxidase, which oxidizes protoporphyrinogen IX to protoporphyrin IX, and ferrochelatase (Ferreira et al., 1988). The occurrence of such an enzyme complex on the mitochondrial membrane suggests that the oxidation of protoporphyrinogen might be coupled to the reduction of iron (Dailey, personal communication), but there is no direct evidence for this attractive hypothesis. Equally hypothetical remains the recent suggestion of Taketani et al. (1986) that ferrochelatase (heart) is associated with complex I of the mitochondrial electron transport system. Although they demonstrated that ferrous iron can be produced by NADH oxidation in complex I and subsequently utilized by ferrochelatase for heme synthesis, the physiological relevance of these observations remains to be established.

Since the transport of iron across biological membranes usually involves a ferric-ferrous transition (Flatmark and Romslo, 1975), the reduction may occur before iron enters mitochondria which are the obvious source of reducing equivalents. However, it is also possible that iron is reduced within endosomes. Evidence for this comes from experiments showing that in reticulocytes specific Fe(II) chelators (bipyridine and phenanthroline type) chelate iron immediately after its release from transferrin, while it is still within endosomes (Morgan, 1983). There is recent evidence that Fe(II) is transported through endosomal membrane into reticulocyte cytosol. Egyed (1988) and Morgan (1988) demonstrated that reticulocytes can transport Fe(II) into cytosol by a carrier-mediated process which is saturable, competitively inhibited by several divalent metals, and which is absent in erythrocytes. This suggests that the same carrier may be utilized by iron after its release from transferrin.

It has been suggested that the uptake of iron (plus protoporphyrin IX) is coupled to the efflux of heme (Romslo, 1983), but such a mechanism can hardly operate in erythroid cells where inhibited heme synthesis leads to iron accumulation within mitochondria (Borova et al., 1983; Ponka et al., 1982b; Adams et al., 1989). On the other hand, Romslo's (1983) hypothesis that the mitochondrial uptake of iron is linked to an antiport for heme may be valid in nonerythroid tissues such as liver, where the mitochondrial iron pool remains constant when ferrochelatase is inhibited (Tangeras, 1986).

IV. Coordination of Heme and Globin Synthesis in Erythroid Cells

Using rabbit reticulocytes, Kruh and Borsook (1956) were the first to show that heme and globin synthesis occurs at parallel and similar rates, an observation which led to the idea that mechanisms must exist for coordinating the synthesis of the protein with that of its prosthetic group. Deprivation of iron leads to a decline in globin synthesis and disaggregation of polysomes in intact cultured reticulocytes and these effects can be reversed by the addition of iron or hemin to the cultures (Bruns and London, 1965; Grayzel et al., 1966; Waxman and Rabinovitz, 1966; Schulman, 1968; Waxman et al., 1977). Thus, the synthesis of hemoglobin components appeared to be coordinated by changes in the intracellular concentration of "free" heme and more direct evidence for this was obtained from experiments with both reticulocytes (Neuwirt et al., 1972; Schulman et al., 1974) and nucleated erythroid cells (Glass et al., 1975).

The development of cell-free protein-synthesizing systems from reticulocytes (Lamfrom and Knopf, 1964; Zucker and Schulman, 1968) which could synthesize globin at rates comparable to those of intact reticulocytes (Zucker and Schulman, 1968; Adamson et al., 1968) and which do not contain mitochondria and, thus, are unable to synthesize heme led to a detailed analysis of the effects of heme on globin synthesis. It was established that heme is required for the initiation of globin mRNA translation but has no effect on polypeptide chain elongation (Zucker and Schulman, 1968). Subsequent investigations showed that in the absence of added heme an inhibitor of chain initiation accumulates in reticulocyte lysates (Maxwell et al., 1971; Legon et al., 1973) and in intact cells deprived of iron (Schulman, 1975).

The mechanism of this translational control by heme has been intensively investigated during the last decade and was recently reviewed by London et al. (1987). The processes involved can be summarized as follows. The inhibitor described in the early experiments is a cyclic AMP-independent protein kinase which in the absence of heme is activated and specifically phosphorylates the α subunit of initiation factor eIF-2. In the initiation of protein synthesis eIF-2 is required for the formation of the complex of eIF-2, GTP, and met-tRNA which binds to the 40-S ribosomal subunit. Inhibition of chain initiation results from the interactions between phosphorylated eIF-2 and another protein which is involved in the recycling of eIF-2. This protein, termed reversing factor, acts by catalyzing the dissociation of GDP from eIF-2, thus rendering it available for binding GTP and entering a new cycle of initiation. The strong association between phosphorylated eIF-2 and reversing factor causes a depletion of reversing factor, resulting in a block in the recycling of eIF-2.

As discussed elsewhere in this chapter, there is compelling evidence showing that the rate-limiting step in heme synthesis in rabbit reticulocytes and differentiating murine Friend erythroleukemia cells is the acquisition of iron from transferrin. Therefore, it seems reasonable to suggest that, in these systems, the overall rate of hemoglobin synthesis is controlled by this process.

V. Control of Heme Biosynthesis in Erythroid Cells: Role of Iron Transport

A. Experimental studies of feedback control

Several groups demonstrated in vitro that incorporation of labeled precursors into heme by erythroid cells may be influenced by experimental changes in intracellular free-heme concentrations (Ponka and Neuwirt, 1969; Neuwirt et al., 1969; Ibrahim et al., 1978). However, the physiological relevance of this phenomenon, as well as the exact mechanism and point of control, have been disputed. The first indirect studies in intact and lysed cells, where hemin inhibited labeled glycine incorporation into heme and had little apparent effect on the incorporation of $4[^{14}C]$-δ-aminolevulinate (ALA), suggested that primary control operated to regulate formation of δ-ALA (Karibian and London, 1965; Ibrahim et al., 1978). These experiments suggested that as in the bacterium *Rhodobacter spheroides* (Burnham and Lascelles, 1963), generation of this first-committed precursor of heme by ALA synthase was subject to direct regulation by a negative allosteric effect. However, these findings have been criticized on the grounds that the concentrations of essential nutrients, especially transferrin iron and the isotopically labeled glycine, were insufficient to allow optimal rates of heme synthesis (Ponka and Schulman, 1985a; Neuwirt and Ponka, 1972) and to make conclusions on heme synthesis regulation. Under conditions of limited iron availability, normal regulatory processes would be disturbed and residual feedback control at the level of ALA formation might become apparent. Further evidence against allosteric inhibition of the enzymatic formation of ALA was provided by studies of the effects of hemin on ALA synthesis in rabbit reticulocytes and on pure enzyme isolated from these cells; the weak inhibitory effects obtained were not comparable to those expected from the observed inhibitory effects of hemin in the intact cell.

1. Effects of heme on iron metabolism.   An attractive solution to these interpretative difficulties has been provided by a series of experiments in which reticulocyte iron metabolism has been examined. Studies by Ponka and his associates have shown that assimilation of transferrin iron by reticulocytes from experimental animals is reduced by heme, whether added exogenously as hemin or increased in these cells by inhibiting globin synthesis (Ponka and Neuwirt, 1969, 1971). This phenomenon has been demonstrated in cells obtained from the mouse (Malik et al., 1979), rat (Ponka and Schulman, 1986), and rabbit (Ponka and Neuwirt, 1969, 1971; Schulman et al., 1974; Ponka and Schulman, 1985b). The experimental demonstration that endogenous or exogenous heme specifically inhibits this rate-limiting step for de novo formation of heme in rabbit reticulocytes indicates that the main pathways of hemoglobin synthesis are coordinated by control of the delivery of iron from transferrin (Ponka and Schulman, 1985a, b, 1986).

Several lines of evidence support this conclusion:

1. Removal of iron from the medium inhibits utilization of glycine for heme synthesis.

2. Addition of ferric acyl-hydrazone chelates, which can donate iron for incorporation into cellular heme independently of the transferrin pathway (Ponka et al., 1982a), stimulate heme synthesis from glycine well above the level seen with saturating concentrations of transferrin (Ponka and Schulman, 1985b, 1986; Laskey et al., 1986) and partially overcome the inhibition of heme formation induced by hemin. Iron incorporation into heme using these chelates as donors is not subject to inhibition by hemin (Ponka and Schulman, 1985a).

3. The rate of heme synthesis from ^{59}Fe-transferrin is not increased by addition of ALA or protoporphyrin and these precursors do not abrogate the inhibitory effects of hemin (Ponka and Schulman, 1985a, b).

4. Hemin inhibits heme synthesis from labeled glycine but no reduction of incorporation of this label into extracted cellular porphyrin was demonstrated (Ponka and Schulman, 1985a). Thus, heme did not appear to affect steps in the synthesis of protoporphyrin between glycine and protoporphyrin.

2. Heme and the transferrin cycle.   Iacopetta and Morgan (1984) studied the effects of modulating the concentration of intracellular heme on internalization of transferrin labeled with ^{125}I and ^{59}Fe. They found a linear relationship between the rate of iron delivery and the initial rate of internalization of the iron-transferrin complex. This relationship pertained in reticulocytes treated with inhibitors of protein synthesis, inhibitors of heme synthesis and exogenous hemin in the concentration range 10 to 50 μM. Other studies, using dual-labeled transferrin-iron complex, also suggested that the effect of heme was to inhibit the initial influx of the transferrin-receptor complex in rabbit reticulocytes (Cox et al., 1985b). More recently, an examination of the effects of hemin indicated that low concentrations of hemin (< 20 μM) inhibit the delivery of iron from transferrin during its intracellular cycle after internalization of the membrane receptor-transferrin complex (Ponka et al., 1988). No effect on the rate of endocytosis was detected at this concentration. It was, therefore, inferred that monoferric transferrin molecules were released into the medium and flux of transferrin through the cycle was reduced by hemin. At higher hemin concentrations (50 μM) the initial rate of transferrin internalization was reduced, but it was suggested that this is probably secondary to heme's primary interaction with a step subsequent to the endocytosis of transferrin-receptor complexes. It is noteworthy that studies using a variety of cell lines have demonstrated that the effects of hemin on iron incorporation were specific for developing erythroid cells (Schulman et al., 1981), indicating restriction of the regulatory effect to cells in which most of the internalized iron is destined for heme synthesis.

3. Control of heme biosynthesis in human erythroid cells. Recently, short-term experiments have been conducted to investigate whether feedback control of heme biosynthesis occurs in human reticulocytes and bone marrow tissue and, if so, how it is regulated (Gardner and Cox, 1988). Incubation of human erythroid cells with ^{59}Fe-labeled transferrin consistently showed that the utilization for heme synthesis of the iron taken up was less than 50% compared with about 80 to 90% in rabbit reticulocytes. Furthermore, unlike rabbit reticulocytes, incubation in the absence of iron had little effect on the rate of incorporation of 2[^{14}C]glycine into heme. Incubation of human erythroid cells with cycloheximide to increase endogenous "free" heme reduced incorporation of labeled glycine and transferrin iron, but not ALA, into cell heme. Incorporation of glycine and iron was sensitive to inhibition by exogenous hematin (K_i 30 and 46 μM). Ferric salicylaldehyde isonicotinoyl hydrazone, which reproducibly stimulates heme synthesis from labeled glycine in rabbit reticulocytes, failed to enhance heme synthesis or modify feedback inhibition in human reticulocytes. In contrast, preincubation of human erythroid cells with unlabeled ALA, protoporphyrin IX, and, to a lesser extent, glycine, stimulated utilization of cellular ^{59}Fe for heme synthesis. These experiments indicate that formation of ALA limits the rate of heme synthesis in the human erythron in contrast with studies carried out under similar conditions with rodent and rabbit erythroid cells. It is not yet clear whether the effects of experimentally increased intracellular heme on formation of ALA reflect bona fide mechanisms which regulate heme synthesis physiologically in humans.

4. Feedback control and the economy of the reticulocyte. The reticulocyte is unique in that it synthesizes heme and proteins but in the absence of a nucleus cannot transcribe RNA: It, thus, lends itself to experimental studies of translational control and direct regulation of heme formation by feedback inhibition. Observations indicate that the complex pathway of heme formation in erythroid cells, like other biosynthetic processes, may be controlled by negative feedback or end-product inhibition. However, with the possible exception of ferrochelatase (Dailey and Fleming, 1983), no defined enzymatic step in this biosynthetic pathway has been shown to be subject to allosteric inhibition. It appears that the cellular uptake and delivery of nutrients (glycine or transferrin iron) to the preheme pool may be specifically regulated. Control of these initial processes required for heme synthesis would preserve the metabolic economy of the cell and would avoid wasteful accumulation of intermediates.

**B. Differentiation in erythroid cell:
comparative aspects**

There is no unifying concept of the signals which mediate proliferation and differentiation in nucleated erythroid progenitor cells. Synthesis of hemoglobin occurs only after multiple nuclear divisions of progenitor cells and morphological evidence of erythroid differentiation precedes formation of heme in the normoblasts. Increased transferrin receptor expression is associated with maximal hemoglobin synthesis (Iacopetta et al., 1982).

The ultimate function of differentiating erythroid cells is the synthesis of large amounts of hemoglobin. Levere and Granick (1965) first examined the appearance of hemoglobin in nucleated erythroid precursor cells in the developing avian blastoderm. Addition of δ-aminolevulinate induced early hemoglobinization and the effects of actinomycin D (to inhibit transcription) and inhibitors of protein synthesis suggested that ALA promotes the appearance of hemoglobin as a result of increased formation of heme. Net stimulation of hemoglobin synthesis in the chick blastoderm occurred apparently as a consequence of increased translation of globin mRNA, as in the rabbit reticulocyte system.

Studies of erythroid differentiation have also been carried out in cultured erythroleukemia cells obtained from mice infected with the Friend virus. The heme concentration in these cells rises up to 50-fold when terminal differentiation is induced by surface-active compounds, for example, dimethyl sulfoxide. Several early studies suggested that this differentiation may be associated with a sequential induction of heme biosynthetic enzymes (Sassa, 1976) and that, as in human K562 cells (Hoffman and Ross, 1980), heme formation was dependent on the induction of appreciable ferrochelatase activity. These findings have been disputed by other workers who found that coordinate induction of several enzymes including ALA synthase occurs simultaneously before heme synthesis can be detected (Beaumont et al., 1984). Addition of ALA to uninduced Friend cells stimulates heme synthesis, suggesting that formation of ALA in the undifferentiated state is rate-limiting (Laskey et al., 1986). Conversely, in cells induced to differentiate terminally, heme synthesis was not influenced by addition of ALA; rather, it could be stimulated by raising the concentration of nonheme intracellular iron (Laskey et al., 1986). Certain Friend cell variants cannot be induced to differentiate with DMSO unless hemin is also added to the culture medium (Mager and Bernstein, 1980). These variants show incomplete expression of cell surface markers of erythroid differentiation, including membrane transferrin receptors (Wilczynska et al., 1984). The precocious synthesis of hemoglobin in DMSO-induced Friend cells on treatment with ferric chelates (which donate iron independently of the transferrin receptor cycle) demonstrates that acquisition of iron via the transferrin receptor pathway is crucial for promoting terminal differentiation in this cellular model (Wilczynska et al., 1984).

Differentiation in chicken erythroid cells transformed with a temperature-sensitive mutant avian erythroblastosis virus has been examined (Schmidt et al., 1986). Cellular iron removal from transferrin was blocked by a monoclonal antibody to the chicken transferrin receptor. The antibody, which had no effect on transferrin binding or internalization, reduced iron uptake and blocked spontaneous and temperature-induced erythroid differentiation at the erythroblast or early reticulocyte stage. Proliferation of noncommitted erythroid cells was unaffected. Addition of succinylacetone, to inhibit heme synthesis, mimicked the effects of antibody and the effects of antibody could be overcome by elevating intracellular iron concentrations.

1. Heme and the program of normal erythroid development. Investigators who have examined the physiological processes which bring about normal differentiation and proliferative responses in erythroid progenitor cells report findings which differ from studies of cultured malignant or transformed cell lines. Erythropoietin (epo) is the physiological inducer of the erythroid differentiation program and its addition to cultures of rat marrow cells stimulates iron uptake and hemoglobin synthesis within a few hours (Beru and Goldwasser, 1985). The activities of δ-ALA synthase and ferrochelatase were unaffected by epo treatment given over several days, whereas that of porphobilinogen (PBG) deaminase was greatly stimulated and rose in parallel to the increased formation of heme. Similar changes were observed in bone marrow cells exposed to epo in vivo and were reversed in cells obtained from animals with suppressed bone marrow activity. Experiments using actinomycin D and cycloheximide suggested that epo-induced stimulation of the enzymatic activity was brought about by transcriptional activation of the gene for PBG deaminase, leading to enhanced enzyme synthesis. These findings are important in that they represent studies of untransformed marrow cells and the influence of a natural determinant of erythropoietic activity; however, insufficient data were presented to give a complete picture of functional differentiation, especially in regard to the iron-transferrin cycle and transferrin receptor expression.

VI. Conclusions

The mechanisms by which heme synthesis is regulated in hemoglobin-synthesizing cells may be discussed from two different perspectives. The first concerns the mechanisms operating during the period when erythroid precursors acquire the machinery for hemoglobin synthesis. While Sassa (1976) reported a sequential induction of the enzymes of heme biosynthesis in differentiating Friend erythroleukemia cells, more recently Beaumont et al. (1984) found that ferrochelatase is induced as early as ALA synthase. Furthermore, they observed that there is a significant delay in the accumulation of heme following ferrochelatase induction, suggesting that the rate-limiting step in heme synthesis during erythroid differentiation might be the capacity of the cells to acquire iron from transferrin (Laskey et al., 1986). There is additional evidence to support this possibility. In epo-responsive Friend cell lines the induction of transferrin receptors clearly precedes the formation of hemoglobin heme (Sawyer and Krantz, 1986), and the noninducibility of heme synthesis by DMSO in some Friend cell variants is accompanied by a lack of induction of transferrin receptors (Wilczynska et al., 1984).

The second aspect concerns the regulation of heme synthesis in erythroid cells after the enzymes of the pathway have been fully induced, such as in erythroblasts and reticulocytes. The rate of heme synthesis in rodent reticulocytes is regulated by iron supply from transferrin which is the rate-limiting step in the heme pathway and is subject to feedback inhibition by heme (Ponka and Schulman, 1985a, b, 1986). In human reticulocytes, formation of ALA seems to be regulated (Gardner and Cox, 1988) and this might at least partially be accomplished by control of the level of intracellular glycine.

Although there is considerable evidence that some aspect of the iron-transferrin cycle controls heme synthesis in erythroid cells (see Chap. 5), to the best of our knowledge, there is no indication for

a role of iron in the regulation of heme synthesis in cells not synthesizing hemoglobin such as lymphoblastoid cell lines (Schulman et al.,
1981), uninduced Friend cells (Laskey et al., 1986), and hepatocytes
(Müller-Eberhardt, personal communication). Therefore, it seems clear
that there might be a specialized intracellular pathway of iron utilization for hemoglobin synthesis.

ACKNOWLEDGMENTS

The authors (P.P. and H.M.S.) are grateful to the Medical Research
Council of Canada for grant support. We thank Sandy Fraiberg for
preparing the manuscript.

REFERENCES

Adams, M. L., Ostapiuk, I., and Grasso, J. A. (1989). The effects of inhibition of heme
synthesis on the intracellular localization of iron in rat reticulocytes, *Biochim. Biophys.
Acta*, **1012**:243–253.

Adamson, S. D., Herbert, E., and Godchaux, W. (1968). Factors affecting the rate of protein
synthesis in lysate systems from reticulocytes, *Arch. Biochem. Biophys.* **125**:671–683.

Aisen, P. (1977). Some physicochemical aspects of iron metabolism. *Iron Metabolism. Ciba
Foundation Symposium*, Elsevier, Amsterdam, Vol. 51 (New Series), pp. 1–17.

Aisen, P., and Leibman, A. (1968). Citrate mediated exchange of Fe^{3+} among transferrin
molecules, *Biochem. Biophys. Res. Comm.* **33**:220–226.

Aisen, P., Leibman, A., and Zweier, J. (1978). Stoichiometric and site characteristics of the
binding of iron to human transferrin, *J. Biol. Chem.* **253**:1930–1937.

Alderton, G., Ward, W. H., and Fevold, H. L. (1946). Identification of the bacteria
inhibiting iron-binding protein of egg white as conalbumin, *Arch. Biochem. Biophys.*
11:9–13.

Anderson, B. F., Baker, H. M., Dodson, E. J., Norris, G. E., Rumball, S. V., Waters, J. M.,
and Baker, E. N. (1987). Structure of human lactoferrin at 3.2-Å resolution, *Proc. Nat.
Acad. Sci. (U.S.A.)* **84**:1769–1773.

Appleton, T. C., Morgan, E., and Baker, E. (1971). A morphological study of transferrin
uptake by reticulocytes, *The Regulation of Erythropoiesis and Haemoglobin Synthesis*
(T. Travnicek and J. Neuwirt, Eds.), Universita Karlova, Prague, pp. 310–315.

Arosio, P., Adelman, T. G., and Drysdale, J. W. (1978). On ferritin heterogeneity. Further
evidence for heteropolymers, *J. Biol. Chem.* **253**:4451–4458.

Aulbert, E., Disselhoff, W., Sorje, H., Schulz, E., and Gericke, D. (1980). Lysosomal
accumulation of 67-Ga-transferrin in malignant tumors in relation to their growth rate,
Eur. J. Cancer **16**:1217–1232.

Aziz, N., and Munro, H. N. (1986). Both subunits of rat liver ferritin are regulated at a
translational level by iron induction, *Nucl. Acid Res.* **14**:915–927.

Bailey-Wood, R., Blayney, L., Muir, J., and Jacobs, A. (1975). The effect of iron deficiency
on rat liver enzymes, *Brit. J. Exp. Pathol.* **56**:193–198.

Bakkeren, D. L., de Jen-Jaspars, C. M. H., Kroos, M. J., and van Eijk, H. G. (1987). Release
of iron from endosomes is an early step in the transferrin cycle, *Int. J. Biochem.*
19:179–186.

Baldwin, D. A., and Egan, T. J. (1987). An inorganic perspective of human serum
transferrin, *S. Afr. J. Sci.* **83**:22–31.

Barnes, D., and Sato, G. (1980). Serum-free cell culture: A unifying approach, *Cell*
22:649–655.

Beamish, M. R., Keay, L., Okigaki, T., and Brown, E. B. (1975). Uptake of transferrin-bound
iron by rat cells in tissue culture, *Brit. J. Haematol.* **31**:479–491.

Beaumont, C., Deybach, J.-C., Grandchamp, B., DaSilva, V., de Verneuil, H., and Nordmann, Y. (1984). Effects of succinylacetone on dimethylsulfoxide mediated induction of heme pathway enzymes in mouse Friend virus-transformed erythroleukemia cells, *Exp. Cell Res.* **154**:474–484.

Bernstein, S. E. (1987). Hereditary hypotransferrinemia with hemosiderosis, a murine disorder resembling human atransferrinemia, *J. Lab. Clin. Med.* **110**:690–705.

Beru, N., and Goldwasser, E. (1985). The regulation of heme biosynthesis during erythropoietin-induced erythroid differentiation, *J. Biol. Chem.* **260**:9251–9257.

Bezkorovainy, A. (1980). *Biochemistry of Non-Heme Iron*, Plenum, New York.

Bezkorovainy, A. (1987). Iron proteins, *Iron and Infection* (J. J. Bullen and E. Griffiths, Eds.), Wiley, New York.

Borova, J., Ponka, P., and Neuwirt, J. (1973). Study of intracellular iron distribution in rabbit reticulocytes with normal and inhibited heme synthesis, *Biochim. Biophys. Acta* **320**:143–156.

Bottomley, S. S. (1982). Sideroblastic anemia, *Clin. Haematol.* **11**:389–409.

Brissot, P., Wright, T. L., Ma, W. L., and Weisiger, R. A. (1985). Efficient clearance of non-transferrin-bound iron by rat liver, *J. Clin. Invest.* **76**:1463–1470.

Brock, J. H., and Stevenson, J. (1987). Replacement of transferrin in serum-free cultures of mitogen-stimulated mouse lymphocytes by a lipophilic iron chelator, *J. Immunol. Lett.* **15**:23–27.

Bruns, G. P., and London, I. M. (1965). The effect of hemin on the synthesis of globin, *Biochem. Biophys. Res. Comm.* **18**:236–242.

Bullen, J. J., and Griffiths, E. (Eds.) (1987). *Iron and Infection*, Wiley, New York.

Burnham, B. F., and Lascelles, J. (1963). Control of porphyrin biosynthesis through a negative feedback mechanism. Studies with preparation of δ-aminolevulinic acid synthetase and δ-aminolevulinic acid dehydratase from *Rhodopseudomonas spheroides*, *Biochem. J.* **87**:462–472.

Cairo, G., Bardella, L., Schiaffonati, L., Arosio, P., Levi, S., and Bernelli-Zazzera, A. (1985). Multiple mechanisms of iron-induced ferritin synthesis in HeLa cells, *Biochem. Biophys. Res. Comm.* **133**:314–321.

Camadro, J. M., Ibraham, N. G., and Levere, R. D. (1984). Kinetic studies of human liver ferrochelatase. Role of endogenous metals, *J. Biol. Chem.* **259**:5678–5682.

Casey, J. L., Di Jeso, B., Rao, K., Rouault, T. A., Klausner, R. D., and Harford, J. B. (1988). Deletional analysis of the promoter region of the human transferrin receptor gene, *Nucl. Acid Res.* **16**:629–646.

Catz, C. S., Juchau, M. R., and Yaffe, S. J. (1970). Effects of iron, riboflavin and iodide deficiencies on hepatic drug-metabolizing enzyme systems, *J. Pharmacol. Exp. Therap.* **174**:197–205.

Chan, R., Schulman, H. M., and Ponka, P. (1989). Distinct controls of transferrin receptor expression in erythroid and non-erythroid cells, *J. Cell. Biochem.* Suppl. **13C**:24.

Chang, C. S., and Sassa, S. (1985). δ-Aminolevulinate dehydratase in human erythroleukemia cells: An immunologically distinct enzyme, *Blood* **65**:939–944.

Choe, H. R., Moseley, S. T., Glass, J., and Nunez, M. T. (1987). Rabbit reticulocyte coated vesicles carrying the transferrin-transferrin receptor complex. I. Purification and partial characterization, *Blood* **70**:1035–1039.

Cole, E. S., and Glass, J. (1983). Transferrin binding and iron uptake in mouse hepatocytes, *Biochim. Biophys. Acta* **762**:102–110.

Costanzo, F., Delius, H., and Cortese, R. (1986). Structure of gene and pseudogenes of human apoferritin, *Nucl. Acid Res.* **14**:721–735.

Cotner, T., Das Gupta, A., Pappayannopoulou, Th., and Stamatoyannopoulos, G. (1989). Characterization of a novel form of transferrin receptor preferentially expressed on normal erythroid progenitors and precursors, *Blood* **73**:214–221.

Cox, T. M., O'Donnell, M. W., Aisen, P., and London, I. M. (1985a). Hemin inhibits internalization of transferrin by reticulocytes and promotes phosphorylation of the membrane transferrin receptor, *Proc. Nat. Acad. Sci. (U.S.A.)* **82**:5170–5174.

Cox, T. M., O'Donnell, M. W., Aisen, P., and London, I. M. (1985b). Biosynthesis of the transferrin receptor in rabbit reticulocytes, *J. Clin. Invest.* **76**:2144–2150.

Craven, C. M., Alexander, T., Eldridge, M., Kushner, J. P., Bernstein, S., and Kaplan, J. (1987). Tissue distribution and clearance kinetics of nontransferrin-bound iron in the hypotransferrinemic mouse: A rodent model for hemochromatosis, *Proc. Nat. Acad. Sci. (U.S.A.)* **84**:3457–3461.

Dailey, H. A., and Fleming, J. E. (1983). Bovine ferrochelatase, *J. Biol. Chem.* **258**:11453–11459.

Dautry-Varsat, A., Ciechanover, A., and Lodish, H. F. (1983). pH and the recycling of transferrin during receptor-mediated endocytosis, *Proc. Nat. Acad. Sci. (U.S.A.)* **80**:2258–2262.

Drysdale, J. W., Adelman, T. G., Arosio, P., Casareale, D., Fitzpatrick, P., Hazard, J. T., and Yokota, M. (1977). Human isoferritins in normal and disease states, *Sem. Hematol.* **14**:71–78.

Ebert, P. S., and Ikawa, Y. (1974). Induction of delta-aminolevulinic acid synthetase during erythroid differentiation of cultured leukemia cells, *Proc. Soc. Exp. Biol. N.Y.* **146**:601–604.

Ecarot-Charrier, B., Grey, V., Wilczynska, A., and Schulman, H. M. (1977). The isolation of transferrin receptors from reticulocyte membranes, *Proteins of Iron Metabolism* (E. B. Brown, P. Aisen, J. Fielding, and R. R. Crichton, Eds.), Grune & Stratton, New York, pp. 291–298.

Ecarot-Charrier, B., Grey, V. L., Wilczynska, A., and Schulman, H. M. (1980). Reticulocyte membrane transferrin receptors, *Canad. J. Biochem.* **58**:418–426.

Egyed, A. (1975). Effect of adenine nucleotides and pyrophosphate on the exchange of transferrin-bound carbonate, *Biochim. Biophys. Acta* **411**:349–356.

Egyed, A. (1988). Carrier mediated iron transport through erythroid cell membrane, *Brit. J. Haematol.* **68**:483–486.

Ehrlich, P. (1881). Bericht über einige Beobachtungen am anämischen Blut, *Ber. Klin. Wochensch.* **18**:43.

Enns, C. A., and Sussman, H. H. (1981). Physical characterization of the transferrin receptor in human placentae, *J. Biol. Chem.* **255**:9820–9823.

Fadigan, A., and Dailey, H. A. (1987). Inhibition of ferrochelatase during differentiation of murine erythroleukemia cells, *Biochem. J.* **243**:419–424.

Faulk, W. P., Hsi, B. L., and Stevens, P. J. (1980). Transferrin and transferrin receptors in carcinoma of the breast, *Lancet* **2**:390–392.

Fava, R. A., Comeau, R. D., and Woodworth, R. C. (1981). Specific membrane receptors for diferric-transferrin in cultured rat skeletal myocytes and chick-embryo cardiac myocytes, *Biosci. Rep.* **1**:377–385.

Ferreira, G. C., Andrew, T. L., Karr, S. W., and Dailey, H. A. (1988). Organization of terminal two enzymes of the heme biosynthetic pathway. Orientation of protoporphyrinogen oxidase and evidence for a membrane complex, *J. Biol. Chem.* **263**:3835–3839.

Fielding, J., and Speyer, B. E. (1974). Iron transport intermediates in human reticulocytes and the membrane binding site of iron transferrin, *Biochim. Biophys. Acta* **363**:387–396.

Flatmark, T., and Romslo, I. (1975). Energy-dependent accumulation of iron by isolated rat liver mitochondria. Requirement for reducing equivalents and evidence for a unidirectional flux of Fe(II) across the inner membrane, *J. Biol. Chem.* **250**:6433–6438.

Frazier, J. L., Caskey, J. H., Yoffe, M., and Seligman, P. A. (1982). Studies of transferrin receptor on both human reticulocytes and nucleated human cell in culture: Comparison of factors regulating receptor density, *J. Clin. Invest.* **69**:853–865.

Friend, C. (1957). Cell-free transmission in adult Swiss mice of a disease having the characteristics of a leukemia, *J. Exp. Med.* **105**:307–318.

Friend, C., Patuleia, S., and de Harven, E. (1966). Erythrocytic maturation in vitro of murine (Friend) virus-induced leukemia cells, *Nat. Cancer Inst. Monogr.* **228**:505–520.

Friend, C., Scher, W., Holland, J. G., and Sato, T. (1971). Hemoglobin synthesis in murine-virus-induced leukemia cells in vitro: Stimulation of erythroid differentiation by dimethylsulfoxide, *Proc. Nat. Acad. Sci. (U.S.A.)* **68**:378–382.

Gardiner, M. E., and Morgan, E. H. (1974). Transferrin and iron uptake by the liver in the rat, *Aust. J. Exp. Biol. Med. Sci.* **57**:723–736.

Gardner, L. C., and Cox, T. M. (1988). Biosynthesis of heme in immature erythroid cells: The regulatory step for heme formation in the human erythron, *J. Biol. Chem.* **263**:6676.

Ghadially, F. N. (1988). *Ultrastructural Pathology of the Cell and Matrix*, Butterworths, London, Vol. 1 (3rd Ed.), pp. 308–310.

Glass, J., Nunez, M., Fisher, S., and Robinson, S. (1978). Transferrin receptors, iron transport and ferritin metabolism in Friend erythroleukemia cells, *Biochim. Biophys. Acta* **542**:154–162.

Glass, J., Nunez, M. T., and Robinson, S. H. (1977). Iron transport from Sepharose-bound transferrin, *Biochem. Biophys. Res. Comm.* **75**:226–232.

Glass, J., Nunez, M. T., and Robinson, S. H. (1980). Transferrin-binding and iron-binding proteins of rabbit reticulocyte plasma membranes. Three distinct protein moieties, *Biochim. Biophys. Acta* **598**:293–304.

Glass, J., Yannoni, C. Z., and Robinson, S. H. (1975). Rapidly synthesized heme: Relationship to erythropoiesis and hemoglobin production, *Blood Cells* **1**:557–571.

Goya, N., Miyazalo, S., Kodate, S., and Ushino, E. (1972). A family of congenital atransferrinemia, *Blood* **40**:239–245.

Grandchamp, B., Beaumont, C., de Verneuil, H., and Nordmann, Y. (1985). Accumulation of porphobilinogen deaminase, uroporphyrinogen decarboxylase, and alpha and beta globin mRNAs during differentiation of mouse erythroleukemic cells, *J. Biol. Chem.* **260**:9630–9635.

Grayzel, A. I., Horchner, P., and London, I. M. (1966). The stimulation of globin synthesis by heme, *Proc. Nat. Acad. Sci.* **55**:650–655.

Greene, F. C., and Feeney, R. (1968). Physical evidence for transferrins a single polypeptide chain, *Biochemistry* **7**:1366.

Grohlich, D., Morley, C. G. D., and Bezkorovainy, A. (1979). Some aspects of iron uptake by rat hepatocytes in suspension, *Int. J. Biochem.* **10**:797–802.

Grohlich, D., Morley, C. G. D., Miller, R. J., and Bezkorovainy, A. (1977). Iron incorporation into isolated rat hepatocytes, *Biochem. Biophys. Res. Comm.* **76**:682–690.

Harbin, B. M., and Dailey, H. A. (1985). Orientation of ferrochelatase in bovine liver mitochondria, *Biochemistry* **24**:366–370.

Harrison, P. M., Clegg, G. A., and May, K. (1980). Ferritin structure and function, *Iron in Biochemistry and Medicine* (A. Jacobs and M. Worwood, Eds.), Academic, London, pp. 131–171.

Heilmeyer, L. (1966). Die atransferrinämien, *Acta Haematol.* **36**:40–49.

Hemmaplardh, D., Kailis, S. G., and Morgan, E. H. (1974). The effects of inhibitors of microtubule and microfilament function on transferrin and iron uptake by rabbit reticulocytes and bone marrow, *Brit. J. Haematol.* **28**:53–65.

Hemmaplardh, D., and Morgan, E. H. (1974). Transferrin and iron uptake by human cells in culture, *Exp. Cell Res.* **87**:207–212.

Hemmaplardh, D., and Morgan, E. H. (1977). The role of endocytosis in transferrin uptake by reticulocytes and bone marrow cells, *Brit. J. Haematol.* **36**:85–96.

Hershko, C., Graham, G., Bates, G. W., and Rachmilewitz, E. A. (1978). Non-specific serum iron in thalassemia: An abnormal serum iron fraction of potential toxicity, *Brit. J. Haematol.* **40**:255–263.

Hoffman, L. M., and Ross, J. (1980). The role of heme in the maturation of erythroblasts. The effects of inhibition of pyridoxal metabolism, *Blood* **55**:762–771.

Hoffman, R., Ibraham, N. G., Murnane, M. J., Diamond, A., Forget, B. G., and Levere, R. D. (1980). Hemin control of heme biosynthesis and catabolism in a human leukemia cell line, *Blood* **56**:567–570.

Holmes, S. D., Bucci, L.R., Lipschultz, L. I., and Smith, R. G. (1983). Transferrin binds specifically to pachytene spermatocytes, *Endocrinology* **113**:1916–1918.

Hosain, F., and Finch, C. A. (1964). Ferrokinetics: A study of transport iron in plasma, *J. Lab. Clin. Med.* **64**:905–912.

Hradilek, J., and Neuwirt, J. (1987). Iron uptake from transferrin and transferrin endocytic cycle in Friend erythroleukemia cells, *J. Cell Physiol.* **133**:192–196.

Hu, H. Y., Gardner, J., Aisen, P., and Skoultchi, A. I. (1977). Inducibility of transferrin receptors of Friend erythroleukemia cells, *Science* **197**:559–561.

Hu, H.-Y. Y., and Aisen, P. (1978). Molecular characteristics of the transferrin-receptor complex of the rabbit reticulocyte, *J. Supramol. Struct.* **8**:349–360.

Huebers, A., Josephson, B., Huebers, E., and Finch, C. A. (1981). Uptake and release of iron from human transferrin, *Proc. Nat. Acad. Sci. (U.S.A.)* **74**:2572–2576.

Iacopetta, B., and Morgan, E. H. (1984). Hemin inhibits transferrin endocytosis in immature erythroid cells, *Biochim. Biophys. Acta* **805**:211–216.

Iacopetta, B. J., and Morgan, E. H. (1983). The kinetics of transferrin endocytosis and iron uptake from transferrin in rabbit reticulocytes, *J. Biol. Chem.* **258**:9108–9115.

Iacopetta, B. J., and Morgan, E. G., and Yeoh, G. C. T. (1982). Transferrin receptors and iron uptake during erythroid cell development, *Biochim. Biophys. Acta* **687**:204–210.

Ibrahim, N. G., Gruenspecht, N. R., and Freeman, M. L. (1978). Hemin feedback inhibition at reticulocyte δ-aminolevulinic acid synthetase and δ-aminolevulinic acid dehydratase, *Biochem. Biophys. Res. Comm.* **80**:722–728.

Jacobs, A. (1977). Low molecular weight intracellular iron transport compounds, *Blood* **50**:433–439.

Jandl, J. H., Inman, J. K., Simmons, R. L., and Allen, D. W. (1959). Transferrin of iron from serum iron-binding protein to human reticulocytes, *J. Clin. Invest.* **38**:161–185.

Karibian, D., and London, I. M. (1965). Control of heme synthesis by feedback inhibition, *Biochem. Biophys. Res. Comm.* **18**:243–249.

Karin, M., and Mintz, B. (1981). Receptor-mediated endocytosis of transferrin in developmentally totipotent mouse teratocarcinoma stem cells, *J. Biol. Chem.* **256**:3245–3252.

Katz, J. H. (1961). Iron and protein kinetics studied by means of a doubly labeled humancrystalline transferrin, *J. Clin. Invest.* **40**:2143–2152.

Keung, W. M., Azari, P., and Phillips, J. L. (1982). Structure and function of ovotransferrin. I. Production of iron-binding fragments from iron-ovotransferrin by the action of immobilized subtilism, *J. Biol. Chem.* **257**:1177–1183.

Klausner, R. D., van Renswoude, J., Ashwell, G., Kempf, C., Schechter, A. N., Dean, A., and Bridges, K. R. (1983). Receptor-mediated endocytosis of transferrin in K562 cells, *J. Biol. Chem.* **258**:4715–4721.

Kondo, H., Saito, K., Grasso, J. P., and Aisen, P. (1988). Iron metabolism in the erythrophagocytosing Kuppfer cell, *Hepatology* **8**:32–38.

Konopka, K. (1978). Differential effects of metal binding agents on the uptake of iron from transferrin by isolated rat liver mitochondria, *FEBS Lett.* **92**:308–312.

Konopka, K., Mareschal, J. C., and Crichton, R. R. (1981). Iron transfer from transferrin to ferritin mediated by polyphosphate compounds, *Biochim. Biophys. Acta* **677**:417–423.

Konopka, K., and Romslo, I. (1981). Studies on the mechanism of pyrophosphate-mediated uptake of iron from transferrin by isolated rat liver mitochondria, *Eur. J. Biochem.* **117**:239–244.

Koury, M. J., Bondurant, M. C., and Roma, S. S. (1987). Changes in erythroid membrane proteins during erythropoietin-mediated terminal differentiation, *J. Cell Physiol.* **133**:438–448.

Koury, M. J., Sawyer, S. T., and Bondurant, M. C. (1984). Splenic erythroblasts in anemia-inducing Friend disease: A source of cells for studies of erythropoietin-mediated differentiation, *J. Cell Physiol.* **121**:526–532.

Kruh, J., and Borsook, H. (1956). Hemoglobin synthesis in rabbit reticulocytes in vitro, *J. Biol. Chem.* **220**:905–915.

Kühn, L. C., McClelland, A., and Ruddle, F. H. (1984). Gene transfer, expression, and molecular cloning of the human transferrin receptor gene, *Cell* **37**:95–103.

Kushner, J. P. and Cartwright, G. E. (1977). Sideroblastic anemia, *Adv. Intern. Med.* **22**:229–249.

Lamfrom, H., and Knopf, P. M. (1964). Initiation of hemoglobin synthesis in cell-free systems, *J. Mol. Biol.* **9**:558–575.

Landschultz, W., Thesleff, I., and Ekblom, P. (1984). A lipophilic iron chelator can replace transferrin as a stimulator of cell proliferation and differentiation, *J. Cell Biol.* **98**:596–601.

Larrick, J. W., and Creswell, P. (1979). Transferrin receptors on human B and T lymphoblastoid cell lines, *Biochim. Biophys. Acta* **583**:483–490.

Laskey, J. D., Ponka, P., and Schulman, H. M. (1986). Control of heme synthesis during Friend cell differentiation: Role of iron and transferrin, *J. Cell Physiol.* **129**:185–192.

Laskey, J., Webb, I., Schulman, H. M., and Ponka, P. (1988). Evidence that transferrin supports cell proliferation by supplying iron for DNA synthesis, *Exp. Cell Res.* **176**:87–95.

Laufberger, V. (1934). O výměně železa, *Biol. Listy* **19**:73.

Laufberger, V. (1937). Sur la cristallisation de la ferritine, *Bull. Soc. Chim. Biol.* **19**:1575–1582.

Laurell, L. C. (1947). Studies on the transportation and metabolism of iron in the body, *Acta Physiol. Scand.* (Suppl.) **46**:1–129.

Legon, S., Jackson, R. J., and Hunt, T. (1973). Control of protein synthesis in reticulocytes by haemin, *Nature New Biol.* **241**:150–152.

Leibman, A., and Aisen, P. (1979). Distribution of iron between the binding sistes of transferrin in serum: Methods and results in normal human subjects, *Blood* **53**:1058–1065.

Leibold, E. A., and Munro, H. N. (1987). Characterization and evolution of the expressed rat ferritin light subunit gene and its pseudogene family, *J. Biol. Chem.* **262**:7335–7341.

Leibold, E. A., and Munro, H. N. (1988). Cytoplasmic protein binds in vitro to a highly conserved sequence in the 5′ untranslated region of ferritin heavy- and light-subunit mRNAs, *Proc. Nat. Acad. Sci.* **85**:2171–2175.

Lesley, J., Hyman, R., Schulte, R., and Trotter, J. (1984). Expression of transferrin receptor on murine hematopoietic progenitors, *Cell. Immunol.* **83**:14–25.

Levere, R. D., and Granick, S. (1965). Control of hemoglobin synthesis in the cultured chick blastoderm by δ-aminolevulinic acid synthetase: Increase in the rate of hemoglobin formation with δ-aminolevulinic acid, *Proc. Nat. Acad. Sci. (U.S.A.)* **54**:2134–2137.

Light, I. A., and Morgan, E. H. (1982). Transferrin endocytosis in reticulocytes. An electron microscopic study using colloidal gold, *Scand. J. Haematol.* **28**:205–214.

Loh, T. T., Yeung, Y. G., and Yeung, D. (1977). Transferrin and iron uptake by rabbit reticulocytes, *Biochim. Biophys. Acta* **471**:118–124.

London, I. M., Levin, D. H., Matts, R. L., Thomas, N. S. B., Petryshyn, R., and Chen, J. J. (1987). Regulation of protein synthesis, *The Enzymes*, (P. D. Boyer, Ed.), Academic, New York, Vol. 18, pp. 359–380.

Lozzio, C. B., and Lozzio, B. B. (1975). Human chronic myelogenous leukemia cell-line with positive Philadelphia chromosome, *Blood* **45**:321–334.

Mack, U., Powell, L. W., and Halliday, J. W. (1983). Detection and isolation of a hepatic membrane receptor for ferritin, *J. Biol. Chem.* **258**:4672–4675.

Mager, D., and Bernstein, A. (1980). The role of heme in the regulation of the late program of Friend cell erythroid differentiation, *J. Cell Physiol.* **100**:467–480.

Makey, D. G., and Seal, U. S. (1976). The detection of four molecular forms of human transferrin during the iron binding process, *Biochim. Biophys. Acta* **453**:250–256.

Malik, Z., Bessler, H., and Djaldetti, M. (1979). The role of hemin in the regulation of heme synthesis by fetal mouse liver erythroblasts in culture, *Exp. Hematol.* **7**:183–188.

Marks, P., and Rifkind, R. (1978). Erythroleukemia differentiation, *Ann. Rev. Biochem.* **47**:419–448.

Martin, A. W., Huebers, E., Huebers, H., Webb, J., and Finch, C. A. (1984). A mono-sited transferrin from a representative deuterostone. The ascidian *Pyura stolonifera* (Subphylum Urochordata), *Blood* **64**:1047–1052.

Martinez-Medellin, J., and Schulman, H. M. (1972). The kinetics of iron and transferrin incorporation into rabbit erythroid cells and the nature of stromal-bound iron, *Biochim. Biophys. Acta.* **264**:272–284.

Martinez-Medellin, J., Schulman, H. M., de Miguel, E., and Benavides, L. (1977). New evidence for the internalization of transferrin in rabbit reticulocytes, *Proteins of Iron Metabolism* (E. B. Brown, P. Aisen, J. Fielding, and R. R. Crichton, Eds.), Gune & Stratton, New York, pp. 305–310.

Mattia, E., Rao, K., Shapiro, D. S., Sussman, H. H., and Klausner, R. D. (1984). Biosynthetic regulation of the human transferrin receptor by desferrioxamine in K562 cells, *J. Biol. Chem.* **259**:2689–2692.

Maxwell, C. R., Kamper, C. S., and Rabinovitz, M. (1971). Hemin control of globin synthesis: An assay for the inhibitor formed in the absence of hemin and some characteristics of its formation, *J. Mol. Biol.* **58**:317–327.

May, A., de Sousa, P., Barnes, S., Kaaba, S., and Jacobs, A. (1982). Erythroblast iron metabolism in sideroblastic marrows, *Brit. J. Haematol.* **52**:611–621.

Mazur, A., and Carleton, A. (1963). Relation of ferritin iron to heme synthesis in marrow and reticulocytes, *J. Biol. Chem.* **238**:1817–1824.

McClelland, A., Kühn, L. C., and Ruddle, F. H. (1984). The human transferrin receptor gene: Genomic organization and the complete primary structure of the receptor deduced from a cDNA sequence, *Cell* **39**:267–274.

Metz-Boutique, M. H., Jolles, J., Mazurier, J., Schoentgen, F., Legrand, D., Spik, G., Montreuil, J., and Jolles, P. (1984). Human lactotransferrin: Amino acid sequence and structural comparisons with other transferrins, *Eur. J. Biochem.* **145**:659–676.

Miskimins, W. K., McClelland, A., Roberts, M. R., and Ruddle, F. H. (1986). Cell proliferation and expression of the transferrin receptor gene: Promoter sequence homologies and protein interactions, *J. Cell. Biol.* **103**:1781–1788.

Miskimins, W. K., Roberts, M. P., McClelland, A., and Ruddle, F. H. (1985). Use of a protein-blocking procedure and a specific cDNA probe to identify nuclear proteins that recognize the promoter region of the transferrin receptor gene, *Proc. Nat. Acad. Sci. (U.S.A.)* **82**:6741–6744.

Morgan, E. H. (1981). Inhibition of reticulocyte iron uptake by NH_4Cl and CH_3NH_2, *Biochim. Biophys. Acta* **642**:119–134.

Morgan, E. H. (1983). Chelator-mediated iron efflux from reticulocytes, *Biochim. Biophys. Acta* **733**:39–50.

Morgan, E. H. (1988). Membrane transport of non-transferrin-bound iron by reticulocytes, *Biochim. Biophys. Acta* **943**:428–439.

Morgan, E. H., and Appleton, T. C. (1969). Autoradiographic localisation of ^{125}I-labelled transferrin in rabbit reticulocytes, *Nature* **223**:1371–1372.

Morgan, E. H., Huehns, E. R., and Finch, C. A. (1966). Iron reflux from reticulocytes and bone marrow cells in vitro, *Amer. J. Physiol.* **210**:579–585.

Morley, C. G. D., and Bezkorovainy, A. (1983). The behavior of transferrin receptors in rat hepatocyte plasma membranes, *Clin. Physiol. Biochem.* **1**:318–328.

Müllner, E. W., and Kühn, L. C. (1988). A stem-loop structure in the 3' nontranslated region mediates iron-dependent regulation of transferrin receptor stability in the cytoplasm, *Cell* **53**:815–825.

Murray, M. T., White, K., and Munro, H. N. (1987). Conservation of ferritin heavy subunit gene structure: Implications for the regulation of ferritin gene expression, *Proc. Nat. Acad. Sci.* **84**:7438–7442.

Najean, Y., Dresch, C., Ardaillon, N., and Bernard, J. (1967). Iron metabolism—a study of different kinetic models in normal conditions, *Amer. J. Physiol.* **213**:533–546.

Neckers, L. M. (1984). Transferrin receptor regulation of proliferation in normal and neoplastic B cells, *Curr. Topics Microbiol. Immunol.* **113**:62–68.

Neilands, J. B. (1981). Microbial iron compounds, *Ann. Rev. Biochem.* **50**:713–731.

Neuwirt, J., and Ponka, P. (1972). The regulation of heme synthesis in erythroid cells by the feedback inhibition of cellular uptake of substrates, *Synthesis, Structure and Function of Haemoglobin* (H. H. Martin and L. Nowicki, Eds.), Lehmann, Munich, pp. 61–66.

Neuwirt, J., Ponka, P., and Borova, J. (1969). The role of heme in the regulation of δ-aminolevulinic acid and heme synthesis in rabbit reticulocytes, *Eur. J. Biochem.* **9**:36–41.

Neuwirt, J., Ponka, P., and Borova, J. (1972). Evidence for the presence of free and protein-bound nonhemoglobin heme in rabbit reticulocytes, *Biochim. Biophys. Acta* **264**:235–244.

Nilsen, T., and Romslo, I. (1984). Transferrin as a donor of iron to mitochondria. Effect of pyrophosphate and relationship to mitochondrial metabolism and heme synthesis, *Biochim. Biophys. Acta* **802**:448–453.

Nilsen, T., and Romslo, I. (1985). Iron uptake and heme synthesis by isolated rat liver mitochondria. Diferric transferrin as iron donor and the effect of pyrophosphate, *Biochim. Biophys. Acta* **842**:162–169.

Omary, M. B., and Trowbridge, I. S. (1981a). Covalent binding of fatty acid to the transferrin receptor in cultured human cells, *J. Biol. Chem.* **256**:4715–4718.

Omary, M. B., and Trowbridge, I. S. (1981b). Biosynthesis of the human transferrin receptor in cultured cells, *J. Biol. Chem.* **256**:12888–12892.

Owen, D., and Kühn, L. C. (1987). Noncoding 3' sequence of the transferrin receptor gene are required for mRNA replication by iron, *EMBO J.* **6**:1287–1293.

Pan, B. T., Blostein, R., and Johnstone, R. M. (1983). Loss of the transferrin receptor during the maturation of sheep reticulocytes in vitro. An immunological approach, *Biochem. J.* **210**:37–47.

Paoletti, C., Durand, M., Gosse, Ch., and Boiron, M. (1958). Absence de consommation de la sidérophiline au cours de la synthèse de l'hémoglobine in vitro, *Rev. Franc. Et. Clin. Biol.* **3**:259–261.

Pelicci, P. G., Tabilio, A., Thomopoulos, P., Titeux, M., Vainchenker, W., Rochant, H., and Testa, U. (1982). Hemin regulates the expression of transferrin receptors in human hematopoietic cell lines, *FEBS Lett.* **145**:350–354.

Pollack, S., and Campana, T. (1980). Low molecular weight nonheme iron and a highly labeled heme pool in the reticulocyte, *Blood* **56**:564–566.

Pollack, S., Campana, T., and Weaver, J. (1985). Low molecular weight iron in guinea pig reticulocytes, *Amer. J. Hematol.* **19**:75–84.

Pollycove, M., and Mortimer, R. (1961). The quantitative determination of iron kinetics and hemoglobin synthesis in human subjects, *J. Clin. Invest.* **40**:753–782.

Ponka, P., Borova, J., Neuwirt, J., Fuchs, O., and Necas, E. (1979). A study of intracellular iron metabolism using pyridoxal isonicotinoyl hydrazone and other synthetic chelating agents, *Biochim. Biophys. Acta* **586**:278–297.

Ponka, P., and Neuwirt, J. (1969). Regulation of iron entry into reticulocytes. I. Feedback inhibition effect of heme on iron entry into reticulocytes and on heme synthesis, *Blood* **33**:690–707.

Ponka, P., and Neuwirt, J. (1971). Regulation of iron entry into reticulocytes. II. Relationship between hemoglobin synthesis and entry of iron into reticulocytes, *Biochim. Biophys. Acta* **230**:381–392.

Ponka, P., Neuwirt, J., Borova, J., and Fuchs, O. (1977). Control of iron delivery to hemoglobin in erythroid cells, *Iron Metabolism. Ciba Foundation Symposium*, Elsevier, Amsterdam, Vol. 51 (New Series), pp. 167–200.

Ponka, P., and Schulman, H. M. (1985a). Regulation of heme synthesis in erythroid cells: Hemin inhibits transferrin iron utilization but not protoporphyrin synthesis, *Blood* **65**:850–857.

Ponka, P., and Schulman, H. M. (1985b). Acquisition of iron from transferrin regulates reticulocyte heme synthesis, *J. Biol. Chem.* **260**:14717–14721.

Ponka, P., and Schulman, H. M. (1986). Regulation of heme synthesis in erythroid cells by iron delivery from transferrin, *Porphyrins and Porphyrias*, (Y. Nordmann, Ed.), John Libbey, London, Colloque INSERM, Vol. 134, pp. 55–67.

Ponka, P., Schulman, H. M., and Martinez-Medellin, J. (1988). Haem inhibits iron uptake subsequent to endocytosis of transferrin in reticulocytes, *Biochem. J.* **251**:105–109.

Ponka, P., Schulman, H. M., and Wilczynska, A. (1982a). Ferric pyridoxal isonicotinoyl hydrazone can provide iron for heme synthesis in reticulocytes, *Biochim. Biophys. Acta* **718**:151–156.

Ponka, P., Wilczynska, A., and Schulman, H. M. (1982b). Iron utilization in rabbit reticulocytes. A study using succinylacetone as an inhibitor of heme synthesis, *Biochim. Biophys. Acta* **720**:96–105.

Porra, R. J., and Jones, O. T. G. (1963). Studies on ferrochelatase. 1. Assay and properties of ferrochelatase from a pig liver mitochondrial extract, *Biochemistry* **87**:181–185.

Princiotto, J. V., and Zapolski, E. J. (1975). Differences between the two iron binding sites of transferrin, *Nature* **255**:87–88.

Rao, K. K., Shapiro, D., Mattia, E., Bridges, K., and Klausner, R. (1985). Effects of alterations in cellular iron on biosynthesis of the transferrin receptor in K562 cells, *Mol. Cell. Biol.* **5**:595–600.

Rapoport, S. M., Rosenthal, S., Schewe, F., Schultze, M., and Müller, M. (1974). The metabolism of the reticulocyte, *Cellular Biology of Erythrocytes* (H. Yoshikawa and S. M. Rappoport, Eds.), University of Tokyo Press, Tokyo, pp. 91–141.

Romslo, I. (1983). Iron uptake by mitochondria, *Structure and Function of Iron Storage and Transport Proteins* (I. Urushizaki, P. Aisen, I. Listowski, and J. W. Drysdale, Eds.), Elsevier, Amsterdam, pp. 493–496.

Ross, J., Ikawa, Y., and Leder, P. (1972). Globin messenger-RNA induction during erythroid differentiation of cultured leukemia cells, *Proc. Nat. Acad. Sci. (U.S.A.)* **69**:3620–3623.

Rothenberger, S., Iacopetta, B. J., and Kühn, L. C. (1987). Endocytosis of the transferrin receptor requires the cytoplasmic domain but not its phosphorylation site, *Cell* **49**:423–431.

Rouault, T., Rao, K., Harford, J., Mattia, E., and Klausner, R. (1985). Hemin, chelatable iron, and the regulation of transferrin receptor biosynthesis, *J. Biol. Chem.* **260**:14862–14866.

Rutherford, T. R., Clegg, J. B., and Weatherall, D. J. (1979). K562 human leukaemic cells synthesize embryonic haemoglobin in response to haemin, *Nature* **280**:164–165.

Santoro, C., Marone, M., Ferrone, M., Costanzo, F., Colombo, M., Minganti, C., Cortese, R., and Silengo, L. (1986). Cloning the gene coding for human L apoferritin, *Nucl. Acid Res.* **14**:2863–2876.

Sassa, S. (1976). Sequential induction of heme pathway enzymes during erythroid differentiation of mouse Friend leukemia virus-infected cells, *J. Exp. Med.* **143**:305–315.

Sawyer, S. T., and Krantz, S. B. (1986). Transferrin receptor number, synthesis, and endocytosis during erythropoietin-induced maturation of Friend virus-infected erythroid cells, *J. Biol. Chem.* **261**:9187–9195.

Schade, A. L., and Caroline, L. (1944). Raw hen egg white and the role of iron in growth inhibition of *Shigella dysenteriae, Staphylococcus aureus, Escherichia coli*, and *Saccharomyces cerevisiae, Science* **100**:14–15.

Schade, A. L., and Caroline, L. (1946). An iron-binding component of human blood plasma, *Science* **104**:340–341.

Schlabach, M. R., and Bates, G. (1975). The synergistic binding of anions and Fe(III) by transferrin, *J. Biol. Chem.* **250**:2182–2188.

Schmidt, J. A., Marshall, J., Hayman, M. J., Ponka, P., and Beug, H. (1986). Control of erythroid differentiation: Possible role of the transferrin cycle, *Cell* **46**:41–51.

Schneider, C. M., Kurkinen, M., and Greaves, M. (1983). Isolation of cDNA clones for the human transferrin receptor, *EMBO J.* **2**:2259–2263.

Schneider, C., Owen, M. J., Banville, D., and Williams, J. G. (1984). Primary structure of human transferrin receptor deduced from the mRNA sequence, *Nature* **311**:675–678.

Schneider, C. R., Sutherland, R., Newman, R., and Greaves, M. (1982). Structural features of the cell surface receptor for transferrin that is recognized by the monoclonal antibody OKT9, *J. Biol. Chem.* **257**:8516–8522.

Schulman, H. M. (1968). Hemoglobin synthesis during rabbit reticulocyte maturation in vitro, *Biochim. Biophys. Acta* **155**:253–261.

Schulman, H. M. (1975). Evidence supporting a physiological role for the hemin-controlled translational repressor of globin synthesis in reticulocytes, *Biochim. Biophys. Acta* **414**:161–166.

Schulman, H. M., Martinez-Medellin, J., and Sidloi, R. (1974). The reticulocyte-mediated release of iron and bicarbonate from transferrin: Effect of metabolic inhibitors, *Biochim. Biophys. Acta* **343**:529–534.

Schulman, H. M., Wilczynska, A., and Ponka, P. (1981). Transferrin and iron uptake by human lymphoblastoid and K-562 cells, *Biochem. Biophys. Res. Comm.* **100**:1523–1530.

Schulman, H. M., Wilczynska, A., and Ponka, P. (1983). Intracellular transferrin and transferrin receptors in reticulocytes, *Structure and Function of Iron Storage and Transport Proteins* (I. Urushizaki, P. Aisen, I. Listowski, and J. W. Drysdale, Eds.), Elsevier, Amsterdam, pp. 305–310.

Shemin, D., and Rittenberg, D. (1946). Biological utilization of glycine for the synthesis of protoporphyrin of hemoglobin, *J. Biol. Chem.* **159**:567.

Sibille, J.-C., Kondo, H., and Aisen, P. (1988). Interactions between isolated hepatocytes and Kupfer cells in iron metabolism: A possible role of ferritin as an iron carrier protein, *Hepatology* **8**:296–301.

Sieff, C., Bicknell, D., Cairne, G., Robinson, J., Lam, G., and Greaves, M. (1982). Changes in cell surface antigen expression during hematopoietic differentiation, *Blood* **60**:703–713.

Speyer, B., and Fielding, J. (1979). Ferritin as a cytosol iron transport intermediate in human reticulocytes, *Brit. J. Haematol.* **42**:255–267.

Stearne, P. A., Pietersz, G. A., and Goding, J. W. (1985). cDNA cloning of the murine transferrin receptor: Sequence of trans-membrane and adjacent regions, *J. Immunol.* **134**:3474–3479.

Sullivan, A. L., Grasso, J. A., and Weintraub, L. R. (1976). Micropinocytosis of transferrin by developing red cells: An electron microscopic study utilizing ferritin-conjugated antibodies to transferrin, *Blood* **47**:133–143.

Surgenor, D. M., Koechlin, B. A., and Strong, L. E. (1949). Chemical, clinical, and immunological studies on the products of human plama fractionation. XXXVII. The metal-combining globulin of human plasma, *J. Clin. Invest.* **28**:73–78.

Sutherland, R., Delia, D., Schneider, C., Newman, R., Kemshead, J., and Greaves, M. (1981). Ubiquitous cell-surface glycoprotein on tumor cells is proliferation-associated receptor for transferrin, *Proc. Nat. Acad. Sci. (U.S.A.)* **78**:4515–4519.

Taketani, S., Tanaka-Yoshioka, A., Masaki, R., Toshiro, Y., and Tokunaga, R. (1986). Association of ferrochelatase with complex I in bovine heart mitochondria, *Biochim. Biophys. Acta* **883**:277–283.

Tangeras, A. (1985). Mitochondrial iron not bound to heme and iron-sulfur centers and its availability for heme synthesis in vitro, *Biochim. Biophys. Acta* **843**:199–207.

Tangeras, A. (1986). Effect of decreased ferrochelatase activity on iron and porphyrin content in mitochondria of mice with porphyria induced by griseofulvin, *Biochim. Biophys. Acta* **882**:77–84.

Tangeras, A., Flatmark, T., Bäckström, D., and Ehrenberg, A. (1980). Mitochondrial iron not bound in heme and iron-sulfur centers. Estimation, compartmentation and redox state, *Biochim. Biophys. Acta* **589**:162–175.

Testa, U., Louache, F., Titeux, M., Thomopoulos, P., and Rochant, H. (1985). The iron-chelating agent picolinic acid enhances transferrin receptor expression in human erythroleukemic cell lines, *Brit. J. Haematol.* **60**:491–502.

Theil, E. C. (1987). Ferritin: Structure, gene regulation, and cellular function in animals, plants, and microorganisms, *Ann. Rev. Biochem.* **56**:289–315.

Theil, E. C., and Aisen, P. (1987). The storage and transport of iron in animal cells, *Iron Transport in Microbes, Plants and Animals* (G. Winkelmann, D. van der Helm, and J. B. Neilands, Eds.), Weinheim, VCH, New York, pp. 491–520.

Thorstensen, K., and Romslo, I. (1984a). Uptake of iron from transferrin by isolated hepatocytes, *Biochim. Biophys. Acta* **804**:200–208.

Thorstensen, K., and Romslo, I. (1984b). Albumin prevents nonspecific transferrin binding and iron uptake by isolated hepatocytes, *Biochim. Biophys. Acta* **804**:393–397.

Thorstensen, K., and Romslo, I. (1987). Uptake of iron from transferrin by isolated hepatocytes. The effect of cellular energy metabolism on the intracellular distribution of iron and transferrin, *Scand. J. Clin. Lab. Invest.* **47**:837–846.

Thorstensen, K., and Romslo, I. (1988). Uptake of iron from transferrin by isolated rat hepatocytes. A redox-mediated plasma membrane process?, *J. Biol. Chem.* **263**:8844–8850.

Trakshel, G. M., Rowley, P. T., and Maines, M. D. (1987). Regulation of the activity of heme degradative enzymes in K562 erythroleukemic cells: Induction by thymidine, *Exp. Hematol.* **15**:859–863.

Trepel, J. B., Colamonici, O. R., Kelly, K., Schwab, G., Watt, R. A., Sausville, E. A., Jaffe, E. S., and Neckers, L. M. (1987). Transcriptional inactivation of c-**mgc** and the transferrin receptor in dibutyryl cyclic AMP-treated HL-60 cells, *Mol. Cell. Biol.* **7**:2644–2648.

Trinder, D., Morgan, E. H., and Baker, E. (1986). The mechanism of iron uptake by fetal rat hepatocytes in culture, *Hepatology* **6**:852–858.

Trinder, D., Morgan, E. H., and Baker, E. (1988). The effects of an antibody to the rat transferrin receptor and of rat serum albumin on the uptake of diferric transferrin by rat hepatocytes, *Biochim. Biophys. Acta* **943**:440–446.

Trowbridge, I. S., and Omary, M. B. (1981). Human cell surface glycoprotein related to cell proliferation is the receptor for transferrin, *Proc. Nat. Acad. Sci. (U.S.A.)* **78**:3039–3043.

Tsao, M.-S., Sanders, G. H. S., and Grisham, J. W. (1987). Regulation of growth of cultured hepatic epithelial cells by transferrin, *Exp. Cell Res.* **171**:52–62.

Ulvik, R. J. (1982). Relevance of ferritin binding sites on isolated mitochondria to the mobilization of iron from ferritin, *Biochim. Biophys. Acta* **715**:42–51.

Ulvik, R. J., and Romslo, I. (1978). Studies on the utilization of ferritin iron in the ferrochelatase reaction of isolated rat liver mitochondria, *Biochim. Biophys. Acta* **541**:251–262.

Ulvik, R. J., and Romslo, I. (1979). Studies on the mobilization of iron from ferritin by isolated rat liver mitochondria, *Biochim. Biophys. Acta* **588**:256–271.

van Renswoude, J., Bridges, K. R., Harford, J. B., and Klausner, R. D. (1982). Receptor-mediated endocytosis of transferrin and the uptake of Fe in K562 cells. Identification of a non-lysosomal acidic compartment, *Proc. Nat. Acad. Sci. (U.S.A.)* **79**:6186–6190.

Walsh, R. J., Thomas, E. D., Chow, S. K., Fluharty, R. G., and Finch, C. A. (1949). Iron metabolism: Heme synthesis in vitro by immature erythrocytes, *Science* **110**:396–398.

Ward, J., Kushner, J., and Kaplan, J. (1982a). Regulation of HeLa Cell transferrin receptors, *J. Biol. Chem.* **257**:10317–10323.

Ward, J. H., Jordan, I., Kushner, J. P., and Kaplan, J. (1984). Heme regulation of HeLa cell transferrin receptor number, *J. Biol. Chem.* **259**:13235–13240.

Ward, J. H., Kushner, J. P., and Kaplan, J. (1982b). Transferrin receptors of human fibroblasts. Analysis of receptor properties and regulation, *Biochem. J.* **208**:19–26.

Watts, C. (1985). Rapid endocytosis of the transferrin receptor in the absence of bound transferrin, *J. Cell Biol.* **100**:633–637.

Waxman, H. S., Freedman, M. L., and Rabinovitz, M. (1967). Studies with Fe-59 labeled hemin on the control of polyribosome formation in rabbit reticulocytes, *Biochim. Biophys. Acta* **145**:353–360.

Waxman, H. S., and Rabinovitz, M. (1966). Control of reticulocyte polyribosome content and hemoglobin synthesis by heme, *Biochim. Biophys. Acta* **129**:369–379.

Wheby, M. S., and Jones, L. (1963). Role of transferrin in iron absorption, *J. Clin. Invest.* **42**:1007–1016.

White, G. P., and Jacobs, A. (1978). Iron uptake by Chang cells from transferrin, nitrilotri-acetate and citrate complexes, *Biochim. Biophys. Acta* **543**:217–225.

White, K., and Munro, H. N. (1988). Induction of ferritin subunit synthesis by iron is regulated at both the transcriptional and translational levels, *J. Biol. Chem.* **263**:8938–8942.

Wilczynska, A., Ponka, P., and Schulman, H. M. (1984). Transferrin receptors and iron utilization in DMSO-inducible and uninducible Friend erythroleukemia cells, *Exp. Cell Res.* **154**:561–566.

Wilczynska, A., and Schulman, H. M. (1980). Friend erythroleukemia cell membrane transferrin receptors, *Canad. J. Biochem.* **58**:935–940.

Williams, J., and Moreton, K. (1980). The distribution of iron between the metal binding sites of transferrin in human serum, *Biochem. J.* **185**:438–448.

Witt, D. P., and Woodworth, R. C. (1978). Identification of the transferrin receptor of the rabbit reticulocyte, *Biochemistry* **17**:3913–3917.

Worwood, M., Dawkins, S., Wagstaff, M., and Jacobs, A. (1976). The purification and properties of ferritin from human serum, *Biochem. J.* **157**:97–103.

Wrigglesworth, J. M., and Baum, H. (1980). The biochemical functions of iron, *Iron in Biochemistry and Medicine* (A. Jacobs and M. Worwood, Eds.), Academic, London, Vol. II, pp. 29–86.

Wright, T. L., Brissot, P., Ma, W. L., and Weisiger, R. A. (1986). Characterization of non-transferrin-bound iron clearance by rat liver, *J. Biol. Chem.* **261**:10909–10914.

Wright, T. L., Fitz, J. G., and Weisiger, R. A. (1988). Non-transferrin-bound iron uptake by rat liver. Role of membrane potential difference, *J. Biol. Chem.* **263**:1842–1847.

Yamamura, T., Hagiwara, S., Nakazato, K., and Satake, K. (1984). Cooper complexes at N- and C-site of ovotransferrin: Quantitative determination and visible absorption spectrum of each complex, *Biochem. Biophys. Res. Comm.* **119**:298–304.

Yeoh, G. C. T., and Morgan, E. H. (1979). Dimethylsulfoxide induction of transferrin receptors on Friend erythroleukemia cells, *Cell Differentiation* **8**:331–343.

Young, S. P. (1982). Evidence for the functional equivalence of the iron-binding sites of rat transferrin, *Biochim. Biophys. Acta* **718**:35–41.

Young, S. P., and Aisen, P. (1980). The interaction of transferrin with isolated hepatocytes, *Biochim. Biophys. Acta* **633**:145–153.

Young, S. P., and Aisen, P. (1981). Transferrin receptors and the uptake and release of iron by isolated hepatocytes, *Heptology* **1**:114–119.

Young, S. P., Bomford, A., and Williams, R. (1984). The effect of the iron saturation of transferrin on its binding and uptake by rabbit reticulocytes, *Biochem. J.* **219**:505–510.

Zahringer, J., Baliga, B. S., and Munro, H. N. (1976). Novel mechanism for translational control in regulation of ferritin synthesis by iron, *Proc. Nat. Acad. Sci. (U.S.A.)* **73**:857–861.

Zak, O., Leibman, A., and Aisen, P. (1983). Metal-binding properties of a single-sited transferrin fragment, *Biochim. Biophys. Acta* **742**:490–495.

Zaman, Z., Heynen, M.-J., and Verwilghen, R. L. (1980). Studies on the mechanism of transferrin iron uptake by rat reticulocytes, *Biochim. Biophys. Acta* **632**:553–561.

Zucker, W. V., and Schulman, H. M. (1968). Stimulation of globin chain initiation by hemin in the reticulocyte cell-free system, *Proc. Nat. Acad. Sci.* **59**:582–589.

Transport of Tetrapyrroles: Mechanisms and Biological and Regulatory Consequences

Ann Smith

I. Introduction

A. General concepts of tetrapyrrole transport

Biological transport processes require a series of ordered interactions to take place, each of which involves molecular recognition. As with most cellular processes these recognition phenomena require the action of specific proteins. Here, the mechanism of the processes involved in transport of tetrapyrroles (when known) will be discussed as well as the ligand-protein interactions necessary for transport. Because heme* is a reactive, lipophilic molecule, several proteins (see Table 9.1) have evolved to direct the chemistry of its reactive iron and to maintain the heme in a

---

*Heme is used here to refer to iron-protoporphyrin. Depending on the valence of the iron, the prefix ferro- for divalent iron and ferri- for trivalent iron will be used. Ferro-protoporphyrin (strictly heme) contains divalent iron but possesses no net charge, whereas ferri-protoporphyrin, or hemin, has a net positive charge, forms salts, and is usually obtained as the chloride (hemin chloride). Free heme in solution is rapidly oxidized to hemin. In the presence of excess alkali, hemin gives rise to a divalent anion of ferri-protoporphyrin hydroxide in which the two propionic acid carboxyl groups are ionized, and the iron is coordinated with the hydroxyl group of the base and to 1 mol of water. If hemin is dissolved in excess alkali and then titrated with acid, the compound precipitates when 2 mol of acid have been added, producing the neutral compound hematin, also called hydroxyhemin or ferri-protoporphyrin hydroxide.

TABLE 9.1   Summary of Mammalian Heme-Proteins and Heme Binding Proteins

Location	Heme-proteins	Heme binding proteins
Serum		Hemopexin
		Albumin
		Histidine-rich glycoprotein
Plasma membrane		MHBP of the HPX system (liver)
		Heme receptor (enterocytes)
		Heme receptor (K562, MEL cells)
		Myelin basic protein*
Cytosol	Hemoglobin	Tryptophan pyrrolase
	Myoglobin	GSH-S transferases
		eIF 2-α kinase
		Guanylate cyclase
		Z class of proteins
		Catalase monomers
Endoplasmic Reticulum	Cytochrome b_5	Heme oxygenase
	Cytochrome P450	
	Prostaglandin H synthase	
Mitochondria	Cytochrome b_2	ALA synthase
	Cytochrome c	Ferrochelatase
	Cytochrome oxidase	
Other organelles	Catalase	?
	Peroxidases	

*The published stoichiometries of one heme bound by more than 6 or 25 myelin basic protein molecules and the admission that most of the protein examined may have been denatured (Morris et al., 1987) makes the claim that this is a heme binding protein somewhat premature.

soluble, monomeric state in aqueous environments. Similarly, tetrapyrrole intermediates in heme metabolism such as the porphyrinogens and their oxidized products, porphyrins, are reactive, lipophilic molecules; and their interaction with proteins guides their movement both inside and outside the cell.

The transport of tetrapyrroles in mammalian cells takes place across many different kinds of membranes via a variety of mechanisms. For example, at the cell surface, receptor-mediated endocytosis of heme-hemopexin is part of the process involved in transporting heme across the plasma membrane of hepatocytes. Intracellularly, transport of heme takes place across mitochondrial membranes during heme synthesis and across the lysosomal membrane during hemoglobin catabolism. Intracellular transport of heme is needed to move heme from intracellular organelles to heme oxygenase in the endoplasmic reticulum, to move heme within the mitochondrial inner membrane space for heme-protein synthesis and from mitochondria to apoproteins in the endoplasmic reticulum, cytosol, and organelles. The intracellular route(s) for heme catabolism and the proteins involved remain to be defined.

Similarly, the mechanism whereby biliverdin reaches cytosolic biliverdin reductase, whereby tetrapyrroles such as bilirubin are excreted from liver parenchymal cells into bile canaliculi, and whereby porphyrins and porphyrinogens overproduced in porphyria reach the gut and kidney are as yet ill-defined. Moreover, when normal metabolic systems are overloaded, heme can even be excreted intact in bile. Bilirubin is also transported *into* hepatocytes for the glucuronidation necessary for its elimination from the body. Another pertinent area is the delineation of the transport route and identification of the proteins involved in the regulation of expression by heme of cellular proteins. For example, it has recently been shown that heme in the nucleus regulates the transcription of heme oxygenase in mammalian cells.

Since the pathways by which heme is synthesized, utilized, or degraded are subject to genetic aberrations or metabolic perturbations, therapies employing analogues of heme and porphyrins have been developed. These include hematin infusion to treat certain forms of porphyria and the use of the heme analogue, Sn-protoporphyrin, to mitigate neonatal jaundice. In addition, the reactivity of porphyrins activated by exposure to light has been exploited to develop a photodynamic therapy of cancer. However, in many instances lack of knowledge concerning the transport of heme, porphyrins, and their analogues and the cellular consequences of this transport has hindered rational development of these therapies.

B. Physiological roles of heme transport

The transport to the liver of heme by hemopexin (Smith and Morgan, 1978, 1979; Davies et al., 1979; Smith and Morgan, 1981) and of hemoglobin by haptoglobin (Higa et al., 1981) are receptor-mediated processes which facilitate the degradation of heme and conservation of its iron. Hemopexin and haptoglobin form important links between heme and iron metabolism. Thus, the transport of heme by hemopexin, of hemoglobin by haptoglobin, and of iron by transferrin can be considered to be functionally related systems which act together to maintain iron homeostasis by the liver (Smith and Ledford, 1988; and see Fig. 9.1).

The hepatic reclamation of heme plays a significant role in three areas: conserving iron, aiding "nutritional immunity," and preventing toxic heme effects. In this regard, it is notable that hemopexin (0.5 to 1.2 g/L), haptoglobin (1.2 to 3 g/L), and transferrin (2 to 4 g/L) together form the third most-abundant group of plasma proteins after albumin (35 to 55 g/L) and the immunoglobulins (8 to 18 g/L). In fact, the circulating levels of the three transport proteins are comparable to those of the protease inhibitors, α_1-antitrypsin (1.9 to 3.5 g/L) and α_2-macroglobulin (1.5 to 3.5 g/L), and of complement C3 (0.6 to 1.2 g/L).

The majority of senescent erythrocytes are taken up by the cells of the reticulo-endothelial system, for example, macrophages and hepatic

Kupffer cells. However, intravascular hemolysis occurs continuously as a result of normal "wear and tear" on the red blood cells and accounts daily for about 10% of red cell breakdown (Garby and Noyes, 1959). This intravascular hemolysis is enhanced in several pathological conditions, for example, in the hemolytic anemias (Muller-Eberhard, 1970), in other hemolytic diseases (Sears, 1968; Muller-Eberhard et al., 1968), in certain viral infections (Sitbon et al., 1986), and in patients with mechanical hemolysis caused by intracardiac prosthetic devices or heart valve dis-

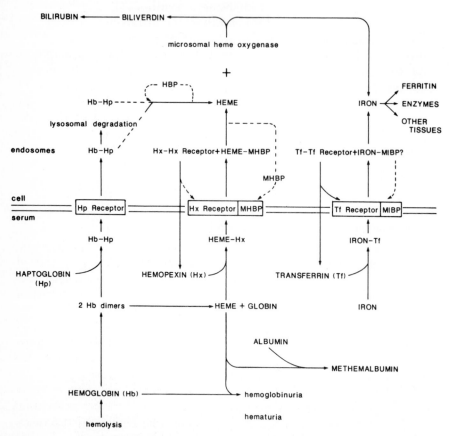

Figure 9.1 Physiological role of hemopexin and haptoglobin in hepatic heme transport and metabolism. This diagram depicts the basic features of the interactions of heme-hemopexin, hemoglobin-haptoglobin, and iron-transferrin with the liver parenchymal cell. It is not known whether heme from hemopexin and heme released from catabolism of hemoglobin-haptoglobin in lysosomes join a common pool, or whether there is an equivalent to MHBP in the haptoglobin system, shown here as HBP. Many details are of necessity omitted from this simplified picture, for example, the subcellular organelles which operate in certain of the steps. MIBP denotes the membrane iron binding protein of Glass et al. (1980).

eases (Eyster et al., 1972). The series of events illustrated in Fig. 9.1 describes the biochemical consequences of intravascular hemolysis and subsequent hepatic transport of heme. This description is supported by clinical observations on patients, by experiments with animals and cells, and by binding studies in vitro using purified proteins. Further details of the transport processes involved are presented in subsequent sections.

After rupture of red blood cells the tetrameric hemoglobin molecules are released and dissociate into two α-β dimers which are then bound to the two β subunits of haptoglobin. The complex interacts through the haptoglobin moiety with a specific receptor on liver parenchymal cells (Kino et al., 1980). After uptake by receptor-mediated endocytosis, the complex is transported to the lysosomes where both hemoglobin and haptoglobin are degraded (Higa et al., 1981). This accounts for the large reduction of serum haptoglobin levels by only mild hemolysis (Hershko, 1975). In fact, the lysis of less than 5 mL of erythrocytes can produce sufficient hemoglobin to exhaust circulating haptoglobin. Haptoglobin depletion can occur much faster than its increase as an acute phase reactant (Warkentin et al., 1987) and allows hemoglobin to circulate as the oxidized form, methemoglobin. Heme dissociates from methemoglobin (K_d 200 nM; Banerjee, 1962) and becomes available for binding by hemopexin and albumin (Hrkal et al., 1974; Muller-Eberhard and Morgan, 1975), the major heme-binding proteins of serum (Table 9.1). Detailed studies in vitro (Bunn and Jandl, 1968; Hrkal et al., 1974; Morgan et al., 1976) have established the relative affinities of globin, hemopexin, and albumin for heme. Albumin binds heme with one high-affinity binding site, K_d 10 nM and two lower-affinity binding sites, K_d ca. 1 μM (Beaven et al., 1974). Heme is bound by hemopexin with a much higher affinity, K_d < 1 pM (Hrkal et al., 1974); and at equilibrium, 50 to 70% of methemoglobin heme is bound to equimolar hemopexin. Even at physiological ratios of albumin and hemopexin (70 albumin : 1 heme : 1 hemopexin), heme is transferred to hemopexin (Morgan et al., 1976; Pasternack et al., 1983). Thus, a complex dynamic redistribution is set up in the circulation as the heme moiety of methemoglobin partitions among globin, hemopexin, and albumin according to the relative affinities of these proteins for heme; but heme-hemopexin formation quickly predominates (Morgan et al., 1976). Albumin appears only to store heme before transport to the liver as heme-hemopexin (Smith and Morgan, 1978, 1979).

Heme-hemopexin complexes interact with a specific receptor on liver parenchymal cells to effect rapid uptake of heme. Whereas there is evidence for hemopexin receptors in human placenta (Taketani et al., 1987a), promyelocytic HL-60 cells (Taketani et al., 1987b), and eythroleukemic K562 cells (Taketani et al., 1986), experiments in vivo demonstrated that hepatic uptake predominates in normal, nonpregnant iron-replete animals (Smith and Morgan, 1979). Heme from hemoglobin-haptoglobin or heme-hemopexin ultimately reaches the endoplasmic reticulum where it is degraded by heme oxygenase. The iron released from heme enters the cellular iron pool (Smith and Ledford, 1988) and, contingent on the iron status of the cell, is re-utilized (Smith and Ledford, 1988) or stored on ferritin (Davies et al., 1979). Depending on the extent of heme uptake, some intact heme reaches the nucleus for transcriptional regulation (Alam et al., 1989, Alam and Smith, 1989). Another suggested fate for heme is incorporation into apoheme-proteins in the endoplasmic reticulum and cytosol (Bhat et al., 1977; Badawy, 1979; Correia et al., 1981).

The importance of iron in the pathogenesis of infection and neoplasia is established (Letendre, 1985). When microorganisms invade the vertebrate host, or when neoplastic cells disseminate, iron availability affects establishment of the diseases. "Nutritional immunity" is the term used to describe sequestration of iron by transferrin (Kochan, 1973) to resist invading organisms (Weinberg, 1984). Binding of heme-iron and its removal from the circulation by haptoglobin (Eaton et al., 1982) is also part of this vital defense system to which hemopexin and membrane heme binding proteins, including that of the hemopexin system (MHBP), can now be added. The role of erythrocyte-hemoglobin and cells of the reticuloendothelial system in these processes is well recognized [for recent reviews see Letendre (1985) and Ward (1986)], but the contribution of the liver to iron sequestration, especially in hemolytic states, is virtually ignored. This is surprising since several strains of virulent *Staphylococci* produce hemolysins as part of their mechanism of infection (Hebert and Hancock, 1985), and certain strains of bacteria such as *Haemophilus influenzae* require heme for growth (Evans et al., 1974). Presumably, hemopexin and haptoglobin evolved in part to help combat this type of infection, and the potential importance of hepatic heme transport in this area is underappreciated.

Furthermore, the hepatic transport mediated by hemopexin and haptoglobin acts to prevent the potentially toxic effects of heme. Heme (ferrous protoporphyrin IX) is a reactive low molecular weight form of iron able to participate in oxygen radical reactions which can lead to the degradation of proteins (Aft and Mueller, 1984), lipids (Tappel, 1955), carbohydrates (Gutteridge, personal communication), and DNA (Aft and Mueller, 1983). Oxidative damage to tissues has been implicated in the pathology of several human diseases and, as a consequence of reperfusion to lung and kidney, also in cerebral trauma or ischemia [for recent reviews, see Halliwell (1987) and Halliwell and Gutteridge (1986)]. Inside cells antioxidant defenses are primarily concerned with removing reactive oxygen species formed during aerobic metabolism. For this purpose the cell relies on superoxide dismutase, glutathione peroxidase, and catalase enzymes. However, in extracellular fluids these enzymes are not present, and different mechanisms from those found inside the cell must be relied on to limit radical reactions (Gutteridge, 1982; Halliwell and Gutteridge, 1986). This is done by converting pro-oxidant forms of iron into less- or nonreactive forms by binding them to proteins. Some of these antioxidants (e.g., haptoglobin) are acute-phase proteins whose metabolism changes in response to tissue damage.

Transferrin (considered an acute-phase plasma protein) and lactoferrin (present in milk, epithelial cell secretions, and mature granulocytes) inhibit iron-catalyzed oxygen radical reactions (Gutteridge et al., 1981). Hemoglobin and other heme-proteins release catalytic iron (heme) in the presence of peroxides (Gutteridge, 1986); and haptoglobin, by binding hemoglobin, prevents this (Gutteridge, 1987). Similarly, heme binding by hemopexin prevents hemin-mediated lipid peroxidation (Gutteridge and Smith, 1988) since hemopexin avidly binds both ferrous and ferric-proto-porphyrin (Morgan and Vickery, 1978). Hemopexin's role as an extracellular antioxidant is supported by its being an acute-phase reactant in rodents (Merriman et al., 1978; Carmel and Gross, 1977; Baumann et al., 1984, 1987; Baumann and Muller-Eberhard, 1987), although not perhaps in humans (Kushner et al., 1972).

Heme's toxic effects are diverse. Heme deposits have been found in kidney and cardiovascular tissues in pathological conditions (Braun et al., 1970; Lips et al., 1978). Direct inhibitory effects of heme have also been shown on mitochondria (Keller and Romslo, 1978), on platelet aggregation and lymphocyte mitogenicity (Malik et al., 1983), and on the activity of thrombin and plasmin (Green et al., 1983). Indirect effects of repeated doses of heme on drug-metabolizing enzymes have also been reported (Muller-Eberhard et al., 1983), and heme has been shown to diminish the structural stability of erythrocyte membrane skeletons, perhaps accounting for the enhanced fragility of erythrocytes in certain hereditary hemolytic anemias (Liu et al., 1985). Ferri-heme is a potent lytic agent for erythrocytes and parasites, probably by a chemiosmotic mechanism (Orjih et al., 1981), and its release upon infection by malarial parasites has been postulated to produce free radicals and other toxic substances (Janney et al., 1986). However, many of these inhibitory effects of heme were found using in vitro assays in the absence of physiological concentrations of hemopexin and albumin, or using heme solutions after storage under conditions (e.g., in aqueous solution in air) known to affect deleteriously the stability of heme (Goetsch and Bissell, 1986), or using concentrated, aggregated stock solutions (e.g., 0.2 to 0.02 M) that even upon dilution do not allow binding by proteins.

The extracellular transport of heme, the requirement for heme-transporting proteins, and the cellular processes involved in the intracellular movement of heme and its metabolites will each be discussed in turn.

II. Heme Transport from Extracellular Sources

A. Receptor-mediated transport of heme

1. Heme-hemopexin. Hemopexin is a single-chain plasma glycoprotein (molecular weight 60,000, Seery et al., 1972) which binds heme tightly in stoichiometric amounts to form a pink-orange-colored complex (Hrkal and Muller-Eberhard, 1971). Heme-hemopexin is a low-spin heme-protein complex (Morgan and Vickery, 1978) in which heme is bound via noncovalent coordination of the heme-iron atom by two histidine residues (Morgan and Muller-Eberhard, 1972; Morgan and Vickery, 1978) as in the so-called b-type cytochromes (Smith and Williams, 1970). However, no amino acid sequence homology of hemopexin with these b-type cytochromes is known. This is not so surprising since the former is a plasma protein, while many of the latter are integral membrane proteins.

The role for hemopexin in heme catabolism was originally proposed from two types of observations: first, the injections of hematin increase the fractional catabolic rate of hemopexin and the plasma clearance of the protein (Lane et al., 1972, 1983; Wochner et al., 1974; Liem et al., 1975); and, second, that in certain human hemolytic states hemopexin concentrations are decreased (Muller-Eberhard et al., 1968; Muller-Eberhard, 1970; Engler and Jayle, 1976), while the catabolism of hemopexin is increased (Wochner et al., 1974; Foidart et al., 1983). However, after injection of hematin, the reported plasma half-clearance times of hemopexin are unusually long, 0.8 days in humans (Wochner et al., 1974), 7 to 8 h in rabbits (Liem et al., 1975), and 5 to 6 h in rats (Liem, 1976), compared with other receptor-mediated processes. For example, clearance times of 10 to 30 min for hemoglobin-haptoglobin (Garby and Noyes, 1959; Freeman, 1964) and 90 to 100 s for asialo-fetuin (LaBadie et al., 1975) have been reported. On the other hand, after separate injection of radiolabeled heme or hemopexin (but not as a complex), radioisotope was found only in liver parenchymal cells (Muller-Eberhard et al., 1970), consistent with the known function of these cells in receptor-mediated uptake.

The first direct evidence for receptor-mediated transport of heme by hemopexin came from studies in rats employing tracer doses of stoichiometric complexes of ^{59}Fe-heme–^{125}I-hemopexin (Smith and Morgan, 1979). It was shown that hemopexin transports heme to the liver in a manner that is rapid and saturable. The association occurs within minutes, on the same time scale as receptor-mediated uptake of iron-transferrin complexes (Gardiner and Morgan, 1974). Furthermore, the association of hemopexin with the liver during heme uptake is a saturable process, indicative of an interaction with a finite number of sites and characteristic of receptor-mediated uptake. Rat ^{59}Fe-heme–^{125}I-hemopexin complexes (700 pmol/rat) associate rapidly and exclusively with the liver after intravenous (IV) injection into anesthetized male rats. However, the two isotopes exhibit different patterns of accumulation. Liver ^{125}I-labeled hemopexin reaches a maximum (20 ± 4.9 pmol/g liver) 10 min after injection and then declines by 2 h to the low values (ca. 3 pmol/g liver) seen after injection of the apoprotein. In contrast, ^{59}Fe-heme accumulates in the liver for at least 2 h, with more than 60% of the injected dose already taken up by 1 h (Smith and Morgan, 1979). Moreover, there is a reciprocal relationship between the liver and serum ^{125}I concentration. Since hemopexin undergoes no extensive proteolysis while transporting, hemopexin was proposed to recycle back to the circulation (Smith and Morgan, 1978, 1979), like transferrin (Morgan, 1964).

These studies have now been extended to include isolated hepatocytes in suspension (Smith and Morgan, 1981), plasma membranes (Tran-Quang et al., 1983; Smith and Morgan, 1984b), and more recently to

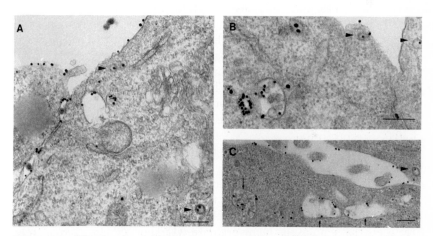

Figure 9.2 Ultrastructural localization of colloidal gold-labeled heme-hemopexin in human Hep G2 cells. Human Hep G2 cells were incubated with a conjugate of heme-hemopexin and colloidal gold (20-nm diameter) for 1 h at 4°C. The cells were then washed free of unbound ligand and warmed at 37°C for 5 (panel A), 10 (panel B), or 40 min (panel C) in the presence of excess unlabeled heme-hemopexin. The cells were then fixed in glutaraldehyde, postfixed in osmium tetroxide, embedded and stained in lead citrate and uranyl acetate. Five minutes after warming, gold-hemopexin is associated with coated vesicles (arrowheads) as well as the cell surface and larger uncoated vesicles. After 10 min, vesicles which are heavily labeled with gold-hemopexin are seen fusing with multivesicular bodies. Arrowheads indicate coated vesicles. After 40 min, some coated vesicles are still taking up gold-hemopexin (arrowheads), which is also associated with large uncoated vesicles withmany (downward arrow) or a few (upward arrows) internal vesicles. Bars are equivalent to 0.25 μm.

cultured hepatoma cells (Smith and Ledford, 1988). In both human Hep
G2 hepatoma and mouse Hepa cells (the parental line derived from the
solid hepatoma BW7756, Bernard et al., 1973), endocytosis of colloidal
gold-labeled heme-hemopexin has been demonstrated by electron microscopy (Fig. 9.2). Hemopexin was found in coated pits, coated endosomes, and multivesicular bodies, all subcellular fractions of the classical
pathway of endocytosis, but was not found in lysosomes (Smith and
Hunt, 1989). Preliminary evidence that heme from heme-hemopexin
reaches endosomes was obtained from a limited series of studies using
isopycnic gradients (Smith, 1985; Smith et al., 1988). Bound hemopexin
is sensitive to pronase after incubation at 4°C, but resistant after
incubation at 37°C, confirming that hemopexin binds to the receptor on
the cell surface at 4°C and the intracellular location of the hemopexin
after endocytosis at 37°C (Smith and Hunt, 1989).

The subcellular distribution and metabolic fate of ^{59}Fe-heme–[125]I-
hemopexin have been examined in rats (Davies et al., 1979; Smith, 1985).
Significant amounts of radiolabel from the heme were found in the
nuclear fraction, increasing slightly over 2 h. Heme was also associated
with the mitochondria and with the microsomal fraction containing
plasma membranes and endoplasmic reticulum (ER). The amount of
both ^{125}I and ^{59}Fe decreased steadily from the microsomal fraction with
time, consistent with a transfer of heme-hemopexin complex, possibly
from the plasma membrane or endosomes. In the cytosol, iron rapidly
accumulated and was incorporated into ferritin within 10 min after IV
injection at a linear rate of 30 pmol/h/g liver. Two additional cytosolic
protein fractions containing at least 50% of the radiolabel as intact
radioactive heme had apparent molecular weights of more than 60,000
and 40,000 respectively.

The influence of hemopexin on the tissue distribution of heme and the
fate of its iron has been extensively studied. However, because of the
dynamic distribution of heme between circulating plasma proteins, there
are problems inherent in attempting to study heme uptake by liver and
pharmacokinetics of heme after injection in vivo of either hematin, the
more recently employed heme-arginate (Linden et al., 1987), free
hemoglobin (Wyman et al., 1986), or heme liposomes (Cannon et al.,
1987). Second, the route of heme administration and dose administered
affect heme metabolism. The results in Table 9.2 are based on a recent
thorough pharmacokinetic analysis of the tissue distribution of radiolabel after administration of [14]C- and ^{59}Fe-labeled heme-arginate either
intravenously or intramuscularly to rabbits (Linden et al., 1987). The IV
route is assumed here to rapidly generate heme-hemopexin. Importantly,
the route clearly alters the distribution of heme to various tissues, the
amount of bilirubin produced, and the amount of iron stored or incorpo-

rated into Hb. For example, after IV injection, more iron is present in the blood, liver, and bone marrow of the sternum than after intramuscular (IM) administration when more iron is present in the spleen. Only 1% of the dose was found in erythrocytes within the first 24 h. The rapid decrease of both isotopes after IV injection, the retention of ^{59}Fe by the liver and excretion of the ^{14}C of the porphyrin ring in the bile, is reminiscent of the distribution of heme seen after intravenous heme-hemopexin in rats (Morgan and Smith, 1979; Davies et al., 1979). Because the dose of heme given to the rabbits was high (5 mg/kg), normal transport and metabolism mechanisms are overloaded, and about 10% of the heme was excreted unchanged in bile, as observed also in rats given 5 to 40 mg heme/kg (Petryka et al., 1977).

Although the available evidence indicates that hemopexin transports heme predominantly to the liver, radioactivity found in the spleen and femur bone marrow is consistent with a low-capacity uptake with recycling of hemopexin (Smith and Morgan, 1979). Hemopexin receptors have been identified in nonhepatic tissues by binding and heme uptake studies in human promyelocytic HL-60 and erythroleukemic K562 cells. HL-60 cells express 42,000 receptors on their surface, K_d 1 nM (Taketani et al., 1987b). K562 cells have only 8000 hemopexin receptors per cell, K_d 5 nM (Taketani et al., 1986), perhaps connected to the fact that K562 cells express high levels of the transferrin receptor (200,000 surface receptors per cell, Hunt et al., 1984). Mouse Hepa cells express 35,000

TABLE 9.2   Effect of Route of Administration of Radiolabeled Heme-Arginate on Subsequent Transport and Metabolism of Its ^{14}C- and ^{59}Fe-Heme

Tissue	Ratio of ^{59}Fe : ^{14}C*	
	Intravenous	Intramuscular
Blood	3.0	1.9
Liver	6.7	1.8
Kidney	3.5	2.1
Bone marrow		
Sternum	4.4	2.7
Femur	5.1	6.8
Spleen	3.5	6.0
Adrenals	2.3	3.1
Heart	2.3	2.8
Brain	1.2	0.8

*These data were recalculated from those presented in Table 4 of Linden et al. (1987). Radioactive heme-arginate was injected into rabbits using a dose of 5 mg heme/kg. Since this compound splits into heme and arginine as soon as it enters the bloodstream and the volume of distribution of the heme after IV injection is that of plasma, these data allow comparison of heme transport and metabolism by heme-HPX (the IV route) with heme administered intramuscularly. The original data were presented as recovered dpm/g/10 μCi dose in each tissue 24 h after injection.

surface hemopexin receptors, K_d 15 nM (Smith and Ledford, 1988). There is also evidence for a hemopexin receptor in human placental tissue (Taketani et al., 1987a), discussed below.

The possibility that hemopexin might act in the transport of heme from other sources (e.g., myoglobin) remains to be fully examined. Serum hemopexin levels are elevated in Duchenne's muscular dystrophy (Adornato et al., 1978), a condition with abnormal myoglobin metabolism. The role of hemopexin in transporting newly synthesized heme from the liver to other tissues (Bissell et al., 1979; Schmid, 1983) such as brain is interesting but unsubstantiated by direct evidence. In fact, negligible levels of either [14]C- or ^{59}Fe-heme were recovered from the brain after intravenous heme-arginate, suggesting poor penetration of heme across the blood brain barrier (Linden et al., 1987), and arguing against a role for hemopexin in transporting heme to the brain.

It was recently suggested that the heme delivered via hemopexin in HL-60 cells is incorporated intact as the prosthetic group of myeloperoxidase (Taketani et al., 1986). However, since the central heme-iron was radiolabeled and not the porphyrin macrocycle, the data are inconclusive. Incorporation of exogenous heme into this enzyme seems unlikely for several reasons. HO in these cells is rapidly induced and reconstitution was examined at times when catabolism could readily have occurred. Furthermore, the two chlorin prosthetic groups of myeloperoxidase (Sibbett and Hurst, 1984) are structurally distinct from Fe-protoporphyrin IX.

Several lines of evidence demonstrate that hemopexin undergoes conformational changes upon binding heme (Morgan, 1976) which are necessary for recognition by its specific receptor. These changes have been shown using absorbance (Morgan et al., 1976) and circular dichroism spectroscopy (Morgan, 1976; Morgan and Vickery, 1978). In addition, binding of heme protects hemopexin from proteolysis by plasmin, trypsin, and other proteases (Morgan and Smith, 1984). Plasmin produces two functional domains from rabbit, but not human, apoprotein (Smith and Morgan, 1984b). The heme binding domain I from the N terminus and domain II, necessary for receptor recognition (Morgan et al., 1988b), are linked by a "hinge" region in the intact protein (Takahashi et al., 1985). The conformational change which plays a pivotal role in hemopexin function requires the bis-histidyl coordination with heme-iron, produces a marked compaction of the heme binding domain I (Smith et al., 1988; Morgan et al., 1988b), and leads to a tighter association between domains I and II (Morgan and Smith, 1984).

At least three conformational changes, designated types I, II, and III, occur in hemopexin upon heme binding (Smith et al., 1988). Type I is associated with alterations in the environment of tryptophan residues and is reflected by characteristic changes in both the absorbance and CD spectra of hemopexin. For this type of change a bis-histidyl coordination complex and an intact hinge region are necessary but not sufficient conditions. This change arises from an interaction between the domains. The type II change confers resistance to proteolysis of the hinge region and is also produced by heme analogues such as Fe-TPPS (Smith et al., 1988) and Sn-PPIX (Morgan et al., 1988a) which do not effect the type I change. This change requires only the coordination of two histidine residues with the metal-porphyrin (Smith et al., 1988). The type III change increases the affinity of hemopexin for its receptor and requires a bis-histidyl coordination of the heme and the compaction of domain I (Smith et al., 1988). For hemopexin to bind to its receptor, both domains and the change in shape of domain I are required but an intact hinge region is not. It should be noted that conformational changes involving release of heme for transport appear to require the hinge region (Morgan et al., 1988b) and that the plasma clearance of isolated domains is rapid (Morgan and Smith, 1984).

Our current view of the reaction sequence of heme with hemopexin and of the complex with the receptor are shown schematically in Fig. 9.3. Upon binding heme, domain I dramatically changes conformation and assumes a more-compact shape which in turn enhances interactions between the two domains, presumably by producing a surface that is complementary with that of domain II. This renders the hinge region inaccessible to plasmin. Both domains of hemopexin contain features

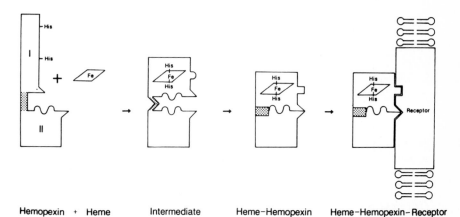

Hemopexin + Heme   Intermediate   Heme-Hemopexin   Heme-Hemopexin-Receptor

Figure 9.3 Schematic representation of the conformational changes which occur in hemopexin upon heme binding resulting in recognition by its specific receptor. Domain I of hemopexin upon binding heme dramatically changes shape and becomes compact. This results in an enhanced interdomain interaction, presumably through complementary surfaces, renders the hinge region between the domains inaccessible to proteases, and stabilizes the protein. Both domains of hemopexin are necessary for full recognition by the receptor. (Reproduced with permission of the *Journal of Biological Chemistry.*)

that are necessary for binding to the hemopexin receptor and heme uptake, as shown by the inhibitory effects on receptor binding of the heme-domain I + II complex and of monoclonal antibodies to either domain (Morgan et al., 1988b).

Two different, but apparently linked, processes of hemopexin-mediated heme uptake have been described in isolated hepatic parenchymal cells and also appear to occur in vivo (Smith and Morgan, 1981). One is defined as the specific transport system. It is saturable, has high affinity, K_d near 50 nM, and exhibits the characteristics of the receptor-mediated system observed in vivo. The second, termed the "selective" transport system, also requires metabolic energy, has a lower affinity, and is not readily saturable. Importantly, it does require hemopexin. Specific and selective hemopexin-mediated heme uptake processes were shown to be distinct by their responses to metabolic inhibitors, and neither mode of heme uptake involved pinocytosis (Smith and Morgan, 1981).

These two uptake processes may reflect two limiting modes of action of the membrane receptor for heme-hemopexin. In the first, the complex bound to the receptor enters the cell via endocytosis (Smith and Hunt, 1989). After transfer of the heme to an intracellular constituent, the apohemopexin recycles to the exterior. In the second mode, the receptor acts at or near the cell surface like an enzyme to catalyze the transfer of heme from hemopexin to a membrane heme binding protein (MHBP) for translocation into the cell. Heme transfer from heme-hemopexin to MHBP takes place in isolated plasma membranes at physiological pH (Smith and Morgan, 1985) and does not require as acidic a pH (5 to 6) as in endosomes.

The smallest heme binding subunit of rabbit liver MHBP has an apparent molecular weight, on SDS-PAGE under reducing conditions, of 17,500 (Smith, 1989a). This protein contains disulfide bonds, has a pI of ca. 5.5, and its amino terminus is blocked. MHBP forms low-spin complexes with heme, as shown by characteristic enhancement and red shift in the α and β bands of its absorbance spectrum upon reduction. Polyclonal, monospecific antibodies to MHBP isolated from rabbit liver plasma membranes inhibit both binding of heme-hemopexin to its receptor and heme uptake in mouse Hepa cells (Smith, 1989a). These goat antibodies cross-react with a heme binding protein in human, mouse, and rat tissues, suggesting that MHBP is highly conserved.

Interestingly, pig liver plasma membranes are reported to contain a 71,000-dalton hemopexin receptor associated with a 16,000-dalton binding subunit (Majuri and Grasbeck, 1986). This receptor migrates as an 80,000-dalton heme binding protein upon gel filtration. The affinity of this receptor for heme-hemopexin is 440 nM. A hemopexin receptor, K_d 66 nM, with an apparent molecular weight of 80,000 on SDS-PAGE under reducing conditions, was isolated from human placenta by cross-linking (Taketani et al., 1987a). Antibodies to this protein inhibit hemopexin binding to HL-60 and K562 cells (Taketani et al., 1987a). Using a variety of hetero-bifunctional cross-linking agents to link iodinated heme-hemopexin complexes to the hemopexin receptor in mouse Hepa cells, evidence was obtained for a 65,000-dalton receptor subunit which may exist as a dimer, under nonreducing conditions (Farooqui et al., 1989). Upon reduction an 18,000-dalton protein remained cross-linked to hemopexin. Whether this 18,000-dalton protein is a small subunit of the hemopexin receptor or MHBP itself is currently under investigation.

Currently, very little is known about the intracellular pathways for guiding heme to heme oxygenase in the endoplasmic reticulum for catabolism. MHBP of the hemopexin transport system appears to play a pivotal role in heme transport (Smith and Morgan, 1985). MHBP-bound heme may be transported in endosomes, since MHBP can still bind heme at pH 5.5 to 6.0 (Smith, 1989a). Certain protein toxins, such as diphtheria toxin, ricin, and abrin, have been shown to penetrate and cross the plasma membrane of cells when the extracellular pH is low (Moskaug et al., 1988), by a process analogous to the normal intracellular release of these toxins after endocytosis and acidification of the maturing endosomes. MHBP may act similarly with a pH-induced conformational change causing release of heme-MHBP into cytosol before interaction with heme oxygenase in the endoplasmic reticulum. Alternatively, uncoated vesicles or multivesicular bodies, still containing heme-MHBP, may ultimately fuse with the endoplasmic reticulum, perhaps after sorting of the vesicles in the Golgi region of the cell. Vesicle fusion is an important route for the transport of many molecules throughout the cell (Rothman and Fine, 1980), and it is tempting to speculate that heme reaches heme oxygenase by fusion of a vesicle with the endoplasmic reticulum. Confinement within vesicles would be an efficient means of compartmentalizing heme. Alternatively, since newly synthesized heme is mobilized from the mitochondria by cytosolic proteins (Israels et al., 1975; Grandchamp et al., 1981; Davies et al., 1982), intracellular transfer of heme for catabolism could be mediated by a cytosolic protein(s) distinct from those transporting newly synthesized heme.

Additional intracellular routes for hemopexin-derived heme exist since, as described in Sect. III-C below, heme delivered via the hemopexin receptor reaches the nucleus for transcriptional regulation of heme oxygenase and, probably, other proteins. Perhaps this intracellular heme pathway is similar to that described for lipophilic glucocorticoids, whereby after binding to cytosolic proteins, translocation to the DNA in the nucleus occurs. These aspects of the intracellular movement of heme via MHBP and other intracellular proteins are currently under investigation.

Hemopexin-mediated heme transport changes in response to cell growth, being significantly greater in the period immediately after seeding and in the early stages of exponential growth (Smith and Ledford, 1988). While the liver is important for iron homeostasis of the body, perhaps cells involved in the immune response, needing to proliferate in rapid response to trauma or infection, express the hemopexin receptor to utilize heme-iron for growth under these pathological conditions when heme-hemopexin is generated. Such cells, possibly monocytes, natural killer cells, and other cells of the immune system, have evolved more than one mechanism to obtain iron and are, in this regard, like pathogenic bacteria which express several mechanisms to absorb iron.

2. Hemoglobin-haptoglobin.   Engulfment of senescent red blood cells by cells of the reticuloendothelial system, including the macrophages of the spleen and lung and the Kupffer cells of the liver, is well recognized as a major route of hemoglobin transport for degradation. However, as mentioned above, intravascular hemolysis of red blood cells occurs in pathological conditions and during the normal wear and tear of red blood cells. Furthermore, hemoglobin is released when tissues are damaged and repair of tissues is continually taking place. Hemoglobin released into the circulation binds immediately with the plasma glycoprotein, haptoglobin, for transport to the liver. One hemoglobin dimer binds to each of the two β subunits of haptoglobin (Higa et al., 1981). Thus, hemoglobin-haptoglobin complexes consist of an α-β (molecular weight 32,000) subunit of hemoglobin bound to each of the β (molecular weight 40,000) subunits of haptoglobin, which are in turn disulfide-linked to the two α subunits (molecular weight 8,900) of haptoglobin (molecular weight 98,000). Although hemoglobin is resistant to proteolysis, haptoglobin can be specifically cleaved by several proteases (Lustbader et al., 1983). However, the stability of haptoglobin to proteases is considerably enhanced when bound to hemoglobin, as is true with many proteins with bound ligand. This enhanced stability in hemoglobin-haptoglobin complexes facilitates the role of haptoglobin as a bacteriostatic agent (Eaton et al., 1982) and extracellular antioxidant (Gutteridge, 1987).

Clearance of ^{125}I-hemoglobin-haptoglobin in rats is rapid, with a plasma half-life of 10 min. Specific receptor-mediated uptake of hemoglobin-haptoglobin complexes occurs exclusively in liver parenchymal cells via interaction of the haptoglobin moiety with its receptor (Kino et al., 1980). The K_d of the association, using isolated rat liver plasma membranes, is 130 nM (Kino et al., 1980). Rapid catabolism of both proteins ensues (Higa et al., 1981). The apparent molecular mass of the degradation products after injection of ^{125}I-[hemoglobin]-haptoglobin or hemoglobin-[125]I-[haptoglobin] into rats suggests that the complexes are cleaved symmetrically into two 82,000-dalton subunits by limited proteolysis in secondary lysosomes before digestion to their constituent amino acids (Higa et al., 1981).

The intracellular path that heme derived from hemoglobin-haptoglobin follows to its site of catabolism is unclear. Density fractionation of liver suggests that haptoglobin-hemoglobin is transferred from low-density vesicles (presumably endosomes) to primary lysosomes by fusion (Higa et al., 1981). The need for an intracellular heme binding protein (HBP, see Fig. 9.1) that targets the heme to heme oxygenase at the endoplasmic reticulum upon its release from hemoglobin-haptoglobin has been postulated (Smith and Ledford, 1988). Whether heme is released from globin at the acidic pH generated during maturation of endosomes or in the lysosomes themselves is unknown. But because of the known stability of hemoglobin to acidic pH, release seems likely to be in the lysosomes. If true, the intracellular pathway of hemoglobin-heme would differ from that of heme delivered by hemopexin.

Though intravenous hemoglobin-haptoglobin is rapidly transported into liver parenchymal cells for degradation, heme delivered by the haptoglobin receptor, like that by the hemopexin receptor (Smith and Ledford, 1988), may have multiple fates, depending on the iron status of the cell. It is also quite possible that at some point the intracellular pathways for heme delivered via the hemopexin and haptoglobin receptors coincide (Fig. 9.1). For example, heme has a role in regulating the expression of heme oxygenase (Alam et al., 1989; Sec. III-C below) and may be incorporated instead of newly synthesized heme to form holo-heme-proteins such as tryptophan pyrrolase and cytochrome P450 (see Sect. III-B and below).

Strong circumstantial evidence for reutilization of hemoglobin-heme by incorporation into hepatic heme proteins has been reported (Wyman et al., 1986). Unfortunately, the role of hemopexin and haptoglobin in the hepatic heme transport processes under investigation were not addressed, hampering interpretation. These investigators injected ^{3}H-hemoglobin or unlabeled hemoglobin mixed with ^{3}H-heme, using the latter mixture as a model for methemoglobin, which they state contains "loosely bound heme." The latter experimental protocol would rapidly produce radiolabeled heme-hemopexin complexes intravenously. In fact, the results show that hepatic uptake of parenterally administered heme (ca. 40 nmol) is more efficient than that of hemoglobin (ca. 450 nmol), whether based on recovery of injected radioactivity, on reconstitution of tryptophan pyrrolase and cytochrome P450 activity, or on incorporation into labeled-allyl-isopropylacetamide-P450-heme-adducts. This supports the reutilization of a portion of the heme after transport to the liver via both the haptoglobin and hemopexin receptors.

3. Heme receptors. Heme receptors from a variety of cell types have been reported but cautious interpretation is required for several reasons. First, binding data per se do not prove the existence of a receptor functioning in transport. Second, heme is not water-soluble (Falk, 1964; Brown et al., 1976; Sievers et al., 1987), readily aggregates in aqueous solutions at micromolar concentrations, and associates nonspecifically with proteins and lipids. Third, the concentrations and affinities of plasma heme binding proteins ensure that there is essentially no free heme in the circulation. Fourth, in vitro even cells known to transport heme by hemopexin receptors (e.g., hepatocytes) avidly accumulate non-protein-bound heme (Smith and Morgan, 1981). This type of heme accumulation occurs not only by diffusion across the membrane, because it takes place at 4°C, but also by processes requiring energy, since heme is concentrated by the cells (Smith and Morgan, 1981). However, other possibilities exist including the sharing of the carrier-mediated system for bilirubin and bile salts (see Sect. III-D below).

One likely candidate for a heme receptor with a clear functional role is the heme binding protein isolated from duodenal mucosal cells (Grasbeck et al., 1982). The dietary sources of iron are heme derived from hemoglobin and myoglobin and inorganic non-heme iron derived mainly from cereals, vegetables, fruits, and diet supplements. Although heme accounts for only 10 to 15% of the total iron intake, even in diets high in meat content, more than 30% of the total daily iron requirement for the average adult is obtained from this source (Hallberg and Solvell, 1967; Bjorn-Rasmussen et al., 1974). This means that the bioavailability of heme-iron is high and that dietary heme is a vital source of iron. The heme moiety appears to be absorbed intact, since iron chelators do not inhibit absorption (Conrad et al., 1966; Brown et al., 1968) and the duodenum is the main site of absorption (Conrad et al., 1966; and see Fig. 9.4).

Rapid uptake and catabolism of heme by duodenal mucosal cells has been shown in a preliminary report (Smith, 1983). After [55]Fe-heme-histidine was injected into the duodenal lumen of anesthetized, iron-replete adult rats, the heme was absorbed within minutes and appeared in the mucosal cells (Table 9.3). [55]Fe levels in the duodenum, liver, and serum were both dose- and time-dependent. After absorption, radiolabeled iron-transferrin was detected in the mesenteric vein draining the duodenum, rather than heme-hemopexin (Smith, 1988b). These observations suggest that duodenal mucosal cells are extremely efficient at taking up the catabolizing heme.

The heme binder from pig and human intestine requires detergent extraction for solubilization, and heme binding is sensitive to trypsin treatment, indicating that they are integral membrane proteins. After isolation by affinity chromatography on hemin-Sepharose, the pig

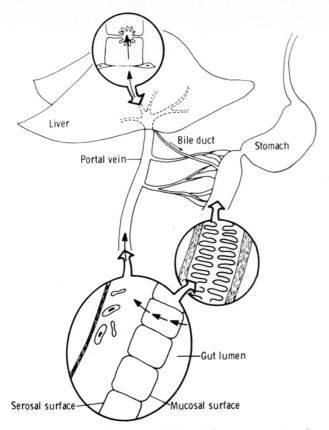

Figure 9.4 Schematic representation of the transport steps involved in absorption of heme by duodenal enterocytes and subsequent distribution of iron to hepatocytes. Receptor-mediated uptake of heme is considered to occur at the surface of mucosal cells lining the microvilli of the duodenum. Catabolism of heme occurs in these cells releasing iron. Whether intact heme reaches the circulation is now yet known. Iron-transferrin reaches the portal vein via blood vessels like the mesenteric vein, which contains nutrients absorbed from this region of the gut. In the liver endothelial cells line hepatic sinusoids and protein-nutrient complexes can pass through pores into the space of Disse to come into contact with microvilli on the sinusoidal surface of the hepatocyte. Heme and iron transport takes place at this plasma membrane surface. In conditions of heme overload, heme is found in bile. Whether transport occurs via passage through the hapatocyte (shown here) or between hepatocytes is not known.

TABLE 9.3   Duodenal Absorption and Distribution in vivo of Heme by Rats*

Administered heme (pmol/100 g body weight)	Time (min)	Serum (pmol heme/mL)	Duodenum (pmol heme/g wet weight)	Liver (pmol heme/mL cytosol)
4.7	30	95	1135	N.D.[†]
4.7	60	80	1900	0.4
47.0	30	1190	3305	1.6

*The distribution of radioactivity in these samples is expressed as picomoles of heme based on the specific activity of the amount of ^{55}Fe-mesoheme loaded into the duodenum. The proportion present as intact heme was not determined.
[†] N.D. = not determined.

heme-binding protein was shown to have an apparent molecular weight of 16,000 on SDS-PAGE (Majuri et al., 1984) and an absorbance maximum at 413 nm (Grasbeck et al., 1982). The K_d for heme binding was estimated to be 1 nM (Grasbeck et al., 1982). In contrast, MHBP has an apparent molecular weight of 17,500 and an absorbance maximum at 417 nm (Smith, unpublished observations).

Because Friend virus-transformed murine erythroleukemia (MEL) cells take up heme from culture medium and incorporate it into newly synthesized hemoglobin (Malik et al., 1979; Ebert et al., 1981), it was suggested that this cell line might express a heme receptor. Although evidence was presented for saturable binding, K_d 0.03 nM with 10,300 sites per cell, the extremely low level of specific binding (< 3% total) and the fact that, of several heme analogues examined, only Sn-PPIX inhibited binding (Galbraith et al., 1985) impede interpretation. However, the lack of competitive inhibition by porphyrins suggest that the central metal atom is important in the binding phenomenon.

Evidence has also been obtained for a heme receptor on human erythroleukemic K562 cells (Majuri and Grasbeck, 1987), using affinity binding to heme immobilized on acrylic microbeads. More than 80% of the K562 cells formed rosettes upon incubation with heme microbeads, whereas mature erythrocytes did not, suggesting that heme binding proteins are not present on the plasma membrane of erythrocytes.

It seems reasonable to speculate that the various heme receptors are either the MHBP of the hemopexin system or proteins closely related to it, since MHBP is a heme-binding protein (Smith and Morgan, 1985). In addition, fluid-phase endocytosis of medium is likely to be one means of acquiring heme in cells incubated in vitro and in cultured cells and would not necessarily require a receptor as has been suggested (Gamberi et al., 1986). In contrast to receptor-mediated endocytosis such uptake would not be saturable.

4. Heme transport by bacteria, parasites, and yeast.   Many elegant studies on the regulation of heme and heme-protein metabolism have been carried out in organisms whose genetic machinery can be more readily manipulated than mammalian cells. In many cases heme is an obligatory requirement for growth in either wild-type or mutant strains, suggesting that these organisms have some mechanism for heme transport. As already mentioned, the ability to acquire iron from the infected host is crucial to the pathogenesis of many bacterial infections. The role of heme and hemoglobin as sources of iron for growth of invading pathogens has until recently been largely ignored, although the obligatory requirement of heme for growth of certain pathogenic organisms such as *Haemophilus influenzae* has been known for over 65 years (Fildes, 1921). Nutritional studies of the *Trypanosomatidae* family demonstrated that hemin or hemoglobin are essential growth factors in certain strains (Lwoff, 1951; Hutner et al., 1979), probably due to a deficiency of ferrochelatase (Biberstein et al., 1965). The source of heme for invasive infections of such organisms in vivo is not yet defined, nor has the intracellular transport and metabolism of heme been delineated. By analogy with iron transport in other organisms, it has generally been assumed that nonprotein-bound heme or hemoglobin is internalized since binding of iron, heme, and hemoglobin by serum proteins is part of the host defense system.

Transport mechanisms for heme and hemoglobin must exist in prokaryotes. For example, the majority of strains of *Gonococci* and *Meningococci* can use free heme (Y and F, M and S) or hemoglobin (Dyer et al., 1987) as a source of iron for growth. Binding of hemoglobin by haptoglobin prevents growth of *Escherichia coli* (Eaton et al., 1982) and of *Neisseria meningitides* and *Neisseria gonorrhoea* (Dyer et al., 1987). Similarly, hemopexin prevents heme being used by these pathogenic *Neisseriae* (Dyer et al., 1987).

Other reports, however, suggest that protein-bound heme can be used to support growth in vitro. *Vibrio vulnificus*, an opportunistic marine pathogen capable of causing fatal septicemia and wound infection in humans, can utilize hemoglobin bound to haptoglobin, phenotypes 1 and 2, but not to haptoglobin 2-1 for growth (Zakaria-Meehan et al., 1988), as can *Vibrio cholerae* (non-Ol), *Staphylococcus aureus*, and *Streptococcus pyogenes* (Francis et al., 1985, and references in Dyer et al., 1987). *H. influenzae* is reported to utilize not only hemoglobin-haptoglobin but also heme from heme-albumin and heme-hemopexin complexes (Stull, 1987). In *H. influenzae* type b, heme is transported actively in the absence of a functional electron transport chain, with the energy coming from the electrical component of the proton motive force (Coulton and Pang, 1983). Because of the known stability to proteases of haptoglobin (Lustbader et al., 1983) and hemopexin (Smith and Morgan, 1984a, b) when ligand is bound, either these organisms secrete powerful proteases or they can internalize intact complexes, or some other factor must be invoked. The presence of binding sites for haptoglobin on certain bacteria, coupled with the fact that proteases from *S. aureus* cleave haptoglobin (Lustbader et al., 1983), help in explaining the ability of certain microorganisms to utilize hemoglobin bound to haptoglobin.

Possible mechanisms of heme or hemoglobin transport include: diffusion of heme through lipid membranes to intracellular binding proteins; facilitated diffusion of heme via membrane heme receptors or carrier molecules; uptake of surrounding medium (in vitro) or serum (in vivo), by fluid-phase endocytosis, as in yeast (Riezman, 1985). In the case of heme-hemopexin or hemoglobin-haptoglobin complexes, phagocytosis or endocytosis by parasites seems likely, similar to the endocytosis of iron-transferrin by the rapidly growing, blood form of *Trypanosoma brucei*, the causative agent of sleeping sickness (Coppens et al., 1987).

Many microorganisms can utilize heme as a sole source of iron for growth. For example, binding of hemin by the *Shigella flexneri* Crb[+] phenotype is thought to occur via a surface molecule which can also bind Congo red (hence the term Crb[+]). Binding of Congo red and hemin can also be used interchangeably in solid media assays to distinguish virulent from nonvirulent strains of *S. flexneri* Crb[+], the causative agent of bacillary dysentery (Payne and Finkelstein, 1977), of *Yersinia pestis* Pgm[+], the plague bacillus (Surgalla and Beesley, 1969), and of the fish pathogen, *Aeromonas salmonicida* (Ishiguro et al., 1985). However, binding of hemin by Crb[+] *S. flexneri* is independent of hemin transport, since both Crb[+] and Crb[−] cells can utilize hemin as a sole source of iron. Likewise in *Yersinia* species, both Pgm[+] and Pgm[−] organisms grow with hemin, although only the Pgm[+] can bind hemin. Thus, this membrane protein appears not to function as a heme receptor for heme transport per se, and *S. flexneri* cells with bound heme were more invasive when tested in the HeLa cell system. Hemin binding to *S. flexneri* Crb[+] may facilitate the attachment of these bacteria to their sites of infection, intestinal epithelial cells (Daskaleros and Payne, 1987). Intriguingly, endocytosis of these organisms may be triggered by binding to the duodenal heme receptor! Alternatively, binding of heme or perhaps other hydrophobic molecules would alter the bacterial surface charge or hydrophobicity and hence the interaction with host cells.

A second possible mechanism for heme uptake is analogous to siderophore production in bacteria, whose response in iron deprivation is not only to increase both the synthesis and secretion of iron binding molecules, siderophores such as enterobactin, but also to amplify the expression on the cell surface of receptors for the iron-siderophore complexes. Some bacteria produce siderophores from genes encoded in a plasmid. For example, plasmid pJM1 allows *Vibrio anquillarum* to grow under iron-deficient conditions by coding for membrane proteins which bind iron chelators (Crosa, 1980), and plasmid Col V is found in pathogenic strains of *E. coli* producing aerobactin, the siderophore associated with disease (Williams, 1979).

Binding of heme to a 49,000-dalton membrane protein, which also binds PPIX (Kay et al., 1985), of the A layer of *A. salmonicida* has been postulated to enable heme-iron acquisition (Daskaleros and Payne, 1987). A heme-repressible 43,000-dalton outer membrane protein in *H. influenzae* type b in ATCC 9795 strain (Coulton and Pang, 1983) and a 38,000-dalton protein (Stull, 1987) detected in heme-restricted organisms (Stull, 1987) have yet to be shown to have roles in heme transport. Presumably, such proteins may in some cases represent heme receptors or, by analogy with the bacterial siderophore system, receptors for newly synthesized "heme-hemophore" complexes.

Presumably, distinct transport systems for hemoglobin exist in hematophagic parasites maintained in the presence of reticulocytes in vitro. Using ^{14}C-aminolevulinate-labeled hemoglobin, Foster and Bogitsh (1986) extracted radiolabeled protein from schistosomules of *Schistosoma mansoni*, providing evidence that both the heme and protein moieties of hemoglobin are degraded and then reutilized by these nematodes. Similar growth-promoting effects of hemoglobin, hematin, or heme have been observed on the larval stages of the nematode *Nippostrongylus brasiliensis* (Bolla et al., 1972).

These nonmammalian systems provide interesting new possibilities for the examination of heme transport mechanisms, but this potential remains largely unexplored.

B. Receptor-mediated transport of heme analogues

Heme analogues have proved to be useful tools to examine structure-function relationships in heme-proteins and to manipulate experimentally the enzymes of heme metabolism. Analogues have also been used to probe the mechanisms of uptake and retention of exogenous porphyrins in porphyrin photodynamic therapy of cancer. In general, the differences in the interaction of heme analogues with proteins arise from the changes in chemistry due to replacement of the central metal iron with divalent tin, cobalt, nickel, and zinc; to modifications of the side chains as in meso- and deuteroheme derivatives; or due to substitutions on the methene-carbons as in Fe-tetraphenylporphine sulfonate (Fe-TPPS).

Examples are abundant. The presence of the central metal iron decreases the affinity of protoporphyrin binding to the peripheral benzodiazepine receptor (Verma et al., 1987; Snyder et al., 1987). Hemopexin binds Sn-PP and Fe-TPPS, but does not undergo a full conformational change (Smith et al., 1988). Ferrochelatase utilizes meso-, deutero- and protoporphyrin IX as substrates, but not analogues with large or ionizable groups in the 2,4 substituent positions (Dailey and Smith, 1984); and heme oxygenase can use a wide variety of heme analogues as substrates (Frydman et al., 1981) but is inhibited strongly by the cobalt analogue (Drummond and Kappas, 1982; Kappas and Drummond, 1986).

Generally, protein binding of heme serves to direct transport through cells. However, such tightly controlled systems are subject to overloading by experimental manipulation, for example, when cells are incubated with high concentrations of δ-aminolevulinate or animals are given heme (5 mg or more/kg). In this condition heme, heme analogues and porphyrins form unusual associations with proteins or reach unusual subcellular locations, for example, biliary excretion of heme (Petryka et al., 1977; Kappas et al., 1985). Similar perturbations occur in conditions of overload such as in the porphyrias after therapeutic administration of hematin, or in neonates after Sn-PPIX therapy.

Space limitations do not permit a complete review of the use of heme analogues, and this section will focus on protein interactions with, and the transport of, heme analogues.

1. Sn-Protoporphyrin in therapy of neonatal jaundice. Sn-Protoporphyrin IX (Sn-PP) is an inhibitor of microsomal heme oxygenase (Drummond and Kappas, 1984) and is being evaluated as a potential therapeutic agent for neonatal hyperbilirubinemia (Kappas et al., 1984). Human serum albumin and myoglobin have been shown to bind Sn-PP (Breslow et al., 1986) and the liver, kidney, and spleen to be major sites of uptake of Sn-PP administered intravenously in rats (Kappas et al., 1984; Anderson et al., 1986). Plasma clearance of Sn-PP is dose-dependent, with a $t_{1/2}$ near 4 h for initial plasma levels of 7 to 15 μM but a $t_{1/2}$ near 15 min for levels of 0.025 to 0.2 μM (Anderson et al., 1986), suggesting that a saturable receptor-mediated process is involved in the transport of Sn-PP.

The interaction of Sn-PP with hemopexin and the role of hemopexin receptors in the hepatic uptake of Sn-PP and the biological consequences to the cells has recently been evaluated (Morgan et al., 1988). The apparent dissociation constant (K_d) and Sn-PP–hemopexin at pH 7.4 is 250 ± 150 nM, but estimation of the K_d is hampered by the fact that at physiological pH Sn-PP exists as monomers and dimers, both of which are bound by hemopexin. Measurements at pH 9.2 (Breslow et al., 1986) have been used to study binding of Sn-PP to HSA (K_d 10 to 30 μM) and myoglobin (K_d "1/200 that of heme"), since dimerization of the tetrapyrrole is decreased at this pH.

Competition experiments at pH 7.4 confirmed that HSA has a significantly lower affinity for Sn-PP (apparent K_d 4 ± 2 μM) than does hemopexin (Morgan et al., 1988a). In the circulation appreciable amounts of Sn-PP (up to 35% in adults and 20% in neonates) would be bound by hemopexin. The remainder would be associated with albumin due to its high serum concentration, but essentially no nonprotein-bound Sn-PP is present. Importantly, Sn-PP–hemopexin binds to the hemopexin receptor on mouse hepatoma cells with an affinity comparable to that of heme-hemopexin, and exposure of these cells to 10 μM Sn-PP–hemopexin, but not Sn-PP alone, causes a rapid 15-fold increase in the steady-state level of heme oxygenase mRNA. Thus, the principle biologically active transporter of Sn-PP in vivo appears to be hemopexin (Morgan et al., 1988a). These observations help explain why, although hepatic heme oxygenase enzymic activity is diminished to 10% of control levels within 30 min of subcutaneous injection of Sn-PP, heme-oxygenase protein has increased 17-fold several hours later (Sardana and Kappas, 1987).

2. Iron-meso-tetra-(4-sulfonatophenyl)-porphine (Fe-TPPS) and other analogues. Another heme analogue iron-meso-tetra-(4-sulfonatophenyl)-porphine, also commonly called iron-tetraphenylporphine sulfonate (Fe-TPPS), has been used together with other metal-TPPS complexes to study the mechanism of porphyrin uptake and retention by normal and cancerous cells in vitro (Winkelman et al., 1967; Carrano et al., 1977, 1978), to examine the heme binding site of GSH-S transferase isozymes (Smith et al., 1985) and to probe the transport and metabolic effects of heme (Smith et al., 1988). Regrettably, often in studies of porphyrin uptake in vitro, the form of the porphyrin in the bloodstream (i.e., bound to protein or lipid) has been ignored.

Fe-TPPS is more symmetrical and water-soluble than the amphipathic, naturally-occurring heme but is bound tightly by hemopexin, K_d below 10 nM (Smith et al., 1988). Importantly, even when such analogues are bound by hemopexin, they may not be transported into liver cells. This is the case for Fe-TPPS (Smith et al., 1988). Although Fe-TPPS–hemopexin interacts nearly normally with the hemopexin receptor, the subsequent events in hemopexin-mediated transport are impaired. Such lack of hepatic transport by hemopexin helps explain the observation that Fe-TPPS, unlike heme and mesoheme, is ineffective at depressing the activity of ALA-S induced in rats by allylisopropylacetamide (Cannon et al., 1985). In these experiments the agents were administered in liposomes, from which hemopexin and albumin rapidly remove heme (Cannon et al., 1984).

III. Intracellular Movement of Tetrapyrroles

A. Transport of pyrroles, porphyrinogens, and porphyrins

As noted above, tetrapyrroles are highly reactive, lipophilic molecules that require proteins to direct the chemical reactions involved in their utilization and metabolism by the cell. In this section the role that enzymes of heme synthesis play in transporting porphyrin metabolites is considered first, and then the transport routes and protein interactions of porphyrins in conditions of porphyrin overload are examined. The disturbances in physiological processes which occur in conditions of porphyrin overload are, not surprisingly, related directly to the physioco-chemical properties of porphyrins. In particular, their lipophilicity which leads to membrane association when the porphyrin concentration is in excess of transporting proteins.

1. In heme metabolism. One of the most intriguing aspects of heme metabolism is the subcellular compartmentalization of the enzymes of heme synthesis and catabolism. Heme synthesis is initiated in the mitochondrion by aminolevulinate synthase, and continues via intermediates synthesized in the cytosol, followed by the return of coproporphyrinogen III to the mitochondrion for the final steps in heme formation. The details of these enzymic steps are covered elsewhere in this book, but this pathway, together with that of heme catabolism, presents an interesting problem in terms of the intracellular movement of pyrrolic compounds. Heme synthesis is rigorously controlled and coordinated with heme-protein synthesis, so that few intermediates of heme metabolism are left free to diffuse through the cell. Rather, the heme-metabolizing enzymes themselves appear to guide the overall transfer. It has even been suggested (Tsai et al., 1987) that the four cytosolic enzymes of heme biosynthesis in eukaryotes may form as a complex to facilitate the sequential reactions and to protect these porphyrinogen intermediates from oxidation to porphyrins. Perhaps these soluble enzymes come together as a complex on a membrane surface as shown for the enzymes of glycolysis.

The question here is how such coordinated transfers take place. Possible answers include binding of intermediates or covalent interaction with proteins, ordered or sequential synthesis of intermediates, associative phenomena of the enzymes, and membrane transport of intermediates. Evidence for all these has been obtained, and specific enzymes will be used as representative examples.

Evidence for enzyme-bound monopyrrole comes from ^{13}C nmr studies of δ-aminolevulinate dehydratase (EC 4.2.1.24), also called porphobilinogen synthase, showing 75% of the species bound to the enzymes under turnover conditions are porphobilinogen (Jaffe and Markham, 1987). Because bound porphobilinogen is displaced by excess free porphobilinogen, this is an example of protein-intermediate binding.

Stable covalent enzyme-pyrrole complexes are formed by human hydroxymethyl bilane synthase (HMB synthase, EC 4.3.1.8), formerly termed porphobilinogen deaminase and uroporphyrinogen I synthase, which can accommodate up to four condensed porphobilinogen units (Anderson and Desnick, 1980). Enzyme-substrate complexes have also been detected with the enzyme from rat spleen, *Euglena gracilis*, and *Rhodobacter spheroides*, but the latter is not a covalent complex (Berry et al., 1981).

Whether the enzymes HMB synthase and uroporphyrinogen III synthase act sequentially with release of product from synthase to provide substrate for cosynthase or act in association as a macromolecular enzyme complex (references in Tsai et al., 1987) remains unknown. Enzyme-bound uroporphyrinogen I has been detected using ^{13}C nmr (Evans et al., 1986a, b) and uroporphyrinogen III synthase can metabolize HMB synthase-bound tetrapyrrole (Battersby et al., 1983). More-detailed descriptions of these enzymes are presented elsewhere in this book.

Transfer of tetrapyrrole intermediates across mitochondrial membranes must occur in the later stages of heme synthesis. For example, the cytosolic location of yeast uroporphyrinogen oxidase implies that its lipophilic product, coproporphyrinogen, must cross the outer mitochondrial membrane to reach its site of oxidation at coproporphyrinogen oxidase in the inner mitochondrial membrane space. Coproporphyrinogen oxidase has also been located in cytosol (Camadro et al., 1986) and may itself interact transiently with the mitochondrial membrane and the next enzyme, protoporphyrinogen oxidase, in subsequent transfer of product (Camadro et al., 1986; Grandchamp et al., 1978). Such interactions are by no means unprecedented and analogies can be made with the proposed movement of protein kinase C from soluble to membrane-associated forms upon calcium/magnesium binding resulting in increased affinity for certain membrane lipids (Ashendel, 1985). In addition, several enzymes, including β-galactosidase-α-2-sialotransferase, β-glucuronidase, dopamine β-hydroxylase, and acetyl cholinesterase, and known to exist in soluble and membrane-bound forms. Perhaps similar mechanisms are involved in the heme synthesis pathway.

In liver cells coproporphyrinogen oxidase is a mitochondrial protein distributed predominantly in the intermembrane space with the remainder of the enzyme associated with the cytosolic side of the inner mitochondrial membrane (Elder and Evans, 1978; Grandchamp et al., 1978). Both protoporphyrinogen oxidase and ferrochelatase are integral membrane proteins of the inner mitochondrial membrane. The active site of protoporphyrinogen oxidase is reported to reside on the cytosolic face of the inner mitochondrial membrane, and ferrochelatase spans the inner mitochondrial membrane lipid bilayer with its active site facing the mitochondrial matrix (Harbin and Dailey, 1965; Dailey, 1985; Ferreira et al., 1988). The apparent K_m for substrate of the oxidase is 5.6 μM (Ferreira and Dailey, 1987) which, like the K_m for many of these mitochondrial enzymes, seems relatively high for substrates with low solubility. It is interesting that calculation of the concentration of one molecule of heme inside a mitochondrion yields an apparent concentration on the order of 1 nM. These three enzymes are stimulated by phospholipids and, with their poorly soluble, highly reactive substrates, may therefore interact together physically, perhaps as a complex spanning the membrane. In such a complex substrates might not be released to other proteins for transport across the membrane to the intermembrane space, but rather channeled from one enzyme active site to the next (Ferreira and Dailey, 1987).

2. In the porphyrias and in porphyrin photodynamic therapy.   To complete this section, the transport routes and interaction of tetrapyrroles with proteins in conditions of porphyrin overload will be addressed. The role of porphyrin-protein interactions in the metabolism of naturally occurring and artificial porphyrins has recently been reviewed (Smith, 1987). The localization of porphyrin(ogens) by binding to cell constituents, principally proteins but also lipids and DNA, plays a major role in determining the cellular effects of porphyrins produced endogenously in excessive amounts in certain porphyrias and of exogenous porphyrins administered for therapeutic reasons. In photodynamic therapy of cancer, artificial porphyrins injected intravenously first encounter plasma proteins, lipoproteins, and the membrane proteins and lipids of circulating cells before reaching the plasma membrane of tissues where uptake occurs. After uptake the intracellular locations of the porphyrins are determined by their interactions with cellular components. Although porphyrin-protein interactions predominate, porphyrins can occupy the lipid phase of membranes, especially in conditions of overload. In porphyric states, whether of genetic or toxic origin, porphyrins have been located in many cellular organelles, including mitochondria and lysosomes (Doiron and Gomer, 1984; Hilf et al., 1984; Tangeras, 1986; Murant et al., 1987) and excreted into the circulation and bile (Kappas et al., 1983).

It is now well established that albumin is the predominant plasma binder of endogenous (Morgan et al., 1980) and exogenous porphyrins (Moan and Christensen, 1981; Reddi et al., 1981; Smith and Neuschatz, 1983) but long-lived associations of these lipophilic compounds occur with circulating lipoproteins. For example, the porphyrins in Photofrin II and hematoporphyrin derivatives used in porphyrin photodynamic therapy are associated with HDL and VLDL (Jori et al., 1984).

There are several means whereby exogenous and endogenous porphyrins can be transported into cells. First, after dissociation from porphyrin-albumin complexes free porphyrin is rapidly taken up by cells by diffusion and binding to intracellular proteins (Kessel, 1981; Smith and Neuschatz, 1983) and by some type of active transport (Smith and Neuschatz, 1983). Certain analogies with the mechanism of linear tetrapyrrole transport described in Sec. III-D may be drawn. Second, endocytosis of HDL and other lipoproteins containing porphyrins will lead to cellular uptake. Which organelles the porphyrins encounter in vivo remains to be established, but the normal destination for lipoproteins is lysosomes. Third, porphyrin uptake may occur by fluid phase endocytosis (pinocytosis) of surrounding medium or plasma containing porphyrin-protein complexes or, in conditions of overload, free porphyrin. Fourth, in vitro in protein-free medium porphyrin aggregates will adhere nonspecifically to plasma membrane of cells and partition between the aqueous phase and membrane lipid as proposed for heme (Rose et al., 1985) and bilirubin dimers and aggregates (Vazquez et al., 1988).

The existence of distinct specific porphyrin receptors on cell plasma membranes seems unlikely in the light of published observations. Porphyrin uptake may be facilitated by carrier molecules of other transport systems including membrane heme-binding proteins or those involved in linear tetrapyrrole transport. However, porphyrins compete only weakly with heme for binding to the heme-binding protein on MEL cells (Galbraith et al., 1985). Porphyrin structure and cell type are important determinants of porphyrin-cell interactions (Kessel, 1981; Moan and Christensen, 1981; Smith and Neuschatz, 1983; Dubbelman and Van Steveninck, 1984), suggesting some degree of specificity in the interaction, although of unknown origin. Perhaps porphyrins, like bilirubin, interact preferentially with certain phospholipids (Vazquez et al., 1988), influencing their membrane location.

Intracellular routes for specific transport of porphyrins to the organelles in which they have been detected are not defined. Endocytosis of porphyrin associated with lipoproteins is one means whereby extracellular porphyrins reach lysosomes. However, abnormal associations of ligand-protein complexes do not ensure cell uptake of ligand. For example, when heme-asialohemopexin interacts with hepatocytes the asialoprotein moiety is efficiently transported to the lysosomes but its heme does not follow the same intracellular route (Smith, 1985). However, lysosomes were the predominant intracellular location of uro- and heptacarboxylic porphyrins in hexachlorobenzene-induced porphyria (Tangeras, 1986). In porphyric states porphyrins are transferred from their sites of synthesis in cytosol and mitochondria to serum and bile. Since bilirubin can be secreted from liver cells before re-uptake for conjugation and biliary excretion, uptake–re-uptake may occur for the more hydrophobic heme intermediates. This may explain why the plasma clearance of uroporphyrin, which is only weakly bound to plasma proteins, differs from that of other porphyrins (Koskelo et al., 1976).

Protoporphyrin generated in excess in the mitochondria in porphyric states seems poised to interact with the newly described "mitochondrial peripheral-type benzodiazepine" (MPTB) receptor, an integral protein of the outer mitochondrial membrane (Snyder et al., 1987). This protein binds protoporphyrin (K_i 15 nM) and heme (K_i 41 nM) tightly and may act to target protoporphyrin to nonhepatic tissues. High levels of MPTB receptors are found in the adrenal cortex, skin, and cardiac muscle, and occupation of MPTB by porphyrin may account for some of the symptoms of erythro-hepatic-protoporphyria (EHPP) and acute intermittent porphyria. Hematin infusion may also result in occupancy of these sites.

Many other proteins have been reported to bind porphyrins or heme in vitro (see Table 9.1) and may influence the transport, accumulation, and biological consequences of porphyrins under conditions of overload. Unfortunately, in many of these studies demonstrating heme-protein interactions, high concentrations of porphyrin and heme and low amounts of protein were used and the effect of competing heme binding proteins likely to be present in vivo was not addressed. Nevertheless, these observations present exciting avenues for future research and pose questions on the many aspects of cell metabolism which could be influenced by the intracellular transport of heme and porphyrins. For example, soluble, but not particulate, guanylate cyclase is activated by protoporphyrin IX and the particulate form is activated 3- to 10-fold by heme. In fact, porphobilinogen and the I isomer of coproporphyrin significantly inhibited the enzyme (Waldman et al, 1984).

The interaction of porphyrins with ferrochelatase has been postulated to be one means for clearance of exogenous porphyrins by cells (Dailey and Smith, 1984). Whether other enzymes of heme synthesis act as carriers for exogenous porphyrins or whether MHBP of the hemopexin transport system has sufficient affinity for porphyrins to act in their transport is not known. Clearly, exogenous porphyrins reach the mitochondrial inner membrane, as shown by porphyrin-mediated damage to cytochrome c oxidase and succinate dehydrogenase enzymes (Hilf et al., 1984; Murant et al., 1987). Pharmacokinetic studies employing radiolabeled porphyrins are needed to trace these compounds as they are transported and metabolized.

Porphyrins are transported across the biliary canalicular membrane as shown by the appearance of porphyrins in bile and feces (Kappas et al., 1983). One consequence of the interaction of protoporphyrin with the perfused liver was a nonspecific inhibition of at least three membrane enzyme activities, namely, Na^+,K^+-ATPase, Mg^{2+}-ATPase, and $5'$-nucleotidase (Avner et al., 1983). Na^+,K^+-ATPase is important for the control of Na^+ concentrations and water transport, major determinants of bile formation, while Mg^{2+}-ATPase is located on basolateral membranes. Since cholestasis occurs in EHPP, reduced clearance of PP from liver could be due to inhibition of biliary excretion, because of ultrastructural abnormalities induced by protoporphyrin within sinusoidal and canalicular membranes.

B. Transport of heme for heme-protein synthesis

While several aspects of heme metabolism are well understood, the intracellular transport of newly synthesized heme is not. Heme-proteins are found in most, if not all, cell compartments, but the final step in heme synthesis is in the intermembrane space of mitochondria. Thus, if heme is to be incorporated, for example, into cytochrome P450 in the endoplasmic reticulm, either an extramitochondrial transit of heme into the cytosol or a membrane fusion event must occur. Unfortunately, only a few studies in this area have been done, limiting the conclusions which can be drawn.

In addition, the incorporation of newly synthesized heme into newly synthesized apoproteins in mammalian systems has rarely been directly addressed. De novo synthesis and intracellular transport of the apocytochromes and of the heme prosthestic group must be well coordinated since neither free heme nor free apoprotein for apocytochrome P450b accumulate during induction. Considerable progress has been made in understanding protein processing and posttranslational modification for the synthesis of mitochondrial cytochromes and other mitochondrial proteins in yeast and in *Neurospora crassa*. An elegant example is the translocation of δ-aminolevulinate synthase to the yeast mitochondrion directed by nine amino acids in its amino terminus (Keng et al., 1986).

Finally, heme itself can affect this process of heme-protein maturation. Binding of small molecules such as heme can alter the conformation of proteins, in turn affecting their ability to move through membranes and decreasing their sensitivity to proteases. Thus, the movement of heme through membranes of subcellular compartments is likely to be coupled with that of proteins as they are processed and move to their site of activity.

1. From the mitochondrion during heme synthesis. The distribution of heme, following radiolabeling with the heme precursor ^{14}C-aminolevulinate (ALA) in rats, showed a rapid, transient peak in the cytosol 10 min after precursor injection (Israels et al., 1975). Heme appeared rapidly in the microsomal fraction which accounted for 70 to 80% of the total radiolabeled heme at 30 min and mitochondria for a further 10%. Essentially, similar subcellular distribution of radioactive heme was found using an elegant dual-labeling technique. Consecutive pulses of ^{3}H- and ^{14}C-ALA given to rats revealed two cytosolic fractions containing heme which appeared to be turning over rapidly (Davies et al., 1982). The fractions contained different proteins separated by gel permeation chromatography, but these were not characterized or identified.

Pulse labeling in primary cultures of hepatocytes using ^{14}C-ALA at concentrations less than or equal to the amount of glycine incorporated to avoid "excess" heme formation led to a complex compartmental model (Grandchamp et al., 1981). An initially labeled cytosolic compartment, considered to be identical with the regulatory or unassigned free-heme pool, exchanges heme with a second cytosolic compartment. One cytosolic compartment was presumed to be associated with heme carrier proteins and the other with tryptophan pyrrolase or soluble catalase monomers. About 20% of the newly formed heme is converted directly to bile pigment and 80% is utilized for formation of cellular heme-proteins. Finally, competition experiments were interpreted as suggesting that exogenous heme can mix with the precursor heme pool for cytochrome formation.

Thus, some experimental evidence supports the concept of cytoplasmic carriers of newly synthesized heme. Arguing against cytosolic carrier or acceptor molecules is the finding that heme addition to cytosol, even at concentrations up to 138 μM, neither reduced the release of heme from isolated mitochondria nor inhibited heme synthesis, as would be predicted (Israels et al., 1975).

From ultrastructural studies, the rough endoplasmic reticulum in adult rat liver is organized as single cisternae intimately associated with mitochondria. These "MITORER" complexes are considered to be the preferred site for synthesis and transport of nuclear-coded cytoplasmic units of mitochondrial cytochrome c oxidase (Parimoo et al., 1982). ^{3}H-ALA was preferentially incorporated into P450b of MITORER complexes at very short labeling periods (2 to 4 min), suggesting that MITORER also has a role in facilitating heme transfer from the mitochondria to the endoplasmic reticulum (Meier et al., 1984). Quantitatively, the rough microsomes were the major site of biosynthesis of P450b at 8 min after injection of precursor, but it is possible that the rate-limiting step had been bypassed by the amount of injected ALA by this time.

To summarize, there is considerable controversy in this area, and much of the experimental evidence is inconclusive. Whether heme is transferred from heme-proteins in the mitochondria to others in the endoplasmic reticulum, what role cytosolic proteins have in this transfer, and whether heme is transferred to the endoplasmic reticulum via direct interaction with the mitochondria remain important questions.

2. In mitochondria. The two mitochondrial membranes produce four compartments: the outer membrane, the inner membrane, the intermembrane space, and the matrix enclosed by the inner membrane. The outer membrane is not particularly rich in proteins. One major component is porin, a protein which forms pores, making the outer membrane permeable to globular molecules of molecular weight 2000 to 6000. Of the few other proteins present, one is a mitochondrial cytochrome b_5 related to microsomal cytochrome b_5 in the endoplasmic reticulum. In contrast, the inner membrane is rich in proteins, is impermeable to charged or polar molecules, and is highly invaginated. Many carrier systems exist in this membrane to allow passage of low molecular weight metabolites required by the enzymes of the mitochondrial matrix. In addition, it contains the enzymes involved in cellular respiration and oxidative phosphorylation. "Translocation contact sites" exist in which the outer and inner membranes come close enough to be spanned by precursor polypeptide chains (Schleyer and Neupert, 1985). The situation is complicated further since mitochondrial proteins are synthesized on free ribosomes in the cytoplasm and have to be selectively translocated across these diverse membranes. There are significant variations in the specific steps depending on whether a polypeptide is transported into the inner-membrane matrix compartment, the intermembrane space, or the outer membrane. Import of polypeptides, such as cytochrome b_2, destined for the mitochondrial intermembrane space, is more complicated than import into the inner-membrane matrix compartment (Gasser et al., 1982) and involves two proteolytic cleavages of membrane-bound intermediates before release of soluble cytochrome into the intermembrane space where, presumably, heme is acquired.

A similar two-step pathway exists for synthesizing yeast cytochrome c_1, located on the outer face of the inner mitochondrial membrane. However, maturation of the intermediate to the mature form requires heme, suggesting synthesis occurs via a heme-containing precursor (Ohashi et al., 1982). Cytochrome c is not made as a larger precursor, but imported as the heme-free apoprotein, which is converted to cytochrome c inside the mitochondrion (Zimmerman et al., 1979) by the covalent attachment of heme in the inner-membrane space by cytochrome c heme lyase (Nicholson et al., 1987).

The mitochondria are the site of heme biosynthesis and the location of the respiratory heme-proteins. Recently, it has been suggested that mitochondria have a heme-degrading system which acts in the regulation of respiratory heme-proteins and in the disposition of aberrant forms of mitochondrial heme-proteins (Kutty and Maines, 1987). As pointed out by these authors such a system would preempt the need for transport of heme complexes from the mitochondria for degradation.

3. In the endoplasmic reticulum. Cytochrome b_5 is synthesized on membrane-bound ribosomes and anchored after synthesis to the smooth endoplasmic reticulum membrane by a sequence of hydrophobic amino acids in its C terminus. Transport of newly synthesized heme from mitochondria to apocytochrome b_5 incorporated in phospholipid vesicles has been reported to be mediated by ligandin (Senjo et al., 1985). The movement of heme from isolated mitochondria to the apoprotein in vesicles required the presence of ligandin, but substantive proof that ligandin and not another protein mediates this process in intact cells is lacking. Cytochrome P450, after synthesis on bound ribosomes, has been proposed to be anchored by two amino-terminal transmembrane helices to the endoplasmic reticulum membrane (Nelson and Strobel, 1988). The heme moiety lies parallel to the membrane surface on the cytoplasmic side of the membrane.

4. In peroxisomes. Peroxisomes, which, like mitochondria, are a major site of oxygen utilization, contain most of the cell's catalase. Catalase consists of four glycoprotein monomers, each of which binds heme. This heme enzyme destroys the potentially lethal oxidant, hydrogen peroxide, generated by other peroxisomal enzymes in the oxidization of a variety of substrates, including phenols, formic acid, formaldehyde, and alcohol. Catalase converts hydrogen peroxide to water and oxygen to prevent the accumulation of this strong oxidizing agent at its site of synthesis.

All peroxisomal proteins must be imported through a single-membrane lipid bilayer. Catalase is not synthesized as a precursor, but is released into the cytosol as apocatalase monomers. Concomitant with transport across the peroxisomal membranes, the chains are assembled into tetramers, and heme transported from the mitochondria is added. The details of this interesting process are not defined.

5. In cytosol. Tryptophan 2,3-dioxygenase (EC 1.13.11.11), commonly called tryptophan pyrrolase, is a soluble, heme-containing enzyme which catalyses the first reaction unique to tryptophan degradation in the liver. Its expression is regulated by tryptophan and by various hormones. Rat liver contains both the active holoenzyme and the heme-free apotryptophan dioxygenase (Fiegelson and Greengard, 1961; Badawy, 1979), and the ratio of holo- to apoenzyme depends on the availability of tryptophan and of heme transported to the cytosol from the mitochondria (Badawy and Evans, 1975). Tryptophan pyrrolase is fully saturated with its heme cofactor in vivo at normal plasma concentrations of 5 to 20 μM tryptophan (Salter and Pogson, 1986).

C. Transport of heme for regulation of expression of enzymes of heme metabolism and cellular proteins

Heme is known in different cell types to regulate cellular processes as varied as differentiation, transcription, and posttranslational processing of proteins. Thus, change in intracellular heme levels can potentially alter the expression of many different proteins. It should be emphasized that the effects of heme on regulation are likely to be modulated by binding of heme or heme-protein complexes to specific regulatory sites, including DNA sequences, after transport to specific tissues and to specific intracellular compartments.

Altered expression of hepatic enzymes has been shown to occur after IV injection of hematin, hemin, or heme-arginate (which immediately splits into heme and arginate in the circulation, Linden et al., 1987). Heme-hemopexin complexes form rapidly in the circulation after IV heme injections (cf., above), and it is certain that many of the effects observed in such studies, although not attributed to hemopexin, are due to heme delivered via the hemopexin receptor to tissues, predominantly the liver, which express the receptor for this protein.

To clarify this issue, a systematic study of the regulation of hepatic proteins by heme-hemopexin has been started in this laboratory, and some early results of this effort are presented below (see Fig. 9.5). The receptor-mediated transport of heme by hemopexin affords a unique opportunity to target heme to specific tissues and to a specific intracellular route for study of the regulatory consequences. For example, only Sn-protoporphyrin IX presented to cells via the hemopexin receptor, but not Sn-protoporphyrin IX alone, caused an increase in heme oxygenase mRNA levels (Morgan et al., 1988a; see Sec. II-2 and below).

In the context of heme regulation, the term "free-heme pool" is often used. In this discussion, free or unassigned heme is negligible, since the affinity and concentration of heme-binding molecules in vivo are considered to preclude "free heme." Heme molecules would be bound either to cellular or regulatory proteins or perhaps even to DNA itself. The intracellular routes whereby newly synthesized heme reaches regulatory sites and the proteins involved remain to be defined. This is also the case for extracellular heme delivered through the hemopexin receptor and for hemoglobin-heme delivered by haptoglobin. However, the MHBP of the hemopexin system appears to be one means to transport heme intracellularly since antibodies to MHBP prevent heme uptake (Smith, 1989).

Other intermediate steps in the path to heme oxygenase in the ER for catabolism or to the nucleus for regulation remain to be elucidated.

Heme has been shown to regulate expression at the transcriptional level (see below); therefore, heme in some form reaches the nucleus. Transcriptional regulation occurs by the binding of specific regulatory proteins to specific DNA sequences. These proteins either enhance or repress transcription by RNA polymerase at specific promotor regions. In turn, the DNA binding activity of such proteins is regulated by synthesis of the regulatory protein, interaction with other proteins, or

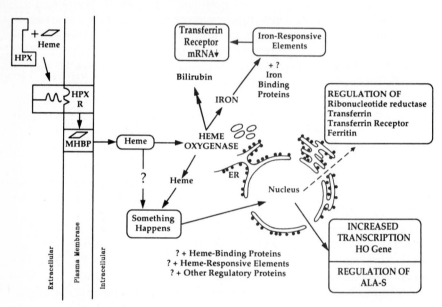

Figure 9.5 Schematic representation of intracellular transport steps and regulatory elements and proteins in the regulation of gene expression after hemopexin-mediated transport of heme.

Heme, like iron, has now been shown to regulate cellular processes involved in its metabolism after specific receptor-mediated transport into mammalian cells (Alam and Smith, 1989). The iron released by heme catabolism regulates the transferrin receptor expression providing additional support for the role of hemopexin in linking heme and iron metabolism. Perhaps heme responsive elements (HREs) are involved in the regulation of mammalian gene expression by heme. In fact, several levels of control can be envisioned involving both heme and iron. Since heme and iron metabolism are linked and since iron has been implicated in the regulation of expression of hepatic ALA-S (Liem et al., 1989), and HRE present in the ALA-S gene may be involved in the repression of ALA-S transcription in nonerythroid tissues, and an iron-responsive element (IRE) may be present in ALA-S mRNA which, like the TfR, has an unusually short half-life (Srivastava et al., 1988). Thus, as levels of intracellular heme rise due to increased heme synthesis, regulation of HRE-responsive genes takes place principally at the transcriptional level. Posttranscriptional regulation of ALA-S and other genes including the TfR may occur principally in response to iron released from heme catabolism by HO in the ER. Additional regulation may occur via heme-responsive RNA elements.

binding of small molecules (e.g., heme) that affect the binding of these proteins to their target DNA sequences. Depending on whether binding of these putative regulatory proteins to DNA results in increased or decreased transcription will determine if these proteins are positive or negative regulators. Finally, binding of heme to other proteins or sites in the cell may alter the expression of regulatory proteins which then migrate to the nucleus, transporting heme there (Fig. 9.5).

Heme may also act at other points of regulation in the cell such as processing of RNA and transport of mRNA to the cytosol, stabilization of mRNA, and so forth. Exogenous hemin has been proposed to affect the processing or transport of globin mRNA and other poly(A)-containing mRNAs from the nucleus to the cytoplasm in murine erythroleukemic Friend cells of the Fw line (Fuchs et al., 1984), but its mode of transport to effect this is unknown.*

Some of the best-known examples of heme regulation are the effects on expression of aminolevulinate synthase and of heme oxygenase, known to be rate-limiting in heme synthesis and catabolism, respectively. In addition, the relationships between heme and iron metabolism which point to coordinated expression of several hepatic proteins including the transferrin receptor (see below) via a common iron pool (Smith and Ledford, 1988) should not be forgotten. Whether heme itself acts as a modulator remains to be demonstrated directly, but this ability seems likely in the case of regulation of heme oxygenase and, by analogy, with the regulation of transferrin by iron, to regulate hemopexin expression. In this regard, it is interesting that IV injection of heme in monkeys altered hemopexin serum levels in a dose-dependent manner (Foidart et al., 1982).

1. Regulation by heme in yeast. Information on regulation of gene expression by heme obtained from yeast mutants also has implications for understanding gene control in eukaryotes. For example, trans-acting factors have been postulated to be the mechanism whereby the four enzymes of heme biosynthesis whose genes are on three different chromosomes may be coordinately expressed during erythroid differentiation (Dubart et al., 1986).

In yeast, heme plays an important regulatory role in biogenesis of the respiratory chain enzymes and is specifically required for transcription of the *CYC1* gene coding for apo-iso-1-cytochrome c (Guarente et al., 1984). One of the two adjacent upstream activation sites of the *CYC1* gene, termed UAS1, is activated by a regulatory protein HAP1 (heme-activat-

---

*The regulation by heme of globin synthesis has been studied in reticulocytes for many years, and details of this are presented elsewhere in this book (Chap. 8).

ing protein; Pfeifer et al., 1987a, b), which is also a positive regulator of at least two other components of the respiratory chain, iso-2-cytochrome c and cytochrome b_2 (Verdiere et al., 1986). Activation via UAS1 is strictly dependent upon the presence of heme, with the low basal activity of UAS1 being induced more than 220-fold by adding heme supplement to heme-deficient cells.

HAP1 binds to region B of UAS1 in vitro; binding is greatly stimulated by heme. A second factor, RC2, present in cells grown under heme-sufficient, but not in heme-deficient, conditions binding to the same DNA sequences as does HAP1. Heme is required for RC2 synthesis or stability, but addition of heme neither stimulates its binding to DNA nor restores activity lost under heme-deficient conditions. Region A of UAS1 binds a second factor (region A factor, RAF) that is distinct from HAP1, and in fact the complex of RAF and HAP1 proteins is required for transcriptional activation. HAP1 also binds to a site in the *CYC7* UAS that bears no obvious sequence similarity to UAS1 of the *CYC1*, gene, and binding of HAP1 to this site is stimulated 10-fold by heme. Thus, both sites mediate activation of transcription in intact cells by HAP1 and heme (Pfeifer et al., 1987a, b).

Experiments in yeast mutants suggested that transcriptional regulation by heme may be a general mechanism for controlling the synthesis of both the heme and nonheme mitochondrial proteins of respiration (Myers et al., 1987). This mechanism is probably restricted to nuclear genes whose products are subunits of respiratory complexes (Myers et al., 1987). The promotors of the genes for subunits of the respiratory complexes are regulated by heme since neither subunit 5 of cytochrome oxidase nor the subunit of coenzyme QH2-cytochrome c reductase are heme-proteins.

2. Heme oxygenase regulation.   Heme oxygenase is an essential enzyme in heme catabolism (see Chap. 10). This enzyme is induced in liver not only by its substrate, heme, but also by a variety of nonheme compounds including metals, drugs, and endotoxin. The route of administration, binding to circulating proteins and transport to tissues, may help explain differences in the effects of metals and metal-porphyrins on heme oxygenase activity reported in the literature. Using mouse Hepa cells, together with the availability of other cell lines which express the hemopexin receptor, enabled a detailed examination to be made of the effects of this heme transport route on regulation. Incubation of hepatoma cells with either heme or heme-hemopexin increases heme oxygenase mRNA levels as judged by Northern blot analysis using the full-length cDNA clone for plasmid pRHO1. Nuclear runoff experiments showed that the mechanism of heme-mediated induction of heme oxygenase mRNA is due to increased transcription of the heme oxygenase gene (Alam et al., 1989; Alam and Smith, 1989). In fact, heme causes a transient increase in transcription of the heme oxygenase gene, reaching a maximum by 2 h, while mRNA levels are maintained for several more hours. The steady-state level of heme oxygenase mRNA is dependent upon the intracellular concentration of heme. This is shown by the fact that incubation with 10 μM heme-hemopexin for 4 h effects a twenty-fold increase in the level of heme oxygenase mRNA over the control level, while 1 to 2 μM "free" heme increases the amount of heme oxygenase mRNA ten- to twentyfold respectively (Alam and Smith, 1988a, b). Over a wide concentration range heme uptake in mouse Hepa cells is fivefold higher after incubation with [^{55}Fe]heme compared with equimolar [^{55}Fe]heme-hemopexin (Fig. 9.6). It should be emphasized that in vivo cells are seldom, if ever, exposed to nonprotein-bound heme. In other experiments, an equivalent dose of cadmium, known to increase heme oxygenase enzymic activity (Maines and Kappas, 1976), produced a 10-fold higher increased rate of transcription of the heme oxygenase gene compared with the increase seen after heme (Alam et al., 1989). The importance of specific transport routes is emphasized by the fact that only when the heme analogue Sn-protoporphyrin IX is presented to hepatocytes bound to hemopexin is heme oxygenase mRNA rapidly

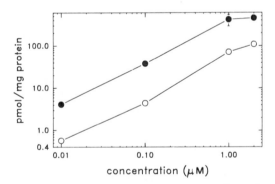

Figure 9.6 Comparison of the amount of cell-associated radioactivity after incubation of mouse Hepa cells with heme-hemopexin or nonprotein-bound heme. Hepa cells, grown in Dulbecco's modified Eagle medium supplemented with 0.35% glucose and 2% calf serum, were incubated at 37°C with the indicated amounts of ^{55}Fe-heme-hemopexin (O) or ^{55}Fe-heme alone (●) in serum-free medium. Heme uptake was measured after 30 min according to the protocol of Smith and Ledford (1988). Data shown are the mean ± standard deviation of triplicate samples from a representative experiment.

induced, whereas Sn-protoporphrin IX alone was without effect (Morgan et al., 1988). It will be of interest to determine if this induction of heme oxygenase mRNA also involves increased transcription of the heme oxygenase gene.

Furthermore, heme-hemopexin also induces heme oxygenase mRNA in nonhepatic cells including the human promyelocytic HL-60 cells (Alam and Smith, 1989), which express the hemopexin receptor (Taketani et al., 1987b). In this case a rapid and extensive 20-fold increase in mRNA levels is seen which is all the more striking compared with mouse Hepa cells because heme oxygenase mRNA is normally present in undetectable levels in HL-60 cells (Alam and Smith, 1989). Differences in the amount of cell-associated heme after incubations with heme-hemopexin or nonprotein-bound heme were also observed in HL-60 cells. In this case threefold higher amounts of heme were found when "free" heme was incubated with cells. However, in contrast to other cell types, the nuclei of HL-60 cells were extremely fragile and even colored red after incubation with levels of "free" heme up to 1 μM, suggesting extensive localization of heme in the nuclei. Thus, the amount of heme uptake and its effects varies for different cell types.

3. Transferrin receptor regulation.   Treatment of cultured cells with exogenous heme or agents known to alter heme synthesis or heme catabolism affect the number of surface transferrin receptors. Whether intracellular heme per se is an important signal for regulating the expression of the transferrin receptor in human hematopoietic, K562 cells (Louache et al., 1984; Rouault et al., 1985) and also in HeLa cells (Ward et al., 1984) remains to be demonstrated directly. Possible mechanisms include regulation by intact heme or heme-protein complexes and such regulation may also be mediated by exogenous heme. Transcriptional regulation by iron of the transferrin receptor has been shown (Rao et al., 1986). Presumably, because of rapid heme catabolism by heme oxygenase, intracellular iron pools are increased in K562 and HeLa cells incubated with heme and the transferrin receptor number decreases. Heme-hemopexin, which delivers heme via a specific intracellular pathway, decreased mRNA levels for the transferrin receptor in mouse Hepa cells (Alam and Smith, 1989), as well as in nonhepatic HL-60 and K562 cells (Alam and Smith, 1989). Presumably here too, the rapid catabolism of heme by heme oxygenase releases iron for this regulatory effect, since the heme-iron has been shown to equilibrate with the iron pool in Hepa cells (Smith and Ledford, 1988). Importantly, cell processes normally considered to be regulated by the iron status of the cell are also likely to be influenced by factors affecting intracellular heme and heme-protein metabolism.

Heme has additional regulatory effects on the transferrin receptor in reticulocytes. Not only does incubation with heme (as hemin) inhibit iron transport and internalization of transferrin, but also promotes phosphorylation of the transferrin receptor causing a redistribution to stromal membranes (Cox et al., 1985). Whether heme exerts these effects by interacting with protein kinase C directly in the plasma membrane or after intracellular transport remains to be determined. However, the effects of hemin vary with cell type and stage of differentiation, suggesting that multiple factors are involved (see Chap. 8).

4. Cytochrome P450 regulation. Heme is a positive regulator of hepatic cytochrome P450(b + e) isozymes, acting on mRNA transcription and/or the immediate events following initiation of transcription (Dwarki et al., 1987). The nuclear heme pool appears to influence this rate of transcription, since addition of heme in vitro to heme-depleted nuclei produced a significant increase in transcription rates for these cytochrome P450 isozymes (Dwarki et al., 1987). Heme also appears to be necessary for stabilization of newly synthesized P450 protein induced by phenobarbital (Dwarki et al., 1987). It will be of interest to learn whether these processes are mediated by a heme-regulator protein binding newly synthesized heme and/or exogenous heme, and whether this protein also interacts with regulatory sequences of other genes (e.g., the heme oxygenase gene), since both these gene products are affected by treatments which alter heme synthesis and catabolism.

D. Transport of linear tetrapyrroles

1. Movement of biliverdin from heme oxygenase to biliverdin reductase. The oxidative cleavage of the heme ring is catalyzed by the combined actions of NADPH-cytochrome c reductase and heme oxygenase, both integral membrane proteins of the endoplasmic reticulum (ER), to yield the linear tetrapyrrole biliverdin IX-α. This bile pigment is then reduced to bilirubin IX-α by the cytosolic enzyme, biliverdin reductase. Heme oxygenase is thought to be located in the ER membrane such that its active site is exposed to the cytoplasmic surface (Hino et al., 1979). This position would facilitate reduction of biliverdin to bilirubin at the ER membrane-cytosol interface. Binary complexes of cytochrome c reductase with heme oxygenase or cytochrome c reductase with biliverdin reductase, as well as ternary complexes of cytochrome reductase, biliverdin reductase, and heme oxygenase were detected in a soluble reconstituted system (Yoshinaga et al., 1982). As mentioned in Sec. III-A, soluble proteins such as protein kinase C can become membrane-associated upon calcium and magnesium binding and other soluble proteins also exist in membrane-bound forms. Perhaps similar mechanisms are involved to alter the cellular location of biliverdin reductase, bringing it close to heme oxygenase. Such multienzyme complexes would facilitate metabolic conversion without the need for extensive intracellular transport of substrates. Thus, biliverdin produced by the membrane-bound NADPH-cytochrome c reductase–heme oxygenase complex could be reduced to bilirubin before the bile pigment leaves the endoplasmic reticulum. The transport route for bilirubin to the ER for conjugation by UDP-glucuronyltransferase is presumed to occur by diffusion through the cytosol. Membrane-membrane collisions rather than by membrane fusion (Whitmer et al., 1987) have also been suggested. UDP-glucuronyltransferase, located primarily in smooth and rough ER, is also found in small amounts in the Golgi membranes and nuclear envelope. Since this enzyme is also membrane-bound in the ER, this opens up the possibility that a certain fraction of heme may undergo metabolic conversion to conjugated bilirubin entirely at the ER membrane-cytosol interface.

Conversely, if the active sites of heme oxygenase and glucuronyltransferase face the lumen of the ER, vesicular transfer of bile pigments through the cell may be important. If the active sites of these enzymes face opposite sides of the ER membrane, additional, even more complex, transport mechanisms must be sought.

2. Cellular uptake of bilirubin. Recent reviews have addressed the hepatic uptake of circulating bilirubin derived from extrahepatic sources (Sorrentino et al., 1987; Berk et al., 1987) and its intracellular transfer to the ER for conjugation (Whitmer et al., 1984). Consequently, discussion here will be confined to transport mechanisms and ligand-protein interactions. Because of its poor water solubility, bilirubin circulates in plasma tightly bound to albumin in equilibrium with its free form (K_d 10 to 100 nM, Sorrentino et al., 1987). Pharmacokinetic studies of the clearance of ^{3}H-bilirubin and ^{125}I-albumin established that bilirubin-albumin is not taken up by liver cells. Rather, bilirubin must first dissociate from albumin before uptake into hepatocytes (references in Sorrentino et al., 1987). Hepatic sinusoids are lined by endothelial cells, in between which large pores allow passage of albumin-bilirubin complexes into the space of Disse. Direct contact of these albumin-ligand complexes occurs with microvilli on the sinusoidal surface of hepatocyte plasma membranes, and dissociation of bilirubin from albumin takes place at, or very near, the surface of the hepatocyte. One mechanism for porphyrin transport from circulating albumin-porphyrin complexes requires dissociation of the porphyrin (Sec. III-B). Thus, certain similarities between the interaction of bilirubin-albumin and porphyrin-albumin complexes with hepatocytes are evident. In addition, as with exogenous porphyrins, significant amounts of bilirubin are bound to high-density lipoproteins in the circulation (Suzuki et al., 1988).

After dissociation from albumin, transport of bilirubin occurs as a result of its specific interaction with a high-affinity membrane carrier protein (Reichen and Berk, 1979; Stremmel et al., 1983). This carrier protein transports other inorganic anions, for example, sulfobromophthalein (BSP) and indocyanine green, but is distinct from the carrier proteins for conjugated bile acids and long-chain, free fatty acids (Stremmel and Berk, 1986). In normal rat liver this carrier protein could be located by immunofluorescence only on surface membranes of hepatocytes, especially those facing the sinusoids. However, after bile duct ligation the protein was also found on the luminal surface of cells lining the bile ducts (Stremmel et al., 1983).

Because the intracellular concentration of free bilirubin exceeds that found in plasma, transport occurs against a chemical gradient. The driving force for bilirubin uptake is not yet established, but the energy for uptake of bile acids derives from the action of Na^+,K^+-ATPase. Two transport models have been proposed: The membrane carrier protein functions alone to move the bilirubin through the membrane by a flip-flop shuttle movement, involving a conformational change in the carrier protein; and second, the transmembrane movement of bilirubin occurs through a two-site pore in the membrane, lined by the carrier protein (Sorrentino et al., 1987). If other membrane proteins are necessary to effect transport, the bilirubin carrier would be more appropriately termed a bilirubin receptor.

Inside the hepatocyte, as in plasma, bilirubin and the other classes of organic anions bind to a specific isozyme of the cytosolic GSH-S-transferases, ligandin (Sorrentino et al., 1987). Binding to ligandin is considered to be one means whereby the diffusion of bilirubin to the endoplasmic reticulum for conjugation is facilitated. Alternative roles for ligandin have been proposed, including diminishing the efflux of bilirubin from hepatocytes to plasma or serving a storage function in conditions of hyperbilirubinemia (Whitmer et al., 1984).

3. Biliary excretion of bilirubin and its conjugates.   Biliary excretion of bilirubin is saturable and a variety of organic anions compete with conjugated bilirubin for biliary excretion. These properties suggest that canalicular excretion of bilirubin and its conjugates is, like sinusoidal uptake of bilirubin, a carrier-mediated process. A passive diffusion component may be involved in addition to secretion against a concentration gradient, but currently, these mechanisms are poorly understood.

IV. Summary and Conclusions

Heme is transported by receptor-mediated endocytosis into hepatocytes by hemopexin receptors and, as hemoglobin, by haptoglobin receptors. Hemopexin receptors are also present in placenta, human erythroleukemic K562 cells, promyelocytic HL-60 cells, and perhaps cells of the immune system and spleen. Heme transport may also occur via specific heme receptors in other cell types such as duodenal enterocytes. Intracellular routes exist, but remain to be elucidated, for heme transfer from the plasma membrane to heme oxygenase in the endoplasmic reticulum, to the nucleus for transcriptional regulation, from sites of synthesis for incorporation into heme-proteins in the inner membrane space of mitochondria and from the mitochondria to apo-proteins in the endoplasmic reticulum, cytosol, and to other organelles. While MHBP of the hemopexin system is required for intracellular heme transport via the hemopexin receptor, any other proteins involved in this or other paths remain to be identified. Proteins active in transcriptional regulation by heme have been isolated from yeast and their counterparts will no doubt soon be found in mammalian cells.

Many pathogenic microorganisms can utilize heme-iron as a sole source of iron for growth, but the mechanism(s) whereby bacteria, yeast, and parasites transport heme and hemoglobin are not yet well defined. In many cases, as in mammalian cells, specific membrane proteins appear to be involved. Hepatoma cells can also utilize heme-iron for growth, and cells of the immune and erythropoietic systems may also express hemopexin receptors to use heme-iron in their proliferative responses to infection and hemolytic conditions.

Proteins are also vital for the transport of porphyrinogens and their oxidation products, porphyrins, inside and outside the cell. The enzymes involved in heme synthesis and catabolism must contribute to the intracellular movement of these reactive lipophilic compounds. Albumin and lipoproteins are the principle transporting molecules of both endogenous and exogenous porphyrins in the circulation.

ACKNOWLEDGMENTS

The author would like to acknowledge Dr. William T. Morgan for his critical review of this manuscript and for his encouragement. Thanks are due to Mrs. Jean Bennett for her technical help and aid in preparing the bibliography and to Ms. Joelle Finlay and Ms. Eileen Cohen for their technical assistance. This work was supported in part by USPHS grants AM27237 and DK37463.

REFERENCES

Adornato, B. T., Engel, W. K., and Foidart-Desalle, M. (1978). Elevations of hemopexin levels in neuromuscular disease, *Arch. Neurol.* **35**:577–580.

Aft, R. L., and Mueller, G. C. (1983). Hemin-mediated DNA strand scission, *J. Biol. Chem.* **258**:12069–12072.

Aft, R. L., and Mueller, G. C. (1984). Hemin-mediated oxidative degradation of proteins, *J. Biol. Chem.* **259**:301–305.

Alam, J., and Smith, A. (1989). Receptor-mediated transport of heme by hemopexin regulates gene expression in mammalian cells, *J. Biol. Chem.*, to appear.

Alam, J., Shibahara, S., and Smith, A. (1989). Transcriptional activation of the heme oxygenase gene by heme and cadmium in mouse hepatoma cells, *J. Biol. Chem.*, **264**:6371–6375.

Anderson, K. E., Simionatto, C. S., Drummond, G. S., and Kappas, A. (1986). Disposition of tin-protoporphyrin and suppression of hyperbilirubinemia in humans, *Clin. Pharmacol. Therap.* **39**:510–520.

Anderson, P. M., and Desnick, R. J. (1980). Purification and properties of uroporphyrinogen I synthase from human erythrocytes. Identification of stable enzyme-substrate intermediates, *J. Biol. Chem.* **255**:1993–1999.

Ashendel, C. L. (1985). The phorbol ester receptor: A phospholipid-regulated protein kinase, *Biochim. Biophys. Acta* **822**:219–242.

Avner, D. L., Larsen, R., and Berenson, M. M. (1983). Inhibition of liver surface membrane Na^+,K^+-adenosine triphosphatase, Mg^{+2}-adenosine triphosphatase and 5′-nucleotidase activities by protoporphyrin, *Gastroenterology* **85**:700–706.

Badawy, A. A.-B. (1979). Central role of tryptophan pyrrolase in haem metabolism, *Biochem. Soc. Trans.* **7**:575–583.

Badawy, A. A.-B., and Evans, M. (1974). Guinea-pig liver tryptophan pyrrolase. Absence of detectable apoenzyme activity and of hormonal induction by cortisol and possible regulation by tryptophan, *Biochem. J.* **138**:445–451.

Badawy, A. A.-B., and Evans, M. (1975). Regulation of rat liver tryptophan pyrrolase by its cofactor haem: Experiments with haematin and 5-aminolaevulinate and comparison with the substrate and hormonal mechanisms, *Biochem. J.* **150**:511–520.

Banerjee, R. (1962). Thermodynamic study of heme-globin association. II. Methemoglobin, *Biochim. Biophys. Acta* **64**:385–395.

Battersby, A. R., Fookes, C. J. R., Hart, G., Matcham, G. W. J., and Pandey, P. S. (1983). Biosynthesis of porphyrins and related macrocycles. 21. The interactions of deaminase and its product (hydroxymethylbilane) and the relationship between deaminase and cosynthetase, *J. Chem. Soc. Perkin Trans.* 1:3041–3047.

Baumann, H., Held, W. A., and Berger, F. G. (1984). The acute phase response of mouse liver, *J. Biol. Chem.* **259**:566–573.

Baumann, H., and Muller-Eberhard, U. (1987). Synthesis of hemopexin and cysteine protease inhibitor is coordinately regulated by HSF-II and interferon-beta 2 in rat hepatoma cells, *Biochim. Biophys. Res. Comm.* **146**:1218–1226.

Baumann, H., Onorato, V., Gauldie, J., and Jahreis, G. P. (1987). Distinct sets of acute phase plasma proteins are stimulated by separate human hepatocyte-stimulating factors and monokines in rat hepatoma cells, *J. Biol. Chem.* **262**:9756–9768.

Beaven, G. H., Chen, S.-H., D'Albis, A., and Gratzer, W. B. (1974). A spectroscopic study of the haemin-human-serum-albumin system, *Eur. J. Biochem.* **41**:539–546.

Berk, P. D., Potter, B. J., and Stremmel, W. (1987). Role of plasma membrane ligand-binding proteins in the hepatocellular uptake of albumin-bound organic anions, *Hepatology* **7**:165–176.

Bernhard, H. P., Darlington, G. J., and Ruddle, F. H. (1973). Expression of liver phenotypes in cultured mouse hepatoma cells: Synthesis and secretion of serum albumin, *Dev. Biol.* **35**:83–96.

Berry, A., Jordan, P. M., and Seehra, J. S. (1981). The isolation and characterization of catalytically competent porphobilinogen deaminase-intermediate complexes, *FEBS Lett.* **129**:220–224.

Bhat, K. S., Sardana, M. K., and Padmanaban, G. (1977). Role of haem in the synthesis and assembly of cytochrome P450, *Biochem J.* **164**:295–303.

Biberstein, E. L., Mini, P. D., Gills, M. G. (1965). Action of Haemophilus cultures on delta-aminolevulinic acid, *J. Bacteriol.* **86**:814–819.

Bissell, D. M., Liem, H. H., and Muller-Eberhard, U. (1979). Secretion of haem by hepatic parenchymal cells, *Biochem. J.* **184**:689–694.

Bjorn-Rasmussen, E., Hallberg, L., Isaksson, B., and Arvidsson, B. (1974). Food iron absorption in man. Applications of the two-pool extrinsic tag method to measure heme and nonheme iron absorption from the whole diet, *J. Clin. Invest.* **53**:247–255.

Bolla, R. I., Weinstein, P. P., Lou, C. (1972). In vitro nutritional requirements of *Nippostrongylus brasiliensis*. I. Effects of sterols, sterol derivatives and heme compounds on the free-living stages, *Comp. Biochem. Physiol.* **43B**:487–501.

Bornheim, L. M., Parish, D. W., Smith, K. M., Litman, D. A., and Correia, M. A. (1986). The influence of side chain modifications of the heme moiety on prosthetic acceptance and function of rat hepatic cytochrome P-450 and tryptophan pyrrolase, *Arch. Biochem. Biophys.* **246**:63–74.

Braun, S. R., Weiss, F. R., Keller, A. I., Ciccone, J. R., and Preuss, H. G. (1970). Evaluation of the renal toxicity of heme proteins and their derivatives: A role in the genesis of acute tubule necrosis, *J. Exp. Med.* **131**:443–460.

Breslow, E., Chandra, R., and Kappas, A. (1986). Biochemical properties of the heme oxygenase inhibitor: Sn-protoporphyrin, *J. Biol. Chem.* **261**:3135–3141.

Brown, E. B., Hwang, Y.-F., Nicol. S., and Ternberg, J. (1968). Absorption of radiation-labeled hemoglobin by dogs, *J. Lab. Clin. Med.* **72**:58–64.

Brown, S. B., Shillcock, M., and Jones, P. (1976). Equilibrium and kinetic studies of the aggregation of porphyrins in aqueous solution, *Biochem. J.* **153**:279–285.

Bunn, H. F., and Jandl, J. H. (1968). Exchange of heme among hemoglobins and between hemoglobin and albumin, *J. Biol. Chem.* **243**:465–475.

Camadro, J.-M., Chambon, H., Jolles, J., and Labbe, P. (1986). Purification and properties of coproporphyrinogen oxidase from the yeast *Saccharomycaes cerevisiae*, *Eur. J. Biochem.* **156**:579–587.

Cannon, J. B., Kuo, F.-S., Pasternack, R. F., Wong, N. M., and Muller-Eberhard, U. (1984). Kinetics of the interaction of hemin liposomes with heme binding proteins, *Biochemistry* **23**:3715–3721.

Cannon, J. B., Kuo, F.-S., Vatandoust, F., Liem, H. H., and Muller-Eberhard, U. (1985). The effect of metalloporphyrins and heme liposomes on delta-aminolevulinate synthase activity in rat liver, *Biochem. Biophys. Res. Comm.* **130**:306–312.

Carmel, N., and Gross, J. (1977). Hemopexin metabolism in mice with transplantable tumors, *Israel J. Med. Sci.* **13**:1182–1190.

Carrano, C. J., Tsutsui, M., and McConnell, S. (1977). Localization of meso-tetra(*p*-sulfophenyl)porphine in murine sarcoma virus-induced tumor-bearing mice, *Cancer Treat. Rep.* **61**:1297–1300.

Carrano, C. J., Tsutsui, M., and McConnell, S. (1978). Tumor localizing agents: The transport of meso-tetra(*p*-sulfophenyl)porphine by Vero and HEp-2 cells in vitro, *Chem. Biol. Interact.* **21**:233–248.

Conrad, M. E., Weintraub, L. R., Sears, D. A., and Crosby, W. H. (1966). Absorption of hemoglobin iron, *Amer. J. Physiol.* **211**:1123–1130.

Coppens, I., Opperdoes, F. R., Courtoy, P. J., and Baudhuin, P. (1987). Receptor-mediated endocytosis in the bloodstream form of *Trypanosoma brucei*, *J. Protozool.* **34**:465–473.

Correia, M. A., Farrell, G. C., Olson, S., Wong, J. S., Schmid, R., Ortiz de Montellano, P. R., Beilan, H. S., Kunze, K. L., and Mico, B. A. (1981). Cytochrome P-450 heme moiety: The specific target in drug-induced heme alkylation, *J. Biol. Chem.* **256**:5466–5470.

Coulton, J. W., and Pang, J. C. S. (1983). Transport of hemin by *Haemophilus influenzae* Type b, *Curr. Microbiol.* **9**:93–98.

Cox, T. M., O'Donnell, M. W., Aisen, P., and London, I. M. (1985). Hemin inhibits internalization of transferrin by reticulocytes and promotes phosphorylation of the membrane transferrin receptor, *Proc. Nat. Acad. Sci. (U.S.A.)* **82**:5170–5174.

Crosa, J. H. (1980). A plasmid associated with virulence in the marine fish pathogen *Vibrio auguillarum* specifies an iron-sequestering system, *Nature* **284**:566–568.

Dailey, H. A. (1985). Spectroscopic examination of the active site of bovine ferrochelatase, *Biochemistry* **24**:1287–1291.

Dailey, H. A., and Fleming, J. E. (1983). Bovine ferrochelatase. Kinetic analysis of inhibition by *N*-methylprotoporphyrin, manganese and heme, *J. Biol. Chem.* **258**:11453–11459.

Dailey, H. A., and Fleming, J. E. (1986). The role of arginyl residues in porphyrin binding to ferrochelatase, *J. Biol. Chem.* **261**:7902–7905.

Dailey, H. A., and Karr, S. W. (1987). Purification and characterization of murine protoporphyrinogen oxidase, *Biochemistry* **26**:2697–2701.

Dailey, H. A., and Smith, A. (1984). Differential interaction of porphyrins used in photoradiation therapy with ferrochelatase, *Biochem. J.* **223**:441–445.

Daskaleros, P. A., and Payne, S. M. (1987). Congo red binding phenotype is associated with hemin binding and increased infectivity of *Shigella flexneri* in the HeLa cell model, *Infect. Immunol.* **55**:1393–1398.

Davies, D. M., Liem, H. H., Johnson, E. F., and Muller-Eberhard, U. (1982). The role of cytosolic proteins in the intracellular transport of haem in rat liver. A dual-label approach, *Biochem. J.* **202**:211–216.

Davies, D. M., Smith, A., Muller-Eberhard, U., and Morgan, W. T. (1979). Hepatic subcellular metabolism of heme from heme-hemopexin: Incorporation of iron into ferritin, *Biochem. Biophys. Res. Comm.* **91**:1504–1511.

Doiron, D. R., and Gomer, C. J. (Eds.) (1984). *Porphyrin Localization and Treatment of Tumors*, Alan R. Liss, New York.

Drummond, G. S., Galbraith, R. A., Sardana, M. K., and Kappas, A. (1987). Reduction of the C_2 and C_4 vinyl groups of Sn-protoporphyrin to form Sn-mesoporphyrin markedly enhances the ability of the metalloporphyrin to inhibit in vivo heme catabolism, *Arch. Biochem. Biophys.* **255**:64–74.

Drummond, G. S., and Kappas, A. (1982). Chemoprevention of neonatal jaundice: Potency of tin-protoporphyrin in an animal model, *Science* **217**:1250–1252.

Drummond, G. S., and Kappas, A. (1984). An experimental model of postnatal jaundice in the suckling rat. Suppression of induced hyperbilirubinemia by Sn-protoporphyrin, *J. Clin. Invest.* **74**:142–149.

Dubart, A., Mattel, M. G., Raich, N., Beaupain, D., Romeo, P. H., Mattei, J. F., and Goossens, M. (1986). Assignment of human uroporphyrinogen decarboxylase (URO-D) to the p34 band of chromosome 1, *Hum. Genet.* **73**:277–279.

Dubbelman, T. M. A. R., and Van Steveninck, J. (1984). Photodynamic effects of hematoporphyrin-derivative on transmembrane transport systems of murine L929 fibroblasts, *Biochim. Biophys. Acta* **771**:201–207.

Dwarki, V. J., Francis, V. N. K., Bhat, G. J., and Padmanaban, G. (1987). Regulation of cytochrome P-450 messenger RNA and apoprotein levels by heme, *J. Biol. Chem.* **262**:16958–16962.

Dyer, D. W., West, E. P., and Sparling, P. F. (1987). Effects of serum carrier proteins on the growth of pathogenic *Neisseriae* with heme-bound iron, *Infect. Immunol.* **55**:2171–2175.

Eaton, J. W., Brandt, P., Mahoney, J. R., and Lee, J. T. (1982). Haptoglobin: A natural bacteriostat, *Science* **215**:691–693.

Ebert, P. S., Frykholm, B. C., Hess, R. A., and Tschudy, D. P. (1981). Uptake of hematin and growth of malignant murine erythroleukemia cells depleted of endogenous heme by succinylacetone, *Cancer Res.* **41**:937–941.

Elder, G. H., and Evans, J. O. (1978). Evidence that the coproporphyrinogen oxidase activity of rat liver is situated in the intermembrane space of mitochondria, *Biochem J.* **172**:345–347.

Engler, R., and Jayle, M. F. (1976). Haptoglobin and hemolysis, *Frontiers in Matrix Biol.* **3**:42–51.

Evans, J. N. S., Burton, G., Fagerness, P. E., Mackenzie, N. E., and Scott, A. I. (1986a). Biosynthesis of porphyrins and corrins. 2. Isolation, purification, and NMR investigations of the porphobilinogen-deaminase covalent complex, *Biochemistry* **25**:905–912.

Evans, J. N. S., Davies, R. C., Boyd, A. S. F., Ichinose, I., Mackenzie, N. E., Scott, A. I., and Baxter, R. L. (1986b). Biosynthesis of porphyrins and corrins. 1. ^{1}H and ^{13}C NMR spectra of (hydroxymethyl)bilane and uroporphyrinogens I and III, *Biochemistry* 25:896–904.

Evans, N. M., Smith, D. D., and Wicken, A. J. (1974). Haemin and nicotinamide adenine dinucleotide requirements of *Haemophilus influenzae* and *Haemophilus parainfluenzae*, *J. Med. Microbiol.* 7:359–365.

Eyster, M. E., Edgington, T. S., Liem, H. H., and Muller-Eberhard, U. (1972). Plasma hemopexin levels following aortic valve replacement. A valuable screening test for assessing the severity of cardiac hemolysis, *J. Lab. Clin. Med.* 80:112–116.

Falk, J. E. (1964). *Porphyrins and Metalloporphyrins*, Elsevier, Amsterdam.

Farooqui, S., Morgan, W. T., and Smith, A. (1989). Investigations on the relationship of the hemopexin receptor with its associated membrane heme-binding protein, manuscript in preparation.

Feigelson, P., and Greengard, O. (1961). A microsomal iron-porphyrin activator of rat liver tryptophan pyrrolase, *J. Biol. Chem.* 236:153–157.

Ferreira, G. C., Andrew, T. L., Karr, S. W., and Dailey, H. A. (1988). Organization of the two terminal enzymes of the heme biosynthetic pathway. Orientation of protoporphyrinogen oxidase and evidence for a membrane complex, *J. Biol. Chem.* 263:3835–3839.

Ferreira, G. C., and Dailey, H. A. (1987). Reconstitution of the two terminal enzymes of the heme biosynthetic pathway into phospholipid vesicles, *J. Biol. Chem.* 262:4407–4412.

Fildes, P. (1921). The nature of the effect of blood-pigment upon the growth of *H. influenzae*, *Brit. J. Exp. Pathol.* 2:16–25.

Foidart, M., Eiseman, J., Engel, W. K., Adornato, B. T., Liem, H. H., and Muller-Eberhard, U. (1982). Effect of heme administration on hemopexin metabolism in the rhesus monkey, *J. Lab. Clin. Med.* 100:451–460.

Foidart, M., Liem, H. H., Adornato, B. T., Engel, W. K., and Muller-Eberhard, U. (1983). Hemopexin metabolism in patients with altered serum levels, *J. Lab. Clin. Med.* 102:838–846.

Foster, L. A., and Bogitsh, B. J. (1986). Utilization of the heme moiety of hemoglobin by *Schistosoma mansoni* schistosomules in vitro, *J. Parasit.* 72:669–676.

Francis, R. T., Jr., Booth, J. W., and Becker, R. R. (1985). Uptake of iron from hemoglobin and the haptoglobin-hemoglobin complex by hemolytic bacteria, *Int. J. Biochem.* 17:767–773.

Freeman, T. (1965). Haptoglobin metabolism in relation to red cell destruction, *Protides Biol. Fluids Proc. Colloq.* 12:344–352.

Frydman, R. B., Tomaro, M. L., Buldain, G., Awruch, J., Diaz, L., and Frydman, B. (1981). Specificity of heme oxygenase: A study with synthetic hemins, *Biochemistry* 20:5177–5182.

Fuchs, O., Hradilek, A., Borova, J., Neuwirt, J., and Travnicek, M. (1984). Effect of hemin on poly(A)-containing RNA synthesis and transport from nucleus into cytoplasm in Friend cells of the Fw line, *Biomed. Biochim. Acta* 43:S94–S97.

Galbraith, R. A., Sassa, S., and Kappas, A. (1985). Heme binding to murine erythroleukemia cells, *J. Biol. Chem.* 260:12198–12202.

Gambari, R., Barbieri, R., Piva, R., Viola, L., Castagnoli, A., and Del Senno, L. (1986). Control of heme internalization and metabolism in tumor cells: Evidence for a heme-receptor?, *Boll. Soc. It. Biol. Sper.* 62:849–852.

Garby, L., and Noyes, W. D. (1959). Studies on hemoglobin metabolism. I. The kinetic properties of the plasma hemoglobin pool in normal man, *J. Clin. Invest.* 38:1479–1483.

Gardiner, M. E., and Morgan, E. H. (1974). Transferrin and iron uptake by the liver in the rat, *Aust. J. Exp. Biol. Med. Sci.* 52:723–736.

Gasser, S. M., Ohashi, A., Daum, G., Bohni, P. C., Gibson, J., Reid, G. A., Yonetani, T., and Schatz, G. (1982). Imported mitochondrial proteins cytochrome b_2 and cytochrome c_1 are processed in two steps, *Proc. Nat. Acad. Sci.* (*U.S.A.*) 79:267–271.

Glass, J., Nunez, M. T., and Robinson, S. H. (1980). Transferrin-binding and iron-binding proteins of rabbit reticulocyte plasma membranes. Three distinct moieties, *Biochim. Biophys. Acta* 598:293–304.

Glueck, R., Green, D., Cohen, I., and Ts'ao, C.-H. (1983). Hematin: Unique effects on hemostasis, *Blood* **61**:243–249.

Goetsch, C. A., and Bissell, D. M. (1986). Instability of hematin used in the treatment of acute hepatic porphyria, *N. Engl. J. Med.* **315**:235–238.

Grandchamp, B., Bissell, D. M., Licko, V., and Schmid, R. (1981). Formation and disposition of newly synthesized heme in adult rat hepatocytes in primary culture, *J. Biol. Chem.* **256**:11677–11683.

Grandchamp, B., Phung, N., and Nordmann, Y. (1978). The mitochondrial localization of coproporphyrinogen III oxidase, *Biochem. J.* **176**:97–102.

Grasbeck, R., Majuri, R., Kouvonen, I., and Tenhunen, R. (1982). Spectral and other studies on the intestinal haem receptor of the pig, *Biochim. Biophys. Acta* **700**:137–142.

Green, D., Reynolds, N., Klein, J., Kohl, H., and Ts'ao, C.-H. (1983). The inactivation of hemostatic factors by hematin, *J. Lab. Clin. Med.* **102**:361–369.

Guarente, L., Lalonde, B., Gifford, P., and Alani, E. (1984). Distinctly regulated tandem upstream activation sites mediate catabolite repression of the *CYC1* gene of *S. cerevisiae*, *Cell* **36**:503–511.

Gutteridge, J. M. C. (1982). Fate of oxygen free radicals in extracellular fluids, *Biochem. Soc. Trans.* **10**:72–73.

Gutteridge, J. M. C. (1986). Iron promotors of the Fenton reaction and lipid peroxidation can be released from haemoglobin by peroxides, *FEBS Lett.* **201**:291–295.

Gutteridge, J. M. C. (1987). The antioxidant activity of haptoglobin towards haemoglobin-stimulated lipid peroxidation, *Biochim. Biophys. Acta* **917**:219–223.

Gutteridge, J. M. C., Paterson, S. K., Segal, A. W., and Halliwell, B. (1981). Inhibition of lipid peroxidation by the iron-binding protein lactoferrin, *Biochem. J.* **199**:259–261.

Gutteridge, J. M. C., and Smith, A. (1988). Antioxidant protection by haemopexin of haem-stimulated lipid peroxidation, *Biochem. J.*, **256**:861–865.

Hallberg, L., and Solvell, L. (1967). Absorption of hemoglobin iron in man, *Acta Med. Scand.* **181**:335–354.

Halliwell, B. (1987). Oxidants and human disease: Some new concepts, *FASEB J.* **1**:358–364.

Halliwell, B., and Gutteridge, J. M. C. (1986). Iron and free radical reactions: Two aspects of antioxidant protection, *TIBS* **11**:372–375.

Harbin, B. M., and Dailey, H. A. (1985). Orientation of ferrochelatase in bovine liver mitochondria, *Biochemistry* **24**:366–370.

Hebert, G. A., and Hancock, G. A. (1985). Synergistic hemolysis exhibited by species of Staphylococci, *J. Clin. Microbiol.* **22**:409–415.

Hennig, B., Koehler, H., and Neupert, W. (1983). Receptor sites involved in posttranslational transport of apocytochrome c into mitochondria: Specificity, affinity and number of sites, *Proc. Nat. Acad. Sci. (U.S.A.)* **80**:4963–4967.

Hennig, B., and Neupert, W. (1981). Assembly of cytochrome c. Apocytochrome c is bound to specific sites on mitochondria before its conversion to holocytochrome c, *Eur. J. Biochem.* **121**:203–212.

Hennig, B., and Neupert, W. (1983). Assembly of mitochondrial proteins, *Horizons in Biochemistry and Biophysics* (A. M. Kroon, Ed.,) Wiley, New York, Vol. 7, pp. 307–346.

Hershko, C. (1975). The fate of circulating haemoglobin, *Brit. J. Haematol.* **29**:199–204.

Higa, Y., Oshiro, S., Kino, K., Tsunoo, H., and Nakajima, H. (1981). Catabolism of globin-haptoglobin in liver cells after intravenous administration of hemoglobin-haptoglobin to rats, *J. Biol. Chem.* **256**:12322–12328.

Hilf, R., Warne, N. W., Smail, D. B., and Gibson, S. L. (1984). Photodynamic inactivation of selected intracellular enzymes by hematoporphyrin derivative and their relationship to tumor cell viability in vitro, *Cancer Lett.* **24**:165–172.

Hino, Y., Asagami, H., Minakami, S. (1979). Topological arrangement in microsomal membranes of hepatic haem oxygenase induced by cobalt chloride, *Biochem. J.* **178**:331–337.

Hrkal, Z., and Muller-Eberhard, U. (1971). Partial characterization of the heme-binding serum glycoproteins rabbit and human hemopexin, *Biochemistry* **10**:1746–1750.

Hrkal, Z., Vodrazka, Z., and Kalousek, I. (1974). Transfer of heme from ferrihemoglobin and ferrihemoglobin isolated chains to hemopexin, *Eur. J. Biochem.* **43**:73–78.

Hunt, R. C., Ruffin, R., and Yang, Y.-S. (1984). Alterations in the transferrin receptor of human erythroleukemic cells after induction of hemoglobin synthesis, *J. Biol. Chem.* **259**:9944–9952.

Hutner, S. H., Bacchi, C. J., and Baker, H. (1979). Nutrition of the Kinetoplastida, *Biology of the Kinetoplastida* (W. H. R. Lumsden and D. A. Evans, Eds.), Academic, New York, No. 2, pp. 654–691.

Ishiguro, E. E., Ainsworth, T., Trust, T. J., and Kay, W. W. (1985). Congo red agar, a differential medium for *Aeromonas salmonicida*, detects the presence of the cell surface protein array involved in virulence, *J. Bacteriol.* **164**:1233–1237.

Ishiguro, T., Imanishi, K., and Suzuki, I. (1984). Hemopexin levels in mice, *Int. J. Immunopharmacol.* **6**:241–244.

Israels, L. G., Yoda, B., and Schacter, B. A. (1975). Heme binding and its possible significance in heme movement and availability in the cell, *Ann. N.Y. Acad. Sci.* **244**:651–661.

Jaffe, E. K., and Markham, G. D. (1987). ^{13}C NMR studies of porphobilinogen synthase: Observation of intermediates bound to a 280000-dalton protein, *Biochemistry* **26**:4258–4264.

Janney, S. K., Joist, J. H., and Fitch, C. D. (1986). Excess release of ferriheme in G6PD-deficient erythrocytes: Possible cause of hemolysis and resistance to malaria, *Blood* **67**:331–333.

Jori, G., Beltramini, M., Reddi, E., Salvato, B., Pagnan, A., Ziron, L., Tomio, L., and Tsanov, T. (1984). Evidence for a major role of plasma lipoproteins as hematoporphyrin carriers in vivo, *Cancer Lett.* **24**:291–297.

Kaplan, K. M., and Oski, F. A. (1980). Anemia with *Haemophilus influenzae* meningitis, *Pediatrics* **65**:1101–1104.

Kappas, A., and Drummond, G. S. (1986). Control of heme metabolism with synthetic metalloporphyrins, *J. Clin. Invest.* **77**:335–339.

Kappas, A., Drummond, G. S., Simionatto, C. S., and Anderson, K. E. (1984). Control of heme oxygenase and plasma levels of bilirubin by a synthetic heme analogue, tin-proto-porphyrin, *Hepatology* **4**:336–341.

Kappas, A., Sassa, S., and Anderson, K. E. (1983). The porphyrias, *The Metabolic Basis of Inherited Diseases* (D. S. Frederickson, J. B. Stanbury, J. B. Wyngaarden, J. C. Goldstein, and M. S. Brown, Eds.), 5th ed., McGraw-Hill, New York, pp. 1301–1384.

Kappas, A., Simionatto, C. S., Drummond, G. S., Sassa, S., and Anderson, K. E. (1985). The liver excretes large amounts of heme into bile when heme oxygenase is inhibited competitively by Sn-protoporphyrins, *Proc. Nat. Acad. Sci. (U.S.A.)* **82**:896–900.

Kay, W. W., Phipps, B. M., Ishiguro, E. E., and Trust, T. T. (1985). Porphyrin binding by surface array virulence protein of *Aeromonas salmonicida*, *J. Bacteriol.* **164**:1332–1336.

Keller, M.-E., and Romslo, I. (1978). Studies on the uptake of porphyrin by isolated rat liver mitochondria, *Biochim. Biophys. Acta* **503**:238–250.

Keng, T., Alani, E., and Guarente, L. (1986). The nine amino-terminal residues of delta-aminolevulinate synthase direct beta-galactosidase into the mitochondrial matrix, *Mol. Cell. Biol.* **6**:355–364.

Kessel, D. R. (1981). Transport and binding of hematoporphyrin derivative and related porphyrins by murine leukemia L1210 cells, *Cancer Res.* **41**:1318–1323.

Kessel, D. R., and Cheng, M.-L. (1985). On the preparation and properties of dihematoporphyrin ether, the tumor-localizing component of HPD, *Photochem. Photobiol.* **41**:277–282.

Kino, K., Tsunoo, H., Higa, Y., Takami, M., Hamaguchi, H., and Nakajima, H. (1980). Hemoglobin-haptoglobin receptor in rat liver plasma membrane, *J. Biol. Chem.* **255**:9616–9620.

Kino, K., Tsunoo, H., Higa, Y., Takami, M., and Nakajima, H. (1982). Kinetic aspects of hemoglobin-haptoglobin-receptor interaction in rat liver plasma membranes, isolated liver cells, and liver cells in primary culture, *J. Biol. Chem.* **257**:4828–4833.

Kochan, I. (1973). The role of iron in bacterial infections, with special consideration of host-tubercle bacillus, *Curr. Topics Microbiol. Immunol.* **60**:1–30.

Koskelo, P., Sunberg, L., and Hakansson, U. (1976). Isolation and partial characterization of rat liver porphyrin binding proteins, *Ann. Clin. Res.* (8 Suppl.) **17**:244–249.

Kushner, I., Edgington, T. S., Trimble, C., Liem, H. H., and Muller-Eberhard, U. (1972). Plasma hemopexin homeostasis during the acute phase response, *J. Lab. Clin. Med.* **80**:18–25.

Kutty, R. K., and Maines, M. D. (1987). Characterization of an NADH-dependent haem-degrading system in ox heart mitochondria, *Biochem. J.* **246**:467–474.

LaBadie, J. A., Chapman, K. P., and Aronson, N. N., Jr. (1975). Glycoprotein catabolism in rat liver, *Biochem. J.* **152**:271–279.

Lane, R. S., Rangeley, D. M., Liem, H. H., Wormsley, S., and Muller-Eberhard, U. (1972). Hemopexin metabolism in the rabbit, *J. Lab. Clin. Med.* **79**:935–941.

Lane, R. S., Rangeley, D. M., Liem, H. H., Wormsley, S., and Muller-Eberhard, U. (1973). Plasma clearance of ^{125}I-labelled haemopexin in normal and haem-loaded rabbits, *Brit. J. Haematol.* **25**:533–540.

Laurell, C.-B., and Nyman, M. (1957). Studies on the serum haptoglobin level in hemoglobinemia and its influence on renal excretion of hemoglobin, *Blood* **12**:493–506.

Letendre, E. D. (1985). The importance of iron in the pathogenesis of infection and neoplasia, *Trends Biochem. Sci.* **10**:166–168.

Liem, H. H. (1976). Catabolism of homologous and heterologous hemopexin in the rat and uptake of hemopexin by isolated perfused rat liver, *Ann. Clin. Res.* (8 Suppl.) **17**:233–238.

Liem, H. H., Smith, A., and Muller-Eberhard, U. (1979). Effect of desferrioxamine and chronic iron deficiency on heme metabolism, *Biochem. Pharmacol.* **28**:1753–1758.

Liem, H. H., Tavassoli, M., and Muller-Eberhard, U. (1975). Cellular and subcellular localization of heme and hemopexin in the rabbit, *Acta Haematol.* **53**:219–225.

Linden, I.-B., Tokola, O., Karlsson, M., and Tenhunen, R. (1987). Fate of haem after parenteral administration of haem arginate to rabbits, *J. Pharm. Pharmacol.* **39**:96–102.

Lips, D. L., Pierach, C. A., and Edwards, P. S. (1978). Hematin toxicity in rats, *Toxicol. Lett.* **2**:329–332.

Liu, S.-C., Zhai, S., Lawler, J., and Palek, J. (1985). Hemin-mediated dissociation of erythrocyte membrane skeletal proteins, *J. Biol. Chem.* **260**:12234–12239.

Louache, F., Testa, U., Pelicci, P., Thomopoulos, P., Titeux, M., and Rochant, H. (1984). Regulation of transferrin receptors in human hematopoietic cell lines, *J. Biol. Chem.* **259**:11576–11582.

Lustbader, J. W., Arcoleo, J. P., Birken, S., and Greer, J. (1983). Hemoglobin-binding site on haptoglobin probed by selective proteolysis, *J. Biol. Chem.* **258**:1227–1234.

Lwoff, M. (1951). The nutrition of parasitic flagellates (*Trypanosomidae, Trichomonadinae*), *Biochemistry and Physiology of Protozoa* (A. Lwoff, Ed.), Academic, New York, pp. 131–182.

Maines, M. D., and Kappas, A. (1976). Studies on the mechanism of induction of haem oxygenase by cobalt and other metal ions, *Biochem. J.* **154**:125–131.

Majuri, R., and Grasbeck, R. (1986). Isolation of the haemopexin-haem receptor from pig liver cells, *FEBS Lett.* **199**:80–84.

Majuri, R., and Grasbeck, R. (1987). A rosette receptor assay with haem-microbeads. Demonstration of a haem receptor on K562 cells, *Eur. J. Haematol.* **38**:21–25.

Majuri, R., Kouvonen, I., and Grasbeck, R. (1984). Purification of the porcine duodenal haem receptor using a new affinity chromatographic medium, *Protides of the Biological Fluids* (H. Peeters, Ed.), Pergamon, Oxford, Vol. 31, pp. 229–232.

Malik, Z., Creter, D., Cohen, A., and Djaldetti, M. (1983). Haemin affects platelet aggregation and lymphocyte mitogenicity in whole blood incubations, *Cytobios* **38**:33–38.

Malik, Z., Halbrecht, I., and Djaldetti, M. (1979). Regulation of hemoglobin synthesis, iron metabolism, and maturation of Friend leukemic cells by 5-amino levulinic acid and hemin, *Differentiation* **13**:71–79.

Meier, P. J., Gasser, R., Hauri, H.-P., Stieger, B., and Meyer, U. A. (1984). Biosynthesis of rat liver cytochrome P-450 in mitochondria-associated rough endoplasmic reticulum and in rough microsomes in vivo, *J. Biol. Chem.* **259**:10194–10200.

Meier, P. J., Spycher, M. A., and Meyer, U. A. (1978). Isolation of a subfraction of rough endoplasmic reticulum closely associated with mitochondria. Evidence for its role in cytochrome P450 synthesis, *Exp. Cell Res.* **111**:479–483.

Merriman, C. R., Upchurch, H. F., and Kampschmidt, R. F. (1978). Effects of leukocytic endogenous mediator on hemopexin, transferrin and liver catalase, *Proc. Soc. Exp. Biol. Med.* **157**:669–671.

Moan, J., and Christensen, T. (1981). Photodynamic effects on human cells exposed to light in the presence of hematoporphyrin. Localization of the active dye, *Cancer Lett.* **11**:209–214.

Morgan, E. H. (1964). The interaction between rabbit, human and rat transferrin and reticulocytes, *Brit. J. Haematol.* **10**:442–452.

Morgan, W. T. (1976). The binding and transport of heme by hemopexin, *Ann. Clin. Res.* (8 Suppl.) **17**:223–232.

Morgan, W. T., Alam, J., Deaciuc, V., Muster, P., Tatum, F., and Smith, A. (1988a). Interaction of hemopexin with Sn-protoporphyrin IX, an inhibitor of heme oxygenase: Role for hemopexin in hepatic uptake of Sn-protoporphyrin IX and induction of mRNA for heme oxygenase, *J. Biol. Chem.*, **263**:8226–8231.

Morgan, W. T., Liem, H. H., Sutor, R. P., and Muller-Eberhard, U. (1976). Transfer of heme from heme-albumin to hemopexin, *Biochim. Biophys. Acta* **444**:435–445.

Morgan, W. T., and Muller-Eberhard, U. (1972), Interactions of porphyrins with rabbit hemopexin, *J. Biol. Chem.* **247**:7181–7187.

Morgan, W. T., Muster, P., Tatum, F. M., McConnell, J., Conway, T. P., Hensley, P., and Smith, A. (1988b). Use of hemopexin domains and monoclonal antibodies to hemopexin to probe the molecular determinants of hemopexin-mediated heme transport, *J. Biol. Chem.*, **263**:8220–8225.

Morgan, W. T., and Smith, A. (1984). Domain structure of hemopexin, *J. Biol. Chem.* **259**:12001–12006.

Morgan, W. T., Smith, A., and Koskelo, P. (1980). The interaction of human serum albumin and hemopexin with porphyrins, *Biochim. Biophys. Acta* **624**:271–285.

Morgan, W. T., Sutor, R. P., Muller-Eberhard, U., and Koskelo, P. (1975). Interaction of rabbit hemopexin with copro- and uroporphyrins, *Biochim. Biophys. Acta* **400**:415–422.

Morgan, W. T., and Vickery, L. E. (1978). Magnetic and natural circular dichroism of metalloporphyrin complexes of human and rabbit hemopexin, *J. Biol. Chem.* **253**:2940–2945.

Morris, S. J., Bradley, D., Campagnoni, A. T., and Stoner, G. L. (1987). Myelin basic protein binds heme at a specific site near the tryptophan residue, *Biochemistry* **26**:2175–2182.

Moskaug, J. O., Sandvig, K., and Olsnes, S. (1988). Low pH-induced release of diphtheria toxin A-fragment in Vero cells, *J. Biol. Chem.* **263**:2518–2525.

Muller-Eberhard, U. (1970). Hemopexin, *N. Engl. J. Med.* **283**:1090–1094.

Muller-Eberhard, U., Bosman, C., and Liem, H. H. (1970). Tissue localization of the heme-hemopexin complex in the rabbit and the rat as studied by light microscopy with the use of radioisotopes, *J. Lab. Clin. Med.***76**:426–431.

Muller-Eberhard, U., Eiseman, J. L., Foidart, M., and Alvares, A. P. (1983). Effect of heme on allylisopropylacetamide-induced changes in heme and drug metabolism in the rhesus monkey (mucaca mulatta), *Biochem. Pharmacol.* **32**:3765–3769.

Muller-Eberhard, U., Javid, J., Liem, H. H., Hanstein, A., and Hanna, M. (1968). Plasma concentrations of hemopexin, haptoglobin and heme in patients with various hemolytic diseases, *Blood* **32**:811–815.

Muller-Eberhard, U., and Morgan, W. T. (1975). Porphyrin-binding proteins in serum, *Ann. N.Y. Acad. Sci.* **244**:624–649.

Murant, R. S., Gibson, S. L., and Hilf, R. (1987). Photosensitizing effects of Photofrin II on the site-selected mitochondrial enzymes adenylate kinase and monoamine oxidase, *Cancer Res.* **47**:4323–4328.

Myers, A. M., Crivellone, M. D., Koerner, T. J., and Tzagoloff, A. (1987). Characterization of the yeast *HEM2* gene and transcriptional regulation of *COX5* and *COR1* by heme, *J. Biol. Chem.* **262**:16822–16829.

Nelson, D. R., and Strobel, H. W. (1988). On the membrane topography of vertibrate cytochrome P450 proteins. *J. Biol. Chem.* **263**:6038–6050.

Nicholson, D. W., Kohler, H., and Neupert, W. (1987). Import of cytochrome c into mitochondria, *Eur. J. Biochem.* **164**:147–157.

Ohashi, A., Gibson, J., Gregor, I., and Schatz, G. (1982). Import of proteins into mitochondria. The precursor of cytochrome c_1 is processed in two steps, one of them heme-dependent, *J. Biol. Chem.* **257**:13042–13047.

Orjih, A. U., Banyal, H. S., Chevil, R., and Fitch, C. D. (1981). Hemin lyses malaria parasites, *Science* **214**:667–669.

Parimoo, S., Rao, N., and Padmanaban, G. (1982). Cytochrome c oxidase is preferentially synthesized in the rough endoplasmic reticulum-mitochondrion complex in rat liver, *Biochem. J.* **208**:505–507.

Pasternack, R. F., Gibbs, E. J., Hoeflin, E., Kosar, W. P., Kubera, G., Skowronek, C. A., Wong, N. M., and Muller-Eberhard, U. (1983). Hemin binding to serum proteins and the catalysis of interprotein transfer, *Biochemistry* **22**:1753–1758.

Pasternack, R. F., Gibbs, E. J., Mauk, A. G., Reid, L. S., Wong, N. M., Kurokawa, K., Hashim, M., and Muller-Eberhard, U. (1985). Kinetics of hemoprotein reduction and interprotein heme transfer, *Biochemistry* **24**:5443–5448.

Payne, S. M., and Finkelstein, R. A. (1977). Detection and differentiation of iron-responsive avirulent mutants on Congo red agar, *Infect. Immunol.* **18**:94–98.

Petryka, Z. J., Pierach, C. A., Smith, A., Goertz, M. N., and Edwards, P. S. (1977). Biliary excretion of exogenous hematin in rats, *Life Sci.* **21**:1015–1020.

Pfeifer, K., Arcangioli, B., and Guarente, L. (1987a). Yeast HAP1 activator competes with the factor RC2 for binding to the upstream activation site UAS1 of the *CYC1* gene, *Cell* **49**:9–18.

Pfeifer, K., Prezant, T., and Guarente, L. (1987b). Yeast HAP1 activator binds to two upstream activation sites of different sequence, *Cell* **49**:19–27.

Rao, K., Harford, J. B., Rouault, T., McClelland, A., Ruddle, F. H., and Klausner, R. D. (1986). Transcriptional regulation by iron of the gene for the transferrin receptor, *Mol. Cell. Biol.* **6**:236–240.

Reddi, E., Ricchelli, F., and Jori, G. (1981). Interaction of human serum albumin with hematoporphyrin and its Zn^{2+}- and Fe^{3+}-derivatives, *Int. J. Peptide Prot. Res.* **18**:402–408.

Reichen, J., and Berk, P. D. (1979). Isolation of an organic anion binding protein from rat liver plasma membrane fractions by affinity chromatography, *Biochem. Biophys. Res. Comm.* **91**:484–489.

Riezman, H. (1985). Endocytosis in yeast: Several of the yeast secretory mutants are defective in endocytosis, *Cell* **40**:1001–1009.

Rose, M. Y., Thompson, R. A., Light, W. R., and Olson, J. S. (1985). Heme transfer between phospholipid membranes and uptake by apohemoglobin, *J. Biol. Chem.* **260**:6632–6640.

Rothman, J. E., and Fine, R. E. (1980). Coated vesicles transport newly synthesized membrane glycoproteins from endoplasmic reticulum to plasma membrane in two successive stages, *Proc. Nat. Acad. Sci. (U.S.A.)* **77**:780–784.

Rouault, T., Rao, K., Harford, J., Mattia, E., and Klausner, R. D. (1985). Hemin, chelatable iron, and the regulation of transferrin receptor biosynthesis, *J. Biol. Chem.* **260**:14862–14866.

Salter, M., and Pogson, C. I. (1986). The role of haem in the regulation of rat liver tryptophan metabolism, *Biochem. J.* **240**:259–263.

Sardana, M. K., and Kappas, A. (1987). Dual control mechanism for heme oxygenase: Tin(IV)-protoporphyrin potently inhibits enzyme activity while markedly increasing content of enzyme protein in liver, *Proc. Nat. Acad. Sci. (U.S.A.)* **84**:2464–2468.

Schenkman, R. (1985). Protein localization and membrane traffic in yeast, *Annual Review of Cell Biology* (G. E. Palade, Ed.), Annual Reviews, Palo Alto, Calif., Vol. 1, pp. 115–143.

Schleyer, M., and Neupert, W. (1985). Transport of proteins into mitochondria: Translocational intermediates spanning contact sites between outer and inner membranes, *Cell* **43**:339–350.

Schmid, R. (1983). Hepatic heme metabolism: New aspects and speculations, *Sem. Liver Dis.* **3**:83–86.

Sears, D. A. (1968). Plasma heme-binding in patients with hemolytic disorders, *J. Lab. Clin. Med.* **71**:484–494.

Seery, V. L., Hathaway, G., and Muller-Eberhard, U. (1972). Hemopexin of human and rabbit: Molecular weight and extinction coefficient, *Arch. Biochem. Biophys.* **150**:269–272.

Senjo, M., Ishibashi, T., and Imai, Y. (1985). Purification and characterization of cytosolic liver protein facilitating heme transport into apocytochrome b5 from mitochondria. Evidence for identifying the heme transfer protein as belonging to a group of glutathione S-transferases, *J. Biol. Chem.* **260**:9191–9196.

Sibbett, S. S., and Hurst, J. K. (1984). Structural analysis of myeloperoxidase by resonance Raman spectroscopy, *Biochemistry* **23**:3007–3013.

Sievers, G., Hakli, H., Luhtala, J., and Tenhunen, R. (1987). Optical and EPR spectroscopy studies on haem arginate, a new compound used for treatment of porphyria, *Chem.-Biol. Interact.* **63**:105–114.

Sitbon, M., Sola, B., Evans, L., Nishio, J., Hayes, S. F., Nathanson, K., Garon, C. F., and Chesebro, B. (1986). Hemolytic anemia and erythroleukemia, two distinct pathogenic effects of Friend MuLV: Mapping of the effects to different regions of the viral genome, *Cell* **47**:851–859.

Smith, A. (1983). Absorption and metabolism of dietary heme-iron, *Fed. Proc.* **42**:2073.

Smith, A. (1985). Intracellular distribution of haem after uptake by different receptors. Haem-haemopexin and haem-asialo-haemopexin, *Biochem. J.* **231**:663–669.

Smith, A. (1987). Mechanisms of toxicity of photoactivated artificial porphyrins, *Ann. N.Y. Acad. Sci.* **514**:309–322.

Smith, A. (1989). Characterization of the hepatic plasma membrane heme-binding protein component of the hemopexin transport system, in preparation.

Smith, A. (1988b). Absorption and metabolism of dietary haem-iron, *Biochem. J.*, manuscript in preparation.

Smith, A., and Hunt, R. C. (1989). Endocytosis of heme-hemopexin: Colocalization with transferrin, *J. Cell. Sci.*, to appear.

Smith, A., and Ledford, B. E. (1988). Expression of haemopexin transport system in cultured mouse hepatoma cells: Links between haemopexin and iron metabolism, *Biochem. J.*, **256**:941–950.

Smith, A., and Morgan, W. T. (1978). Transport of heme by hemopexin to the liver: Evidence for receptor-mediated uptake, *Biochem. Biophys. Res. Comm.* **84**:151–157.

Smith, A., and Morgan, W. T. (1979). Haem transport to the liver by haemopexin. Receptor-mediated uptake with recycling of the protein, *Biochem. J.* **182**:47–54.

Smith, A., and Morgan, W. T. (1981). Hemopexin-mediated transport of heme into isolated rat hepatocytes, *J. Biol. Chem.* **256**:10902–10909.

Smith, A., and Morgan, W. T. (1984a). Cleavage of rabbit hemopexin by plasmin and isolation of two glycopeptides, *Protides of the Biological Fluids* (H. Peeters, Ed.), Pergamon, Oxford, Vol. 31, pp. 219–224.

Smith, A., and Morgan, W. T. (1984b). Hemopexin-mediated heme uptake by liver. Characterization of the interaction of heme-hemopexin with isolated rabbit liver plasma membranes, *J. Biol. Chem.* **259**:12049–12053.

Smith, A., and Morgan, W. T. (1985). Hemopexin-mediated heme transport to the liver. Evidence for a heme-binding protein in liver plasma membranes, *J. Biol. Chem.* **260**:8325–8329.

Smith, A., and Neuschatz, T. (1983). Haematoporphyrin and *OO'*-diacetylhaematoporphyrin binding by serum and cellular proteins, *Biochem. J.* **214**:503–509.

Smith, A., Nuiry, I., and Awasthi, Y. C. (1985). Interactions with glutathione S-transferases of porphyrins used in photodynamic therapy and naturally occurring porphyrins, *Biochem. J.* **229**:823–831.

Smith, A., Tatum, F. M., Muster, P., Burch, M. K., and Morgan, W. T. (1988). Importance of ligand-induced conformational changes in hemopexin for receptor-mediated heme transport, *J. Biol. Chem.*, **263**:5224–5229.

Smith, D. W., and Williams, R. J. P. (1970). The spectra of ferric haems and haemoproteins, *Structure and Bonding*, Springer-Verlag, N.Y., Vol. 7, pp. 1–45.

Snyder, S. H., Verma, A., and Trifiletti, R. R. (1987). The peripheral-type benzodiazepine receptor: A protein of mitochondrial outer membranes utilizing porphyrins as endogenous ligands, *FASEB J.* **1**:282–288.

Sorrentino, D., Stremmel, W., and Berk, P. D. (1987). The hepatocellular uptake of bilirubin: Current concepts and controversies, *Mol. Aspects Med.* **9**:405–428.

Stremmel, W., and Berk, P. D. (1986). Hepatocellular influx of [^{14}C] oleate reflects membrane transport rather than intracellular metabolism of binding, *Proc. Nat. Acad. Sci. (U.S.A.)* **83**:3086–3090.

Stremmel, W., Gerber, M. A., Glezerov, V., Thung, S. N., Kochwa, S., and Berk, P. D. (1983). Physicochemical and immunohistological studies of a sulfobromophthalein- and bilirubin-binding protein from rat liver plasma membranes, *J. Clin. Invest.* **71**:1796–1805.

Stull, T. L. (1987). Protein sources of heme for *Haemophilus influenzae. Infect. Immunol.* **55**:148–153.

Surgalla, M. J., and Beesley, E. D. (1969). Congo red agar plating medium for detecting pigmentation of *Pasteurella pestis, Appl. Microbiol.* **18**:834–837.

Suzuki, N., Yamaguchi, T., and Nakajima, H. (1988). Role of high-density lipoproteins in transport of circulating bilirubin in rats, *J. Biol. Chem.* **263**:5037–5043.

Takahashi, N., Takahashi, Y., and Putnam, F. W. (1985). Complete amino acid sequence of human hemopexin, the heme-binding protein of serum, *Proc. Nat. Acad. Sci. (U.S.A.)* **82**:73–77.

Taketani, S., Kohno, H., Naitoh, Y., and Tokunaga, R. (1987a). Isolation and characterization of the hemopexin receptor from human placenta, *J. Biol. Chem.* **262**:8668–8671.

Taketani, S., Kohno, H., and Tokunaga, R. (1986). Receptor-mediated heme uptake from hemopexin by human erythroleukemia K562 cells, *Biochem. Int.* **13**:307–312.

Taketani, S., Kohno, H., and Tokunaga, R. (1987b). Cell surface receptor for hemopexin in human leukemia HL60 cells: Specific binding, affinity labeling and fate of heme, *J. Biol. Chem.* **262**:4639–4643.

Tangeras, A. (1986). Lysosomes, but not mitochondria, accumulate iron and porphyrins in porphyria induced by hexachlorobenzene, *Biochem. J.* **235**:671–675.

Tappel, A. L. (1955). Unsaturated lipid oxidation catalyzed by hematin compounds, *J. Biol. Chem.* **217**:721–733.

Tokola, O. (1987). Effects of repeated intravenous administration of haem arginate upon hepatic metabolism of foreign compounds in rats and dogs, *Brit. J. Pharmacol.* **90**:661–668.

Tran-Quang, N., Bernard, N., Higa, Y., and Engler, R. (1983). In vitro studies on some parameters of the binding of the rat hemopexin-heme complex with the hepatic membrane receptor, *FEBS Lett.* **159**:161–166.

Tsai, S.-F., Bishop, D. F., and Desnick, R. J. (1987). Purification and properties of uroporphyrinogen III synthase from human erythrocytes, *J. Biol. Chem.* **262**:1268–1273.

Vazquez, J., Garcia-Calvo, M., Valdivieso, F., Mayor, F., and Mayor, F., Jr. (1988). Interaction of bilirubin with the synaptosomal plasma membrane, *J. Biol. Chem.* **263**:1255–1265.

Verdiere, J., Greusot, F., Guarente, L., and Slonimski, P. (1986). The overproducing *CYP1* and the underproducing *hap1* mutations are alleles of the same gene which regulates in trans the expression of the structural genes encoding the iso-cytochrome c, *Curr. Genet.* **10**:339–342.

Verma, A., Nye, J. S., and Snyder, S. H. (1987). Porphyrins are endogenous ligands for the mitochondrial (peripheral-type) benzodiazepine receptor, *Proc. Nat. Acad. Sci. (U.S.A.)* **84**:2256–2260.

Verweij-Van Vught, A. M. J. J., Otto, B. R., Namavar, F., Sparrius, M., and Maclaren, D. M. (1988). Ability of bacteroides species to obtain iron from iron salts haem-compounds and transferrin, *FEMS Microbiol. Lett.* **49**:223–228.

Waldman, S. A., Sinacore, M. S., Lewicki, J. A., Chang, L. Y., and Murad, F. (1984). Selective activation of particulate guanylate cyclase by a specific class of porphyrins, *J. Biol. Chem.* **259**:4038–4042.

Ward, C. G. (1986). Influence of iron on infection, *Amer. J. Surg.* **151**:291–295.

Ward, J. H., Jordan, I., Kushner, J. P., and Kaplan, J. (1984). Heme regulation of HeLa cell transferrin receptor number, *J. Biol Chem.* **259**:13235–13240.

Warkentin, D. L., Marchand, A., and Van Lente, F. (1987). Serum haptoglobin concentrations in concurrent hemolysis and acute-phase reaction, *Clin. Chem.* **33**:1265–1266.

Weinberg, E. D. (1984). Iron withholding: A defense against infection and neoplasia, *Physiol. Rev.* **64**:65–102.

Whitmer, D. I., Hauser, S. C., and Gollan, J. L. (1984). Mechanisms of formation, hepatic transport, and metabolism of bile pigments, *Intrahepatic Calculi, Progress in Clinical and Biological Research*, Alan R. Liss, New York, Vol. 152, pp. 29–52.

Whitmer, D. I., Russell, P. E., and Gollan, J. L. (1987). Membrane-membrane interactions associated with rapid transfer of liposomal bilirubin to microsomal UDP-glucuronyltransferase, *Biochem. J.* **244**:41–47.

Williams, P. H. (1979). Novel iron uptake system specified by Col V plasmids: An important component in the virulence of invasive strains of *Escherichia coli, Infect. Immunol.* **26**:925–932.

Winkelman, J. G., Slater, G., and Grossman, J. (1967). The concentration in tumor and other tissues of parenterally administered tritium and ^{14}C-labeled tetraphenylporphine-sulfonate, *Cancer Res.* **27**:2060–2064.

Wochner, R. D., Spilberg, I., Iio, A., Liem, H. H., Muller-Eberhard, U. (1974). Hemopexin metabolism in sickle-cell disease, porphyrias and control subjects—effects of heme injection, *N. Engl. J. Med.* **290**:822–826.

Wyman, J. F., Gollan, J. L., Settle, W., and Farrell, G. C. (1986). Incorporation of haemoglobin haem into the rat hepatic haemoproteins tryptophan pyrrolase and cyto-chome P-450, *Biochem. J.* **238**:837–846.

Yoda, B., and Israels, L. G. (1972). Transfer of heme from mitochondria in rat liver cells, *Canad. J. Biochem.* **50**:633–637.

Yoshinaga, T., Sassa, S., and Kappas, A. (1982). Purification and properties of bovine spleen heme oxygenase. Amino acid composition and sites of action of inhibitors of heme oxidation, *J. Biol. Chem.* **257**:7778–7785.

Zakaria-Meehan, Z., Massad, G., Simpson, L. M., Travis, J. C., and Oliver J. D. (1988). Ability of *Vibrio vulnificus* to obtain iron from hemoglobin-haptoglobin complexes, *Infect. Immunol.* **56**:275–277.

Zimmermann, R., Paluck, U., Neupert, W. (1979). Cell-free synthesis of cytochrome c, *FEBS Lett.* **108**:141–146.

Human Hereditary Porphyrias

Yves Nordmann

Jean-Charles Deybach

I. Introduction

The porphyrias are a group of disorders of heme biosynthesis in which specific patterns of overproduction of heme precursors are associated with characteristic clinical features. Each type of porphyria is the result of a specific decrease in the activity of one of the enzymes of heme biosynthesis.

Porphyrias as clinical entities were recognized and described at the end of the nineteenth century and the beginning of the twentieth century (Günther, 1911). This recognition was clearly linked to the appearance on the market of hypnotics such as sulphonal and barbiturates. The history of porphyrias cannot be dissociated from the evolution of knowledge on porphyrin biochemistry and the heme biosynthetic pathway (see Chap. 1).

In 1968 Levin demonstrated that the primary mechanism of bovine and human congenital erythropoietic porphyrias (Levin, 1968; Romeo and Levin, 1969) relies on a deficiency of the activity of the uroporphyrin cosynthase. Between 1969 and 1980, the enzymic deficiency of all of the porphyrias was described (see below). In 1987, for the first time, the nature of the genic mutation of a porphyria was described (de Verneuil, et al., 1986b) and it is likely that several other molecular descriptions will soon follow.

A. Classification and inheritance

Porphyrias are presently classified as *erythropoietic* or *hepatic* in type depending on the primary organ in which excess production of porphyrins or precursors takes place (Sassa and Kappas, 1981) (Table 10.1).

Two types of clinical syndromes occur in the porphyrias: skin lesions in areas exposed to light, and attacks of acute porphyria. The former occurs in all types of porphyria except acute intermittent porphyria. Four hepatic porphyrias out of five may be provoked into an acute attack with abdominal pains and sometimes a neuropsychiatric syndrome: these are called acute porphyrias (Table 10.1). However, in most patients who have inherited an enzyme defect the condition remains latent throughout life [except for congenital erythropoietic porphyria (CEP)]. It is clear that factors other than the decrease in enzyme activity must be important in determining the clinical manifestations (see below). The porphyrias are inherited as dominant-autosomal characters, except CEP and Doss porphyria (both extremely rare) which are inherited as recessive-autosomal characters.

B. Standard methods used in the author's laboratory

A convenient summary of the standard methods for measurement of ALA, PBG, and porphyrins is available in several reviews (Bissell, 1982;

TABLE 10.1   Classification of Inherited Human Porphyrias

Classification	Inheritance	Deficient enzyme
I. Hepatic porphyrias		
1. Acute porphyrias		
Acute intermittent porphyria	Autosomal dominant	PBG* deaminase
Hereditary coproporphyria[†]	Autosomal dominant	Coproporphyrinogen oxidase
Variegate porphyria[†]	Autosomal dominant	Protoporphyrinogen oxidase
Doss porphyria	Autosomal recessive	ALA* dehydrase
2. Porphyria cutanea[†] symptomatica (familial type)	Autosomal dominant	Uroporphyrinogen decarboxylase
II. Erythropoietic porphyrias		
Congenital erythropoietic porphyria (Günther's disease)	Autosomal recessive	Uroporphyrinogen III cosynthetase
Erythropoietic protoporphyria[†]	Autosomal dominant	Ferrochelatase

*ALA, δ-aminolevulinic acid; PBG, porphobilinogen.
[†]Homozygous variant has been described (see text).

Elder, 1980; Moore et al., 1987). We will just describe briefly the methods used in the authors' laboratory: qualitative screenings are not used, because we think that several errors of interpretation are unavoidable, even for very well trained biochemists. In urine, ALA and PBG are quantitated by coupled ion exchange column chromatography, as described by Mauzerall and Granick (1956). This method (available as a kit from Biorad Laboratories) is very easy and does not require special training. Finding a high level of precursors is the best way for a physician to discover if a patient with acute abdominal pains has a porphyria.

Our routine approach for urinary porphyrins is differential solvent extraction and quantitation of absorption; calculation of results is based on the correction formulas derived by Rimington (1960). Study of porphyrins, isomers I and III, is realized by reverse-phase high-pressure liquid chromatography (HPLC) on C_{18} columns (Lim et al., 1986); detection is by spectrofluorimetry. When a precise profile of urinary porphyrins is needed, HPLC of esterified porphyrins is carried out and detection is also by spectrofluorimetry (excitation of 405 nm; emission at 630 nm).

The standard approach for fecal porphyrins relies on the same techniques (differential solvent extraction or HPLC).

The routine quantitation of erythrocyte porphyrins is carried out by differential extraction in HCl after global extraction in ethyl acetate/acetic acid (3:1). Plasma porphyrins are measured by a technique described by Grandchamp et al. (1980). All the enzymes of the heme biosynthetic pathway are measured either from erythrocytes for cytoplasmic enzymes (ALA dehydrase, PBG deaminase, uroporphyrinogen cosynthase, and uroporphyrinogen decarboxylase) or from lymphocytes for mitochondrial enzymes (ALA synthase, coproporphyrinogen oxidase, protoporphyrinogen oxidase, and ferrochelatase). All of the techniques used have been described previously [see Bishop and Desnick (1982)].

II. Hepatic Porphyrias

A. Acute hepatic porphyrias

Identical acute attacks of porphyria occur in four of the hepatic porphyrias—acute intermittent porphyria (AIP), hereditary coproporphyria (HC), variegate porphyria (VP), and Doss porphyria (DP).

1. Clinical features have recently been reviewed by several authors such as Sassa and Kappas (1981), Moore et al. (1987), Meyer and Schmid (1978), and Kappas et al. (1988) and we will only briefly summarize the most-common symptoms (Table 10.2).

Typically, the attacks consist of acute abdominal pain with vomiting and constipation and are associated with psychiatric manifestations such as anxiety, depression, disorientation, confusion, and delirium, and neurological manifestations such as peripheral neuropathy with occasional cranial nerve involvement, respiratory embarrassment, grand mal seizures, and so forth. In most of these cases neurological manifestations should be considered as complications still, too often, linked to therapeutic errors. Despite the autosomic character of the traits of acute porphyrias, more than 80% of the patients showing acute attacks are females (18 to 45 years old), and, in fact, sex steroids are among the most important factors that result in clinical expression of acute porphyrias (Kappas et al., 1983a).

It is extremely difficult for the physician to know precisely the type of acute porphyria following the clinical examination: darkening coloration (attributed to nonenzymatic conversion of PBG to a porphyrin-like compound) of urine is common to all porphyrias, except protoporphyria. Patients with AIP never show cutaneous features, but very often VP or HC may also be present without manifestations of skin photosensitivity (which will be described with porphyria cutanea tarda). Of course, the association—abdominal pain plus cutaneous features—is suggestive of VP but is also sometimes found in HC.

2. Classical biologic data. An increase in the intracellular concentration of the substrate of each defective enzyme gives rise to a characteristic pattern of tissue accumulation and excretion of heme precursors. Table 10.3 summarizes these patterns. Elder (1986) and Elder and Path (1982) suggested that the characteristic increase of precursor excretion during attacks of acute porphyrias is linked to a rapid leakage of porphyrins

TABLE 10.2 Incidence of Clinical Symptoms* and Signs in Patients with Acute Intermittent Porphyria [from Walddenström (1957)]

Abdominal pain	85%
Vomiting	59%
Psychiatric features[†]	55%
Constipation	48%
Paresis/paralysis	42%
Hypertension	40%
Fever	37%
Tachycardia	28%
Convulsions	10%
Transient amaurosis	4%
Jaundice	3%

*Muscle pain is missing in this list (50% in our patients).
[†] Depression, delirium, disorientation.

and/or precursors from the hepatocyte; thus, the substrate concentration is prevented from increasing sufficiently before PBG deaminase becomes rate-limiting. In nonacute porphyrias (i.e., porphyria cutanea symptomatica) the rate of substrate loss from the cell is very slow; consequently, intracellular substrate concentrations may attain a level compensating the enzyme defects before PBG supply becomes rate-limiting.

a. Acute intermittent porphyria. During acute attacks, patients with AIP excrete large amounts of PBG and ALA (20 to 200-fold elevated above normal levels). Uro- and coproporphyrin are usually moderately increased (uroporphyrin is often the result of a nonenzymatic reaction favored by light and/or heat). Let us once more emphasize the use of precursors (mostly PBG) as a diagnostic tool, whereas urinary porphyrin could be increased in several other conditions and therefore lacks diagnostic specificity.

About one-third of clinically asymptomatic carriers shows an abnormal excretion of PBG (two- to fivefold above the normal level), but the others show normal excretion of this precursor.

Stool porphyrins are normal or moderately increased in this porphyria. Excess PBG and ALA have been found in the liver and kidneys after death. During acute attack, PBG is much more increased in plasma than ALA.

b. Hereditary coproporphyria. During acute attacks of HC, the profile of urine porphyrins and precursors is similar to that in AIP; however, sometimes coproporphyrin is dramatically increased. Stool porphyrins usually allow typing of the porphyria, the characteristic abnormality being a large excess of coproporphyrin, contrasted with normal protoporphyrin. Approximately 20 to 30% of asymptomatic carriers show this typical fecal profile (and often a normal urinary profile) after puberty.

TABLE 10.3   Acute Hepatic Porphyrias: Biochemical Features

	n	Urine			Feces		
		PRE	U	C	U	C	P
Acute intermittent	1*	+++	++	++	++	+	
porphyria	2*	++		±			
Hereditary	1	+++	++	+++	++	++++	+
coproporphyria	2	+		+		+++	
Variegate	1	+++	++	+++	+	++	+++
porphyria	2	+		+		+	++

*1, during attack; 2, during remission.
U = Uroporphyrin; C = Coproporphyrin; P = Protoporphyrin; PRE = Precursor.

c. Variegate porphyria. During acute attacks of VP, urinary data are identical to those in AIP and HC. Carriers with only chronic cutaneous manifestations or even asymptomatic carriers often show a slight increase of precursors.

The characteristic finding is elevated fecal protoporphyrin and, to a lesser degree (at least when measurement is carried out using the differential extraction method), coproporphyrin; HPLC of fecal porphyrins usually shows only an isolated peak of protoporphyrin. A heterogeneous group of porphyrin-peptide conjugates called X porphyrins (Rimington et al., 1968; Elder, 1974) which are ether-insoluble porphyrins is also increased in VP. In plasma, Day et al. (1978) and Longas and Poh-Fitzpatrick (1982) have also described an increased level of porphyrin which is not extracted by the normal methods, but remains bound to the protein fraction. A plasma fluorescence emission maxi- mum at 626 nm has been described as a diagnostic marker for VP (Poh-Fitzpatrick, 1980). The significance of the porphyrin-protein complex remains unknown; however, the porphyrin X fraction "is no longer considered of diagnostic importance in VP since raised levels of similar conjugates have been detected in the feces of porphyria cutanea tarda" (Day, 1986).

d. Doss porphyria (ALA dehydrase deficiency). Doss et al. (1979) recently described two cases of young adults with a new acute hepatic porphyria, characterized by a large increase of excretion of ALA and coproporphyrin (mainly isomer type III) in urine; PBG was only moderately elevated; fecal excretion of porphyrins was normal, but erythrocyte porphyrins were slightly increased (three times the normal level). Thunell et al. (1987) also described a case of this new porphyria; the only differences with the two cases of Doss were the age of the patient (a very young child with several attacks including nervous palsy during the two first years of life) and a moderate increase of fecal porphyrins (mainly harderoporphyrin, i.e., a tricarboxyporphyrin which is an intermediate step between coproporphyrin and protoporphyrin).

In Doss porphyria, the pattern of overproduction of heme precursors closely resembles that of severe lead poisoning; however, some features allow one to refute this diagnosis. These are normal urinary and blood levels of lead or the activity of ALA dehydrase which is not restored by dithiothreitol.

3. Enzymatic abnormalities and genetic defects. Increased hepatic *ALA synthase* activity was described during acute attacks in AIP, HC, and VP patients (Sweeney et al., 1970; Tschudy et al., 1965; Dowdle et al., 1967) and it was initially postulated that induction of ALA synthase might represent the primary enzyme abnormality in all of these diseases

(Tschudy et al., 1965), notwithstanding the differences between patterns of porphyrin excretion (or the absence of cutaneous features in AIP, contrasted with VP or HC). As will be discussed later in connection with the mechanism of acute attacks, it is now admitted that ALA synthase induction is a secondary phenomenon.

Moreover, the compensatory changes in ALA synthase activity are restricted to certain tissues such as liver (Meyer and Schmid, 1978), intestinal tract, and kidney (Day et al., 1981); increased ALA synthase activity has also been detected in peripheral blood leukocytes (Brodie et al., 1977a). However, in AIP, ALA synthase activity is not increased in lymphocytes (Sassa et al., 1978) or skin fibroblasts (Meyer, 1973).

a. Acute intermittent porphyria. PBG deaminase deficiency (50% of normal activity) has been demonstrated in all examined tissues (Strand et al., 1970; Meyer et al., 1972; Meyer, 1973; Sassa et al., 1978; Sassa et al., 1975). Measurement in erythrocytes is now widely used not only to

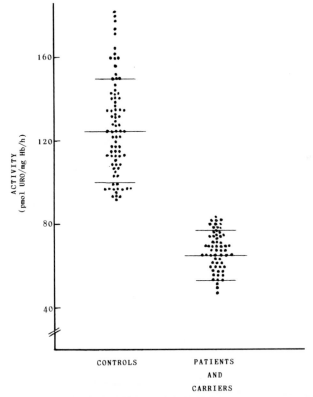

Figure 10.1 PBG-D activity in AIP patients. Normal controls: 125 ± 40 units; patients and carriers: 65 ± 15 units.

confirm the type of porphyria, but also to detect the clinically latent individuals who often do not show evidence of heme precursor overproduction (Fig. 10.1).

Analysis of PBG deaminase measurement has to be done carefully: several sources of error have been described such as increased activity during or just after an acute attack (Kostrzewska and Gregor, 1986), when blood reticulocytes are higher than normal (Meyer and Schmid, 1978), when a baby is under 6 months old (Nordmann et al., 1976), or in liver disease (Ostrowski, 1987) and in lymphoproliferative disease (Epstein et al., 1983). Some overlap may occur between the normal and AIP groups (Kappas et al., 1983b); in these cases it could be interesting to measure simultaneously ALA synthase in leukocytes (McColl et al., 1982) or PBG deaminase in mitogen-stimulated lymphocytes (Sassa et al., 1975) because there would be less overlap. If the precise nature of the enzyme deficiency remains obscure, genetic heterogeneity of AIP is already well known: Mustajoki (1981) and later Wilson et al. (1986) described families each of whom included subjects with the usual phenotypic expression of AIP but with normal activity of PBG deaminase in erythrocytes.

Using antibodies against PBG deaminase, Anderson et al. (1981), Desnick et al. (1985), and Mustajoki and Desnick (1985) showed that at least four genetic variants of AIP exist (Table 10.4): In the majority of families studied, the amount of immunoreactive enzyme proteins corresponded to the amount of enzymatic activity (50% of normal level). These families are CRIM (cross-reacting immunologic material)-negative; another type of CRIM-negative subject was found in the families described by Mustajoki (1981) and Wilson et al. (1986), with a normal amount of enzymatic activity and also of CRIM in erythrocytes (but not in liver as will be shown later). On the other hand, two types of CRIM-positive mutations were identified with a CRIM/activity ratio of 1.7 and 5.7, respectively. Desnick et al. (1985) and Wilson et al. (1986) suggested that the CRIM-positive mutations resulted from the enhanced

TABLE 10.4   PBG Deaminase Mutant Classes (in Erythrocytes)

	Activity (%)	CRIM (%)	CRIM activity	
Control	100	100	1	CRIM-negative
Type 1 (AIP)	50	50	1	
Type 2 ("Finnish")	100	100	1	
Type 3	50	85	1.7	CRIM-positive
Type 4	50	280	5.7	

binding and/or defective release of substrate molecules, rendering the complexes more resistant to intraerythrocyte proteolysis.

Recently, it has been shown by Grandchamp et al. (1987) that PBG deaminase from human nonerythropoietic sources (i.e., liver, lymphocytes) displays a different molecular mass (39,220 daltons) from its erythropoietic counterpart (37,627 daltons). The protein sequence of both isoforms is identical, except for an additional stretch of 17 amino acids at the NH_2 terminus of the nonerythropoietic enzyme. This difference is due to the existence of two distinct tissue-specific mRNAs differing by their 5' extremity: both mRNAs are generated from a single gene through alternative splicing of two primary transcripts arising from two promoters separated by 3 kb (Chretien et al., 1989). If in some families with AIP, the PBG deaminase deficiency appears to be restricted to nonerythropoietic tissues, it seemed logical to look for a molecular defect lying within sequences of the PBG deaminase gene which are specifically expressed in nonerythropoietic cells. Grandchamp et al. (1989) investigated one Dutch family with this subtype of AIP. Using the recently described restriction fragment length polymorphisms (RFLP) of the human PBG deaminase gene (Llewellyn et al., 1987), they found a strong linkage (Lod score 3.2) between one haplotype and the AIP phenotype: This finding suggested that the mutation was lying within the AIP gene and involved the nonerythropoietic-specific sequence of the gene, keeping in mind the normal activity of erythrocyte PBG deaminase of these patients. Cloning and sequencing of the nonerythropoietic part of the PBG deaminase gene from an affected individual revealed a $G \rightarrow A$ transition at the first position of the first intron. Similar mutations have previously been shown to completely abolish normal splicing (DiLella et al., 1986). Normal erythrocyte PBG deaminase activity is expected in these patients, since transcription in erythropoietic cells starts 2.8 kb downstream from the identified mutation (Fig. 10.2). In a second family with the same subtype of AIP previously described by Mustajoki (1981), a different point mutation was identified in the nonerythroid exon of the PBG deaminase gene (manuscript in preparation). These observations provide new diagnostic tools for detecting asymptomatic carriers of the mutated gene in the affected families

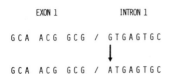

Figure 10.2 Type of mutation in a Dutch family with AIP but normal erythrocyte PBG deaminase activity.

(namely the direct detection of the base change using mutation-specific oligonucleotides).

In the usual subtype of AIP the nature of mutation(s) is still unknown; lack of homozygous cases is one of the valuable explanations of the difficulties to progress in this field.

b. Hereditary coproporphyria. In coproporphyria, coproporphyrinogen oxidase (Copro-ox) is decreased to around 50% of normal in liver (Hawk et al., 1978), fibroblasts (Elder et al., 1976), lymphocytes (Grandchamp and Nordmann, 1977), and leukocytes (Brodie et al., 1977c). Considerable excess of copro-ox activity in liver cells probably explains why patients with acute attacks are rare, whereas several asymptomatic carriers are found in their kindred when copro-ox is measured (Andrews et al., 1984).

Two different types of homozygous cases have been described, both with a deficiency of copro-ox activity about 90% of normal. In the first type (Grandchamp et al., 1977), the patient was very small (140 cm at 20 years), showed skin photosensitivity, and had several acute attacks since the age of 5 years. Her feces and urine contained a large amount of coproporphyrin. The residual lymphocyte copro-ox showed a normal K_m with coproporphyrinogen and normal thermosensitivity. This case is very similar to the case described by Berger and Goldberg (1955).

The other type of homozygous coproporphyria was found in children with intense jaundice and hemolytic anemia at birth (Nordmann et al., 1983). The pattern of fecal porphyrin excretion was atypical for coproporphyria because the major porphyrin was harderoporphyrin ($> 60\%$; normal $< 20\%$): This variant was called "harderoporphyria." Harderoporphyrin is the natural intermediate between copro- and protoporphyrinogen. The kinetic parameters of copro-ox were clearly modified, with a K_m 15-fold higher than normal values when using coproporphyrinogen or harderoporphyrinogen as substrates. Maximal velocity was half the normal value, and a marked sensitivity to thermal denaturation was observed. This mutation was markedly different from the other one, underlining once more the heterogeneity among each inherited disease.

c. Variegate porphyria. Several studies have shown a 50% deficiency in the activity of protoporphyrinogen oxidase (proto-ox) in VP (Brenner and Bloomer, 1980; Deybach et al., 1981a; Viljoen et al., 1983; Meissner et al., 1986). This genetic defect has always been found in one parent and some offspring in families of patients with VP in the authors' laboratory. If the evidence confirms that overproduction of protoporphyrinogen is the primary metabolic disturbance, it should, however, be noted that other enzymatic abnormalities have been described, such as decrease as ferrochelatase activity (Becker et al., 1977; Viljoen et al., 1979) or association of proto-ox and ferrochelatase deficiencies (Siepker and

Kramer, 1985; Viljoen et al., 1983) or association of proto-ox and PBG deaminase deficiencies (Meissner et al., 1986). Knowledge of homozygous cases (see below) with more than 90% of deficiency of proto-ox allows one to state that the mutation is lying in the proto-ox gene and to suggest that the abnormalities of other enzymes are epiphenomenons.

Four homozygous cases of VP have been described (Kordac et al., 1984; Murphy et al., 1986; Mustajoki et al., 1987). All of the patients showed a severe lifelong photosensitivity, a more or less decreased growth rate, and an increased erythrocyte protoporphyrin. Both patients of Kordac et al. (1984) showed neurologic symptoms; onset was in childhood in all cases. All of the parents were apparently healthy in spite of a 50% decrease of proto-ox. The mechanism underlying the accumulation of protoporphyrin in the red blood cells of the patients is still unexplained, but it seems to be common to all homozygous cases of hepatic porphyrias (Kordac et al., 1985).

Other variants of VP have been described.

1. Day (1986) and Day et al. (1982) found in 25 patients (from families with a well-known VP porphyrin profile) isomer composition and 7-5-carboxyl porphyrin fractions indistinguishable from those found in overt porphyria cutanea tarda (PCT): The overall biochemical picture was that of PCT superimposed on VP ("dual porphyria"), as was described previously by Watson et al. (1975). The activities of proto-ox and uroporphyrinogen decarboxylase were not measured and no clear inheritance pattern for dual porphyria emerged. Additional investigations are clearly needed.

2. McColl et al. (1985) described another dual porphyria, the "Chester porphyria": members of the same family (from Chester, UK) presented with typical attacks of AIP; some individuals had a pattern of porphyrin excretion typical of AIP, others showed that of VP, and some had an intermediate pattern. All of the patients showed a dual enzyme deficiency in leukocytes (reduced activity of both PBG deaminase and proto-ox). It is presently not known if the Chester family represents double heterozygotes or if one of both enzyme deficiencies is only a secondary phenomenon.

d. Doss porphyria. This porphyria has an autosomal-recessive pattern of inheritance and ALA dehydrase activity shows in erythrocytes and bone marrow cells (Doss et al., 1982; Thunell et al., 1987) a dramatic decrease as expected for homozygotes (1% of mean control), with approximately 50% decrease in the activities of parents. The same decrease (50%) was also found in erythrocytes of the heterozygous case described by Bird et al. (1979). All cases of Doss porphyria were CRIM-positive (de Verneuil et al., 1985; Fujita et al., 1987), suggesting that a structural mutation is in a coding sequence of the ALA dehydrase gene; the molecular weight and the isoelectric point of ALA dehydrase of the mutants of Doss did not show any difference by comparison with the normal enzyme (de Verneuil et al., 1985).

4. Prevalence of acute hepatic porphyrias. The high incidence of latent cases of AIP, HC, and VP allows only rough approximation of the prevalence of these autosomal-dominant porphyrias. Most of the estimates of AIP [cf. Waldenstrom and Haeger-Aronson (1967)] were established by screening populations for urinary porphyrin precursors and are, therefore, underestimated; they ranged from 1 to 8 per 100,000. The incidence of VP of 3 per 1000 in South Africa (Eales et al., 1980) is higher than elsewhere; in Finland, it has been reported at 1.3 per 100,000 (Mustajoki, 1980). The incidence of HC was estimated by With (1983) at 2 per million. Tishler et al. (1985) measured PBG deaminase activity in a psychiatric patient population and found an overall prevalence of 2%. Epidemiological studies of a healthy population with measurement of PBG deaminase activity are presently not available; they will be complicated by the overlapping values between normal and porphyric patients (Sassa et al., 1974). In all acute porphyrias onset is usually delayed until after infancy, except in homozygous cases; furthermore, probably at least 80% of individuals who inherit a gene for one of the autosomal-dominant porphyrias remain asymptomatic throughout life (Elder, 1986); 66% of latent porphyrics have normal precursor and porphyrin excretion (this percentage is almost 100% before puberty). Among 301 acute attacks studied in the authors' laboratory, 200 (66%) were AIP, 41 (14%) were HC, and 60 (20%) VP. In AIP, acute attacks are more common in women than in men; the important role of endocrine factors (Kappas et al., 1983a) will be discussed later.

5. Pathogenesis of the acute attack

a. Neuropathy. It is largely admitted that the symptoms of acute attacks of porphyria are due to the effects of the disease on the nervous system. Excellent reviews have recently been written on this subject (Moore et al., 1987; Kappas et al., 1983b; Bonkowsky and Schady, 1982) describing histological changes in peripheral and autonomic nerves as well as changes in central nervous system or electrodiagnostic findings. Among several hypotheses for the precise mechanism of neurologic lesions still debated, two are presently favored. One involves the deficiency of heme synthesis in neural tissues; the other involves the neurotoxicity of the precursors of heme, mainly ALA. The first hypothesis is obviously of great importance but only scarce data support it: It has been shown that the rodent brain synthesizes heme and cytochrome P450 (Gibson and Goldberg, 1970; Percy and Shanley, 1979; Cohn et al., 1977); however, porphyrinogenic chemicals (sulfonamides, etc.) that reach the brain do not induce ALA synthase, at least not in the rat (Percy and Shanley, 1979; Feuer et al., 1971; Nabeshima et al., 1981). Therefore, it is difficult to accept a significant deficiency in heme biosynthesis in neural tissues as the central factor of acute crises if accumulation of porphyrins and precursors arising on nervous tissue is not demonstrable.

An indirect metabolic consequence of relative hepatic heme deficiency could be the reduced activity of tryptophan pyrrolase (TP), a heme-dependent enzyme which converts tryptophan to kynurenine; if in acute attacks of porphyria there is decreased activity of TP, increases in the concentration of tryptophan and 510H tryptamine (serotonin) would be observed. Experimental data in rodents (Litman and Correia, 1983) support this hypothesis.

Presently, the neurotoxicity of ALA (mainly synthesized in liver) is the more-favored hypothesis for the following reasons. First, symptoms of acute attacks never occur when excretion of porphyrin precursors is normal. Second, typical neurologic manifestations have been observed in patients with abnormalities who overproduce ALA but not PBG such as Doss porphyria, lead intoxication, or tyrosinemia (Gentz et al., 1969). If ALA is synthesized mostly in the liver, it has to cross the blood-brain barrier to exert a neurotoxic effect. Brain uptake of ALA has been demonstrated in rodents (Shanley et al., 1975; McGillian et al., 1975) and both precursors have been found in the cerebrospinal fluid of patients during acute attacks of AIP and VP (Bonkowsky et al., 1971; Percy and Shanley, 1977). Unfortunately, the results of in vivo or in vitro experimental assays of ALA toxicity are still unimpressive (Moore et al., 1987) mostly because parameters such as species used or ALA concentration are too different from the human features.

b. Precipitating factors. Subjects with latent or clinically expressed acute porphyria may be precipitated into an acute attack by several factors such as sex steroid hormones, drugs, alcohol, stress, infectious diseases, and reducing diet. We will concentrate only on drugs and sex steroid hormones. However, most (if not all) of these factors precipitate acute attacks because they are related to an increase in the metabolic demand for heme in the liver; the ensuing induction of ALA synthase renders the deficient enzyme rate-limiting, with accumulation of precursors (and of porphyrins) resulting in the neurologic lesions of acute attacks.

i. Endocrine factors. The major role of endocrine factors is very well known: 80% of the patients with acute attacks are women between puberty and menopause and the attacks generally occur during the week preceding the menses; synthetic estrogens and progesterone of oral contraceptives have clearly been reported to induce acute attacks (Lamon et al., 1979a; Moore and Disler, 1983). Surprisingly, most of the women with acute porphyria display normal gestation when they are not treated with porphyrinogenic drugs (Mustajoki, 1986; Doss, 1986); however, mild attacks have been observed in early pregnancy (Brodie et al., 1977b).

The 5β epimers are more porphyrinogenic than the 5α. Anderson et al. (1979) found a ratio of 5β to 5α metabolites of testosterone higher in a group with clinically expressed AIP as compared with a group with latent AIP; it would be an impaired (and acquired) 5α reduction of steroid hormones in the group with clinical expression of the disorder (Kappas et al., 1971, 1972; Bradlow et al., 1973).

ii. Drugs.   Before describing the role of drugs as precipitating factors, it seems useful to recall some data concerning the regulation of the hepatic heme biosynthetic pathway. As previously shown in Chap. 4, the rate of flux through the heme synthetic pathway is under the control of its end-product heme, which exerts a negative feedback effect on the limiting enzyme ALA synthase.

Inhibition of the enzymatic activity occurs at high and nonphysiological concentration of heme (10^{-4} M). On the contrary, repression of the synthesis of the enzyme appears physiologically at low levels of heme concentration (10^{-8} to 10^{-9} M) and at two main stages: heme inhibits the maturation of a precursor of ALA synthase and the incorporation of the mature enzyme into the mitochondrial matrix (Hayashi et al., 1983; Srivastava et al., 1983). Recent experiments have shown that heme was able to prevent accumulation of ALA synthase mRNA (Ades et al., 1987). The stages of heme biosynthetic regulation are shown in the Fig. 10.3; the heme concentration of the so-called "regulatory heme pool" may decrease as a result of increased breakdown or decreased production. Impaired heme synthesis may occur when the activity of one of the

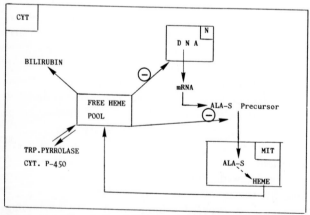

Figure 10.3   Regulation of sites of ALA synthase (ALA-S) activity through the regulatory free-heme pool. Cyt, cytochrome; N, nucleus; Mit, mitochondria; TRP, tryptophan.

enzymes along the pathway is decreased either genetically (case of the porphyrias) or by external factors (i.e., lead intoxication). The partial defect in heme synthesis in acute hepatic porphyrias results in increased ALA synthase activity through negative feedback regulation. The resulting increase in PBG production may be sufficient to compensate for the defect in heme synthesis. Thus, the effective heme concentration may approach a normal level, provided ALA synthase remains induced. Such a compensation may reflect the situation in patients with "latent" porphyria where clinical symptoms are absent. Drugs may upset this balance at several stages. Very few chemicals are known to be porphyrinogenic in normal individuals.

Allyl-containing acetamides [e.g., allyl isopropyl acetamide (AIA)] cause massive degradation of the heme moiety of cytochrome P450 and a resulting stress of heme synthesis. Diethoxy dicarbethoxy collidine (DDC) and griseofulvine both decrease heme synthesis through specific inhibition of ferrochelatase (De Matteis, 1978). Hexachlorobenzene, well known for its role in the epidemic PCT in Turkey, inhibits URO decarboxylase (Elder, 1978); however, numerous drugs such as barbiturates and sulfonamides are porphyrinogenic only if a genetic defect in porphyrin metabolism is already present.

The large heterogeneity of these compounds should be emphasized since they share little chemical features apart from lipid solubility. The way in which they interfere with heme synthesis is not completely clear. Some drugs may directly activate synthesis of ALA synthase (De Matteis, 1978), but there is evidence that lipid-soluble drugs induce a further depletion of the hepatic heme pool by stimulating synthesis of cytochrome P450 apoprotein, thereby increasing the demand for heme from a pathway whose capacity is already limited by the inherited

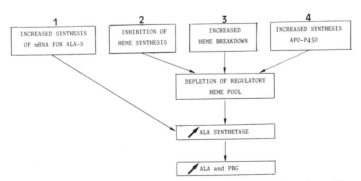

Figure 10.4 Different ways to produce stimulation of ALA synthase. The nonspecific pathways 1 and 4 are produced by many lipid-soluble drugs. The specific pathways 2 and 3 are produced by a few porphyrinogenic drugs (AIA, DDC).

enzymatic defect; this leads to the accumulation of precursors (ALA and PBG) and intermediate porphyrins and the offset of clinical symptoms of acute crises. The different ways to stimulate ALA and PBG accumulations are summarized in Fig. 10.4.

One, of course, should select drugs which are unable to induce the enzymes of the heme biosynthetic pathway when considering drugs for treatment of porphyric individuals. This is generally achieved through the prior testing of drugs in animal models either in vivo (rats, mice, chicken embryos) or in vitro (chick embryo liver cells in culture).

The inducing effects of drugs on heme synthesis are usually followed by measurements of ALA synthase activity, porphyrin concentrations, and/or cytochrome P450 levels. In the most-sensitive models, partial blocks in the heme pathway are first produced by appropriate chemical means in order to mimic the hereditary enzymatic defects found in

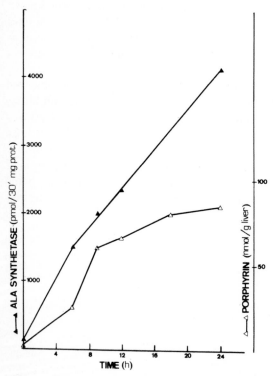

Figure 10.5 Time course of effects of Phenobarbital (4 mg/egg) + DDC (0.25 mg/egg) on liver ALA synthase activity and total porphyrin concentration. Values represent the average of four independent determinations made on six pooled livers from 18-day-old chick embryos.

hepatic porphyrias: for example, DDC produces a rapid and effective inhibition of ferrochelatase activity. As shown by Anderson (1978) and our team (de Verneuil et al., 1983a), the use of a small "priming" dose of DDC in the chick embryo system in ovo allows one to test drug porphyrinogenicity under the condition of an experimental block in heme synthesis (i.e., porphyria-like situation) and to simplify drug testing. In this system a high correlation was found between ALA synthase induction and liver porphyrin accumulation using drugs such as phenobarbital (Fig. 10.5). The inducing effects of drugs can be detected only by measurement of liver porphyrin accumulation.

Because of its good predictive value and ease of handling, we used the DDC-primed chick embryo system in order to test a large set of drugs. For easier clinical use, the drugs have been classified as nonporphyrinogenic (safe) and porphyrinogenic (unsafe) (Table 10.5). This list is in addition to the drugs which are already well known as inducers: barbiturates, sulfonamides, antiepileptic drugs, and so forth.

The danger of any untested medication for porphyric patients is obvious and cannot be easily predicted. Medical practitioners must base their therapy of affected individuals on lists of drugs whose porphyrinogenicity has been established in several ways on different animal models. At this time all drugs clearly involved in the onset of acute attacks in humans were found to be porphyrinogenic in the chicken embryo system in ovo.

6. Treatment of acute attacks.   Before describing the so-called "specific" therapies (acting on the biosynthetic pathway), we will focus on a few points: As soon as an attack has been diagnosed, a careful search should be made for any precipitating factor, especially drugs (including oral contraceptives), underlying infection, and hypocaloric diet. Agitation and other psychiatric manifestations are usually controlled with chlorpromazine. Treatment of severe pain requires morphine-like drugs such as pethidine, but the danger of addiction (in patients experiencing frequent attacks) has always to be kept in mind. We usually combine chlorpromazine with pethidine and leave the patient in a quiet room.

Specific therapies are now superseded by glucose and hematin (Kappas et al., 1988; Pierach, 1982, 1986b): The "glucose effect" frequently leads to a reduction in urinary porphyrin precursor excretion by a mechanism which is not certain (Bonkowsky et al., 1976; Doss et al., 1985). It is well known that a poor carbohydrate intake aggravates the attack and, therefore, an adequate administration is needed (300 to 400 g per day), usually by slow intravenous perfusion.

The treatment of a porphyric attack has been greatly improved with the introduction of hematin (Bonkowsky et al., 1971). Earlier observa-

TABLE 10.5 Drug Porphyrinogenicity (DDC-primed Chicken Embryo Liver System in Ovo)

Nonporphyrinogenic			Porphyrinogenic
Ac. acetylsalicylique	Digoxine	Ac. mefenamique	Clorazepate
Ac. clavulanique	Diltiazem	Ac. nalidixique	Clotiazepam
Ac. niflumique	Diphenhydramine	Ac. pipemidique	Dexfenfluramine
Ac. oxolinique	Dipyridamole	Alcool	Dextromoramide
Ac. tiaprofenique	Doxycycline	Alcuronium	Dextropropoxyphene
Ac. tienilique	Droperidol	Alfadolone-alfaxolone	Diazepam
Ac. tranexamique	EDTA	Allopurinol	Disopyramide
Acetazolamide	Estazolam	Alprazolam	Enflurane
Aciclovir	Ether	Amidopyrine	Ergotamine + derivatives
Acth	Etybenzatropine	Amineptine	Erythromycine
Adrenaline	Fentanyl	Amiodarone	Etamsylate
Alimemazine	Flucytosine	Amobarbital	Etidocaine
Amitriptyline	Flumazenil	Androgenes	Etomidate
Amoxicilline	Flunitrazepam	Articaine	Fenofibrate
Amphotericine B	Fluphenazine	Astemizole	Fenoverine
Atropine	Furosemide	Barbituriques	Floctafenine
Beta-alanine	Gentamycine	Barclofene	Flumequine
Bromazepam	Glafenine	Basdene	Flunarizine
Bromure	Glucagon	Benzbromarone	Fluorbiprophene
Buflomedil	Guanethidine	Bepridil	Glutethimide
Butacaine	Guanfacine	Beta-histine	Griseofulvine
Carpipramine	Haloperidol	Bromocriptine	Halothane
Chloral hydrate	Heparine	Bupivacaine	Hexapropymate
Chlordiazepoxide	Heptaminol	Captopril	Hydantoines
Chlorpromazine	Hydrochlorothiazide	Carbamazepine	Hydralazine
Cimetidine	Imipramine	Carisoprodol	Hydroxyzine
Clomipramine	Indometacine	Chloramphenicol	IMAO
Clonazepam	Insuline	Chlormezanone	Isoniazide
Codeine	Josamycine	Chloroquine	Kebuzone
Dexchlorpheniramine	Ketoprofene	Clobazam	Ketamine
Diazoxide	Ketotifene	Clometacine	Ketoconazole
Diclofenac	Labetalol	Clomethiazole	Lidocaine
Dicoumarol	Levomepromazine	Clomifene	Loprazolam
Digitoxine	Loperamide	Clonidine	Loxapine

Lorazepam
Maprotiline
Meclofenoxate
Mefloquine
Mequitazine
Metapramine
Metoclopramide
Metopimazine
Metoprolol
Midazolam
Minaprine
Minocycline
Morphine
Naftidrofuryl
Naproxene
Nefopam
Netilmicine
Nicergoline
Nifuroxazide
Nitroprussiate
Noradrenaline
Norfloxacine
Ofloxacine
Organon
Oxazepam
Oxybate de sodium
Oxybuprocaine
Oxyphenbutazone
Pancuronium
Parapenzolate
Peflacine
Pencilline
Perhexiline
Pethidine

Phenoperidine
Pipotiazine
Piracetam
Piroxicam
Pivampicilline
Prazosine
Probucol
Procainamide
Procaine
Promethazine
Propanidide
Propanolol
Propericiazine
Propoxyphene
Proxymetacaine
Reserpine
Salbutamol
Succinylcholine
Sulbutiamine
Sulindac
Terfenadine
Tetracaine
Thyroxine
Timolol
Triamterene
Trihexyphenidyle
Trimebutine
Trimetazidine
Trinitrine
Troleandomycine
Tubocurarine
Verapamil
Vitamines

Mebeverine
Mebubarbital
Mephenesine
Mepivacaine
Meprobamate
Methyldopa
Methylergometrine
Methyprilone
Metronidazole
Mianserine
Miconazole
Nifedipine
Nitrazepam
Noramydopyrine
Nordazepam
Oestro-Progestatifs
Oestrogenes
Oxybutynine
Paracetamol
Pargyline
Pentazocine
Pentoxifyline
Phenacetine
Phenazone
Phenobarbital
Phenoxybenzamine
Phenylbutazone
Pipebuzone
Prazepam
Prenylamine
Prilocaine
Primidone
Probenecide
Progabide

Progestatifs
Propantheline
Propofol
Pyrazinamide
Pyrrocaine
Quinine
Ranitidine
Rifampicine
Secobarbital
Spironolactone
Succinimides
Sulfamides
Sulfinpyrazone
Sulpiride
Sultopride
Tamoxifene
Tetrazepam
Theophylline
Ticlopidine
Tinidazole
Trazodone
Triazolam
Trimethadione
Trimipramine
Valproate de Sodium
Valpromide
Veralipride
Viloxazine

The spelling of the drug names is taken from Index Nominum (Switzerland).

tions (Watson et al., 1978) showed the superiority of hematin over glucose: Most of the patients responded favorably to hematin, whereas several were recalcitrant to glucose. Hematin is given intravenously in doses up to 3 to 4 mg/kg body weight/24 h, usually during 4 days. It has been demonstrated that heme finds access to the hepatocyte (Wyman et al., 1986; Linden et al., 1987) and, therefore, probably refurnishes the depleted heme pool; urinary ALA (and PBG) decreases dramatically in 2 to 3 days, showing that the feedback control of ALA synthase became efficient. The side effects of hematin such as coagulopathy (Morris et al., 1981) or phlebitis (Lamon et al., 1979b) have never been associated with real hemorrhage; however, hematin should not be used in conjunction with anticoagulant therapy (and the vein for infusion has to be changed each day). Stable preparations of hematin are now available (i.e., heme-arginate, Medica, Finland) and the side effects are practically excluded (Goetsch and Bissel, 1986; Mustajoki et al., 1986). Recently, women with cyclical perimenstrual acute attacks have benefitted from administration of agonists of luteinizing hormone-releasing hormone (LHRH). These factors allow one to inhibit ovulation and are perfectly tolerated by the patients; acute attacks soon disappear (Anderson et al., 1984, 1986). Other encouraging treatments have been proposed, such as beta adrenergic blocking agents (Douer et al., 1978) or resin hemoperfusions such as charcoal (Laiwah et al., 1983) or amberlite (Tishler et al., 1982; Martasek et al., 1986). All of the described treatments have to be used early in the attack before any nervous or respiratory complication arises, otherwise a biochemical response without concomitant clinical amelioration may be the only result (Pierach, 1986a).

B. Porphyria cutanea symptomatica (porphyria cutanea tarda) and hepatoerythropoietic porphyria

1. Porphyria cutanea symptomatica. Porphyria cutanea symptomatica (PCS) is the most-common form of porphyria; cutaneous photosensitivity is the predominating clinical feature; acute attacks with abdominal pain, psychiatric, and/or neurological manifestations are never observed. PCS is a heterogeneous group including at least two types: (1) The sporadic type (or type I) classically more often observed in male patients (40 to 50 years old) without a family history of the disease; its development appears related to some inducing compounds such as alcohol. (2) The familial type (rarer) has an earlier onset (sometimes before puberty) and is observed equally in both genders; other members of the kindred may have overt PCS. In the sporadic type, uroporphyrinogen decarboxylase (URO-D) activity is deficient only in the liver (50% reduction); in familial PCS, there is a 50% reduction of URO-D activity in all tissues and this is inherited in an autosomal-dominant pattern. PCS has not been well characterized in terms of its incidence; it has been found in all parts of the world, with perhaps a higher frequency among the Bantus in South Africa (Eales et al., 1975). In our files, among 681 patients, 576 (85%) show a sporadic type and 105 (15%) a familial type with a 50% decrease of URO-D activity in erythrocytes; the percentage of familial type seems higher in the United States (Kushner, 1982).

   a. Clinical features. Skin lesions have been described in several recent reviews (Kappas et al., 1983b; Pimstone, 1982; Mascaro et al., 1986; Moore et al., 1987). The lesions of photosensitivity involve the light-exposed areas such as the backs of the hands, face, and neck, and also in women the legs and backs of the feet. Skin fragility is perhaps the most specific feature: A minimal trauma is followed by a superficial erosion soon covered by a crust. Bullae (vesicles) usually appear after sun exposure and take several weeks to heal, leaving hypo- or hyperpigmented atrophic scars. White papules (milia) may develop in areas of the bullae, particularly the backs of the hands. Hypertrichosis is often found in the upper part of the cheeks (malar area) and sometimes also in the ears and arms. Increased uniform pigmentation of sun-exposed areas is common. Alopecia and hypopigmented scleroderma-like lesions of the skin are rarer. All of these skin lesions are similar to those seen in VP and HC.

   Variable degrees of liver dysfunction are common among PCS patients, particularly in association with excessive alcohol intake (Bruguera, 1986; Mayer and Schmid, 1978). However, it is not clear to what extent liver cell injury is important in the expression of the PCS syndrome. It is well known that in patients with typical cirrhosis PCS is very rare. Taddeini and Watson (1968) suggested that in patients with PCS there may be an underlying constitutional abnormality which might enhance the liability of the liver to develop PCS. Needlelike inclusions have been found in the cytoplasm of hepatocytes (Cortes et al., 1980; Waldo and Tobias, 1973). These inclusions are probably composed of uroporphyrin which could promote progressive liver damage (Bruguera, 1986). The incidence of hepatic cancer among PCS patients seems to be greater than in the general population, but the published results are very different, from 47% in Czechoslovak series (Kordak, 1972) to 0% in Italy (Topi et al., 1980). Sometimes, the onset of skin pigmentation occurred simultaneously with the development of the hepatic tumor; fluorescence was present in the tumor, indicating its porphyrin content (Tio et al., 1959).

   b. Precipitating factors. Among the precipitating factors, *alcohol, estrogens*, and *iron* are the most frequently incriminated: If alcohol consumption is often acknowledged, the mechanisms by which it exacerbates PCS are unclear: URO-D and ALA-D (Doss et al., 1981; Kondo et al., 1983) have been shown to be decreased by alcohol, whereas ALA synthase would be stimulated by alcohol (Shanley et al., 1969) in the livers of PCS patients. Sinclair et al. (1981) have demonstrated that ethanol increases cytochrome P450 in cultured hepatocytes; they have also shown the role of the higher chain (3 to 5 carbon) alcohols on the induction of ALA synthase and cytochrome P450 in primary cultures of chick embryo hepatocytes. The higher-chain alcohols are often included in commercial alcoholic beverages, and may contribute to the exacerbation of PCS.

Estrogen-containing oral contraceptives have increased the prevalence of PCS in women (Malina and Chlumsky, 1975; Sixel-Dietrich and Doss, 1985); the role of estrogen was already well known in male patients treated with stilbestrol for prostatic cancer (White, 1977).

It should be emphasized that in our patients most of the drugs classified as porphyrinogenic (i.e., unsafe for use in acute porphyrias, Table 10.5) have been found to precipitate or exacerbate PCS; as in any hepatic porphyria, most of the patients may have used these drugs (or alcohol) during several years before developing PCS.

Abnormal *iron* metabolism appears to be another precipitating factor of the clinical onset of PCS: serum iron is frequently elevated in PCS patients; a mild hepatic siderosis has been described in at least 80% of the patients (Grossman et al., 1979; Lundvall et al., 1970). However, other authors found a normal total body iron store in most of the patients studied (Sweeney, 1986). Iron removal by phlebotomy is a highly effective treatment of PCS (Ippen, 1977). Several conflicting results have been published concerning the effects of iron on URO-D activity in vitro. Whereas some authors claim that iron inhibits URO-D (Kushner et al., 1975, 1985; Straka and Kushner, 1983; Mukerji et al., 1984), others have reported that iron either activates (Blekkenhorst et al., 1979) or has no effect (Woods et al., 1981; de Verneuil et al., 1983b). In vivo, URO-D of patients with PCS seems to have a specific sensitivity to iron because no reduced activity of URO-D has been found in iron-overloaded livers such as those of patients with hemochromatosis or alcohol-related liver diseases (Felsher et al., 1982). Presently, the iron-mediated induction of a free radical system seems to be the more-popular proposal to explain the effect of iron on uroporphyrinogen metabolism in PCS (Elder et al., 1986). Smith and Francis (1983) showed that mice given both iron and hexachlorobenzene became porphyric: Iron would exert its synergistic action through the formation of highly reactive hydroxyl radicals which in turn would cause site-selective URO-D damage without any decrease in the concentration of immunoreactive enzyme (Elder and Sheppard, 1982).

The cause of the iron overload is still unknown; Kushner et al. (1985) suggested that patients with PCS are heterozygous for the hemochromatosis allele. In one patient's family they found the presence of a HLA-A$_3$-B$_7$ haplotype among the patient and four other members of the family, confirming the presence of a hemochromatosis allele; Llorente et al. (1980) and Kuntz et al. (1981) also found a high incidence of HAL-A$_3$ in PCS patients. However, Beaumont et al. (1987) working on 69 PCS patients (42 had the sporadic type and 27, unrelated, had the familial one) found the same incidence (24%) of HLA-A$_3$ antigen (the best marker of hemochromatosis) in each type of PCS and in the controls. If a systematic association between hemochromatosis and PCS seems ruled out, some random association can occur which would probably favor the clinical manifestations of PCS.

Polyhalogenated hydrocarbons (PHCs) have been found to be porphyrinogenic in humans and in animals (rodents); the first identified was hexachlorobenzene, which precipitated a massive outbreak of about 4000 cases of PCS in Turkey (from 1956 to 1961) following the ingestion of hexachlorobenzene-treated wheat (Schmid, 1960; Dogramici, 1962). The animals exposed to hexachlorobenzene show a pattern of porphyrin excretion closely resembling that seen in human PCS with a diminished hepatic URO-D activity (we have already discussed the synergistic effect of iron, Smith and Francis, 1983). However, PHCs do not induce clinical features of PCS in experimental animals.

Several other PHCs, such as tetrachloro-dibenzo-*p*-dioxin (TCDD), 2,4-dichlorophenol, and 2,4,5-trichlorophenol, were incriminated in the development of PCS in industrial workers (Pazderova-Vejlupkova et al., 1981; Poland et al., 1971). Doss et al. (1984) found slight abnormalities in urinary porphyrin excretion among 13 workers exposed to TCDD in an Italian industrial plant; two siblings with a familial type developed a clinically manifest PCS. TCDD is highly porphyrinogenic; however, if URO-D activity is strongly decreased, the immunoreactive protein is unchanged (Elder and Sheppard, 1982), suggesting that only the catalytic sites of the enzyme have been modified. de Verneuil et al. (1983b) showed that TCDD directly added to homogenates from chick embryo liver cells did not inhibit URO-D; they suggested that inhibitory substances might be metabolites generated in the liver from parent hydrocarbons. Smith et al. (1986) suggested that the inhibition of hepatic URO-D requires a specific cytochrome P450 isoenzyme and an unknown iron species.

c. **Classical biologic data.** Urine contains an increased concentration of uroporphyrin (mainly isomer I) and 7-carboxylic porphyrin (mainly isomer III); coproporphyrin, 5- and 6-carboxylic porphyrins are moderately increased (Elder, 1977). Both precursors are usually normal but the accompanying liver disease may indicate a minor increase of δ-aminole-vulinate (ALA) excretion (Elder, 1977).

In feces, the dominant porphyrin excreted is often the isocopropor-phyrin (Elder, 1974) (see Fig. 10.6). However, coproporphyrin, 7-car-boxylic porphyrin, uroporphyrin, and X porphyrin concentrations (ether-insoluble fraction) may all be enhanced in PCS (Elder, 1977). During clinical remission, total porphyrin excretion decreases progres-sively and measurement of urinary porphyrins is one of the best methods to follow the effects of the treatment (usually repeated phlebotomy). After a few months, urinary porphyrin patterns look normal, but in the feces copro- and isocoproporphyrin may remain increased for a long time.

An additional characteristic feature of PCS is the accumulation of large quantities of porphyrin in the liver (Doss et al., 1971), mostly URO and 7-carboxyl porphyrin (hydrophilic porphyrins). The same por-phyrins are also found in plasma (Moore et al., 1973; Kalb et al., 1985). Serum iron and ferritin levels are frequently increased (see above).

d. Enzymatic abnormalities. Uroporphyrinogen decarboxylase (URO-D) is decreased in the liver of all patients with PCS (Kushner et al., 1976; Elder et al., 1978); it is also reduced in the livers of animals fed with polyhalogenated hydrocarbons (Taljaard et al., 1971). In familial PCS, URO-D has been found to be decreased by 50% in all tissues, including erythrocytes (de Verneuil et al., 1978; Elder et al., 1980). Kindred studies of erythrocyte URO-D deficiency have demonstrated the autosomal-dominant pattern of inheritance (Fig. 10.7) and allowed detection of latent carriers without biochemical abnormalities. Familial PCS is not rare (15 to 20% of PCS) but it is not uncommon to find several patients in the same family with the latent carriers being predominant. Using

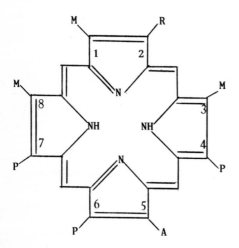

Figure 10.6 Isocoproporphyrin (iso C). A, acetyl; M, methyl; P, propionyl. R $=$ —CH_2—CH_3, iso C; R $=$ —CH$=$$CH_2$, dehydro iso C; R $=$ —H, deethyl iso C; R $=$ —CHOH—CH_3, hydrox-yethyl iso C.

specific antibodies, Elder et al. (1983) and de Verneuil et al. (1984a) showed that in patients with familial PCS erythrocyte immunoreactive URO-D protein was decreased to the same extent as catalytic activity (CRIM-negative), whereas in sporadic PCS both measurements were normal. In 1985 Elder et al. measured both catalytic and immunoreactive URO-D protein in the liver of sporadic PCS patients. They found the ratio of catalytic activity to immunoreactive protein lower in patients in whom the disease was active; during remission following venesection, enzyme activity and immunoreactive enzyme concentration were normal. These findings were consistent with the view that sporadic PCS is an acquired disorder. As Moore et al. (1987) have written, "though there appears to be no genetic deficiency of URO-D enzyme protein in sporadic PCS, there may still be some hereditary predisposition to damage at the catalytic site of URO-D. The fact that only a minority of patients with iron overload and alcoholic liver disease develop PCS favors the existence of such a predisposition." In the authors' laboratory two brothers both had an overt PCS (clinical features and biochemical data were typical); however, erythrocyte URO-D activity was normal. These patients were, therefore, indistinguishable from sporadic cases of PCS. Roberts et al. (1988) found identical cases in four families; URO-D activities were normal in erythrocytes, fibroblasts, and, after prolonged remission, in liver. If a liver-specific mutation for this form of PCS seems, therefore, not plausible, a mutation at some other locus predisposing individuals to develop PCS in response to acquired factors (alcohol, drugs, etc.) is likely.

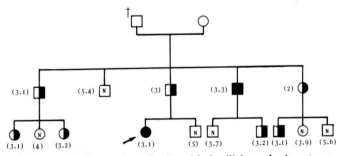

Figure 10.7 Pedigree of one family with familial porphyria cutanea. Numbers in parentheses give erythrocyte URO decarboxylase activity, expressed as nmol coproporphyrin formed/mg protein/h at 37°C.

Male	Female	
□	○	Not investigated
■	●	Patient
◨	◑	Asymptomatic carriers
N̲	Ⓝ	Normal
	↗	Propositus

e. Variants

- *Hemodialysis and pseudoporphyria cutanea.* Some patients on hemodialysis show cutaneous lesions that clinically and histologically are similar to those seen in PCS (Korting, 1975); the diagnosis rests on demonstrating markedly elevated plasma levels of uroporphyrin (Seubert et al., 1985; Thivolet et al., 1977; Poh-Fitzpatrick, 1980, 1982). Patients can be divided in two groups: Group 1 consists of patients with mildly elevated plasma porphyrins. This mild elevation is linked to renal failure and the relevance of this to the skin lesions is unclear; the name "pseudoporphyria" is therefore, appropriate. Group 2 includes patients with strongly elevated plasma porphyrins: They have a real PCS in addition to their renal disease.
- Associations of PCS with several other diseases have been reported (Kappas et al., 1988). No genetic reason for this association has been found (the development of hepato cellular carcinoma has already been discussed).
- *Hepatoerythropoietic porphyria.*   (See below.)

f. Treatment   First, all patients with PCS should be advised to avoid the precipitating factors (alcohol, pills, drugs, etc.) and also exposure to sunlight until clinical and biological remissions have been obtained by treatment.

Presently, phlebotomy (Ippen, 1961, 1977) is the treatment of choice in PCS, even when serum iron or ferritin levels are not increased. Venesections of 300 ml spaced at 10 to 12 day intervals are continued during 2 months until the serum iron level falls to 60 to 70% of its original value. Urine porphyrin levels are monitored each month: Clinical and biological remissions are usually obtained within 6 months.

When phlebotomy is contraindicated (anemia, cardiac or pulmonary disorders, age), low-dose chloroquine therapy (250 mg weekly) is the favored alternate therapy (Kordac and Semradova, 1974; Kowertz, 1975). Duration of treatment and relapse rate are only marginally greater than with venesection (Ashton et al., 1984; Malina, 1986). High-dose therapy has to be avoided because it causes a hepatitis-like syndrome in PCS patients (Felsher and Redeker, 1966).

Topi et al. (1984) reported 16 cases of PCS treated with success only by avoidance of hepatic toxins. Rocchi et al. (1986) tested the efficacy of long-term subcutaneous infusion of desferrioxamine. They recommend it when severe associated diseases contraindicate venesection; this treatment emphasizes the role of iron in the pathogenesis of PCS.

2. Hepatoerythropoietic porphyria.

Hepatoerythropoietic porphyria (HEP) is a very rare porphyria resulting from a homozygous defect in URO-D activity. Clinically, it is very similar to congenital erythropoietic porphyria (CEP) with a severe photosensitivity usually beginning in early infancy (Pinol-Aguadé et al., 1969; Hofstad et al., 1973; Simon et al., 1977; Czarnecki, 1980; Lim and Poh-Fitzpatrick, 1984; Sfar et al., 1985; Smith, 1986; Toback et al., 1987).

a. Clinical findings are described with CEP; a difference with CEP consists in the absence of erythrodontia (Mascaro et al., 1986). Another difference is the usual absence of hemolytic anemia, which is often very severe in CEP.

b. Biochemical findings. Patterns of urine and fecal porphyrin excretions are similar to those found in PCS. A comparison of the data obtained in patients with CEP or HEP is shown in Table 10.6. As in other homozygous cases of porphyrias, increased Zn-protoporphyrin is found in erythrocytes.

c. Enzymatic features and molecular biology. Elder et al. (1981) described a severely deficient (7% of normal activity) URO-D activity in patients with HEP, suggesting that these patients are homozygous for the gene that causes PCS. Several other studies (Lazaro et al., 1984; de Verneuil et al., 1984a; Toback et al., 1987) confirmed the homozygous inheritance of a defect of the URO-D gene and also showed a 50% reduction of URO-D activity in parents and in children of the patient (parents and children being asymptomatic).

Immunological studies on URO-D in HEP patients showed that there were two groups of patients, one displaying the enzyme deficiency with CRIM-positive mutation (Sassa et al., 1983) and the other with CRIM-negative mutation (de Verneuil et al., 1984a). This heterogeneity of the CRIM-negative group has been shown by immunochemical study of the

TABLE 10.6 Porphyrin Excretion in Hepatoerythropoietic Porphyria (HEP) and Congenital Erythropoietic Porphyria (CEP)

| | Porphyrins (percentage total recovered) | | | | | |
| | Urine | | | Feces | | |
	CEP (patient 1)	HEP	Normal	CEP (patient 1)	HEP	Normal
Coproporphyrin	14	4	81	96	20	97
Isocoproporphyrin series	—	1	—	—	39	Traces
5-Carboxyl	3	5	2	4	26	Traces
6-Carboxyl	1	4	1	Traces	9	—
7-Carboxyl	2	33	1	—	5	—
Uroporphyrin	80	53	15	—	1	—

The high pressure liquid chromatography profile of urinary and fecal porphyrins from CEP patients is very different from the profile obtained from the excreta of patients with HEP.

HEP patient described by Toback et al. (1987). Fujita et al. (1987) found that erythrocyte URO-D activity was disproportionately elevated (16% of normal control) in comparison to its immunoreactive material (under 7% of normal control). de Verneuil et al. (1986a) also described the molecular heterogeneity of URO-D deficiency in HEP: One patient had a URO-D with a half-life 12 times shorter than URO-D of control cell lines; URO-D of another patient was characterized by a higher molecular weight; URO-D of the third patient showed decreased synthesis and increased degradation rates of the protein.

The recent availability of a human uroporphyrinogen decarboxylase cDNA clone (Romeo et al., 1986) allowed de Verneuil et al. (1986c) to investigate the mutant gene and its expression in lymphoblastoid cell lines from a family with two cases of HEP. Southern analysis after digestion of genomic DNA showed the same restriction fragments in DNA isolated from a normal cell line or from both patients, excluding large deletion or rearrangements in the mutant gene. Northern and dot

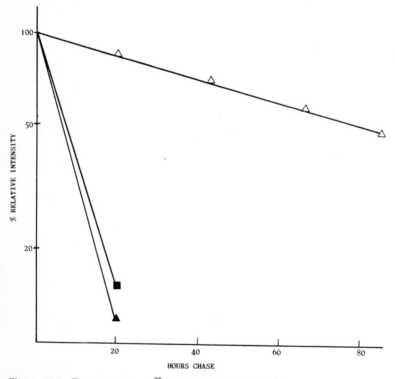

Figure 10.8 Turnover rate of ^{35}S methionine-labeled URO decarboxylase. The percentage of integrated values (relative to the 0-h chase time point) vs. hours of chase is shown as a semilog plot. △, normal cell line; ■, patient 1 cell line; ▲, patient 2 cell line.

blot analysis demonstrated that the concentration of mRNA was very similar in cell lines from controls, heterozygous parents, or homozygous patients. Study of in vitro translation products of uroporphyrinogen decarboxylase mRNA showed a normal amount of immuno-precipitable uroporphyrinogen decarboxylase in all cell lines. The size and molecular weight of the protein were identical to those of the marker enzyme. The only explanation of the very low level of uroporphyrinogen decarboxylase protein in cells (5% of control value) was given by study of the half-life of the enzyme: Whereas in control cells $t_{1/2}$ was 82 h, it was only 7 h in the patient cells (Fig. 10.8); the enzyme defect results from rapid degradation in vivo of an unstable protein.

Cloning and sequencing of a cDNA for the mutated gene in one patient from that family (de Verneuil et al., 1986b) has revealed the nature of the mutation which consists of a G to A change at nucleotide 860 in cDNA sequence leading to a Gly (GGG) to Glu (GAG) change in the amino acid sequence at position 281. In vitro experiments revealed that the cDNA with this mutation encoded a polypeptide product that was very rapidly degraded (when compared with the polypeptide encoded by the normal cDNA) in the presence of cell lysate. This observation was consistent with the decreased stability of the mutant protein in vivo.

The prevalence of the 281 (Gly → Glu) mutation in HEP was investigated by the use of hybridization with a synthetic oligonucleotide probe (de Verneuil et al., 1988). The mutation was found in HEP-affected members of two unrelated families from Spain, but was absent in two other patients from Italy and Portugal; moreover, this mutation was not detected in 13 unrelated cases of familial PCS. It is still not known if some cases of HEP are due to homozygosity for the same mutation responsible for familial PCS; heterogeneity of PCS may explain why no mutation similar to HEP has been found in a small number of tested subjects. On the other hand, HEP may be a specific recessive disease entirely distinct from PCS.

III. Erythropoietic Porphyrias

Erythropoietic porphyrias have few features in common other than solar photosensitivity. *Congenital erythropoietic porphyria* is very rare and follows an autosomal-recessive mode of inheritance; clinical manifestations are usually very spectacular. *Erythropoietic protoporphyria* is more frequent and follows an autosomal-dominant mode of inheritance. Clinical manifestations are usually modest. In these forms of porphyria, patients do not experience acute attacks and do not need a list of porphyrinogenic agents.

A. Congenital erythropoietic porphyria

Congenital erythropoietic porphyria (CEP), or Günther's disease, is one
of the rarest inherited porphyrias (less than 200 cases have been reported
in the literature); CEP was, however, the first porphyria described
(Schultz, 1874) and the first porphyria in which a specific enzyme defect
has been demonstrated (uroporphyrinogen III cosynthase) (Levin, 1968;
Romeo and Levin, 1969); it is a porphyria with a recessive mode of
transmittance.

1. Clinical features. The predominant site of metabolic expression of
CEP is the erythropoietic system. The highly abnormal accumulation of
porphyrins in bone marrow, peripheral blood, and other organs leads to
the three main manifestations: chronic photodermatitis with photosensitivity, massive porphyrinuria, and hematologic alterations.

Generally, one or all of these pathologic changes occur at birth or
during early infancy. Alterations can be observed before birth (Nitowsky
et al., 1978) and a few cases have been reported in patients with late
onset of photosensitivity (Deybach et al., 1981b; Nordmann and
Deybach, 1986).

In infants, the first symptom suggesting CEP is usually the excretion
of red urine with pink staining of the diapers. The red discoloration
depends on the amount of porphyrins excreted and in all reported cases
is subject to large fluctuations: from pink to dark reddish brown.

Photosensitivity is manifested when the child is in sunlight. A vesicular or bullous eruption may follow exposure, with effects on the face and
the back of the hands. The vesicles contain a serous fluid that may
exhibit a red fluorescence under ultraviolet (uv) light. Often the vesicles
lead to erosions and impetiginous infection and heal slowly, leaving
pigmented or even depigmented scars. Scarring due to severe infection
may give the skin a pinched appearance.

The repetition of bullous eruptions, minor injuries, and infections may
lead to severe mutilation of ears, nose cartilage, and digits. Fortunately,
modern medical treatment can greatly reduce the severity of secondary
infections and the severe scarring described in the older literature should
thereby be avoided. Nevertheless, all exposed or already affected areas of
the skin of patients remain more sensitive to slight injury, and a diffuse
thickening of the skin (pseudoscleroderma) is a common feature after
several years. Hypertrichosis appears in most patients; it also affects the
exposed areas, especially the upper arm and the face on the temple and
malar region. The additional hair is typically blond, downy, and of
lanugo type, but may be coarse and dark. There may also be loss of
cranial hair that occurs as a "scarring alopecia" in the scalp. Fingernails
are often dystrophically altered (koilonychia).

Erythrodontia is reported in almost all cases and, if present, is pathognomonic of CEP. The teeth, deciduous and/or permanent, may exhibit a red or usually dirty-brown discoloration under normal light and a red fluorescence under uv light. This is due to the deposit of large amounts of porphyrins in the dentine. The discoloration of the deciduous teeth suggests that porphyrin overproduction begins in the fetus. Such deposits of porphyrins, mainly uroporphyrin, have been found in bones and other calcium-containing structures and may be due to the affinity of higher carboxylated porphyrins for calcium phosphate (Kappas et al., 1983b; Sveinsson et al., 1949). Splenomegaly is another feature commonly reported in patients. It has been found at birth or soon after birth in a few cases, but it usually appears as the disease progresses and in relation to the hemolytic activity in most cases. The eyes may be afflicted in the form of severe ulcerations, ectropion, or cataract, with ensuing blindness; in all instances extreme care should be taken with such patients.

Finally, CEP patients never exhibit the abdominal or neuropsychiatric symptoms observed in the acute hepatic porphyrias.

2. Hematologic findings. The hematologic features in CEP have long been the subject of investigation and controversy (Kappas et al., 1983b).

An increased hemolytic activity was found in the majority of previously reported cases (Kappas et al., 1983b; Goldberg and Rimington, 1962; Schmid et al., 1955) and also in every one of our seven patients.

The intermittent nature of the course of the hemolytic process is a striking and specific feature of CEP. At times a patient may manifest an obvious hemolytic anemia and at other times only slight, subdetectable hemolysis. This feature has to be kept in mind when reviewing the data available on hemolysis in CEP. In most patients, the anemia is only slight and the hemolytic process well compensated by heightened erythrocyte production. In some cases anemia is, at times, very severe, requiring multiple transfusions. Early death due to anemia has been reported (Sato and Takahasi, 1926; Simard et al., 1972).

Red blood cell survival has been the subject of conflicting reports. Although closely associated with porphyrin overproduction, the mechanism responsible for the hemolytic process in CEP is still under investigation (Nordmann and Deybach, 1986).

Fluorescence of a large proportion of the normoblasts is readily demonstrable in the bone marrow of all patients with CEP (Kappas et al., 1983b; Varadi, 1958). Fluorescence is principally localized in the nuclei of the cells (Schmid et al., 1955; Varadi, 1958). Fluorescent normoblasts were morphologically abnormal (Schmid et al., 1955); heme deposition has been demonstrated within the vacuoles of nuclei in these fluorescent erythroblasts (Schmid et al., 1955). Not all of the more mature normoblasts were fluorescent, and the nonfluorescent normoblasts did not exhibit abnormal morphology (Schmid et al., 1955). This suggests, at least, that the underlying defect does not express itself with the same intensity in all erythroid cells.

3. Biochemical findings (Table 10.7)

a. Urine. The urine always contains large amounts of uroporphyrin and, to a lesser extent, coproporphyrin, but with daily and seasonal fluctuations. Smaller amounts of 7-, 6-, and 5-carboxylic porphyrins are also extracted, but their pattern of excretion is quite different from that found in porphyria cutanea symptomatica (PCS). The major fraction of urinary uroporphyrin and coproporphyrin is of isomeric series I (> 80%), but there is an absolute increase in uroporphyrin III in all patients. ALA is usually found within normal limits or only slightly increased in some cases. PBG is normal in most cases.

b. Feces. Feces contain large amounts of coproporphyrin and only slight amounts of uroporphyrin. Most of the fecal porphyrins belong to the isomeric series I as in urine. The protoporphyrin levels are usually within the normal range.

Of interest is the pattern of fecal porphyrin excretion in CEP as compared with HEP (Table 10.6). The absence of the isocoproporphyrin series and the normal level of 5-carboxylic porphyrin excretion in feces from CEP patients should be underlined for distinction between hepatoerythropoietic porphyria (HEP) and CEP.

c. Plasma. The plasma also contains large amounts of uroporphyrin and (less) coporporphyrin, both belonging to the isomeric series I (> 80%). They are thought to be derived from porphyrins eluted from the red blood cells into plasma (see before) but the hemolytic process probably accounts for a part of the increase in porphyrin content of plasma (Schmid et al., 1955; Heilmeyer et al., 1963).

TABLE 10.7   Erythropoietic Porphyrias: Biochemical Features

	Urine			Feces			Erythrocytes			
	PRE	U	C	U	C	P	U	C	P	Fluorescence
Erythropoietic protoporphyria					±	+++		+	++++	+
Congenital erythropoietic porphyria	Type I +++	Type I +++	Type I ++	Type I +++		+	Type I +++	Type I ++	++	+++

U = Uroporphyrin; C = Coproporphyrin; P = Protoporphyrin; PRE = Precursor

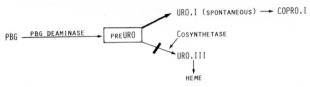

Figure 10.9 Congenital erythropoietic porphyria: primary deficiency of cosynthase.

d. Erythrocytes. Red blood cells contain variable, but always increased,
concentrations of uroporphyrin and coproporphyrin I. The values for
protoporphyrin are usually not higher than those found in other
hemolytic conditions.

4. Porphyria overproduction and enzyme defect in CEP. A genetic defect
resulting in *a primary deficiency of the activity of uroporphyrinogen III
cosynthase* is now widely accepted and documented (Fig. 10.9): A 10 to
30% residual cosynthase activity has been demonstrated by Levin (1968)
in hemolysates from porphyric cattle, then by Romeo and Levin (1969)
in human patient eythrocytes, and finally by Romeo et al., (1970) in
cultured skin fibroblasts from these patients.

Several family studies (Romeo and Levin, 1969; Deybach et al., 1981b;
Tsai et al., 1987) have shown that presumed heterozygotes (cattle and
human beings) have, in their erythrocytes, cosynthase activity that is
between that of porphyrics and controls (Table 10.8). However, heterozygotes always have normal PBG deaminase activity, which is not compatible with a primary increase of this enzyme activity (Watson et al., 1964;
Miyagi et al., 1976). Normal PBG deaminase activity does not correlate
with the hypothesis that decreased cosynthase activity found in all cells
is secondary to the observed inactivation (in vitro) as the synthesis of
uroporphyrinogen I occurs (Miyagi et al., 1976). It has also been shown
that in normal fibroblasts the cosynthase activity is of the same order of
magnitude as in erythrocytes (Grandchamp et al., 1980), in contrast to
the specific activity of PBG deaminase, which is very low in fibroblasts
as compared with erythrocytes (Sassa et al., 1975). These findings explain the fact that only in erythropoietic tissue is the rate of porphyrin
synthesis great enough to exceed the reduced capacity of the residual
cosynthase.

The normal supply of heme might be obtained through an increase of
ALA synthase and PBG deaminase activities, as these enzymes were
shown to be inducible in erythroid tissue (Beaumont et al., 1984). The
consequent imbalance between cosynthase and PBG deaminase activity
in erythroid cells explains the appearance of porphyrins of series I.

Among the practical implications of a defective cosynthase activity as the primary defect, it is interesting to note the possibility of the prenatal diagnosis of the disease. The prenatal exclusion of CEP has already been done in a fetus at risk (Deybach et al., 1980). Cosynthase was measured in amniotic cells and found to be normal when compared to control cells. These data were confirmed by the normal level of porphyrins in amniotic fluid. Furthermore, the porphyrin was found to be only coproporphyrin, whereas in one case of a fetus with CEP described by Nitowsky et al. (1978), a high level of uroporphyrin I was found in amniotic fluid. Postnatal studies of cosynthase activity in the latter infant's erythrocytes confirmed that he was not a carrier.

5. Variants of CEP

a. Late onset CEP. Since 1965 five cases of late onset CEP have been described (Kramer et al., 1965; Deybach et al., 1981b; Pain et al., 1975; Weston et al., 1978) with clinical features similar to sporadic porphyria cutanea occurring in adulthood. However, biologic data confirmed that these cases were CEP. Pain et al. (1975) suggested that late manifestation may represent the heterozygous state, but Deybach et al. (1981b) showed that the blood cosynthase of two patients was very low when compared with the enzyme activity of presumed heterozygotes and not significantly different from the activity of homozygous patients. Furthermore, familial studies of cosynthase activity showed that all the children of one patient were heterozygous (Nordmann and Deybach, 1986). Although the mechanism of late onset is presently unknown, the mild cases force one to admit the heterogeneity of CEP. However, the observed cosynthase activities are quite homogeneous and do not appear to explain the differences found between mild and severe cases.

TABLE 10.8   **Levels of Erythrocyte Uroporphyrinogen III Cosynthase and PBG Deaminase Activity from CEP Patients and Obligatory Carriers**

	Cosynthase[*]			PBG deaminase[†]		
	Number of subjects	Mean ± standard deviation	Range	Number of subjects	Mean ± standard deviation	Range
Controls	12	6.0 ± 1.1	4.1–7.9	50	150 ± 40	105–195
Obligatory carriers	7	2.8 ± 0.6[‡]	2.0–3.1	7	154 ± 27	107–190
Patients	6	1.05± 0.5[‡]	0.1–1.6	6	358 ± 153	180–620

[*]Units of cosynthase/mg of protein.
[†]Picomoles of uroporphyrin/mg of protein/30 min.
[‡]$p < 0.001$ for carriers vs. normal controls and also for patients vs. carriers.

6. Inheritance. All formal genetic data on CEP were consistent with an autosomal-recessive mode of inheritance in which male and female are equally afflicted (Kappas et al., 1983b).

Direct biochemical evidence concerning the inheritance of CEP is now available. Romeo et al. (1970) first demonstrated that parents and offspring of porphyric individuals and other obligatory carriers, have erythrocyte cosynthase activities between those of normal and porphyric subjects. Similar results have been obtained from our laboratory (Deybach et al., 1981b).

7. Therapy. No important advances have been made in the treatment of CEP. General treatment includes minimal exposure to the sun, avoidance of trauma to the skin, and careful treatment of any skin infection. Oral carotenoids undoubtedly decrease the photosensitivity of patients (Gajdos et al., 1977; Jung, 1977; Seip et al., 1974; Sneddon and Stretcher, 1978).

Several methods have been proposed to try to decrease excessive production of porphyrins: Administration of purines such as inosine (Haining et al., 1968) or adenylic acid (Gajdos and Gajdos-Torok, 1962) is ineffective in most cases. Use of glucocorticoids has been reported (Chatterjea, 1964), but the effectiveness of these drugs remains questionable, and the danger of a long-term steroid therapy is well known. Pimstone et al. (1987) obtained a complete clinical remission during therapy by orally administred sorbent (charcoal).

Packed erythrocyte transfusions markedly reduce excessive hemolysis and its stimulation of increased erythropoiesis. It also decreases porphyrin excretion (Haining et al., 1970); however, it is well known that multiple transfusions can be harmful. Continuous medical care is required to maintain the iron load of the patients at a sufficiently low level to prevent serious damage to the heart, liver, and endocrine organs (Piomelli et al., 1986).

To avoid the dangers of multiple transfusions, Watson et al. (1974) have proposed the intravenous administration of hematin. Heme produces, at least in the liver, a negative feedback repression of porphyrin biosynthesis (Ibrahim et al., 1978). Hematin was found to produce a reduction of porphyrin formation of the same order of magnitude but of shorter duration than erythrocyte transfusion.

Splenectomy is not necessarily recommended. A few reports indicate that after splenectomy there is a lessening of porphyrin excretion, a diminution is skin manifestations and in hemolytic anemia (Aldrich et al., 1951; Varadi, 1958). For some authors, however, there seems to be little evidence for specific, long-term improvement (Gray and Neuberger, 1952; Gross, 1964). The decision for or against splenectomy would seem to depend on an evaluation of the degree of hypersplenism (very large spleen, short red cell life span, sometimes thrombocytopenia).

B. Erythropoietic protoporphyria

Erythropoietic protoporphyria (EPP) is a porphyria involving a partial defect of ferrochelatase activity; it is inherited in an autosomal-dominant manner; there is no racial or sexual predilection.

1. Clinical features. Photosensitivity is the major clinical manifestation in EPP (Magnus et al., 1961): Short exposure to sunlight induces painful burning sensations in the skin sun-exposed areas; these symptoms occur without any immediately observable change in the appearance of the skin but several hours later they are usually followed by edema and erythema; vesicles, bullae, and crusting rarely occur. Chronic skin changes may develop which consist of thickening of skin areas that are most exposed to sunlight (backs of the hands, face). More typically, facial skin appears normal; however, it bears a few shallow, circular scars often scattered over the bridge of the nose, forehead, and cheeks (Poh-Fitzpatrick, 1986); onset of cutaneous symptoms is usually in early childhood (3 to 5 years); however, penetrance of EPP is variable: Several subjects carrying the abnormal gene remain asymptomatic, whereas a few other patients show only a mild photosensitivity and EPP is detected sometimes in late adulthood (Murphy et al. 1985).

EPP is generally a benign disease although a number of cases associated with abnormalities of the biliary tract and/or the liver have been reported (De Leo et al., 1976): Cholelithiasis often requires cholecystectomy (Mathews-Roth, 1977); chemical analysis of the gallstones reveals high levels of protopophyrin (De Leo et al., 1976). In rare cases (1 out of 56 patients in our study) fatal liver disease with cirrhosis may develop (Barnes et al., 1968; Donaldson et al., 1971; Bloomer, 1982); massive deposition of protoporphyrin was revealed by microscopic examination of liver biopsy specimens from these patients. However, protoporphyrin deposition has often been described in liver biopsy specimens from patients with EPP and normal liver function studies (Cripps and Scheuer, 1965).

2. Pathogenesis of skin lesions. The high levels of protoporphyrin present in the erythrocytes or extracellular fluid of the skin (Van Gog and Schothorst, 1973) can be stimulated to an excited state by absorption of light energy (the wavelengths producing peak reactivity, 400 to 410 nm, parallel the Soret band of porphyrin absorption spectra). The excited protoporphyrin may either destroy cellular components directly (i.e., lysosomes, Allison et al., 1966) or may react with molecular oxygen to form singlet oxygen or other "toxic oxygen" species such as superoxide anion or hydroxyl radicals (Poh-Fitzpatrick, 1986) which can be highly damaging to cellular components [i.e., peroxidation of cell membrane lipids (Goldstein and Harber, 1972) cross-linking of intracellular proteins (Schothorst et al., 1972), disruption of intracellular organelles, etc.].

No photosensitivity is observed in two other pathological circumstances (lead intoxication and iron deficiency anemia) associated with a high level of protoporphyrin in erythrocytes; Piomelli et al. (1975) have shown that in EPP the protoporphyrin is accumulated mostly as a free base, whereas in lead intoxication or iron deficiency anemia the porphyrin is present in erythrocytes as Zn-protoporphyrin. A significant amount of free protoporphyrin diffuses very rapidly from the erythrocytes of EPP patients through the plasma into the skin. On the contrary, Zn-protoporphyrin remains bound at heme binding sites in erythrocytes; there is no diffusion into the plasma and hence no photosensitivity.

3. Biochemical findings. EPP is characterized by an elevated level of protoporphyrin in erythrocytes and plasma; fecal protoporphyrin is often (but not always) abnormally increased; urinary porphyrin excretion is normal, except in rare cases with deteriorated hepatic function who show an increased porphyrinuria (mostly coproporphyrin), whereas baseline levels of protoporphyrin rise in erythrocytes and decrease in feces (Poh-Fitzpatrick, 1986). On the other hand, several asymptomatic patients are detected only by measurement of ferrochelatase activity.

4. Enzymatic abnormalities. The primary defect of EPP is the deficiency of the mitochondrial enzyme ferrochelatase (heme synthetase). This defect has been found in all studied tissues including liver (Bonkowsky et al., 1975), bone marrow cells (Bottomley et al., 1975), peripheral blood

TABLE 10.9 Erythropoietic Protoporphyria: Lymphocyte Ferrochelatase Activity

	Lymphocyte ferrochelatase activity*
Patients	3.58 ± 1.05[†] $(n = 33)$
Asymptomatic carriers	5.29 ± 1.08[†] $(n = 61)$
Normal controls	13.0 ± 2.0[‡] $(n = 58)$

*nmol mesoheme/h/mg protein at 37°C.
[†]Patients vs. carriers $p < 0.001$ (Student t test).
[‡]Patients or carriers vs. controls $p < 0.001$ (Student t test).

cells (de Goeij et al., 1975), skin fibroblasts (Bloomer et al., 1976), and lymphocytes (Deybach et al., 1981a).

For some unknown reason, the activity of ferrochelatase in EPP patients was found to be lower than 50% of normal levels (usually between 10 and 30%). However, Sassa et al. (1982) found an average defect of 42% of ferrochelatase activity by measuring protoporphyrin accumulated in mitogen-stimulated lymphocytes. These data are consistent with the heterozygous status of these patients for the gene defect of this disease. Table 10.9 shows our data on lymphocyte ferrochelatase activity [the technique used has been described by Deybach et al. (1981a)] of 33 patients with EPP and 60 asymptomatic carriers. Whereas EPP carriers show a mean defect of 44%, patients show a mean defect of 30%. This difference is highly significant ($p < 0.001$) but no clear-cut explanation is presently known: Inhibition of ferrochelatase by protoporphyrin is unlikely because protoporphyrin is not measurable in EPP patient lymphocytes (Deybach et al., unpublished). As suggested by Sassa et al. (1982), "some additional factor(s) (to a single gene mutation) is probably required for full clinical expression of the gene lesion in this disorder."

Recently, Deybach et al. (1986) described the first homozygous case of EPP: The clinical features of the proband were similar to those of other EPP patients. However, lymphocyte ferrochelatase activity of the patient was only 6.5% of the mean normal, whereas activity of both parents

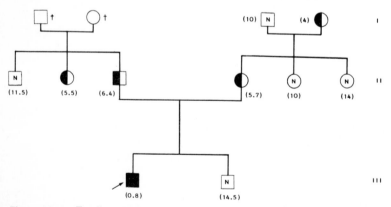

Figure 10.10   Family tree of a homozygous case of EPP. In parentheses: lymphocyte ferrochelatase activity expressed as nmol mesoheme/mg protein/h at 37°C.

Male	Female	
□	○	Not investigated
■	●	Patient
◖	◑	Asymptomatic carriers
□	○	Normal
↗		Propositus
†		Deceased

was around 50%. Cases with a similar defect were found in both parent families (Fig. 10.10). Further work is needed to discover if this case is either a homozygous form of the usual dominant EPP or a variant of EPP with a recessive mode of inheritance, as has been described in cattle (Ruth et al., 1977).

In most patients, erythropoietic tissue is the main source of the excess protoporphyrin (Bloomer, 1982). Protoporphyrin accumulates during the late stages of red cell maturation (Piomelli et al., 1975). When erythrocytes enter the circulation, protoporphyrin diffuses across the cell membrane and binds to plasma proteins (Seery and Muller-Eberhard, 1973). The youngest cells contain most of the protoporphyrin, whereas old cells contain little or none (Clark and Nicholson, 1971). The rate of loss of protoporphyrin from erythrocytes can account for the amount of protoporphyrin excreted in feces without invoking any additional contribution from hepatic source of protoporphyrin overproduction in these patients (Lamola et al., 1975). Bloomer (1982) accurately described the indirect lines of evidence, suggesting that the liver may contribute in some patients to the excessive amount of protoporphyrin that is excreted in the feces; however, the aforementioned studies (Lamon et al., 1980; Scholnick et al., 1971) are only suggestive, since the erythropoietic and hepatic production of protoporphyrin cannot be quantitated separately. On the other hand, Samuel et al. (1988) recently described a patient with EPP complicated by severe cirrhosis in whom liver transplantation was successfully performed: The level of protoporphyrin in erythrocytes decreased rapidly from 100,000 nmol/L to 20,000 nmol/L (normal level: 750 ± 250 nmol/L) and remained constant at least for 2 years between 20,000 and 30,000 nmol/L which is the usual level in uncomplicated EPP. This case supports the view that in EPP the relative part of the liver in protoporphyrin overproduction is very small.

5. Treatment. Oral administration of beta carotene may afford photoprotection resulting in improved tolerance to the sun (Mathews-Roth et al., 1974); however, results are variable. Whereas several patients report increased tolerance to light, a few patients (around 20%) seem to receive no improvement. Beta carotene would prevent the photosensitivity reaction by quenching the singlet oxygen or the triplet states of protoporphyrin (porphyrin concentrations remain unchanged).

The therapy of liver disease in EPP included several trials such as ingestion of cholestyramin resin (Bloomer, 1979) to try to interrupt the enterohepatic recirculation of protoporphyrin to the liver or administration of bile salts to mobilize protoporphyrin directly from the liver (Avner and Berenson, 1979; Poh-Fitzpatrick et al., 1983). Liver transplantation is the therapy of last resort in irreversible liver damage.

REFERENCES

Ades, I. Z., Stevens, T. M., and Drew, P. D. (1987). Biogenesis of embryonic chick liver delta aminolevulinate synthase: Regulation of the level of mRNA by hemin, *Arch. Biochem. Biophys.* **253**:297–304.

Aldrich, R. A., Hawkinson, V., Grinstein, M., and Watson, C. J. (1951). Photosensitive or congenital porphyria with hemolytic anemia. I. Clinical and fundamental studies before and after splenectomy, *Blood* **6**:685–698.

Allison, A. C., Magnus, I. A., and Young, M. R. (1966). Role of lysosomes and of cell membranes in photosensitization, *Nature* **209**:874–878.

Anderson, K. E. (1978). Effects of antihypertensive drugs on hepatic heme biosynthesis and evaluation of ferrochelatase inhibitors to simplify testing of drugs for heme pathway induction, *Biochim. Biophys. Acta* **543**:313–327.

Anderson, K. E., Bradlow, H. L., Sassa, S., and Kappas, A. (1979). Studies in porphyria. VIII. Relationship of the 5 alpha reductive metabolism of steroid hormones to the clinical expression of the genetic defect in acute intermittent porphyria, *Amer. J. Med.* **66**:644–650.

Anderson, K. E., Spitz, I. M., Sassa, S., Bardin, W., and Kappas, A. (1984). Prevention of cyclical attacks of acute intermittent porphyria with a long-acting agonist of luteinising hormone releasing hormone, *N. Engl. J. Med.* **311**:643–645.

Anderson, K. E., Spitz, I. M., Sassa, S., Bardin, W., and Kappas, A. (1986). Intranasal luteinising hormone-releasing hormone agonist for prevention of cyclical attacks of acute intermittent porphyria, *Porphyrins and Porphyrias* (Y. Nordmann, Ed.), John Libbey, Paris, Vol. 134, pp. 225–231.

Anderson, P. M., Reddy, R. M., Anderson, K. E., and Desnick, R. J. (1981). Characterization of the porphobilinogen deaminase deficiency in acute intermittent porphyria, *J. Clin. Invest.* **68**:1–12.

Andrews, J., Erdument, H., and Nicholson, D. C. (1984). Hereditary coproporphyria: Incidence in a large English family, *J. Med. Genet.* **21**:341–349.

Ashton, R. E., Hawk, J. L., and Magnus, I. A. (1984). Low dose oral chloroquine in the treatment of porphyria cutanea tarda, *Brit. J. Dermatol.* **11**:609–613.

Avner, D. L., and Berenson, M. M. (1979). Bile acid-dependent biliary protoporphyrin excretion, *Gastroenterology* **77**:A2.

Barnes, H. D., Hurworth, E., and Millar, J. H. (1968). Erythropoietic porphyrin hepatitis, *J. Clin. Pathol.* **21**:157–159.

Beaumont, C., Deybach, J. C., Grandchamp, B., Da Silva, V., de Verneuil, H., and Nordmann, Y. (1984). Effects of succinylacetone on dimethylsulfoxide-mediated induction of heme pathway enzymes in mouse Friend virus-transformed erythroleukemia cells, *Exp. Cell Res.* **154**:474–484.

Beaumont, C., Fauchet, R., Phung, L. N., de Verneuil, H., Gueguen, M., and Nordmann, Y. (1987). Porphyria cutanea tarda and HLA-linked hemochromatosis: Evidence against a systematic association, *Gastroenterology* **92**:1833–1838.

Becker, D. M., Viljoen, J. D., Katz, J., and Kramer, S. (1977). Reduced ferrochelatase activity: A defect common to porphyria variegata and protoporphyria, *Brit. J. Haematol.* **36**:171–179.

Berger, H., and Goldberg, A. (1955). Hereditary coproporphyria, *Brit. Med. J.* **2**:85–87.

Bird, T. D., Hamernyik, P., Nutter, J. Y., and Labbe, R. F. (1979). Inherited deficiency of delta aminolevulinic acid dehydratase, *Amer. J. Hum. Genet.* **31**:662–668.

Bishop, D. F., and Desnick, R. J. (1982). Assays of the haem biosynthetic enzymes, *Enzyme* **28**:91–231.

Bissell, D. M. (1982). Laboratory evaluation in porphyria, *Sem. Liver Dis.* **2**:100–107.

Blekkenhorst, G. H., Eales, L., and Pimstone, N. R. (1979). Activation of uroporphyrinogen decarboxylase by ferrous iron in porphyria cutanea tarda, *S. Afr. Med. J.* **56**:918–920.

Bloomer, J. R. (1979). Pathogenesis and therapy of liver disease in protoporphyria, *Yale J. Biol. Med.* **52**:39–48.

Bloomer, J. R. (1982). Protoporphyria, *Sem. Liver Dis.* **2**:143–153.

Bloomer, J. R., Bonkowsky, H., Ebert, P. S., and Mahoney, M. J. (1976). Inheritance in protoporphyria. Comparison of haem synthase activity in skin fibroblasts with clinical features, *Lancet* ii:226–228.

Bonkowsky, H., Bloomer, J., and Ebert, P. (1975). Heme synthetase deficiency in human protoporphyria, *J. Clin. Invest.* **56**:1139–1148.

Bonkowsky, H. L., Magnussen, C. R., Collins, A. R., Doherty, J., Hess, R. A., and Tschudy, D. P. (1976). Comparative effects of glycerol and dextrose on porphyrin precursor excretion in acute intermittent porphyria, *Metabolism* **25**:405–414.

Bonkowsky, H. L., and Schady, W. (1982). Neurological manifestations of acute porphyria, *Sem. Liver Dis.* **2**:108–124.

Bonkowsky, H. L., Tschudy, D. P., Collins, A., Doherty, J., Bossenmaier, I., Cardinal, R., and Watson, C. J. (1971). Repression of the overproduction of porphyrin precursors in acute intermittent porphyria by intravenous infusion of hematin, *Proc. Nat. Acad. Sci. (U.S.A.)* **68**:2725–2729.

Bottomley, S. S., Tanaka, M., and Everett, M. A. (1975). Diminished erythroid ferrochelatase activity in protoporphyria, *J. Lab. Clin. Med.* **86**:126–131.

Bradlow, H. L., Gillette, P. N., Gallagher, T. F., and Kappas, A. (1973). Studies in porphyria. II. Evidence for a deficiency of steroid delta 4-5 alpha reductase activity in acute intermittent porphyria, *J. Exp. Med.* **138**:754–763.

Brenner, D. A., and Bloomer, J. R. (1980). The enzymatic defect in variegate porphyria, *N. Engl. J. Med.* **302**:765–769.

Brodie, M. J., Moore, M. R., and Goldberg, A. (1977a). Enzyme abnormalities in the porphyrias, *Lancet* **2**:699–701.

Brodie, M. J., Moore, M. R., Thompson, G. G., and Goldberg, A. (1977b). Pregnancy and the acute porphyrias, *Brit. J. Obstet. Gynaecol.* **84**:726–731.

Brodie, M. J., Thompson, G. G., Moore, M. R., Beattie, A. D., and Goldberg, A. (1977c). Hereditary coproporphyria, *Quart. J. Med.* **46**:229–241.

Bruguera, M. (1986). Liver involvement in porphyria, *Sem. Dermatol.* **5**:178–185.

Chatterjea, J. B. (1964). Erythropoietic porphyria, *Blood* **24**:806–807.

Chretien, S., Dubart, A., Beaupain, D., Raich, N., Grandchamp, B., Rosa, J., Goossens, M., and Romeo, P. H. (1988). Alternative transcription and splicing of the human porphobilinogen deaminase gene result either in tissue-specific or in housekeeping expression, *Proc. Nat. Acad. Sci. (U.S.A.)* **85**:6–10.

Clark, K. G., and Nicholson, D. C. (1971). Erythrocyte protoporphyrin and iron uptake in erythropoietic protoporphyria, *Clin. Sci.* **41**:363–370.

Cohn, J. A., Alvares, A. P., and Kappas, A. (1977). On the occurrence of cytochrome P-450 and aryl hydrocarbon hydroxylase activity in rat brain, *J. Exp. Med.* **145**:1607–1611.

Cortes, J. M., Oliva, H., Paradinas, F. J., and Hernandez-Guio, C. (1980). The pathology of the liver in porphyria cutanea tarda, *Histopathology* **4**:471–485.

Cripps, D. J., and Scheuer, P. J. (1965). Hepatobiliary changes in erythropoietic protoporphyria, *Arch. Pathol.* **80**:500–508.

Czarnecki, D. B. (1980). Hepatoerythropoietic porphyria, *Arch. Dermatol.* **116**:307–313.

Day, R. S. (1986). Variegate porphyria, *Sem. Dermatol.* **5**:138–154.

Day, R. S., and Eales, L. (1980). Porphyrins in chronic renal failure, *Nephron* **26**:90–95.

Day, R. S., Eales, L., and Disler, P. B. (1981). Porphyrias and the kidney, *Nephron* **28**:261–267.

Day, R. S., Eales, L., and Meissner, D. (1982). Coexistent variegate porphyria and porphyria cutanea tarda, *N. Engl. J. Med.* **307**:36–41.

Day, R. S., Pimstone, N. R., and Eales, L. (1978). The diagnostic value of blood plasma porphyrin methyl ester profiles produced by quantitative TLC, *Int. J. Biochem.* **9**:897–904.

De Goeij, A., Christianse, K., and Van Steveninck, I. (1975). Decreased haem synthetase activity in blood cells of patients with erythropoietic protoporphyria, *Eur. J. Clin. Invest.* **5**:397–400.

De Leo, V. A., Poh-Fitzpatrick, M., Mathews-Roth, M. M., and Harber, L. C. (1976). Erythropoietic protoporphyria. 10 years experience, *Amer. J. Med.* **60**:8–22.

De Matteis, F. (1978). Hepatic porphyrias, *Heme and Hemoproteins* (F. De Matteis and W. N. Aldridge, Eds.), Springer, New York, pp. 129–155.

Desnick, R. J., Ostasiewicz, L. T., Tishler, P. A., and Mustajoki, P. (1985). Acute intermittent porphyria: Characterization of a novel mutation in the structural gene for porphobilinogen deaminase, *J. Clin. Invest.* **76**:865–874.

de Verneuil, H., Aitken, G., and Nordmann, Y. (1978). Familial and sporadic porphyria cutanea tarda: Two different diseases, *Hum. Genet.* **44**:145.

de Verneuil, H., Beaumont, C., Deybach, J. C., Nordmann, Y., Sfar, Z., and Kastally, R. (1984a). Enzymatic and immunological studies of uroporphyrinogen decarboxylase in familial porphyria cutanea tarda and hepatoerythropoietic porphyria, *Amer. J. Hum. Genet.* **36**:613–622.

de Verneuil, H., Beaumont, C., Grandchamp, B., Phung, L. N., and Nordmann, Y. (1986a). Molecular heterogeneity of uroporphyrinogen decarboxylase deficiency in hepatoerythropoietic porphyria, *Porphyrins and Porphyrias* (Y. Nordmann, Ed.), John Libbey, Paris, Vol. 134, pp. 201–208.

de Verneuil, H., Deybach, J. C., Phung, L. N., Grelier, M., and Nordmann, Y. (1983a). Study of anaesthetic agents for their ability to elicit porphyrin biosynthesis in chick embryo liver, *Biochem. Pharmacol.* **32**:1011–1018.

de Verneuil, H., Doss, M., Brusco, N., Beaumont, C., and Nordmann, Y. (1985). Hereditary hepatic porphyria with delta aminolevulinic dehydrase deficiency. Immunologic characterization of the non-catalytic enzyme, *Hum. Genet.* **69**:174–177.

de Verneuil, H., Grandchamp, B., Beaumont, C., Picat, C., and Nordmann, Y. (1986b). Uroporphyrinogen decarboxylase structural mutant (Gly 281 Glu) in a case of porphyria, *Science* **234**:732–734.

de Verneuil, H., Grandchamp, B., Foubert, C., Weil, D., N'Guyen, V. C., Gross, M. S., Sassa, S., and Nordmann, Y. (1984b). Assignment of the gene for uroporphyrinogen decarboxylase to human chromosome 1 by somatic cell hybridization and specific enzyme immunoassay, *Hum. Genet.* **66**:202–205.

de Verneuil,, H., Grandchamp, B., Romeo, P. H., Raich, N., Beaumont, C., Goossens, M., Nicolas, H., and Nordmann, Y. (1986c). Molecular analysis of uroporphyrinogen decarboxylase deficiency in a family with two cases of hepatoerythropoeitic porphyria, *J. Clin. Invest.* **77**:431–435.

de Verneuil, H.,. Hansen, J., Picat, C., Grandchamp, B., Kushner, J., Roberts, A., Elder, G. H., and Nordmann, Y. (1988). Prevalence of the 281 (Gly-Glu) mutation in hepatoerythropoietic porphyria and porphyria cutanea tarda, *Hum. Genet.* **78**:101–102.

de Verneuil, H., Sassa, S., and Kappas, A. (1983b). Effects of polychlorinated biphenyl compounds, 2,3,7,8-tetrachlorodibenzo-p-dioxin, phenobarbital and iron on hepatic uroporphyrinogen decarboxylase, *Biochem. J.* **214**:145–151.

Deybach, J. C., Da Silva, V., Pasquier, Y., and Nordmann, Y. (1986). Ferrochelatase in human erythropoietic protoporphyria: The first case of a homozygous form of the enzyme deficiency, *Porphyrins and Porphyrias* (Y. Nordmann, Ed.), John Libbey, Paris, pp. 163–173.

Deybach, J. C., de Verneuil, H., and Nordmann, Y. (1981a). The inherited enzymatic defect in porphyria variegata, *Hum. Genet.* **58**:425–428.

Deybach, J. C., de Verneuil, H., Phung, N., Nordmann, Y., Puissant, A., and Boffety, B. (1981b). Congenital erythropoietic porphyria (Gunther's disease): Enzymatic studies on two cases of late onset, *J. Lab. Clin. Med.* **97**:551–558.

Deybach, J. C., Grandchamp, B., Grelier, M., Nordmann, Y., Boué, J., Boué, A., and de Berranger, P. (1980). Prenatal exclusion of congenital erythropoietic porphyria (Gunther's disease) in a fetus at risk, *Hum. Genet.* **53**:217–221.

DiLella, A. G., Marvit, J., Lidsky, A. S., Guttler, F., and Woo, S. L. (1986). Tight linkage between a splicing mutation and a specific DNA haplotype in phenylketonuria, *Nature* **322**:799–803.

Dogramaci, I. (1962). Porphyria turcica (cutaneous porphyria) in southeastern Turkey. General considerations, *Turk. J. Pediatr.* **4**:129–131.

Donaldson, E. M., McCall, A. J., and Magnus, I. A. (1971). Erythropoietic protoporphyria: Two deaths from hepatic cirrhosis, *Brit. J. Dermatol.* **84**:14–24.

Doss, M. (1986). Diagnosis and therapy of acute porphyrias: State of art, *New Therapeutic Approach to Hepatic Porphyria* (P. Mustajoki, Ed.), Leiras Medica, Finland, pp. 19–29.

Doss, M., Meinhof, W., Look, D., Henning, H., Nawrocki, P., Dolle, W., Strohmeyer, G., and Filippini, L. (1971). Porphyrins in liver and urine in acute intermittent and chronic hepatic porphyrias, *S. Afr. J. Lab. Clin. Med.* **17**:50–54.

Doss, M., Sauer, H., Von Tiepermann, R., and Colombi, A. M. (1984). Development of chronic hepatic porphyria (porphyria cutanea tarda) with inherited uroporphyrinogen decarboxylase deficiency under exposure to dioxin, *Int. J. Biochem.* **16**:369–373.

Doss, M., Schneider, J., Von Tiepermann, R., and Brandt, A. (1982). A new type of acute porphyria with porphobilinogen synthase defect in the homozygous state, *Clin. Biochem.* **15**:52–55.

Doss, M., Sixel-Dietrich, F., and Verspohl, F. (1985). "Glucose effect" and rate limiting function of uroporphyrinogen synthase on porphyrin metabolism in hepatocyte culture: Relationship with human acute hepatic porphyrias, *J. Clin. Chem. Clin. Biochem.* **23**:505–513.

Doss, M., Von Tiepermann, R., Schneider, J., and Schmid, H. (1979). New type of hepatic porphyria with porphobilinogen synthase defect and intermittent acute clinical manifestation, *Klin. Wochensch.* **57**:1123–1127.

Doss, M., Von Tiepermann, R., Stutz, G., and Teschke, R. (1981). Alcohol-induced decrease in uroporphyrinogen decarboxylase activity in rat liver and spleen, *Enzyme* **26**:24–31.

Douer, D., Schoenfeld, N., Weinberger, A., Pinkhas, J., and Atsmon, A. (1978). Favourable effect of intravenous propranolol in acute intermittent porphyria, *Monogr. Hum. Genet.* **10**:223–226.

Dowdle, E. B., Mustard, P., and Eales, L. (1967). Delta aminolevulinic acid synthetase activity in normal and porphyric human livers, *S. Afr. Med. J.* **41**:1093–1097.

Eales, L., Day, R. S., and Blekkenhorst, G. H. (1980). The clinical and biochemical features of variegate porphyria. An analysis of 300 cases studied at Groote Schuur Hospital, Cape Town, *Int. J. Biochem.* **12**:837–853.

Eales, L., Grosser, T., and Sears, W. G. (1975). The clinical biochemistry of the human hepatocutaneous porphyrias in the light of recent studies of newly identified intermediates and porphyrin derivatives, *Ann. N.Y. Acad. Sci.* **244**:441–471.

Elder, G. H. (1974). The metabolism of porphyrins of the isocoproporphyrin series, *Enzyme* **17**:61–68.

Elder, G. H. (1977). Porphyrin metabolism in porphyria cutanea tarda, *Seminars in Hematology* (U. Muller-Eberhard, Ed.), Grune & Stratton, New York, Vol. 14, pp. 227–242.

Elder, G. H. (1978). Porphyria caused by hexachlorobenzene and other polyhalogenated aromatic hydrocarbons, *Heme and Hemoproteins* (F. De Matteis and W. N. Aldridge, Eds.), Springer, New York, pp. 157–170.

Elder, G. H. (1980). Haem synthesis and breakdown, *Iron in Biochemistry and Medicine* (A. Jacobs and M. Worwood, Eds.), Academic, London, pp. 245–285.

Elder, G. H. (1986). Metabolic abnormalities in the porphyrias, *Sem. Dermatol.* **5**:88–98.

Elder, G. H., De Salamanca, R. E., Urqhart, A. J., Munoz, J. J., and Bonkowsky, H. L. (1985). Immunoreactive uroporphyrinogen decarboxylase in the liver in porphyria cutanea tarda, *Lancet* **ii**:229–233.

Elder, G. H., Evans, J. O., Thomas, N., Cox, R., Brodie, M. J., Moore, M. R., Goldberg, A., and Nicholson, D. C. (1976). The primary enzyme defect in hereditary coproporphyria, *Lancet* **2**:217–219.

Elder, G. H., Lee, G. B., and Tovey, J. A. (1978). Decreased activity of hepatic uroporphyrinogen decarboxylase in sporadic porphyria cutanea tarda, *N. Engl. J. Med.* **299**:274–278.

Elder, G. H., Magnus, I. A., and Handa, F. (1974). Fecal "X-porphyrin" in the hepatic porphyrias, *Enzyme* **17**:29–38.

Elder, G. H., and Path, F. R. C. (1982). Enzymatic defects in porphyria: An overview, *Sem. Liver Dis.* **2**:87–99.

Elder, G. H., Roberts, A. G., and Urquhart, A. J. (1986). Acquired uroporphyrinogen decarboxylase defects: Molecular mechanisms, *Porphyrins and Porphyrias* (Y. Nordmann, Ed.), John Libbey, Paris, Vol. 134, pp. 147–153.

Elder, G. H., and Sheppard, D. M. (1982). Immunoreactive uroporphyrinogen decarboxylase is unchanged in porphyria caused by TCDD and hexachlorobenzene, *Biochem. Biophys. Res. Comm.* **109**:113–120.

Elder, G. H., Sheppard, D. M., De Salamanca, R. E., and Olmos, A. (1980). Identification of two types of porphyria cutanea tarda by measurement of erythrocyte uroporphyrinogen decarboxylase, *Clin. Sci.* **58**:477–484.

Elder, G. H., Sheppard, D., Tovey, J., and Urquhart, A. (1983). Immuno-reactive uroporphyrinogen decarboxylase in porphyria cutanea tarda, *Lancet* **i**:1301–1304.

Elder, G. H., Smith, S. G., Herrero, C., Mascaro, J. M., Lecha, M., Muniesca, A. M., Czarnecki, D. B., Brenan, J., Poulos, V., and De Salamanca, R. E. (1981). Hepatoerythropoietic porphyria: A new uroporphyrinogen decarboxylase defect of homozygous porphyria cutanea tarda, *Lancet* **i**:916–919.

Epstein, O., Lahav, M., Schoenfeld, N., Nemesh, L., Shaklai, M., and Atsmon, A. (1983). Erythrocyte uroporphyrinogen synthase activity as a possible diagnostic aid in the diagnosis of lymphoproliferative diseases, *Cancer* **52**:828–832.

Felsher, B. F., Carpio, N. M., Engleking, D. W., and Nunn, A. T. (1982). Decreased hepatic uroporphyrinogen decarboxylase activity in porphyria cutanea tarda, *N. Engl. J. Med.* **306**:766–769.

Felsher, B. F., and Redeker, A. G. (1966). Effect of chloroquine on hepatic uroporphyrin metabolism in patients with porphyria cutanea tarda, *Medicine* **45**:575–583.

Feuer, G., Sosa-Lucero, J. C., Lund, G., and Moddel, G. (1971). Failure of various drugs to induce drug-metabolizing enzymes in extrahepatic tissues of the rat, *Toxicol. Appl. Pharmacol.* **19**:579–589.

Fujita, H., Sassa, S., Lundgren, J., Holmberg, L., Thunell, S., and Kappas, A. (1987). Enzymatic defect in a child with hereditary hepatic porphyria due to homozygous delta aminolevulinic acid dehydratase deficiency: Immunochemical studies, *Pediatrics* **80**:880–885.

Gajdos, A., de Paillerets, F., Bouygues, D., and Nordmann, Y. (1977). Un cas de porphyrie erythropoietique congenitale (maladie de Gunther) traité par le béta carotène, *Nouv. Presse Med.* **6**:2345.

Gajdos, A., and Gajdos-Torok, M. (1962). Clinical and experimental trial of adenosine 5 monophosphoric acid in porphyria, *Panminerva Med.* **4**:332–339.

Gentz, J., Johanssonn, S., Lindstedt, S., and Zetterstrom, R. (1969). Excretion of delta aminolevulinic acid in hereditary tyrosinemia, *Clin. Chim. Acta* **23**:257–263.

Gibson, S. L., and Goldberg, A. (1970). Defects in haem synthesis in mammalian tissues in experimental lead poisoning and experimental porphyria, *Clin. Sci.* **38**:63.

Goetsch, C. A., and Bissell, D. M. (1986). Instability of hematin used in the treatment of acute hepatic porphyria, *N. Engl. J. Med.* **315**:235–238.

Goldberg, A., and Rimington, C. (1962). *Diseases of Porphyrin Metabolism*, Charles C. Thomas, Springfield, Ill.

Goldstein, B. D., and Harber, L. C. (1972). Erythropoietic protoporphyria: Lipid peroxidation and red cell membrane damage associated with photohaemolysis, *J. Clin. Invest.* **51**:892–902.

Grandchamp, B., de Verneuil, H., Beaumont, C., Chrétien, S., Walter, O. and Nordmann, Y. (1987). Tissue-specific expression of porphobilinogen deaminase: Two isoenzymes from a single gene, *Eur. J. Biochem.* **162**:105–110.

Grandchamp, B., Deybach, J. C., Grelier, M., de Verneuil, H., and Nordmann, Y. (1980). Studies of porphyrin synthesis in fibroblasts of patients with congenital erythropoietic porphyria and of a case of homozygous coproporphyria, *Biochim. Biophys. Acta* **629**:577–586.

Grandchamp, B., and Nordmann, Y. (1977). Decreased lymphocyte coproporphyrinogen III oxidase activity in hereditary coproporphyria, *Biochem. Biophys. Res. Comm.* **74**:1089–1095.

Grandchamp, B., Phung, L. N., and Nordmann, Y. (1977). Homozygous case of hereditary coproporphyria, *Lancet* **i**:1348–1349.

Grandchamp, B., Picat, C., Mignotte, V., Wilson, J. H. P., Te Velde, K., Sandkuyl, L., Romeo, P. H., Goossens, M., and Nordmann, Y. (1989). Tissue-specific splice junction mutation in acute intermittent porphyria, *Proc. Nat. Acad. Sci. (U.S.A.)*, **74**:661–664.

Gray, C. H., and Neuberger, A. (1952). Effect of splenectomy in a case of congenital porphyria, *Lancet* i:851–854.

Gross, S. (1964). Hematologic studies on erythropoietic porphyria: A new case with severe hemolysis, chronic thrombocytopenia and folic acid deficiency, *Blood* 23:762–775.

Grossman, M. E., Bickers, D. R., Poh-Fitzpatrick, M. D., Deleo, V. A., and Harber, L. C. (1979). Porphyria cutanea tarda, *Amer. J. Med.* 67:277–286.

Günther, H. (1911). Die haematoporphyrie, *Deutsch. Arch. Klin. Med.* 105:89–146.

Haining, R. C., Cowger, M. L., and Labbe, R. F. (1970). Congenital erythropoietic porphyria. II. The effects of induced polycythemia, *Blood* 36:297–309.

Haining, R. C., Cowger, M. L., and Shurtleff, D. B., and Labbe, R. F. (1968). Congenital erythropoietic porphyria. I. Case report, special studies and therapy, *Amer. J. Med.* 45:624–637.

Hawk, J. L., Magnus, I. A., Parkes, A., Elder, G. H., and Doyle, M. (1978). Deficiency of hepatic coproporphyrinogen oxidase in hereditary coproporphyria, *J. Roy. Soc. Med.* 71:775–777.

Hayashi, N., Wanatabe, N., and Kikuchi, G. (1983). Inhibition by hemin of in vivo translocation of chicken liver 5-aminolaevulinate synthase into mitochondria, *Biochem. Biophys. Res. Comm.* 115:700–706.

Heilmeyer, L. E., Clotten, R., and Kerp, L. (1963). Porphyria erythropoietic congenita Gunther: Bericht uber zwei familien mit erfassung der Merkmalsträger, *Deutsch. Med. Wochensch.* 88:2449–2456.

Hofstad, F., Seip, M., and Eriksen, L. (1973). Congenital erythropoietic porphyria with a hitherto undescribed porphyrin pattern, *Acta Paediatr. Scand.* 62:380–384.

Ibrahim, N. G., Gruenspecht, N. R., and Freedman, M. L. (1978). Hemin feedback inhibition of reticulocyte delta aminolevulinic acid synthetase and delta aminolevulinic acid dehydratase, *Biochem. Biophys. Res. Comm.* 80:722–728.

Ippen, H. (1961). Allgemeine symptome der spaten hautporphyrie (porphyria cutanea tarda) als hinweise fur deren Behandlung, *Deutsch Med. Woschensch.* 86:127–133.

Ippen, H. (1977). Treatment of porphyria cutanea tarda by phlebotomy in iron excess, *Seminars in Hematology* (U. Muller-Eberhard, Ed.), Grune & Stratton, New York, Vol. 14, pp. 253–259.

Jung, E. G. (1977). Porphyria erythropoietica congenita Gunther, *Deutsch. Med. Wochensch*, 102:279–280.

Kalb, R. E., Grossman, M. E., and Poh-Fitzpatrick, M. B. (1985). Correlation of serum and urinary porphyrin levels in porphyria cutanea tarda, *Arch. Dermatol.* 121:1289–1291.

Kappas, A., Anderson, K. E., Conney, A. H., Pantuck, E. J., Fishman, J., and Bradlow, H. L. (1983a). Nutrition-endocrine interaction: Induction of reciprocal changes in the delta 4-5 alpha-reduction of testosterone and the cytochrome P-450 dependent oxidation of estradiol by dietary macronutrients in man, *Proc. Nat. Acad. Sci. (U.S.A.)* 80:7646.

Kappas, A., Bradlow, H. L., Gillette, P. N., and Gallagher, T. F. (1971). Abnormal steroid hormone metabolism in the genetic liver disease, acute intermittent porphyria, *Ann. N.Y. Acad. Sci.* 179:611–624.

Kappas, A., Bradlow, H. L., Gillette, P. N., and Gallagher, T. F. (1972). A defect of steroid metabolism in acute intermittent porphyria, *Fed. Proc.* 31:1293–1297.

Kappas, A., Sassa, S., and Anderson, K. (1983b). The porphyrias, *The Metabolic Basis of Inherited Diseases* (J. B. Stanbury, Ed.), 5th ed., McGraw-Hill, New York, pp. 1301–1384.

Kappas, A., Sassa, S., Galbraith, R. A., and Nordmann, Y. (1989). The porphyrias, *The Metabolic Basis of Inherited Diseases* (J. B. Stanbury, Ed.), 6th ed., McGraw-Hill, New York, in press.

Kondo, M., Urata, G., and Shimizu, Y. (1983). Decreased liver delta-aminolevulinate dehydratase activity in porphyria cutanea tarda and in alcoholism, *Clin. Sci.* 65:423–428.

Kordac, V. (1972). Frequency of occurrence of hepatocellular carcinoma in patients with porphyria cutanea tarda in long-term followup, *Neoplasma* 19:135–139.

Kordac, V., Deybach, J. C., Martasek, P., Seman, J., Da Silva, V., Nordmann, Y., Houstkova, H., Rubin, A., and Holub, J. (1984). Homozygous variegate porphyria, *Lancet* i:851.

Kordac, V., Martasek, P., Zeman, J., and Rubin, A. (1985). Increased erythrocyte protoporphyrin in homozygous variegate porphyria, *Photodermatology* **2**:257–259.

Kordac, V., and Semradova, M. (1974). Treatment of porphyria cutanea tarda with chloroquine, *Brit. J. Dermatol.* **90**:95–100.

Korting, K. W. (1975). Uber porphyria cutanea tarda artige hautveranderungen bei langzeithamodialyse patienten, *Dermatology* **150**:58–61.

Kostrzewska, E., and Gregor, A. (1986). Increased activity of porphobilinogen deaminase in erythrocytes during attacks of acute intermittent porphyria, *Ann. Clin. Res.* **18**:195–198.

Kowertz, M. J. (1975). Retreatment with chloroquine in porphyria cutanea tarda, *J. Amer. Med. Assoc.* **233**:22.

Kramer, S., Viljoen, E., Meyer, A. M., and Metz, J. (1965). The anemia of erythropoietic porphyria with the first description of the disease in an elderly patient, *Brit. J. Haematol.* **11**:666–675.

Kuntz, B. M. E., Goerz, G., Sonneborn, H. H., and Lissner, R. (1981). HLA-types in porphyria cutanea tarda, *Lancet* **i**:155.

Kushner, J. P. (1982). The enzymatic defect in porphyria cutanea tarda, *N. Engl. J. Med.* **306**:799–800.

Kushner, J., Barbuto, A., and Lee, G. (1976). An inherited enzymatic defect in porphyria cutanea tarda. Decreased uroporphyrinogen decarboxylase activity, *J. Clin. Invest.* **58**:1089–1097.

Kushner, J. P., Edwards, C. Q., Dadone, M. M., and Skolnick, M. H. (1985). Heterozygosity of HLA-linked hemochromatosis as a likely cause of the hepatic siderosis associated with sporadic porphyria cutanea tarda, *Gastroenterology* **88**:1232–1238.

Kushner, J., Steinmuller, P., and Lee, G. R. (1975). The role of iron in the pathogenesis of porphyria cutanea tarda. II. Inhibition of uroporphyrinogen decarboxylase, *J. Clin. Invest.* **56**:661–667.

Laiwah, C. Y., Junor, B., Macphee, G. J. A., Thompson, G. G., and McColl, K. E. L. (1983). Charcoal haemoperfusion and haemodialysis in acute intermittent porphyria, *Brit. Med. J.* **287**:1746–1747.

Lamola, A. A., Piomelli, S., and Poh-Fitzpatrick, M. B. (1975). Erythropoietic protoporphyria and Pb intoxication: The molecular basis for difference in cutaneous photosensitivity, *J. Clin. Invest.* **56**:1528–1525.

Lamon, J. M., Frykholm, B. C., Herrera, W., and Tschudy, P. D. (1979a). Danazol administration to females with menses-associated exacerbation of acute intermittent porphyria, *J. Clin. Endochrinol. Metab.* **48**:123–126.

Lamon, J. M., Frykholm, B. C., Hess, R. A., and Tschudy, P. D. (1979b). Hematin therapy for acute porphyria, *Medicine* **58**:252–269.

Lamon, J. M., Poh-Fitzpatrick, M. B., Lamola, A. A., Frykholm, B. C., Freeman, M. L., and Doleiden, F. H. (1980). Hepatic protoporphyria production in human protoporphyria, *Gastroenterology* **79**:115–125.

Lazaro, P., De Salamanca, R. E., Elder, G. H., Villaseca, M. L., Chinarro, S., and Jacquetti, G. (1984). Is hepatoerythropoietic porphyria a homozygous form of porphyria cutanea tarda? Inheritance of uroporphyrinogen decarboxylase deficiency in a Spanish family, *Brit. J. Dermatol.* **110**:613–617.

Levin, E. Y. (1968). Uroporphyrinogen III cosynthetase in bovine erythropoietic porphyria, *Science* **161**:907–908.

Lim, C. K., Li, F., and Peters, T. J. (1986). High performance liquid chromatography of uroporphyrinogen and coproporphyrinogen isomers with amperometric detection, *Biochem. J.* **234**:629–633.

Lim, H. W., Poh-Fitzpatrick, M. B. (1984). Hepatoerythropoietic porphyria. A variant of childhood onset porphyria cutanea tarda. Porphyrin profiles and enzymatic studies of two cases in a family, *J. Amer. Acad. Dermatol.* **11**:1103–1111.

Linden, J. B., Tokola, O., Karlsson, M., and Tenhunen, R. (1987). Rate of haem after parenteral administration of haem arginate to rabbits, *J. Pharm. Pharmacol.* **39**:96–102.

Litman, D. A., and Correia, M. A. (1983). L-Tryptophan. A common denominator of biochemical and neurological events of acute hepatic porphyria, *Science* **222**:1031–1033.

Litman, D. A., and Correia, M. A. (1985). Elevated brain tryptophan and enhanced 5-hydroxy-tryptamine turnover in acute hepatic heme deficiency: Clinical implications, *J. Pharmacol. Exp. Therap.* **232**:337–345.

Llewellyn, D. H., Elder, G. H., Kalsheker, N. A., and Marsh, O. W. M. (1987). DNA polymorphism of human porphobilinogen deaminase gene in acute intermittent porphyria, *Lancet* i:706–708.

Llorente, L., De Salamanca, E., Campillo, F., and Pena, M. L. (1980). HLA and porphyria cutanea tarda, *Arch. Dermatol. Res.* **269**:209–210.

Longas, M. O., and Poh-Fitzpatrick, M. B. (1982). A tightly bound protein porphyrin complex isolated from the plasma of a patient with variegate porphyria, *Clin. Chim. Acta* **118**:219–228.

Lundvall, O., Weinfeld, A., and Lundin, P. (1970). Iron storage in porphyria cutanea tarda, *Acta Med. Scand.* **188**:37–53.

Magnus, I., Jarret, A., Prankerd, T., and Rimington, C. (1961). Erythropoietic protoporphyria: A new porphyria syndrome with solar urticaria due to protoporphyrinaemia, *Lancet* ii:448–451.

Malina, L. (1986). Treatment of chronic hepatic porphyria (PCT), *Photodermatology,* **3**:113–121.

Malina, L., and Chlumsky, J. (1975). Oestrogen-induced familial porphyria cutanea tarda, *Brit. J. Dermatol.* **92**:707–709.

Martasek, P., Kordac, V., Kotal, P., Vacek, J., Jirsa, M., Horak, J., and Tomasek, R. (1986). Recovery from a severe attack of acute intermittent porphyria during coated-resin hemoperfusion, *Int. J. Art. Organs* **9**:117–118.

Mascaro, J. M., Herrero, C., Lecha, M., and Muniesa, A. M. (1986). Uroporphyrinogen decarboxylase deficiencies. Porphyria cutanea tarda and related conditions, *Sem. Dermatol.* **5**:114–124.

Mathews-Roth, M. M. (1977). Erythropoietic protoporphyria. Diagnosis and treatment, *N. Engl. J. Med.* **287**:98–100.

Mathews-Roth, M. M., Pathak, M. A., Fitzpatrick, T. B., Harber, L. H., and Kass, E. H. (1974). Beta carotene as an oral photoprotective agent in erythropoietic protoporphyria, *J. Amer. Med. Assoc.* **228**:1004–1008.

Mauzerall, D., and Granick, S. (1956). The occurrence and determination of 5-aminolaevulinic acid and porphobilinogen in urine, *J. Biol. Chem.* **219**:435–446.

McColl, K. E. L., Moore, M. R., Thompson, G. C., and Goldberg, A. (1982). Screening for latent acute intermittent porphyria: The value of measuring both leucocyte delta-aminolaevulinic acid synthase and uroporphyrinogen I synthase, *J. Med. Genet.* **19**:271–276.

McColl, K. E. L., Moore, M. R., Thompson, G. C., Goldberg, A., Church, S. E., Quadiri, M. R., and Youngs, G. R. (1985). Chester porphyria. Biochemical studies of a new form of acute porphyria, *Lancet* ii:796–799.

McGillian, F. B., Moore, M. R., and Goldberg, A. (1975). Some pharmacological effects of delta-aminolevulinic acid on blood pressure in the rat and on rabbit isolated ear arteries, *Clin. Exp. Pharmacol. Physiol.* **2**:365–371.

Meissner, P. N., Day, R. S., Moore, M. R. , Disler, P. B., and Harley, E. (1986). Protoporphyrinogen oxidase and porphobilinogen deaminase in variegate porphyria, *Eur. J. Clin. Invest.* **16**:257–261.

Meyer, U. A. (1973). Intermittent acute porphyria: Clinical and biochemical studies of disordered heme biosynthesis, *Enzyme* **16**:334–342.

Meyer, U. A., and Schmid, R. (1978). The porphyrias, *The Metabolic Basis of Inherited Disease* (J. B. Stanbury, Ed.), 4th ed., McGraw-Hill, New York, pp. 1166–1220.

Meyer, U. A., Strand, L., Doss, M., Rees, A. C., and Marver, H. S. (1972). Intermittent acute porphyria. Demonstration of a genetic defect in porphobilinogen metabolism, *N. Engl. J. Med.* **286**:1277–1282.

Miyagi, K., Petryka, Z. J., and Bossenmaier, I. (1976). The activities of uroporphyrinogen synthetase and cosynthetase in congenital erythropoietic porphyria (CEP), *Amer. J. Hematol.* **1**:3–21.

Moore, M. R., and Disler, P. B. (1983). Drug induction of the acute porphyrias, *Adverse Drug Reaction–Acute Poison Review* **2**:149–189.

Moore, M. R., McColl, K. E., Rimington, C., and Goldberg, A. (1987). *Disorders of Porphyrin Metabolism*, Plenum, New York.

Moore, M. R., Thompson, G. G., Allen, B. R., Hunter, J. A. A., and Parker, S. (1973). Plasma porphyrin concentrations in porphyria cutanea tarda, *Clin. Sci. Mol. Med.* 45:711–714.

Morris, D. L., Dudley, M. D., and Pearson, R. D. (1981). Coagulopathy associated with hematin treatment for acute intermittent porphyria, *Ann. Intern. Med.* 95:700–701.

Mukerji, S. K., Pimstone, N. R., and Burns, M. (1984). Dual mechanism of inhibition of rat liver uroporphyrinogen decarboxylase activity by ferrous iron. Its potential role in the genesis of porphyria cutanea tarda, *Gastroenterology* 87:1248–1254.

Murphy, G. M., Hawk, J. L., and Magnus, I. A. (1985). Late-onset erythropoietic protoporphyria with unusual cutaneous features, *Arch. Dermatol.* 121:1309–1312.

Murphy, G. M., Hawk, J. L., Magnus, I. A., Barrett, D. F., Elder, G. H., and Smith, S. G. (1986). Homozygous variegate porphyria. Two similar cases in unrelated families, *J. Roy. Soc. Med.* 79:361–363.

Mustajoki, P. (1980). Variegate porphyria. Twelve years' experience in Finland, *Quart. J. Med.* 194:191–203.

Mustajoki, P. (1981). Normal erythrocyte uroporphyrinogen I synthase in a kindred with acute intermittent porphyria, *Ann. Intern. Med.* 95:162–166.

Mustajoki, P. (Ed.) (1986). Heme arginate for acute porphyric attacks: Experience with Finnish patients, *New Therapeutic Approach to Hepatic Porphyrias*, Leiras Medica, Finland, pp. 51–55.

Mustajoki, P., and Desnick, R. J. (1985). Genetic heterogeneity in acute intermittent porphyria: Characterisation and frequency of porphobilinogen deaminase mutations in Finland, *Brit. Med. J.* 291:505–509.

Mustajoki, P., Tenhunen, R., Niemi, K. M., Nordmann, Y., Kaariainen, H., and Norio, R. (1987). Homozygous variegate porphyria. A severe skin disease of infancy, *Clin. Genet.* 32:300–305.

Mustajoki, P., Tenhunen, R., Tokola, O., and Gothoni, G. (1986). Haem arginate in the treatment of acute hepatic porphyrias, *Brit. Med. J.* 293:538–539.

Nabeshima, T., Fontenot, J., and Ho, J. K. (1981). Effects of chronic administration of phenobarbital or morphine on the brain microsomal cytochrome P-450 system, *Biochem. Pharmacol.* 30:1142–1145.

Nitowsky, H. M., Sassa, S., Nakagawa, M., and Jagani, N. (1978). Prenatal diagnosis of congenital erythropoietic porphyria (Abstract), *Pediatr. Res.* 12:455.

Nordmann, Y., and Deybach, J. C. (1986). Congenital erythropoietic porphyria, *Sem. Dermatol.* 5:106–114.

Nordmann, Y., Grandchamp, B., de Verneuil, H., Phung, L. N., Cartigny, B., and Fontaine, G. (1983). Harderoporphyria. A rare variant hereditary coproporphyria, *J. Clin. Invest.* 72:1139–1149.

Nordmann, Y., Grandchamp, B., Grelier, M. Phung, L. N., and de Verneuil, H. (1976). Detection of intermittent acute porphyria trait in children, *Lancet* 2:201–202.

Ostrowski, J. (1987). Erythrocyte porphobilinogen deaminase: Activity in liver disease, *Gastroenterology* 92:845–851.

Pain, R. W., Welch, F. W., and Woodroffe, A. J. (1975). Erythropoietic uroporphyria of Gunther first presenting at 58 years with positive family studies, *Brit. Med. J.* 3:621–623.

Pazderova-Vejlupkova, J., Nemcova, N., Pickova, J., Jirasek, L., and Lukos, E. (1981). The development and prognosis of chronic intoxication by tetrachlorodibenzo-*p*-dioxin in man, *Arch. Environ. Health* 36:5.

Percy, V. A., and Shanley, B. C. (1977). Porphyrin precursors in blood, urine and cerebrospinal fluid in acute porphyria, *S. Afr. Med. J.* 52:219–222.

Percy, V. A., and Shanley, B. C. (1979). Studies on haem biosynthesis in rat brain, *J. Neurochem.* 33:1267–1274.

Pierach, C. A. (1982). Hematin therapy for the porphyric attack, *Sem. Liver Dis.* 2:125–131.

Pierach, C. A. (1986a). The treatment of the porphyric attack with hematin, *Porphyrins and Porphyrias* (Y. Nordmann, Ed.), John Libbey, Paris, Vol. 134, pp. 217–224.

Pierach, C. A. (1986b). Treatment of the acute porphyric attack, *New Therapeutic Approach to Hepatic Porphyrias* (P. Mustajoki, Ed.), Leiras Medica, Finland, pp. 30–35.

Pimstone, N. R. (1982). Porphyria cutanea tarda, *Sem. Liver Dis.* **2**:132–142.

Pimstone, N. R., Gandhi, S. N., and Mukerji, S. K. (1987). Therapeutic efficacy of oral charcoal in congenital erythropoietic porphyria, *N. Engl. J. Med.* **316**:390–393.

Pinol-Aguade, J., Castells, A., Indocochea, A., and Rodes, J. (1969). A case of biochemically unclassifiable hepatic porphyria, *Brit. J. Dermatol.* **81**:270–275.

Piomelli, S., Lamola, A. A., Poh-Fitzpatrick, M. B., Seaman, C., and Harber, L. C. (1975). Erythropoietic protoporphyria and lead intoxication. The molecular basis for differences in cutaneous photosensitivity, *J. Clin. Invest.* **56**:1519–1527.

Piomelli, S., Poh-Fitzpatrick, M. B., Seaman, C., Skolnick, L. M., and Berdon, W. E. (1986). Complete suppression of the symptoms of congenital erythropoietic porphyria by longterm treatment with high-level transfusions, *N. Engl. J. Med.* **314**:1029–1031.

Poh-Fitzpatrick, M. B. (1980). A plasma porphyrin fluorescence marker for variegate porphyria, *Arch. Dermatol.* **116**:543–547.

Poh-Fitzpatrick, M. B. (1982). Porphyrin levels in plasma and erythrocytes of chronic haemodialysis patients, *J. Amer. Acad. Dermatol.* **7**:100–104.

Poh-Fitzpatrick, M. B. (1986). Erythropoietic protoporphyria, *Sem. Dermatol.* **5**:88–105.

Poh-Fitzpatrick, M. B., Sklar, J. A., Goldsman, C., and Lefkowitch, J. A. (1983). Protoporphyrin hepatopathy. Effects of cholic acid ingestion in murine griseofulvin-induced protoporphyria, *J. Clin. Invest.* **72**:1449–1458.

Poland, A. P., Smith, D., Metter, G., and Possick, P. (1971). A health survey of workers in a 2,4-D and 2,4,5-T plant, *Arch. Environ. Health* **22**:316–327.

Rimington, C. (1960). Spectral-absorption coefficient of some porphyrins in the Soret band region, *Biochem. J.* **75**:620–623.

Rimington, C., Lockwood, W. H., and Belcher, R. V. (1968). The excretion of porphyrin-peptide conjugates in porphyria variegata, *Clin. Sci.* **35**:211–247.

Roberts, A. G., Elder, G. H., Newcombe, R. G., DeSalamanca, R. E., and Munoz, J. J. (1988). Heterogeneity of familial porphyria cutanea tarda, *J. Med. Genet.* **10**:669–676.

Rocchi, E., Gibertini, P., Cassanelli, M., Pietrangelo, A., Borghi, A., Pantaleoni, M., Jensen, J., and Ventura, E. (1986). Iron removal therapy in porphyria cutanea tarda: Phlebotomy versus slow subcutaneous desferrioxamine infusion, *Brit. J. Dermatol.* **114**:621–629.

Romeo, G., Glenn, B. L., and Levin, E. Y. (1970). Uroporphyrinogen III cosynthetase in asymptomatic carriers of congenital erythropoietic porphyria, *Biochem. Genet.* **4**:719–726.

Romeo, G., and Levin, E. Y. (1969). Uroporphyrinogen III cosynthetase in human congenital erythropoietic porphyria, *Proc. Nat. Acad. Sci.* **63**:856–863.

Romeo, P. H., Raich, N., Dubart, A., Beaupain, D., Pryor, M., Kushner, J., Cohen-Solal, M., and Goossens, M. (1986). Molecular cloning and nucleotide sequence of a complete human uroporphyrinogen decarboxylase cDNA, *J. Biol. Chem.* **261**:9825–9830.

Ruth, G. R., Schwartz, S., and Stephenson, B. (1977). Bovine protoporphyria: The first non-human model of this hereditary photosensitizing disease, *Science* **198**:199–201.

Samuel, D., Boboc, B., Bernuau, J., Bismuth, H., and Benhamou, J. P. (1988). Liver transplantation for protoporphyria, *Gastroenterology* **95**:816–819.

Sassa, S., de Verneuil, H., Anderson, K. E., and Kappas, A. (1983). Purification and properties of human erythrocyte uroporphyrinogen decarboxylase: Immunological demonstration of the enzyme defect in porphyria cutanea tarda, *Trans. Assoc. Amer. Physicians* **96**:65–75.

Sassa, S., Granick, S., Bickers, D. S., Bradlow, H. L., and Kappas, A. (1974). A microassay for uroporphyrinogen I synthase, one of three abnormal enzyme activities in acute intermittent porphyria, and its application to the study of the genetics of this disease, *Proc. Nat. Acad. Sci.* **71**:732–736.

Sassa, S., and Kappas, A. (1981). The porphyrias, *Advances in Human Genetics* (H. Harris, Ed.), Plenum, New York, Vol. 11.

Sassa, S., Solish, G., Levere, R. D., and Kappas, A. (1975). Studies in porphyria. IV. Expression of the gene defect of acute intermittent porphyria in cultured human skin fibroblasts and amniotic cells: Prenatal diagnosis of the porphyric trait, *J. Exp. Med.* **142**:722–731.

Sassa, S., Zalar, G. L., and Kappas, A. (1978). Studies in porphyria. VII. Induction of uroporphyrinogen 1 synthase and expression of the gene defect of acute intermittent porphyria in mitogen-stimulated human lymphocytes, *J. Clin. Invest.* **61**:499–508.

Sassa, S., Zalar, G. L., Poh-Fitzpatrick, M. B., Anderson, K. E., and Kappas, A. (1982). Studies in porphyria. Functional evidence for a partial deficiency of ferrochelatase activity in mitogen-stimulated lymphocytes from patients with erythropoietic protoporphyria, *J. Clin. Invest.* **69**:809–815.

Sato, A., and Takahasi, N. (1926). A new form of congenital hematoporphyria: Oligochromemia porphyrinuria (megalosplenica congenita), *Amer. J. Dis. Child.* **32**:325–333.

Schmid, R. (1960). Cutaneous porphyria in Turkey, *N. Engl. J. Med.* **263**:397–398.

Schmid, R., Schwartz, D., and Sundberg, D. (1955). Erythropoietic (congenital) porphyria. A rare abnormality of the normoblasts, *Blood* **10**:416–428.

Scholnick, P., Marver, H. S., and Schmid, R. (1971). Erythropoietic protoporphyria: Evidence for multiple sites of excess protoporphyrin formation, *J. Clin. Invest.* **50**:203–207.

Schothorst, A. A., Van Steveninck, J., Went, L. N., and Suurmond, D. (1972). Photodynamic damage of the erythrocyte membrane caused by protoporphyrin in protoporphyria and in normal red blood cells, *Clin. Chim. Acta* **39**:161–170.

Schultz, J. H. (1874). Ein fall von pemphigus leprosus, kompliziert durch Lepra visceralis. Inaugural Dissertation, Greifswald.

Seery, V. L., and Muller-Eberhard, U. (1973). Binding of porphyrins to rabbit hemopexin and albumin, *J. Biol. Chem.* **248**:3796–3800.

Seip, M., Thune, P. O., and Eriksen, L. (1974). Treatment of photosensitivity in congenital erythropoietic porphyria with beta carotene, *Acta Dermatol Venereol.* **54**:239–240.

Seubert, S., Seubert, A., Rumpf, K., and Kiffe, H. (1985). A porphyria cutanea tarda like distribution pattern of porphyrins in plasma hemodialysate hemofiltrate in urine of patients on chronic hemodialysis, *J. Invest. Dermatol.* **85**:107–109.

Sfar, Z., Kamoun, M. R., Kastally, R., de Verneuil, H., and Nordmann, Y. (1985). Porphyrie hépato-érythrocytaire chez deux soeurs jumelles, *Ann. Dermatol. Venereol.* **112**:453–456.

Shanley, B. C., Neethling, A. C., Percy, V. A., and Carstens, H. (1975). Neurochemical aspects of porphyrias. I. Studies on the possible neurotoxicity of delta aminolevulinic acid, *S. Afr. Med. J.* **49**:576–680.

Shanley, B. C., Zail, S. S., and Joubert, S. M. (1969). Effect of ethanol on liver delta-aminolevulinate synthetase activity and urinary porphyrin excretion in symptomatic porphyria, *Brit. J. Haematol.* **17**:389.

Siepker, L. J., and Kramer, S. (1985). Protoporphyrin accumulation by mitogen stimulated lymphocytes and protoporphyrinogen oxidase activity in patients with porphyria variegata and erythropoietic protoporphyria, *Brit. J. Haematol.* **60**:65–74.

Simard, H., Barry, A., and Villeneuve, B. (1972). Porphyrie erythropoietique congenitale, *Canad. Med. Assoc. J.* **106**:1002–1004.

Simon, N., Berko, G., and Schneider, I. (1977). Hepato-erythropoietic porphyria presenting as scleroderma and acrosclerosis in a sibling pair, *Brit. J. Dermatol.* **96**:663–668.

Sinclair, J. F., Sinclair, P., Smith, E., Bement, W., Pomeroy, J., and Bonkowsky, H. (1981). Ethanol-mediated increased in cytochrome P-450 in cultured hepatocytes, *Biochem. Pharmacol.* **30**:2805.

Sinclair, J. F., Zaitlin, L. M., Smith, E. L., Howell, S. K., Bonkowsky, H. L., and Sinclair, P. R. (1986). Induction of delta aminolevulinate synthase and changes in porphyrin patterns caused by 2- to 5-carbon alcohols: Possible risk factors in patients with hepatic porphyrias, *Porphyrins and Porphyrias* (Y. Nordmann, Ed.), John Libbey, Paris, Vol. 134, pp. 137–146.

Sixel-Dietrich, F., and Doss, M. (1985). Hereditary uroporphyrinogen-decarboxylase deficiency predisposing porphyria cutanea tarda (chronic hepatic porphyria) in females after oral contraceptive medication, *Arch. Dermatol. Res.* **278**:13–16.

Smith, A. G. (1986). Hepatoerythropoietic porphyria, *Sem. Dermatol.* **5**:125–137.

Smith, A. G., and Francis, J. E. (1983). Synergism of iron and hexachlorobenzene inhibits hepatic uroporphyrinogen decarboxylase in inbred mice, *Biochem. J.* **214**:909–913.

Smith, A. G., Francis, J. E., Kay, S. J., Greig, J. B., and Stewart, F. P. (1986). Mechanistic studies of the inhibition of hepatic uroporphyrinogen decarboxylase in C57BL/10 mice by iron-hexachlorobenzene synergism, *Biochem. J.* **238**:871–878.

Sneddon, I. B., and Stretcher, G. S. (1978). Beta carotene in congenital porphyria, *Arch. Dermatol.* **114**:1242–1243.

Srivastava, G., Borthwick, I. A., Brooker, J. D., Wallace, J. C., May, B. K., and Elliot, W. H. (1983). Hemin inhibits transfer of pre 5-aminolaevulinate synthase into chick liver mitochondria, *Biochem. Biophys. Res. Comm.* **117**:344–349.

Straka, J. C., and Kushner, J. (1983). Purification and characterization of bovine hepatic uroporphyrinogen decarboxylase, *Biochemistry* **22**:4664–4672.

Strand, L. J., Felsher, B. F., Redeker, A. G., and Marver, H. S. (1970). Heme biosynthesis in acute intermittent porphyria: Decreased hepatic conversion of porphobilinogen to porphyrin and increased delta aminolaevulinic acid synthetase activity, *Proc. Nat. Acad. Sci.* **67**:1315–1320.

Sveinsson, S. L., Rimington, C., and Barnes, H. D. (1949). Complete porphyrin analysis of pathological urines, *Scand. J. Clin. Lab. Invest.* **1**:2–11.

Sweeney, G. D. (1986). Porphyria cutanea tarda, or the uroporphyrinogen decarboxylase deficiency diseases, *Clin. Biochem.* **19**:3–15.

Sweeney, V. P., Pathak, M. A., and Asbury, A. K. (1970). Acute intermittent porphyria: Increased ALA-synthetase activity during an attack, *Brain* **93**:369–380.

Taddeini, L., and Watson, C. J. (1968). The clinical porphyrias, *Sem. Hematol.* **5**:335–369.

Taljaard, J. J., Shanley, B. C., and Joubert, S. M. (1971). Decreased uroporphyrinogen decarboxylase activity in experimental symptomatic porphyria, *Life Sci.* **10**:887–893.

Thivolet, J., Euvrard, S., Perrot, H., and Nordmann, Y. (1977). La pseudo-porphyrie cutanée tardive des hemodialyses, *Ann. Dermatol. Venereol.* **104**:12–17.

Thunell, S., Holmberg, L., and Lundgren, J. (1987). Aminolaevulinate dehydratase porphyria in infancy. A clinical and biochemical study, *J. Clin. Chem. Clin. Biochem.* **25**:5–14.

Tio, T. H., Leijnse, B., Jarrett, A., and Rimington, C. (1959). Acquired porphyria from a liver tumor, *Clin. Sci. Mol. Med.* **16**:517.

Tishler, P. V., Gordon, B. J., and O'Connor, J. (1982). The absorption of porphyrins and porphyrin precursors by sorbents: A potential therapy for the porphyrias, *Meth. Find Exp. Clin. Pharmacol.* **4**:125–131.

Tishler, P. V., Woodward, B., O'Connor, J., Holbrook, D. A., Seidman, L. J., Hallett, M., and Knighton, D. J. (1985). High prevalence of intermittent acute porphyria in a psychiatric patient population, *Amer. J. Psych.* **142**:1430–1436.

Toback, A. C., Sassa, S., Poh-Fitzpatrick, M. B., Schacter, J., Zaider, E., Harber, L. C., and Kappas, A. (1987). Hepatoerythropoietic porphyria: Clinical, biochemical and enzymatic studies in a three-generation family lineage, *N. Engl. J. Med.* **36**:613–622.

Topi, G. C., Amantea, A., and Griso, D. (1984). Recovery from porphyria cutanea tarda with no specific therapy other than avoidance of hepatic toxins, *Brit. J. Dermatol.* **111**:75–82.

Topi, G. C., D'Alessandro, G. L., Griso, D., and Morini, S. (1980). Porphyria cutanea tarda and hepatocellular carcinoma, *Int. J. Biochem.* **12**:883–885.

Tsai, S. F., Bishop, D. F., and Desnick, R. J. (1987). Coupled-enzyme and direct assays for uroporphyrinogen III synthase activity in human erythrocytes and cultured-lymphoblasts, *Anal. Biochem.* **166**:120–133.

Tschudy, D. P., Perlroth, M. G., Marver, H. S., Collins, A., Hunter, G., Jr., and Rechcigl, M., Jr. (1965). Acute intermittent porphyria: The first "overproduction disease" localized to a specific enzyme, *Proc. Nat. Acad. Sci. (U.S.A.)* **53**:841–846.

Van Gog, H., and Schothorst, A. A. (1973). Determination of very small amounts of protoporphyrin in epidermis, plasma and blister fluids, *J. Invest. Dermatol.* **61**:42–45.

Varadi, S. (1958). Haematological aspects in a case of erythropoietic porphyria, *Brit. J. Haematol.* **4**:270–280.

Viljoen, D. J., Cayanis, F., Becker, D. A., Kramer, S., Dawson, B., and Bernstein, R. (1979). Reduced ferrochelatase activity in fibroblasts from patients with porphyria variegata, *Amer. J. Hematol.* **6**:185–190.

Viljoen, D. J., Cummins, R., Alexopoulos, J., and Kramer, S. (1983). Protoporphyrinogen oxidase and ferrochelatase in porphyria variegata, *Eur. J. Clin. Invest.* **13**:283–287.

Waldenstrom, J., and Haeger-Aronsen, B. (1967). The porphyrias: A genetic problem, *Progress in Medical Genetics* (A. G. Steinberg, Ed.), Grune & Stratton, New York, Vol. 5.

Waldo, E. D., and Tobias, H. (1973). Needle-like cytoplasmic inclusions in the liver in porphyria cutanea tarda, *Arch. Pathol.* **96**:368–371.

Watson, C. J., Bossenmaier, I., Cardinal, R., and Petryka, Z. J. (1974). Repression by hematin of porphyrin biosynthesis in erythrocyte precursors in congenital erythropoietic porphyria, *Proc. Nat. Acad. Sci. (U.S.A.)* **71**:278–282.

Watson, C. J., Cardinal, R. A., Bossenmaier, I., and Petryka, Z. J. (1975). Porphyria variegata and porphyria cutanea tarda in siblings: Chemical and genetic aspects, *Proc. Nat. Acad. Sci.* **72**:5126–5129.

Watson, C. J., Pierach, C. A., Bossenmaier, I., and Cardinal, R. (1978). Use of hematin in the acute attack of the "inducible" hepatic porphyrias, *Adv. Intern. Med.* **23**:265–286.

Watson, C. J., Runge, W., and Taddeini, L. (1964). A suggested control gene mechanism for the excessive production of types I and III porphyrins in congenital erythropoietic porphyria, *Proc. Nat. Acad. Sci.* **52**:478–485.

Weston, M. J., Nicholson, D. C., and Lim, C. K. (1978). Congenital erythropoietic uroporphyria (Gunther's disease) presenting in a middle aged man, *Int. J. Biochem.* **9**:921–926.

White, M. I. (1977). Porphyria cutanea tarda induced by oestrogen therapy, *Brit. J. Urol.* **49**:468.

Wilson, J. H. P., De Rooy, F. W. M., and Te Velde, K. (1986). Acute intermittent porphyria in the Netherlands. Heterogeneity of the enzyme porphobilinogen deaminase, *Neth. J. Med.* **29**:393–399.

With, T. K. (1983). Hereditary coproporphyria and variegate porphyria in Denmark, *Dan. Med. Bull.* **30**:106–112.

Woods, J. S., Kardish, R., and Fowler, B. A. (1981). Studies on the action of porphyrinogenic trace metals on the activity of hepatic uroporphyrinogen decarboxylase, *Biochem. Biophys. Res. Comm.* **103**:264–271.

Wyman, J. F., Gollan, J. L., Settle, W., Farrell, G. C., and Correia, M. A. (1986). Incorporation of haemoglobin haem into the rat hepatic haemoproteins tryptophan pyrrolase and cytochrome P-450, *Biochem. J.* **238**:837–846.

11

Heme Degradation and Biosynthesis of Bilins

Stanley B. Brown

Jennifer D. Houghton

Angela Wilks

I. Introduction

Most studies of the metabolism of functional groups are primarily concerned with biosynthesis and much less with breakdown. For example, the biosynthesis of carotenoids and chlorophyll are now well understood, but relatively little is known of their breakdown. In the case of heme, however, whereas its biosynthesis has been widely studied and is the subject of much of this book, its breakdown has also been investigated in detail. The reason for this is twofold. First, the heme breakdown process has important medical implications and this has been a strong driving force for many studies. Second, whereas in mammals heme conversion to bile pigments has no functional implications other than providing a pathway for the elimination of unwanted heme, in plant systems the same pathway is biosynthetic, leading to the chromophore of phycobiliproteins such as phytochrome and phycocyanin (see chap. 7).

The subject of heme metabolism has been reviewed often [see, e.g., Schmid and McDonagh (1975, 1979) and Brown and Troxler (1982)] and the details of earlier work will not be repeated here. This chapter focuses on recent work and, in particular, how enzymic heme degradation may be viewed in relation to other processes involving hemoproteins. We will use the term *heme* to signify protoheme; other substituted hemes will be referred to by their commonly accepted trivial names (e.g., mesoheme).

A. Systems in which heme and porphyrins may be degraded

Because of their extensive highly delocalized electron systems, hemes and porphyrins are relatively stable molecules so far as the macrocyclic ring system is concerned. For example, the heme of hemoglobin is stable throughout the lifetime of the red blood cell. Also, porphyrins are found in many types of geological deposits of great age and laboratory samples of hemes and porphyrins prepared many decades ago are often found when analyzed to be almost unchanged from their original specification. Nevertheless, degradation of the heme and porphyrin macrocycle does occur in both biological and nonbiological systems; indeed, this process is a vital one in many, if not all, living organisms.

1. Biological degradation to bile pigments. The most important functional pathway by which heme is broken down in living systems is its conversion to the bile pigment (bilin) biliverdin as shown in Fig. 11.1. In some organisms, the further conversion of biliverdin to the yellow bile pigment bilirubin occurs (see Fig. 11.1). It is this process which is most important in the physiological breakdown of heme and, as will be seen later, in the biosynthesis of important functional bile pigments in plants. We will, therefore, concentrate on the biochemical and physiological aspects of this pathway of heme degradation.

Nevertheless, several other routes for the breakdown of the porphyrin macrocycle do exist and some of these may have biological or medical significance under certain circumstances. These are considered very briefly below.

2. Coupled oxidation. Treatment of heme derivatives with a reductant such as ascorbate or hydrazine in the presence of molecular oxygen leads

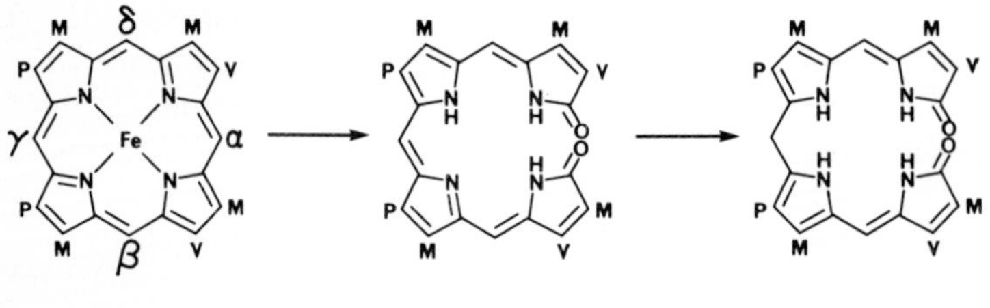

Heme   Biliverdin   Bilirubin

Figure 11.1 Structure of the pigments involved in the catabolism of heme. (M, $-CH_3$; V, $-CH=CH_2$; P, $-CH_2CH_2CH_2CO_2H$.)

to rapid breakdown of the macrocycle to produce the corresponding biliverdin. This process is known as coupled oxidation because both the heme and the reductant are simultaneously oxidized by molecular oxygen. The reducing agent is essential for the reaction, that is, heme is not attacked by molecular oxygen alone and metal-free porphyrins do not undergo coupled oxidation. The stoichiometry and mechanism of coupled oxidation is so closely allied to that of biological heme breakdown that the process has often been studied as a model for the biological reaction and, for this reason, it is considered in more detail later in this chapter.

3. Biological conversion of heme to *N*-substituted porphyrins.   When experimental animals are treated with allylisopropylacetamide (AIA) or a number of other drugs, green pigments often accumulate in the liver. These are now known to be *N*-alkyl-substituted porphyrins, formed by the action of the drugs on cytochrome P450 heme. Whereas such reactions do not fit into the category of degradation of the heme macrocycle, the heme is, in effect, irreversibly degraded and these reactions have been extensively studied in relation to the function and structure of cytochrome P450 [for a review, see Ortiz de Montellano (1986)].

4. Chemical degradation to mono- and dipyrroles.   Certain oxidizing agents are able to attack the heme macrocycle with the loss of iron and degradation to mono- or dipyrrolic fragments. For example, addition of hydrogen peroxide to a solution of heme in aqueous alkali results in the rapid bleaching of the heme to dipyrroles known as propent dyopents, so-called because on reduction with dithionite they yield red-orange pigments with an absorption peak at 525 nm (Gray, 1953). Although early literature suggested that this reaction proceeded via the intermediacy of biliverdin, this bile pigment has never been isolated or directly demonstrated in this system. Indeed, even attempts to show indirectly the intermediacy of biliverdin (e.g., by carrying out the reaction in the presence of biliverdin reductase when conversion to bilirubin might have been expected) have been unsuccessful and it seems likely that the oxidation of heme by hydrogen peroxide does not involve the formation of biliverdin. Stronger oxidizing agents such as chromic acid convert heme to a mixture of mono- and dipyrroles and methods have been developed to use this process to characterize structurally heme and porphyrin derivatives (Rudiger, 1968).

5. Photochemical reactions.   Hemes (i.e., iron-porphyrins) are neither photosensitive nor photosensitizing and are stable in the presence of light for long periods. By contrast, the metal-free porphyrins are associated with a great deal of photochemistry. They fluoresce strongly, they are able to photosensitize oxidations of other substances (as for example in the newly developing technique of photochemotherapy for cancer treatment), and they are relatively unstable in the light, probably due to a self-photosensitization.

B. Chemistry of heme breakdown to bile pigments

Although the conversion of heme to biliverdin is depicted in Fig. 11.1 as a single process, the reaction is clearly a complex one and must take place in a series of steps with a corresponding series of intermediates. A novel feature of this reaction is the elimination of a methene bridge carbon atom as carbon monoxide. The reaction also involves elimination of the iron atom and the insertion of two oxygen atoms into the product bile pigment. The conversion of biliverdin to bilirubin requires reduction at the central methene bridge, thus formally breaking the conjugation. Although biliverdin and bilirubin have been drawn in Fig. 11.1 in a manner to emphasize their origin from heme, their actual conformations are rather different. Indeed, the conformation adopted by bilirubin is such as to maximize intramolecular hydrogen bonding (Bonnett and McDonagh, 1973) and this leads to its remarkably high lipophilicity and, hence, its potential toxicity. The methyl propionyl and vinyl side chains of heme are unchanged on its degradation to biliverdin or bilirubin.

Because of the asymmetrical arrangement of these side chains around the periphery of the heme molecule (Fig. 11.1), the four methene bridge carbon atoms, designated α, β, γ, and δ are not equivalent. In principle, degradation can, therefore, lead to four possible biliverdin isomers and, hence, bilirubin isomers according to whether the α, β, γ, or δ methene bridges are attacked. However, the bilirubin found in mammalian bile consists almost exclusively of the α isomer as shown in Fig. 11.1. Since it is known that there is little intrinsic difference in reactivity between the four methene bridge carbon atoms, the selectivity (sometimes termed regioselectivity) must clearly be biologically directed.

II. Mammalian Heme Breakdown

A. Hemoprotein turnover

Heme, in association with various proteins, plays a remarkably versatile set of roles in biology. In hemoglobin and myoglobin, which are concerned with oxygen transport and storage, it is essential that the iron atom of the heme is maintained formally in the $+2$ oxidation state in order that the heme may bind oxygen. In the cytochromes, almost the reverse criterion applies, that is, there is a positive requirement that the heme must shuttle between the $+2$ and $+3$ oxidation states. Cytochrome P450 is, in one sense, intermediate in function because it must both permit its iron to oscillate between $+2$ and $+3$, and it must accommodate the binding of oxygen while the iron is in the $+2$ oxidation state. Other hemoproteins include catalase, peroxidase, and tryptophan-dioxygenase.

Although hemoproteins carry out such a variety of functions, in mammals by far the great majority of the heme (probably more than 95%) resides in the hemoglobin contained in the circulating erythrocytes. In considering the flux of heme degradation, however, not only must the abundance of a particular hemoprotein component be taken into account, but also its turnover rate. For hemoglobin, little or no degradation occurs in the circulating erythrocyte and no significant heme degradation occurs during the life span of its host red cell, that is, about 125 days in humans (Shemin and Rittenburg, 1946). At the end of this period hemoglobin degradation is rapid and this implies that rather less than 1% of hemoglobin is degraded each day. However, turnover of liver hemoproteins, principally cytochrome P450, is relatively fast and they make a contribution to heme degradation which is disproportionately high compared with their abundance.

Early experiments, particularly those using ^{15}N-labeled glycine, laid the basis for distinguishing between metabolism of liver heme and metabolism of erythrocyte heme (Gray et al., 1950; Berlin et al., 1956; Robinson, 1975). Administration of ^{15}N-glycine to a normal human and subsequent measurement of the isotopic enrichment in the fecal stercobilin (derived from bilirubin) gave an initial peak after 8 days followed by a much lower plateau region with a further peak after 135 days. The isotopic enrichment in the heme of hemoglobin increased over the first 14 days during hemoglobin synthesis, remained steady for about 100 days, and then decreased as the cohort of labeled cells were removed from the circulation. The main conclusions from such experiments were that the initial peak or "early labeled peak," corresponding to about 10 to 15% of the label, arose from the rapid turnover of liver hemoproteins, mainly cytochrome P450 and possibly also of a labile protein-free heme pool. The plateau region in ^{15}N excretion in fecal stercobilin probably represents degradation of the heme of hemoproteins such as catalase and myoglobin and the large peak at about 135 days corresponds to the lifetime of the human red cell.

Turnover of hemoproteins in the normal adult human involves production of about 0.4 bilirubin per day and about 15 cm^3 of carbon monoxide measured at STP. This carbon monoxide accounts for about 1 to 2 ppm of exhaled gases, a level which is easily measured. Measurement of exhaled carbon monoxide has been used to detect hemolytic states, for example, to distinguish between hemolytic and hepatic jaundice (see below). Carbon monoxide formed by heme breakdown does not present significant toxicity problems since the oxygen concentration in air is about 200,000 ppm and effectively swamps the carbon monoxide in terms of binding to hemoproteins, in spite of the latter's greater affinity.

Whereas carbon monoxide and bilirubin are eliminated from the body following heme degradation, the third product, iron, is not eliminated but is retained in the iron pool and reutilized. It is sometimes useful to consider the heme synthetic and degradation pathways as in "iron cycle" as shown in Fig. 11.2.

B. Free-heme pool

There has been considerable debate as to the existence and size of a "free-heme pool" in the liver or elsewhere. Whereas free heme must exist, at least transiently, in the course of incorporation into hemoproteins, the contribution of such a pool to heme degradation and to regulation of heme metabolism is not yet clear. Studies on rat liver hepatocytes in primary culture suggested that newly formed heme exists transiently in a small pool which turns over rapidly (Grandchamp et al., 1981). It was further suggested that this same pool, or one very similar in nature, represents heme in transit to apoprotein acceptors and may act as an inhibitor of ALA synthase (EC 2.3.1.37), while inducing heme oxygenase (EC 1.14.99.3) (Bissell and Hammaker, 1977), and an increase in tryptophan dioxygenase (EC 1.13.11.11) (Badawy and Evans, 1975). Contraction of the heme pool may conversely result in the induction of ALA synthase and the concomitant synthesis of heme transporting proteins in order to obtain heme extracellularly or to shift the heme distribution within the cell (Foidart et al., 1982).

When intravenously injected in small amounts, heme may give rise to increased production of the serum binding protein hemopexin (Foidart

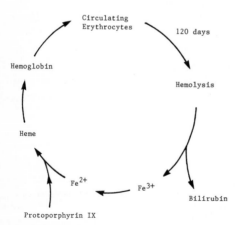

Figure 11.2 Representation of the biosynthesis and metabolism of heme as an iron cycle.

et al., 1982). Similar injection can, shortly after administration, replenish the drug-induced cytochrome P450 function in the rat (Farrell and Correia, 1980; Ortiz de Montellano and Correia, 1983). It has been shown recently that hemoglobin heme can be incorporated into hepatic tryptophan dioxygenase, as well as restoring cytochrome P450 content and its mixed-function oxidase activity, following substrate-induced destruction of the P450 heme moiety (Wyman et al., 1986).

The whole question of the size and function of the heme pool and the effect on such a pool of administration of exogenous heme is of some importance, not only to the understanding of heme metabolism and its regulation, but also because administration of heme is used clinically in the treatment of porphyria. However, the complexities in the subcellular and intracellular distribution of heme and its relationship to various hemoproteins are not yet well understood.

C. Sites of mammalian heme breakdown

A large number of tissues and organs contain systems capable of degrading heme. The most visually striking example is in the progress of a subcutaneous bruise which displays the characteristic color changes from purple (heme) through blue-green (biliverdin) to yellow (bilirubin). However, in quantitative terms, the spleen has a high specific activity in terms of heme degradation in vitro and, since it is the organ normally responsible for removal of senescent red blood cells, it appears that the majority of normal heme degradation occurs in this organ. However, because of its greater size, the liver has an overall heme degrading activity comparable to that of the spleen, and it is thought that the liver takes over the heme degradation function following splenectomy.

Little or no heme degradation takes place while hemoglobin is contained within the red blood cell and, normally, cell-free hemoglobin does not occur at significant levels in the blood. However, in abnormal situations when significant levels of plasma hemoglobin are reached (e.g., following intravascular hemolysis or intravenous hemoglobin administration), it has been shown that the hepatic parenchymal cells and the renal tubes are important sites of heme breakdown (Pimstone et al., 1971a). It seems likely that whereas the spleen is responsible for the majority of heme breakdown on a quantitative basis, the liver probably plays a more-sophisticated role in the regulation of heme metabolism.

D. Enzymology of heme breakdown

1. Heme macrocycle cleavage step. In 1968 Schmid and co-workers first described the discovery of an enzyme system, named heme oxygenase, which appeared to catalyze specifically the degradation of heme to biliverdin and carbon monoxide (Tenhunen et al., 1968). The kinetics and tissue distribution of the enzyme suggested that it was of major importance in the physiological degradation of the heme of hemoglobin and other hemoproteins to bile pigments. Some 20 years later, following a good deal of intensive study, it is now known that heme oxygenase is the enzyme primarily responsible for the degradation of the heme macrocycle, not only in mammals, but also in other species. The enzyme is located in the microsomal fraction of a variety of tissues, in particular spleen, liver, bone marrow, kidney, and macrophages. In order to carry out its heme cleaving function, heme oxygenase requires an electron transport system and depends upon the microsomal enzyme NADPH-cytochrome P450 reductase for activity. A detailed discussion of heme oxygenase and its relationship to NADPH-cytochrome P450 reductase is given in the sections which follow.

2. Biliverdin reductase.   In mammals, the immediate heme breakdown product, biliverdin, does not accumulate and is reduced to the yellow bile pigment, bilirubin, by the enzyme biliverdin reductase (EC 1.3.1.24). This enzyme, first described by Lemberg and Wyndham (1936), is cytosolic and requires NADPH as a source of electrons. Biliverdin reductase appears to have a wide distribution in mammals, being present in liver, kidney, spleen, brain, and muscle. It is generally assumed that spleen biliverdin reductase is responsible for most of the physiological conversion of biliverdin to bilirubin, but this is not known with certainty and, in any event, the liver must take over this function following a splenectomy. The enzyme is either absent or present at only very low levels in birds, reptiles, and amphibia, where biliverdin is the end product of heme degradation.

In early work the enzyme was partially purified from rat kidney and from guinea pig liver (Tenhunen et al., 1970b; O'Carra and Colleran, 1971; Colleran and O'Carra, 1975) and appeared to show a molecular weight of about 70,000. More recently, bilirubin reductase has been purified to homogeneity from rat liver and pig spleen (Noguchi et al., 1979; Kutty and Maines, 1981) and has been shown to have a minimum molecular weight on SDS-polyacrylamide gel electrophoresis of 32,000. Although NADH can act as an electron donor in vitro, NADPH is preferred, and since the enzyme is cytosolic it is assumed that this is the source of reducing power in vivo.

The isomer selectivity of biliverdin reductase (i.e., whether there is a preference for α, β, γ, or δ biliverdin isomers as substrate) has been of some interest. This is partly because of the possibility, in principle, that the absolute selectivity for formation of bilirubin IXα in vivo might be due to the specificity of biliverdin reductase. Several studies have shown that the purified enzyme has a marked preference for the α isomer of biliverdin, although it is clear that reduction of non-α-isomers does occur in vivo. This is confirmed by the fact that intravenous injection of ^{14}C-labeled biliverdin IXβ, -γ, and -δ into the rat, give rapid and quantitative conversion of the isomers to the respective bilirubin isomers (Brown and Troxler, 1982). A possible explanation for the ability of mammals to reduce all four biliverdin isomers may come from recent evidence describing the existence of different molecular forms of the rat hepatic biliverdin reductase in vivo (Frydman et al., 1984; Awruch et al., 1984). Under normal circumstances, it is reported that there is a predominant species (designated molecular form 1), the chief characteristic of which is the high reduction rate of biliverdin IXα. The minor species (molecular form 2) has a similar rate for both the α and β isomers. Apparently, a third molecular form is induced by cobalt chloride or phenylhydrazine treatment and is produced by transformation of molecular form 1. The net effect of the conversion of molecular form 1 to molecular form 3 is an increased activity toward biliverdin IXα (Frydman et al., 1984). It was suggested that the in vivo transformation of molecular form 1 to molecular form 3 is carried out by a peroxisomal dehydrogenase, isolatable from rat liver (Frydman et al., 1984). In view of the strict α selectivity of heme oxygenase itself (see below), the need for an enzyme capable of reducing β, δ, or γ isomers is not obvious and it is not clear at present whether the activity in vivo toward non-α isomers reflects a specific functional role or whether such activity is a secondary consequence of the primary α-selective activity.

3. Bilirubin UDP glucuronyltransferase.

It has already been mentioned that bilirubin free acid is an extremely lipophilic, water-insoluble compound. In order to permit its secretion into the bile, it must, therefore, be rendered water-soluble and this is done by conjugation usually with glucuronic acid. This reaction is controlled by the enzyme bilirubin-UDP-glucuronyltransferase (EC 2.4.1.17), which is specifically found in the liver and not in the spleen. The detailed properties and mechanisms of action of this enzyme are important clinically, but are considered beyond the scope of the present account. [For a detailed review, see Billing (1982).]

E. Clinical aspects of heme breakdown

The clinical consequences of deficiencies in the process of heme biosynthesis are considered in detail in other parts of this book. In terms of heme breakdown, the most important abnormality is hyperbilirubinemia, which may result in deposition of bilirubin in the skin, leading to the characteristic yellow pigmentation associated with jaundice. Jaundice is not in itself harmful, but it is a symptom of the underlying hyperbilirubinemia which is itself a symptom of an underlying clinical problem. Broadly, jaundice and hyperbilirubinemia may arise either as a result of increased hemolysis with normal liver function (hemolytic jaundice) or as a result of the inability of the body to handle normal bilirubin production. Since the latter is almost always due to a malfunction of the liver, this is known as hepatic jaundice.

Hemolytic jaundice arises as a result of a reduced red cell lifetime, which may be due to a genetic lesion or to the effect of extrinsic factors. Hepatic jaundice occurs because of the impairment of the conjugating system by which bilirubin is rendered water-soluble for excretion into the bile. The causes include hepatitis, liver tumors, and inherited deficiency in glucuronyltransferase, the enzyme responsible for bilirubin conjugation. The very common neonatal jaundice which often occurs transiently following birth is due to delay in the production of glucuronyltransferase in the neonate following birth. In most cases, this enzyme reaches normal levels in the first few days of life, and the jaundice disappears. However, because of the risk of the toxic effects of bilirubin on the brain of neonates (kernicterus), bilirubin levels in newborns are carefully monitored and corrective action taken where appropriate.

III. Heme Oxygenase

A. Properties of the enzyme

1. Subcellular location and function. Heme oxygenase is found in the microsomal fraction of cells from a variety of tissues and has a requirement for molecular oxygen and NADPH (Tenhunen et al., 1968). It is, therefore, typical of the group of enzymes known as monooxygenases or mixed-function oxygenases requiring both molecular oxygen and a reducing agent. The enzyme is difficult to purify with retention of activity and most of the early characterization work was carried out on a postmitochondrial supernatant, rich in microsomes, which also contains NADPH-cytochrome P450 reductase, which is required for electron transfer to heme oxygenase.

2. Assay of the enzyme. Since the postmitochondrial supernatant also contains the cytosolic enzyme biliverdin reductase, the bile pigment which accumulates in this system following addition of heme is bilirubin, which may be assayed at 468 nm. In the standard assay, heme is added as a complex with serum albumin (known as methemalbumin), and this yields activities about twice those observed when heme is used alone. Other substituted hemes such as meso-, deutero-, and coproheme are also substrates for the enzyme, though its activity is less toward these compounds than toward the naturally occurring protoheme (Tenhunen et al., 1969). Iron-free protoporphyrin IX is not a substrate for heme oxygenase, the iron atom being essential for degradation. Hemoproteins themselves are not substrates for heme oxygenase, except insofar as their heme may be transferred to the enzyme. Thus, oxyhemoglobin and carboxyhemoglobin, where heme is tightly bound, show little or no activity with the enzyme, whereas methemoglobin, from which the heme readily dissociates, gives about the same activity as protoheme itself (Tenhunen et al., 1969).

It is not clear why serum albumin should enhance the activity of heme oxygenase toward protoheme but this could have no significance in vivo, serum albumin being an extracellular protein. One role of the albumin may be to prevent dimerization of the heme, which occurs very readily and which would be expected to prevent binding of the heme to heme oxygenase. It may be easier to transfer monomeric heme for methemalbumin to heme oxygenase than for heme oxygenase to combine directly with the very low concentration of monomeric heme present in aqueous heme solutions. Whereas serum albumin itself can play no physiological role in heme breakdown, a corresponding role may be played by intracellular proteins. Alternatively, the enhancing ability of serum albumin toward heme oxygenase activity may be due to an interaction between albumin and the membrane-bound heme oxygenase in microsomal preparations.

3. Stoichiometry of the heme oxygenase reaction. As will be seen, it is a matter of some debate as to whether heme oxygenase acts only to hydroxylate the α-methene bridge position of heme, the rest of the reaction sequence to biliverin occurring spontaneously and nonenzymically, or whether the enzyme is required also for these additional steps in the reaction to biliverdin. For the first step, 1 mol of heme would be expected to require 1 mol of molecular oxygen and 1 mol of NADPH for hydroxylation. At least 1 mol more of molecular oxygen is clearly required for biliverdin formation.

The accurate experimental measurement of the stoichiometry of molecular oxygen and NADPH in the heme oxygenase reaction has proved to be very difficult. For the spleen enzyme, it was shown that for every mol of heme degraded, at least 3 mol of molecular oxygen and up to 6 mol of NADPH was utilized (Tenhunen et al., 1969, 1970a). In these measurements, which were carried out on microsomal preparations, the utilization of molecular oxygen and NADPH by enzymes other than heme oxygenase clearly cannot be ruled out. More recently, ^{18}O-labeling experiments (Brown and King, 1975, 1976) have confirmed that 3 mol of oxygen is required.

4. Relationship of heme oxygenase to cytochrome P450. In functional terms, the cytochrome P450 enzymes are closely related to heme oxygenase. Both enzymes are microsomal, requiring molecular oxygen and NADPH to carry out hydroxylation reactions, both use protoheme to activate molecular oxygen, and both use the same electron transport system via NADPH-cytochrome P450 reductase. Of course, the roles of the heme in the two enzymes are somewhat different. In the case of cytochrome P450, the heme is a prosthetic group in the enzyme which activates molecular oxygen in order to oxidize another substrate. In the case of heme oxygenase, the enzyme itself does not contain heme, but binds the heme which becomes both a prosthetic group and a substrate in a suicide-type reaction. At one time, it was thought that heme oxygenase activity might be directly linked to cytochrome P450 (i.e., that the enzyme might be a specific form of P450). However, there is now abundant evidence that heme oxygenase is a specific heme degrading protein, quite distinct from P450, and it is also probable that the mechanisms by which the two enzymes work are also somewhat different.

B. Purification of heme oxygenase

1. Methods of purification. Purification of heme oxygenase has proved to be a difficult, time-consuming, and unpredictable procedure. The difficulties are largely associated with the detergent solubilization steps necessary for extraction of the enzyme from microsomes.

The partial purification of heme oxygenase (Yoshida et al., 1974; Maines et al., 1977) was not described until some 10 years after its initial discovery by Tenhunen et al., (1968). The complete purification of the enzyme from pig spleen, rat liver, and bovine spleen was subsequently reported by Yoshida and Kikuchi (1978, 1979) and Yoshinaga et al. (1982). Microsomes were prepared by centrifuging the postmitochondrial supernatant from spleen for 2 h at $56,000 \times g$. Heme oxygenase was solubilized from the microsome fraction by the addition of sodium cholate and the enzyme was precipitated by addition of ammonium sulphate (40% saturation). The crude precipitated enzyme was resuspended in buffer containing sodium cholate and Triton X100 and subjected to DEAE cellulose chromatography at pH 7.4. Final purification was carried out using Sephadex G-200 gel exclusion chromatography.

The assay of heme oxygenase activity during purification procedures requires the addition of purified preparations of NADPH-cytochrome P450 reductase and biliverdin reductase in order to yield bilirubin measurable at 468 nm. Clearly, in such a coupled assay, biliverdin reductase must be added in excess to be sure that the activity being measured is truly that of heme oxygenase and not that of the biliverdin reductase. The dependence of the assay on the amount of NADPH-cytochrome P450 reductase added is less simple, since the reductase and heme oxygenase act in a concerted, rather than in a consecutive, manner. The relationship between the apparent activity of the heme oxygenase system and the amount of NADPH-cytochrome P450 reductase added to reconstitute it has recently been investigated by Wilks (1987), who found that it was necessary to add considerably higher activity of the reductase than had been used in previous studies, in order to achieve maximum heme oxygenase activities. This work also showed that the use of highly purified NADPH-cytochrome P450 reductase and highly purified biliverdin reductase to reconstitute the heme oxygenase system resulted in complete loss of activity. It was necessary to have at least one of the enzymes in only a partially purified form in order to observe normal activity. It is possible that purification of the enzymes results in the loss of a factor required for successful reconstitution, possibly a lipid component, although it has been reported that detergents such as Triton X100 can substitute for lipid in such systems (Lu et al., 1974). The activity of NADPH-cytochrome P450 reductase is usually measured in terms of the reduction of cytochrome c, which is also an in vitro substrate for the enzyme. However, there is evidence that the activity of the enzyme toward cytochrome c does not necessarily parallel its activity toward cytochrome P450 or heme oxygenase. This was shown by experiments in which controlled tryptic digestion of the reductase in a protein reduced from molecular weight 78,000 to 68,000, following which the reductase showed an enhanced cytochrome c reducing activity but a virtual abolition of its ability to reconstitute either heme oxygenase or the cytochrome P450 system (Yoshinaga et al., 1982).

A novel modification in the purification procedure for heme oxygenase was recently introduced by Wilks and Brown (1988), using chromatofocusing. The introduction of this higher-resolution technique gave a purification factor of ×6 after this one step and removed the need for a second ion exchange column as described in earlier procedures. This technique also revealed the presence, in some preparations, of two peaks of heme oxygenase activity, designated F1 and F2. The approximate pI values were 5.9 and 5.7 for F1 and F2, respectively. In other experiments, only a single peak corresponding to F1 was observed. In these cases SDS-polyacrylamide gel electrophoresis showed a homogeneous protein of molecular weight 32,000. However, the observation of two peaks on chromatofocusing coincided with the appearance of second band running at a molecular weight of 28,000 in the F2 fraction. Purification via chromatofocusing is, therefore, able to separate the two heme oxygenase fractions which, by previous techniques, had not readily been distinguishable, though Yoshida and Kikuchi (1978), during purification of heme oxygenase from pig spleen, observed bands on SDS-polyacrylamide gel electrophoresis of molecular weight 32,000 and 26,000, both of which represented heme oxygenase activity. The significance of the relationship of the 28,000 dalton species to the 32,000-dalton species will be discussed further below.

2. Properties of the purified enzyme. The molecular weight of the purified enzyme has been reported to be 32,000 (Yoshida and Kikuchi, 1979; Wilks and Brown, 1988) and 31,000 (Yoshinaga et al., 1982). The latter authors reported a K_m for heme of 0.93 μM and a specific activity of 6770 units per milligram of protein. This compares with the value for K_m of 1 μM obtained by Wilks and Brown (1988) using the chromatofocusing purification technique.

The activity of purified bovine heme oxygenase toward a variety of substrates was examined by Wilks (1987) and is shown in Table 11.1. Protoheme, in the form of methemalbumin, gave the greatest activity in the heme oxygenase reaction as had previously been determined for the partially purified rat spleen enzyme (Tenhunen et al., 1969). The enzyme also shows reduced activity toward hemes having substituted side groups such as deutero-, meso-, and coproheme, showing that the activity of the enzyme does not depend critically on the side chains of the heme. Although the order of activity for the substituted hemes was found to be the same for the purified bovine enzyme as for the crude rat spleen enzyme, the relative activities (compared with protohemes) were somewhat less than in the earlier work. Table 11.1 also shows that both the α and β chains of hemoglobin, in the met form, may act as substrates for

TABLE 11.1   Relative Activity of Various Substrates for Purified Bovine Heme Oxygenase

Substrate	Heme oxygenase activity (nmol/h)	Relative activity (to methemalbumin)
Protohemin (methemalbumin)	45	100
Mesohemin	65	30
Deuterohemin	24	10.8
Coprohemin	10	4.5
Methemoglobin α chain	30	13.5
Methemoglobin β chain	15	6.8

All assays contained 5 μg of heme oxygenase as purified protein. In the case of meso-, deutero-, and coproheme, 1 μM bovine serum albumin was included in the assay.

heme oxygenase, though interestingly they have somewhat different activities from one another.

C. Regulation of heme oxygenase

A full understanding of the regulatory aspects of heme oxygenase in vivo has not yet been achieved, though it may be expected that rapid progress will now be made following the isolation of the cDNA for the enzyme (Shibahara et al., 1985) and the application of the techniques of molecular biology. That the enzyme is subject to sophisticated metabolic regulation is apparent from the variety of compounds which cause either its induction or its inhibition. Perhaps most significant is the marked enhancement of enzyme activity in animals given heme or hemoglobin (Pimstone et al., 1971b; Tenhunen et al., 1970a; Gemsa et al., 1973).

Heme oxygenase has been shown to be induced in vivo by a number of metals and synthetic metalloporphyrins [reviewed by Kikuchi and Yoshida (1983)]. The best-known metal inducer of heme oxygenase is cobalt (Maines and Kappas, 1974), but other metals such as cadmium, zinc, tin, mercury, and lead have also been shown to induce the enzyme. The effect of these metals is reported to vary between tissues. For example, in the liver the most potent inducers appear to be cobalt and cadmium, and in the kidney tin and nickel gave the greatest induction of the enzyme (Maines and Kappas, 1975). Metal-porphyrin complexes also have marked but varying effects on heme oxygenase, which often contrasts with those of the metal alone. For example, Sn-protoporphyrin, unlike uncomplexed tin ions, is a potent inhibitor of heme oxygenase both in vivo and in vitro (Yoshinaga et al., 1982) and this compound is now in trial use therapeutically to prevent jaundice by reducing heme degradation. In contrast, Co-protoporphyrin maintains a long induction effect on heme oxygenase in vivo, while in vitro it acts as a competitive inhibitor of the enzyme (Yoshinaga et al., 1982).

As well as metal inducers of heme oxygenase, compounds such as bromobenzene, phenylhydrazine, and trinitrotoluene have been shown to induce hepatic and renal heme oxygenase (Guzellian and Elshourbagy, 1979; Maines and Veltman, 1984; Tenhunen et al., 1984). It was also reported that the administration of insulin or epinephrine also induced heme oxygenase in rat liver, probably via an increase in the liver heme pool (Bakken et al., 1972).

Two different molecular forms of heme oxygenase, designated HO-1 and HO-2, have been reported in rat liver, testis, and spleen (Maines et al., 1986; Trakshel et al., 1986; Braggins et al., 1986). It was reported that the minimum molecular weights of HO-1 and HO-2 in the rat testis were 30,000 and 36,000, respectively. It was further reported that the liver (HO-1) enzyme was inducible by heme and by agents such as cobalt chloride. More recent work by Cruse and Maines (1988) has put forward evidence suggesting that the two forms of heme oxygenase are products of different genes. Further studies showed that there was no detectable activity of the inducible form HO-1 in rat brain (Trakshel et al., 1988).

D. Structural studies on heme oxygenase

Heme oxygenase, or more strictly heme-heme oxygenase, is a particularly interesting enzyme because in many ways it is intermediate in structure and function between hemoglobin and cytochrome P450.

1. Primary structure.   The greatest achievement so far in studies on the structure of heme oxygenase has been the isolation of the cDNA and the elucidation of its sequence (Shibahara et al., 1985). The deduced amino acid sequence for rat heme oxygenase is shown in Fig. 11.3 and the sequence for the human enzyme has also been reported recently (Yoshida et al., 1988). Although these authors reported no significant homology between heme oxygenase and other hemoproteins, detailed examination of the structure by Wilks (1987) has shown that such homology undoubtedly exists. Residues 106 to 135 and 181 to 205 in heme oxygenase show close homology with the hemoglobin α chain and with myoglobin as shown in Fig. 11.4. On closer examination of these homologous regions between heme oxygenase on the one hand and hemoglobin and myoglobin on the other hand, it is apparent that the two sequences are important functional regions of the hemoproteins. They do, in fact, form the heme binding pocket and it is interesting to record that the residues that have been shown to be invariant in all vertebrate globins so far examined are retained in the heme oxygenase protein (Fig. 11.4). By comparison, it is, therefore, very likely that histidine 132 in heme oxygenase corresponds to the distal histidine in myoglobin at residue 93 and it seems likely that the heme binding site in heme oxygenase is very similar in three-dimensional structure to that of hemoglobin and myoglobin, thus explaining the great similarity in absorption spectra and in EPR properties (see below).

2. Three-dimensional structure.   An especially significant property of the enzyme is that the heme-heme oxygenase complex is able to reversibly bind molecular oxygen when the iron is in the $+2$ oxidation state (Yoshida et al., 1980). The absorption spectrum of this oxyhemoprotein is remarkably similar to that of oxyhemoglobin or oxymyoglobin and, moreover, the spectra of the carbonmonoxy complex of heme-heme oxygenase and the metheme-heme oxygenase parallel those of carbonmonoxy hemoglobin and methemoglobin. This implies that the heme binding site in heme oxygenase is similar to that in hemoglobin.

However, unlike oxyhemoglobin and oxymyoglobin, the oxyheme-heme oxygenase complex is relatively unstable, oxidizing back to the met derivative within 30 min of standing in air.

The EPR spectra of the various complexes of heme-heme oxygenase have been studied by Wilks (1987). The spectrum of the metheme-heme oxygenase complex is typical of the corresponding derivatives of other oxygen binding proteins (Feher et al., 1973). On the addition of cyanide, the peak at $G = 6.02$ was lost, corresponding to a change of spin from the high-spin iron III to the low-spin iron III state, again characteristic of the oxygen binding hemoprotein. The quiet spectra recorded for the iron II derivatives are indicative of the low-spin state. These EPR studies, therefore, support the view that the heme binding site in heme oxygenase is very similar to that of the globins. Further EPR studies are

```
MetGluArgProGlnLeuAspSerMetSerGlnAspLeuSerGluAlaLeuLys
1                           10
GluAlaThrLysGluValHisIleArgAlaGluAsnSerGluPheMetArgAsnPheGln
20                          30
LysGlyGlnValSerArgGluGlyPheLysLeuValMetAlaSerLeuTyrHisIleTyr
40                          50
ThrAlaLeuGluGluGluIleGluArgAsnLysGlnAsnProValTyrAlaProLeuTyr
60                          70
PheProGluGluLeuHisArgArgAlaAlaLeuGluGlnAspMetAlaPheTrpTyrGly
80                          90
ProHisTrpGlnGluAlaIleProTyrThrProAlaThrGlnHisTyrValLysArgLeu
100                         110
HisGluValGlyGlyThrHisProGluLeuLeuValAlaHisAlaTyrThrAgrTyrLeu
120                         130
GlyAspLeuSerGlyGlyGlnValLeuLysLysIleAlaGlnLysAlaMetAlaLeuPro
140                         150
SerSerGlyGluGlyLeuAlaPhePheThrPheProSerIleAspAsnProThrLysPhe
160                         170
LysGlnLeuTyrArgAlaArgMetAsnThrLeuGluMetThrProGluValLysHisArg
180                         190
ValThrGluGluAlaLysThrAlaPheLeuLeuAsnIleGluLeuPheGluGluLeuGln
200                         210
AlaLeuLeuThrGluGluHisLysAspGlnSerProSerGlnThrGluPheLeuArgGln
220                         230
ArgProAlaSerLeuValGlnAspThrThrSerAlaGluThrProArgGlyLysSerGln
240                         250
IleSerThrSerSerSerGlnThrProLeuLeuArgTrpValLeuThrLeuSerPheLeu
260                         270
LeuAlaThrValAlaValGlyIleTyrAlaMet
280                         289
```

Figure 11.3   Deduced amino acid sequence of rat heme oxygenase [from Shibahara et al. (1985)].

Myoglobin (Man)

```
                                                                              96            *→
32 L K F G H P E T L E K F D K F K H L K S E D E M K A S E D L K K H G A T V L T A L G G I L K K K G H H E A E I K P L A Q S H A T K
```

Hemoglobin Man (α-chain)

```
   M F L S F P T T K T Y F P H F – D L S H          G S A Q V K G H G K K V A D A L T N A V A H V D D M P N A L S A L S D L H A H K
```

Hemoglobin Zeta Chain

```
                                                                                                                       135
   L F L S H P Q T K T Y F P H F – D L H P              G S R E L R A H G S K V V A A V G D A V K S I D D L V G G L A S L S E L H A Y K
```

Heme Oxygenase

```
181                              205                106
   L Y R A R M N T L E M T P E V K R H R V T E E A K    P Y T P A T Q H Y V K R L H E V G G T H P E L L V A H A Y T
```

Figure 11.4 Sequence comparison of heme oxygenase with other hemoproteins. Bars surrounding amino acids indicate positions that are invariant in all known vertebrate globins. *Histidine residue (His-F8) which binds the Fe of the heme in hemoglobin and myoglobin.

desirable to probe the nature of the heme-protein interaction, but it would be necessary to use larger quantities of the enzyme than were available in the above work.

Titration of heme against heme oxygenase indicates, as expected, a molar ratio of heme to heme oxygenase of 1 : 1 (Yoshida and Kikuchi, 1978; Wilks, 1987). Wilks also measured the rate of heme exchange between heme-heme oxygenase and free heme in solution. This was found to be relatively rapid, 50% exchange having occurred within 5 min at 37°C. However, the rate of exchange of heme between methemalbumin and heme-heme oxygenase was slower with 50% heme exchange being achieved in approximately 25 min. This is comparable with the rate of heme exchange observed between methemoglobin and methemalbumin which reached 50% completion in approximately 42 min.

In summary, there is now a growing body of sequence, spectroscopic, and kinetic evidence that the heme binding site in heme oxygenase is very similar to that in the well-characterized oxygen binding hemoproteins.

3. Immunological studies. Further structural characterization of heme oxygenase has been carried out by Wilks and Brown (1988) using an antibody raised against purified heme oxygenase (F1, 32,000-dalton fraction, as discussed previously). This antibody cross-reacted with the major protein found in the F2 fraction, (28,000 daltons) as observed by Western immunoblotting. Since the F2 fraction had a similar specific activity to that of the F1 fraction, and both reacted with the same antibody, it seems likely that the F2 fraction is a proteolytic fragment derived from the F1 fraction. This is supported by experiments in which the conditions of purification were varied and which revealed that the F2 fraction was not formed in preparations that were rapidly carried through to the final purification stage without intermediate freezing. It seems likely, therefore, that there is no connection between the two fractions observed by Wilks and Brown (1988) and the two different molecular forms, HO-1 and HO-2, described by Maines and co-workers.

The sensitivity of heme oxygenase to proteolytic cleavage has been further investigated by Wilks (1987) and Wilks and Brown (1988) who showed that treatment of purified native heme oxygenase with trypsin produced a 28,000-dalton fragment which cross-reacted with an antibody raised to the original protein. On controlled tryptic cleavage of whole microsomes, followed by SDS-polyacrylamide gel electrophoresis and Western blotting, a progressive shift in molecular weight from 32,000 to 28,000 was also observed (Houghton et al., 1988a, b), but no lower molecular weight material was seen even after prolonged exposure to trypsin. These results show that heme oxygenase is readily cleaved by trypsin to a 28,000-dalton fragment, which is remarkably resistant to further tryptic cleavage. It seems likely that these observations correspond to the cleavage of a transmembrane segment of heme oxygenase, similar to the tryptic proteolysis previously reported by NADPH-cytochrome P450 reductase (Pederson et al., 1973) and for cytochrome b_5 (Mathews et al., 1979). Examination of the amino acid sequence suggests that this transmembrane segment corresponds to residues 263 to 289. These results also suggested that the 28,000-dalton component of the F2 fraction which showed enzyme activity might be the same as the 28,000-dalton band observed following tryptic cleavage.

Recently, Houghton et al. (1988a, b) have attempted to use the sensitivity of heme oxygenase to trypsin to prepare a solubilized, active form of the enzyme. Postmitochondrial preparations of the enzyme were exposed to varying levels of trypsin, at various time intervals up to 1 h. Samples were subjected to SDS-polyacrylamide gel electrophoresis and Western immunoblotting, which revealed a progressive loss in 32,000 daltons and a corresponding increase in the cross-reacting 28,000-dalton band. Surprisingly, however, in view of the observed activity of the F2 fraction, the activity of the samples fell in proportion to the level of the 32,000-dalton protein, suggesting that the 28,000-dalton protein was not active. The reason for this is not clear, but it is, of course, possible that the 28,000-dalton F2 fraction (which is active) is different from the 28,000-dalton tryptic cleavage fraction (which is inactive).

IV. Coupled Oxidation as a Model for Biological Heme Breakdown

Studies more than 50 years ago (Warburg and Negelein, 1930) showed that heme in solutions of pyridine-water mixtures were degraded by reaction with hydrazine in the presence of molecular oxygen to yield a green product, which they referred to as "green-hemin." This coupled oxidation reaction was found to occur more rapidly with the use of ascorbate rather than hydrazine as a reductant (Lemberg, 1935). Since the green product was readily convertible to biliverdin and since carbon monoxide was released concomitantly, it was clear that coupled oxidation reactions might be useful model systems for biological heme breakdown.

The initial green product was clearly not biliverdin itself, since it retained an iron atom, but it could be readily converted to biliverdin under hydrolytic conditions. The initial product from coupled oxidation was termed verdohemin or, in the presence of pyridine, it was called pyridine verdohemochrome. Since this material is readily converted into bile pigment, it has long been considered as a possible intermediate in the breakdown of heme in vivo. However, there has been a good deal of confusion about the precise structure of verdoheme and some debate as to its role in physiological heme breakdown. This question is considered more fully in the following section.

The determination of the isomeric nature of the biliverdin produced following coupled oxidation reactions has been particularly useful in the understanding of the mechanism of heme breakdown and in relating model systems to biological heme degradation. The quantitative separation of all four biliverdin isomers is clearly important in this regard. Separation of the biliverdin free acids is not easy and most approaches have used either TLC or HPLC of the biliverdin dimethylesters (Bonnett and McDonagh, 1973; O'Carra and Colleran, 1970; Rüdiger, 1968; Rasmussen et al., 1980). Clearly, the isomer formed reflects the particular methene bridge carbon atom which is attacked during the initial step of heme degradation. For the coupled oxidation of protein-free heme (e.g., heme in the pyridine-water solution), it was shown that an almost equimolar mixture of all four isomers was produced (O'Carra and Colleran, 1969, as shown in Table 11.2).

A feature which makes these systems particularly suitable as models for biological heme degradation is the fact that coupled oxidation may also be applied directly to the heme of hemoproteins (e.g., hemoglobin and myoglobin). When these are treated with ascorbate in the presence of molecular oxygen in aqueous solution they are readily degraded to biliverdin. TLC analysis of the isomers produced showed that, in these heme protein systems, there was a high degree of selectivity in the biliverdin isomers formed. Some examples are shown in Table 11.2, from which it is clear that myoglobin yields exclusively the α isomer of biliverdin, whereas hemoglobin yields both α and β isomers in the ratio of about $2:1$. Neither hemoprotein yields any γ or δ isomer. The results with protein-free heme clearly show that there is no marked selectivity for any particular methene bridge intrinsic to the heme molecule itself. It follows, therefore, that the high degree of selectivity observed with hemoproteins must be due to the influence of the protein environment upon the heme during coupled oxidation. This adds further weight to the

TABLE 11.2   Coupled Oxidation of Heme Derivatives

Heme derivative	Percentage biliverdin isomers			
Pyridine hemochrome	32	25	23	20
Hemoglobin (human)	65	35	0	0
Myoglobin	100	0	0	0
Catalase	48	52	0	0
Myoglobin (8 M urea)	32	21	25	22
Hemoglobin (8 M urea)	33	21	25	21
Methemalbumin	28	21	31	20

Data taken from O'Carra and Colleran (1969).

view that coupled oxidation of hemoproteins represents a good model for biological heme cleavage.

V. Mechanism of Heme Degradation

Whereas much progress has been made in determining the mechanism of heme degradation (which on the basis of evidence considered above is likely to be essentially the same in biological systems and in coupled oxidation systems), some details are not yet well understood. In this regard, our knowledge of the detailed mechanism of heme oxygenase action is rather poor compared to that for cytochrome P450 or horseradish peroxidase. Detailed mechanistic analyses have been presented in earlier reviews (Schmid and McDonagh, 1975, 1979; Brown and Troxler, 1982) and only a summary and some recent findings are outlined here. The main approaches to studies of the mechanism have been the use of ^{18}O labeling and the isolation and identification of intermediates.

A. Mesohydroxylation

It is now well established that the first step in the heme degradation sequence, whether in biological or coupled oxidation systems, involves the hydroxylation of one of the four methene bridges, leading to a so-called mesohydroxylated heme derivative as shown in Fig. 11.5. Although it is difficult to isolate mesohydroxyprotoheme from either biological or coupled oxidation systems, it is possible to synthesize analogues of these compounds by iron insertion into oxophlorins. The synthetic mesohydroxymesoheme has been shown to be readily converted to bile pigment either in vivo (Kondo et al., 1971) or in vitro (Jackson et al., 1978).

An important question which is not yet fully resolved is whether the role of heme oxygenase is complete once mesohydroxyheme is formed, the rest of the degradation sequence being nonenzymically controlled, or alternatively, whether heme oxygenase is necessary for the further

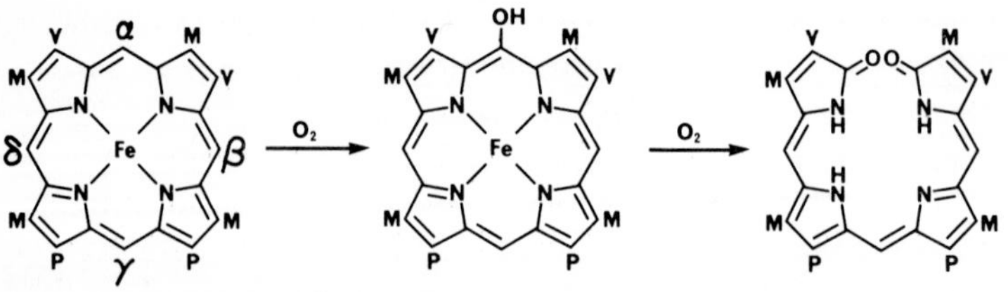

Figure 11.5 Structures showing the mesohydroxylation of heme and subsequent cleavage to form biliverdin IX. (M, $-CH_3$; V, $-CH=CH_2$; P, $-CH_2CH_2CO_2H$.)

breakdown of the mesohydroxyheme intermediate. Of course, the selectivity of methene bridge attack and, hence, the isomeric nature of the biliverdin and bilirubin ultimately produced is already completely determined once the mesohydroxyheme has been formed. In the sense of specificity, therefore, the role of heme oxygenase is complete with the formation of the mesohydroxyheme intermediate. However, there is growing evidence that the enzyme is needed for further conversion of mesohydroxyheme to biliverdin. The iron atom is essential for further reaction; iron-free oxophlorins are not degraded either by coupled oxidation systems or biological systems. Also, whereas mesohydroxyheme does react slowly and in poor yield with oxygen in the absence of reducing agent to give biliverdin, the rate of reaction and yield of biliverdin is greatly increased by the addition of ascorbate. The requirement for iron and the enhancement by reducing agent suggests that iron-mediated oxygen activation, similar to that occurring in the initial step from heme to mesohydroxyheme, is required for its further breakdown. The effect of the purified reconstituted heme oxygenase system on mesohydroxyheme does not appear to have been studied.

B. Macrocyclic ring cleavage step

Following formation of mesohydroxyheme, the next stage involves cleavage of the macrocycle, elimination of the methene bridge carbon atom as carbon monoxide, and insertion of two oxygen atoms which become the lactam oxygen atoms of biliverdin (Fig. 11.5). The chemistry of this sequence is not easy to account for, and there is still some debate as to the intermediates involved. Detailed mechanistic studies have been carried out by using ^{18}O labeling, followed by mass spectrometric analysis of the bile pigments produced. The first such experiments were carried out by Anan and Mason (1961) who studied the coupled oxidation of hemoglobin under an atmosphere containing $^{18,18}O_2$. The immediate product was hydrolyzed to yield biliverdin which contained only one atom of labeled oxygen. Correspondingly, the biliverdin also contained only one atom of ^{18}O when the reaction was performed in $H_2{}^{18}O$ under an atmosphere of $^{16,16}O_2$. It is now known that the incorporation of an atom of oxygen from water into the product bile pigment reflects an artifact of the work-up procedure, which involves exchange of solvent oxygen under the hydrolytic conditions used.

The foundations for more recent labeling studies were laid by Tenhunen et al. (1972), who showed that formation of bilirubin by the crude postmitochondrial heme oxygenase system, in the presence of $^{18,18}O_2$, resulted in the labeling of both lactam oxygen atoms of the bile pigment. Correspondingly, when the reaction was carried out in $H_2{}^{18}O$ under an atmosphere of $^{16,16}O_2$, no label appeared in the product bile pigment. It was, thus, established that both lactam oxygen atoms in bile pigments are derived from molecular oxygen during the degradation of heme. More-detailed and extensive studies have been carried out by Brown and co-workers in order to determine more precisely the origin of the lactam oxygen atoms.

Assuming that the oxygen atoms incorporated into biliverdin are derived from molecular oxygen, two possible mechanisms may be defined. The first, designated the one-molecule mechanism, involves incorporation of both atoms of oxygen from a single-oxygen molecule. In the second process, designated the two-molecule mechanism, again both oxygen atoms are derived from molecular oxygen, but each originates in a different molecule of molecular oxygen. By carrying out heme degradation studies under an atmosphere containing $^{18,18}O_2$ and $^{16,16}O_2$, but none of the mixed species $^{18,16}O_2$, it was possible to distinguish between these two mechanisms. In a variety of systems including living rats, the crude postmitochondrial heme oxygenase system, the purified reconstituted heme oxygenase system, the coupled oxidation of hemoproteins, and the coupled oxidation of protein-free heme (Brown and King, 1975; King and Brown, 1978; Docherty et al., 1984; Chaney and Brown, 1978), it was shown that heme degradation always occurs via the two-molecule mechanism. Further work showed that the oxygen of the carbon monoxide eliminated during heme degradation was also derived from molecular oxygen and, moreover, that it was derived from yet a third molecule of molecular oxygen, presumably that used in the initial hydroxylation step.

The experimental data are, therefore, very clear and the problem is that of deducing the mechanism to fit the data. Initially, it was thought that the observation of the two-molecule mechanism eliminated the possibility that verdoheme (Fig. 11.6) might be an intermediate since it was assumed that the conversion of verdoheme to biliverdin would require a hydrolytic process, with insertion of an atom of oxygen from water. Certainly, it is known that such hydrolytic conversion of verdoheme to biliverdin can occur (Jackson, 1974). However, the whole question of the possible involvement of verdoheme was reopened by the studies of Itano and co-workers (Saito and Itano, 1982, 1986; Itano and

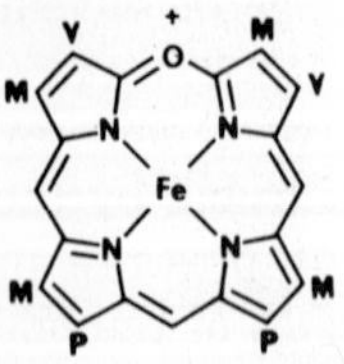

Figure 11.6   Structure of verdoheme. (M, $-CH_3$; V, $-CH=CH_2$; P, $-CH_2CH_2CO_2H$.)

Hirota, 1985), which showed that verdoheme could also be oxidatively converted to biliverdin with incorporation of an additional oxygen atom from molecular oxygen. This observation has, therefore, had the effect of reinstating verdoheme or a similar compound as a possible intermediate in the heme cleavage step.

An alternative approach to determination of the mechanism of the heme cleavage step is to attempt to isolate and identify intermediates. Yoshida et al. (1980) described a new intermediate of heme degradation found in the heme-heme oxygenase and the NADPH-cytochrome P450 reductase system. The intermediate showed an absorption peak at 688 nm and its carbon monoxide complex gave a peak at 638 nm. These workers reported that it was possible to almost completely stop the degradation sequence at the level of the 638-nm substance by performing the reaction under a mixture of carbon monoxide and air. The carbon monoxide complex of the 688-nm substance was easily and quantitatively converted to biliverdin-iron complex when exposed to air. Whereas the heme moiety of the 688-nm substance had similarities to verdoheme, the precise structural nature of this intermediate was not established. However, by using ^{14}C labeling, Yoshida et al. (1982) showed that the methene bridge carbon atom was liberated as carbon monoxide during formation of the 688-nm compound. Other studies by Sano et al. (1986) suggested that the 688-nm compound contains only one oxygen atom and that its conversion to the iron-biliverdin complex involves insertion of an additional oxygen atom from molecular oxygen. The intermediate would, therefore, be fully consistent with the observation of the two-molecule mechanism.

In conclusion, recent evidence tends to favor the formation of a verdoheme-like intermediate during both coupled oxidation and biological heme cleavage, though the issue cannot yet be considered to be completely resolved.

C. Regioselectivity

Following the observations referred to earlier, that coupled oxidation of hemoproteins led to directed selectivity of heme cleavage, the question arose as to how precisely the apoprotein was able to direct this selectivity. In the cases of hemoglobin and myoglobin where the three-dimensional structures were accurately known, this question could be approached in terms of the precise structure of the proteins. An examination of these structures posed the immediate paradox that the α methene bridge, which is exposed to solvent and external reagents, is not attacked, whereas the γ bridge, which is the main site of reaction, is buried within the hydrophobic interior of the protein and thereby shielded from attack by reagents in solution.

There is now a good deal of evidence [reviewed by Brown and Troxler (1982)] to suggest that the initial hydroxylation step in heme breakdown is an intramolecular reaction in which an iron-bound oxygen molecule attacks its own porphyrin periphery as envisaged in Fig. 11.7. On the basis of such a mechanism, Brown (1976) suggested that it might be more important to consider the accessibility of the various methene bridge carbon atoms to an iron-bound molecule rather than to the external medium. In protein-free heme there would be equal accessibility to each methene bridge and this would account for the almost equal distribution of all four isomers observed on coupled oxidation of heme in pyridine-water mixtures. However, in hemoproteins it would be expected that accessibility to some of the bridges might be restricted. Following examination of the heme pocket structures of hemoglobin and myoglobin, it was found that the observed methene bridge selectivity in coupled oxidation could be accurately accounted for on the basis of the steric hindrance imposed by specific amino acid residues in the protein (Brown, 1976). On this basis, it would be expected that any change in the residues causing such hindrance might lead to a different isomer pattern and this was shown to be the case in studies involving appropriate abnormal hemoglobins (Brown and Docherty, 1978). Assuming that the same criteria applied to determination of selectivity in the action of heme oxygenase in vivo, this would require that the heme binding site in heme oxygenase was similar to that in myoglobin and hemoglobin which is consistent with the various observations discussed earlier.

D. Summary of mechanism

An overall scheme for the heme oxygenase catalyzed breakdown of heme, as it occurs in vivo is shown in Fig. 11.8. The heme leaves its apoprotein (e.g., hemoglobin or cytochrome P450) to form a complex with heme oxygenase which, so far as the heme binding site is concerned, very

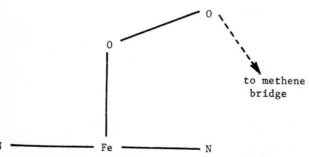

Figure 11.7   Possible scheme for the intramolecular hydroxylation of heme.

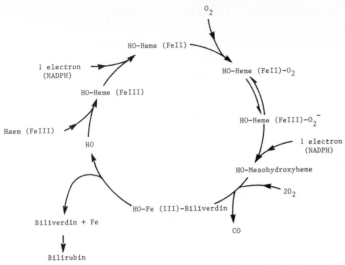

Figure 11.8 Scheme for the conversion of heme to bilirubin by the action of heme oxygenase (HO).

closely resembles that of hemoglobin and myoglobin. However, the heme oxygenase protein must also have the ability to interact with NADPH-cytochrome P450 reductase, in order to reduce the iron atom so that the oxygen may be bound and mesohydroxylation may occur. The next stage probably also takes place with the mesohydroxylated heme still bound to heme oxygenase and involves release of carbon monoxide and insertion of two oxygen atoms to yield an iron-biliverdin complex which may still be bound to the heme oxygenase. Biliverdin would then be formed by the removal of the iron atom and by the release of the pigment from the enzyme.

VI. Heme Breakdown in Plants: Biosynthesis of Phycobiliproteins

A. Formation of the chromophore of phycobiliproteins

In mammals, bile pigments play no functional role other than in providing a pathway for the elimination of unwanted heme. In plants, however, bile pigments very similar in structure to biliverdin play vital roles in photosynthesis and photomorphogenesis. In blue-green algae (Cyanobacteria) and in red algae (Rhodophyta) the photosynthetic antenna pigments are proteins with covalently linked chromophores known as phycocyanobilin and phycoerythrobilin, as shown in Fig. 11.9. In higher plants the important regulatory pigment phytochrome is also a biliprotein with the chromophore structure shown in Fig. 11.9. It is highly significant that, like the mammalian bile pigments, those found in plants and cyanobacteria are also IXα isomers. The biosynthetic pathway by which these chromophores are formed remained in some doubt until relatively recently, when Brown et al. (1981) demonstrated directly that heme was a biosynthetic precursor of phycocyanobilin. It was also shown (Brown et al., 1980; Troxler et al., 1979), using ^{18}O labeling, that the biosynthesis of phycocyanobilin followed a two-molecule mechanism, in exactly the same way as biliverdin is formed from heme. The intermediacy of heme in the biosynthesis of these pigments implies that plants must also contain heme oxygenase. Further confirmation of this was obtained by Brown and Holroyd (1984), who showed that administration of mesoheme to algal cells resulted in its conversion to mesobiliverdin, presumably because the mesoheme was acting as a substrate for the algal heme oxygenase.

The formation of heme in plant systems also requires ferrochelatase (EC 4.99.1.1), the enzyme responsible for insertion of iron into protoporphyrin IX. The existence of this enzyme in the rhodophyte *Cyanidium caldarium* has been demonstrated both directly by enzyme assay (Brown et al., 1984) and also by implication, since administration of *N*-methylprotoporphyrin IX, a potent and specific inhibitor of ferrochelatase, resulted in marked inhibition of phycocyanobilin synthesis (Brown et al., 1982).

The direct assay of heme oxygenase in algal systems is not easy. Nevertheless, Beale and co-workers have demonstrated enzyme activity

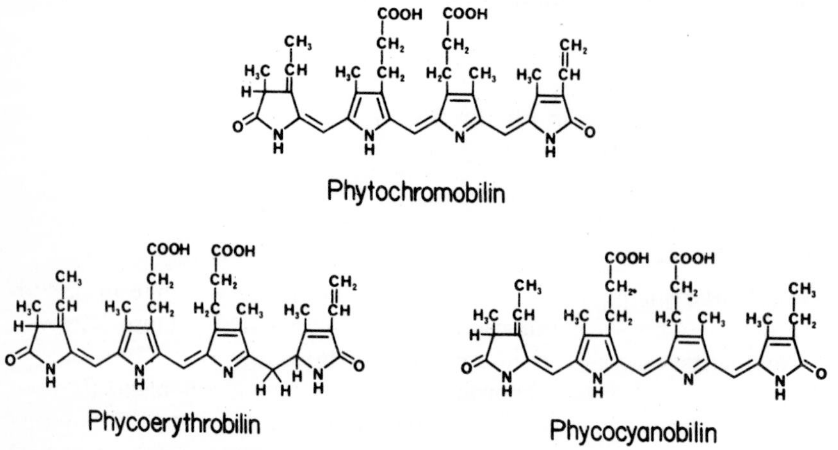

Phytochromobilin

Phycoerythrobilin

Phycocyanobilin

Figure 11.9 Chemical structures of three plant bile pigments.

in homogenates of *C. caldarium* and have partially characterized the enzyme. This work is considered at length in Chap. 7.

Using the antibody raised against purified beef spleen heme oxygenase, Houghton et al. (1988a, b) have demonstrated cross reactivity with an algal protein of molecular weight 32,000. Furthermore, the crossreacting species in *C. caldarium* was induced by exposure of dark-grown cells to light, prior to the formation of phycobiliproteins, and in parallel to the induction of ferrochelatase. These results strongly suggest that the antibody is cross-reacting with the algal heme oxygenase, which implies that the enzyme must be strongly conserved, bearing in mind the wide divergence of species being studied.

ACKNOWLEDGMENTS

We wish to thank the Medical Research Council, the Science and Engineering Research Council, and the Yorkshire Cancer Research Campaign for financial support.

REFERENCES

Anan, F. K., and Mason, H. S. (1961). An ^{18}O study of the haemoglobin degradation to biliverdin in the model reaction, *J. Biochem. (Tokyo)* **49**:765–771.

Awruch, J., Tomaro, M. L., Frydman, R. B., and Frydman, B. (1984). The specificity of biliverdin reductase. The reduction of biliverdin XIII isomers, *Biochim. Biophys. Acta.* **787**:146–151.

Badawy, A.-B. A., and Evans, M. (1975). The regulation of rat liver tryptophan pyrrolase by its cofactor haem, *Biochem. J.* **150**:511–520.

Bakken, A. A., Thaler, M. M., and Schmid, R. (1972). Metabolic regulation of heme catabolism and biliverdin production, *J. Clin. Invest.* **51**:530–536.

Berlin, N. I., Neuberger, A., and Scott, J. J. (1956). The metabolism of δ-aminolaevulinic acid II: Normal pathways studied with the aid of ^{14}C, *Biochem. J.* **64**:90–100.

Billing, B. H. (1982). The role of conjugating enzymes in the biliary excretion of bilirubin, *Bilirubin* (K. P. M. Heirwegh and S. B. Brown, Eds.), CRC Press, Boca Raton, Fla., Vol. II, pp. 85–102.

Bissell, D. M., and Hammaker, L. E. (1977). Effect of endotoxin on tryptophan pyrrolase and aminolaevulinate synthase: Evidence for an endogenous regulatory haem fraction in rat liver, *Biochem. J.* **166**:301–304.

Bonnett, R., and McDonagh, A. F. (1973). The meso-reactivity of porphyrins and related compounds. VI. Oxidative cleavage of the haem system. The four isomeric biliverdins of the IX series, *J. Chem. Soc. Perkin Trans. I* 881–888.

Braggins, P. E., Trakshel, M. E., Kutty, K. R., and Maines, M. D. (1986). Characterisation of two heme oxygenase isoforms in rat spleen: Comparison with the hematin-induced and constitutive isoforms of the liver, *Biochem. Biophys. Res. Comm.* **141**:528–533.

Brown, S. B. (1976). Stereospecific haem cleavage. A model for the formation of bile pigment isomers in vivo and in vitro, *Biochem. J.* **159**:23–27.

Brown, S. B., and Docherty, J. C. (1978). Haem degradation in abnormal haemoglobins, *Biochem. J.* **173**:985–987.

Brown, S. B., and Holroyd, J. A. (1984). Biosynthesis of the chromophore of phycobiliproteins: A study of mesohaem and mesobiliverdin as possible intermediates and further evidence for an algal haem oxygenase, *Biochem. J.* **217**:265–272.

Brown, S. B., Holroyd, J. A., and Troxler, R. F. (1980). Mechanism of bile pigment synthesis in algae. ^{18}O incorporation into phycocyanobilin in the unicellular rhodophyte, *Cyanidium caldarium*, *Biochem. J.* **190**:445–449.

Brown, S. B., Holroyd, J. A., Troxler, R. F., and Offner, G. D. (1981). Bile pigment synthesis in plants: Incorporation of haem into phycocyanobilin and phycobiliproteins in *Cyanidium caldarium*, *Biochem. J.* **194**:137–147.

Brown, S. B., Holroyd, J. A., Vernon, D. I., and Jones, O. T. G. (1984). Ferrochelatase activity in the photosynthetic alga *Cyanidium caldarium*, *Biochem. J.* **220**:861–863.

Brown, S. B., Holroyd, J. A., Vernon, D. I., Troxler, R. F., and Smith, K. M. (1982). The effect of *N*-methyl protoporphyrin IX on the synthesis of photosynthetic pigments in *Cyanidium caldarium*, *Biochem. J.* **208**:487–491.

Brown, S. B., and King, R. F. G. J. (1975). An ^{18}O double labelling study of haem catabolism in the rat, *Biochem. J.* **150**:565–567.

Brown, S. B., and King, R. F. G. J. (1976). ^{18}O studies of haem catabolism, *Biochem. Soc. Trans.* **4**:197–201.

Brown, S. B., and Troxler, R. F. (1982). Heme degradation and bilirubin formation, *Bilirubin* (K. P. M. Heirwegh and S. B. Brown, Eds.), CRC Press, Boca Raton, Fla., Vol. II, pp. 11–38.

Chaney, B. D., and Brown, S. B. (1978). The mechanism of coupled oxidation of octaethyl-haem to octaethylbiliverdin, *Biochem. Soc. Trans.* **6**:419–421.

Colleran, E., and O'Carra, P. (1975). Physiologic purpose of biliverdin reduction, *Chemistry and Physiology of Bile Pigments* (P. D. Berk and N. I. Berlin, Eds.), U.S. Department of Health, Education, and Welfare, Washington, D.C., pp. 69–80.

Cruse, I., and Maines, M. D. (1988). Evidence suggesting that the two forms of heme oxygenase are products of different genes, *J. Biol. Chem.* **263**:3348–3353.

Docherty, J. C., Schacter, B. A., Firneisz, G. D., and Brown, S. B. (1984). Mechanism of action of haem oxygenase: A study of haem degradation to bile pigment by ^{18}O labelling, *J. Biol. Chem.* **259**:13066–13069.

Farrell, G. C., and Correia, M. A. (1980). Structural and functional reconstitution of hepatic cytochrome P450 in vivo, *J. Biol. Chem.* **255**:10128–10133.

Feher, G., Isaacson, R. A., Scholes, C. P., and Nagel, R. (1973). Electron nuclear double resonance (ENDOR) investigation on myoglobin and haemoglobin, *Ana. N.Y. Acad. Sci.* **222**:86–101.

Foidart, M., Eisman, J., Engel, W. K., Adoranto, B. T., Liem, H. H., and Muller-Eberhard, U. (1982). Effect of heme administration on hemopexin metabolism in the rhesus monkey, *J. Lab. Clin. Med.* **100**:457–460.

Frydman, R. B., Tomaro, M. L., Awruch, J., and Frydman, B. (1984). Isolation from rat liver of a peroxisomal enzyme which converts molecular form 1 of biliverdin reductase into molecular form 3, *Biochem. Biophys. Res. Comm.* **121**:249–254.

Gemsa, D., Woo, C. H., Fudenberg, H. H., and Schmid, R. (1973). Erythrocyte catabolism by macrophages in vitro. The effect of hydrocortisone on erythrophagocytosis and on the induction of haem oxygenase, *J. Clin. Invest.* **52**:812–822.

Grandchamp, B., Bissel, D. M., Licko, V., and Schmid, R. (1981). Formation and disposition of newly synthesised heme in adult rat hepatocytes in primary culture, *J. Biol. Chem.* **256**:11677–11683.

Gray, C. H. (1953). *The Bile Pigments*, Methuen, London.

Gray, C. H., Neuberger, A., and Sneath, P. H. A. (1950). Studies in congenital porphyria II: Incorporation of ^{15}N in the stercobilin in the normal and in the porphyric, *Biochem. J.* **47**:87–92.

Guzellian, P. S., and Elshourbagy, N. A. (1979). Induction of hepatic heme oxygenase activity by bromobenzene, *Arch. Biochem. Biophys.* **196**:178–185.

Houghton, J. D., Holroyd, J. A., Wilks, A., and Brown, S. B. (1988a). In preparation.

Houghton, J. D., Wilks, A., and Brown, S. B. (1988b). In preparation.

Itano, H. A., and Hirota, T. (1985). A two-molecule mechanism of heme degradation, *Biochem. J.* **226**:767–771.

Jackson, A. H. (1974). Heme catabolism, *Iron in Biochemistry and Medicine* (A. Jacobs, and M. Worwood, Eds.), Academic, New York, pp. 145–182.

Jackson, A. H., Lee, M. G., Jenkins, R. T., Brown, S. B., and Chaney, B. D. (1978). Oxidative ring opening of octaethylchlorohaemin and its mesohydroxy derivatives to octaethylbiliverdin. *Tet. Lett.* **51**:5135–5138.

Kikuchi, G., and Yoshida, T. (1983). Function and induction of the microsomal heme oxygenase, *Mol. Cell. Biochem.* **53 / 54**:163–183.

King, R. F. G. J., and Brown, S. B. (1978). The mechanism of haem catabolism. A study of haem breakdown in spleen microsomal fraction and in a model system of ^{18}O labelling and metal substitution, *Biochem. J.* **174**:103–109.

Kondo, T., Nicholson, P. C., Jackson, A. H., and Kenner, G. W. (1971). Isotopic studies of the conversion of oxophlorins and their ferrihaems into bile pigments in the rat, *Biochem. J.* **121**:601–607.

Kutty, K. R., and Maines, M. D. (1981). Purification and characterisation of biliverdin reductase from rat liver, *J. Biol. Chem.* **256**:3956–3962.

Lemberg, R. (1935). Transformation of hemins into bile pigments, *Biochem. J.* **29**:1322–1336.

Lemberg, R., and Wyndham, R. A. (1936). Reduction of biliverdin to bilirubin in tissues, *Biochem. J.* **30**:1147–1170.

Lu, A. Y. H., Levine, W., and Kuntznan, R. (1974). Reconstituted liver microsomal enzyme system that hydroxylates drugs, other foreign compounds and endogenous substrates, *Biochem. Biophys. Res. Comm.* **60**:266–272.

Maines, M. D., Ibrahim, N. G., and Kappas, A. (1977). Solubilisation and partial purification of heme oxygenase from rat liver, *J. Biol. Chem.* **252**:5900–5903.

Maines, M. D., and Kappas, A. (1974). Cobalt induction of hepatic heme oxygenase; with evidence that cytochrome P450 is not essential for this enzyme activity, *Proc. Nat. Acad. Sci. (U.S.A.)* **71**:4293–4297.

Maines, M. D., and Kappas, A. (1975). Cobalt stimulation of heme degradation in the liver, *J. Biol. Chem.* **250**:4171–4177.

Maines, M. D., Trakshel, G. M., and Kutty, K. R. (1986). Characterisation of two constitutive forms of rat liver microsomal heme oxygenase, *J. Biol. Chem.* **261**:411–419.

Maines, M. D., and Veltman, J. C. (1984). Phenylhydrazine-mediated induction of heme oxygenase activity in rat liver and kidney and development of hyperbilirubinaemia, *Biochem. J.* **217**:409–417.

Mathews, F. S., Czerwinski, E. W., and Argos, P. (1979). The X-ray crystallographic structure of calf liver cytochrome b_5, *The Porphyrins* (D. Dolphin, Ed.), Academic, New York, Vol. VII, pp. 107–147.

Noguchi, M., Yoshida, T., and Kikuchi, G. (1979). Purification and properties of biliverdin reductases from pig spleen and rat liver. *J. Biochem. (Tokyo)* **86**:833–848.

O'Carra, P., and Colleran, E. (1969). Haem catabolism and coupled oxidation of haemoproteins, *FEBS Lett.* **5**:295–298.

O'Carra, P., and Colleran, E. (1970). Separation and identification of biliverdin isomers and isomer analysis of phycobilins and bilirubin, *J. Chromatog.* **50**:458–468.

O'Carra, P., and Colleran, E. (1971). Properties and kinetics of biliverdin reductase, *Biochem. J.* **125**:110p.

Ortiz de Montellano, P. R. (Ed.) (1986). Cytochrome P450: *Structure, Mechanism and Biochemistry*, Plenum, New York.

Ortiz de Montellano, P. R., and Correia, M. A. (1983). Suicidal destruction of cytochrome P-450 during oxidative drug metabolism, *Ann. Rev. Pharmacol. Toxicol.* **23**:481–503.

Pederson, T. C., Buege, J. A., and Aust, S. D. (1973). Microsomal electron transport: The role of reduced nicotinamide adenine dinucleotide phosphate-cytochrome c reductase in liver microsomal lipid peroxidation, *J. Biol. Chem.* **248**:7134–7141.

Pimstone, N. R., Engel, P., Tenhunen, R., Seitz, P., Marver, S. H., and Schmid, R. (1971a). Inducible haem oxygenase in the kidney: A model for the homeostatic control of haemoglobin catabolism, *J. Clin. Invest.* **50**:2042–2050.

Pimstone, N. R., Tenhunen, R., Seitz, P. T., Marver, S., and Schmid, R. (1971b). The enzymatic degradation of haemoglobin to bile pigments by macrophages, *J. Exp. Med.* **133**:1264–1281.

Rasmussen, R. D., Yokoyama, W. H., Blumenthal, S. G., Bergstrom, D. E., and Ruebner, B. H. (1980). High performance liquid chromatographic separation and quantification of the four biliverdin dimethyl ester isomers of the IX series, *Anal. Biochem.* **101**:66–74.

Robinson, S. H. (1975). Origins of the early-labelled peak, *Chemistry and Physiology of Bile Pigments* (P. D. Berk and N. I. Berlin, Eds.), U.S. Department of Health, Education, and Welfare, Washington, D.C., pp. 175–188.

Rudiger, W. (1968). Bile pigments: A new degradation technique and its application, *Porphyrins and Related Compounds* (T. W. Goodwin, Ed.) (*Biochem. Soc. Symp.*, No. 28), Academic, London, pp. 121–130.

Saito, S., and Itano, H. A. (1982). Verdohemochrome IX: Preparation and oxidoreductive cleavage to biliverdin IX, *Proc. Nat. Acad. Sci. (U.S.A.)* **79**:1393–1397.

Saito, S., and Itano, H. A. (1986). Cyclization of biliverdins to verdohemochromes, *J. Chem. Soc. 'Perkin Trans. I* 1–7.

Sano, S., Sano, T., Morishima, I., Shiro, Y., and Maeda, Y. (1986). On the mechanism of the chemical and enzymic oxygenations of -oxyprotohemin IX to Fe-biliverdin IX, *Proc. Nat. Acad. Sci. (U.S.A.)* **83**:531–535.

Schmid, R., and McDonagh, A. F. (1975). The enzymatic formation of bilirubin, *Ann. N.Y. Acad. Sci.* **244**:533–552.

Schmid, R., and McDonagh, A. F. (1979). Formation and metabolism of bile pigments in vivo, *The Porphyrins* (D. Dolphin, Ed.), Academic, New York, Vol. VI, pp. 257–292.

Shemin, D., and Rittenberg, D. (1946). The life span of the human red blood cell, *J. Biol. Chem.* **166**:627–636.

Shibahara, S., Muller, R., Taguchi, H., and Yoshida, T. (1985). Cloning and expression of cDNA for rat heme oxygenase, *Proc. Nat. Acad. Sci. (U.S.A.)* **82**:7865–7869.

Tenhunen, R., Marver, H. S., Pimstone, N. R., Trager, W. F., Cooper, D. Y., and Schmid, R. (1972). Enzymatic degradation of heme. Oxygenative cleavage requiring cytochrome P_{450}, *Biochemistry* **11**:1716–1720.

Tenhunen, R., Marver, H. S., and Schmid, R. (1968). The enzymatic conversion of haem to biliverdin by microsomal haem oxygenase, *Proc. Nat. Acad. Sci. (U.S.A.)* **61**:748–755.

Tenhunen, R., Marver, H. S., and Schmid, R. (1969). Microsomal haem oxygenase: Characterisation of the enzyme, *J. Biol. Chem.* **244**:6388–6394.

Tenhunen, R., Marver, H., and Schmid, R. (1970a). The enzymatic catabolism of haemoglobin: Stimulation of microsomal haem oxygenase by haemin, *J. Lab. Clin. Med.* **75**:410–421.

Tenhunen, R., Ross, M. E., Marver, H. S., and Schmid, R. (1970b). Reduced nicotinamide adenine dinucleotide dependent biliverdin reductase: Partial purification and characterisation, *Biochemistry* **9**:298–303.

Tenhunen, R., Zitting, A., Nickels, J., and Savolainen, H. (1984). Trinitrotoluene-induced effects on rat haem metabolism, *Exp. Mol. Pathol.* **40**:362–366.

Trakshel, G. M., Kutty, K. R., and Maines, M. D. (1986). Purification and characterisation of the major constitutive form of testicular heme oxygenase, *J. Biol. Chem.* **261**:11131–11137.

Trakshel, G. M., Kutty, K. R., and Maines, M. D. (1988). Resolution of the rat brain heme oxygenase activity: Absence of a detectable amount of the inducible form HO-1, *Arch. Biochem. Biophys.* **260**:732–739.

Troxler, R. F., Brown, A. S., and Brown, S. B. (1979). Bile pigment synthesis in plants. Mechanism of ^{18}O incorporation into phycocyanobilin in the unicellular rhodophyte, *Cyanidium caldarium*, *J. Biol. Chem.* **254**:3411–3418.

Warburg, O., and Negelein, E. (1930). Grunes Haemin aus Blast-haemin, *Chem. Ber.* **63**:1816–1819.

Wilks, A. (1987). Ph.D. Thesis, University of Leeds, England.

Wilks, A., and Brown, S. B. (1988). Purification of bovine spleen haem oxygenase and susceptibility to proteolytic cleavage, *Biochem. J.*, to appear.

Wyman, J. F., Gollan, J. L., Settle, W., Farrell, G. C., and Correia, M. A. (1986). Incorporation of hemoglobin heme into the rat hepatic hemoproteins, tryptophan pyrrolase and cytochrome P450, *Biochem. J.* **238**:837–846.

Yoshida, T., Biro, P., Cohen, T., Müller, R. M., and Shibahara, S. (1988). Human heme oxygenase cDNA and induction of its mRNA by hemin, *Eur. J. Biochem.* **171**:457–461.

Yoshida, T., and Kikuchi, G. (1978). Purification and properties of heme oxygenase from pig spleen microsomes, *J. Biol. Chem.* **253**:4224–4229.

Yoshida, T., and Kikuchi, G. (1979). Purification and properties of heme oxygenase from rat liver microsomes, *J. Biol. Chem.* **254**:4487–4491.

Yoshida, T., Noguchi, M., and Kikuchi, G. (1980). Oxygenated form of heme: Oxygenase complex and requirement for second electron to initiate heme degradation from the oxygenated complex, *J. Biol. Chem.* **255**:4418–4420.

Yoshida, T., Noguchi, M., and Kikuchi, G. (1982). The step of carbon monoxide liberation in the sequence of heme degradation catalyzed by the reconstituted microsomal heme oxygenase system, *J. Biol. Chem.* **257**:9345–9348.

Yoshida, T., Takahashi, S., and Kikuchi, G. (1974). Partial purification and reconstitution of the heme oxygenase system from pig spleen microsomes, *J. Biochem. (Tokyo)* **75**:1187–1191.

Yoshinaga, T., Sassa, S., and Kappas, A. (1982). Purification and properties of bovine spleen heme oxygenase: Amino acid composition and sites of action of inhibitors of heme oxidation, *J. Biol. Chem.* **257**:7778–7785.

INDEX

Page references in *italic* refer to illustrations.

DATE DUE